Fundamentals of Cancer Prevention

David S. Alberts · Lisa M. Hess (Editors)

Fundamentals of Cancer Prevention

With 37 Figures

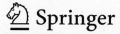 Springer

Editors

David S. Alberts
Lisa M. Hess
Arizona Cancer Center
Cancer Prevention and Control
1515 N. Campbell Avenue
PO Box 245 024
Tuscon, AZ 85724

ISBN-10 3-540-24212-0 Springer Berlin Heidelberg New York
ISBN-13 978-3-540-24212-3 Springer Berlin Heidelberg New York

Library of Congress Control Number: 2005920701

A catalog record for this book is available from Library of Congress.

Bibliographic information published by Die Deutsche Bibliothek.
Die Deutsche Bibliothek lists this publication in the Deutsche Nationalbibliografie;
detailed bibliographic data is available in the Internet at http://dnb.ddb.de

Springer is a part of Springer Science+Business Media
springeronline.com

© Springer Berlin Heidelberg 2005
Printed in Germany

Editor: Dr. Ute Heilmann, Heidelberg, Germany
Desk Editor: Meike Stoeck, Heidelberg, Germany
Production: PRO EDIT GmbH, Heidelberg, Germany
Cover Design: Frido Steinen-Broo, eStudio Calamar, Spain
Typesetting: K + V Fotosatz GmbH, Beerfelden, Germany

Printed on acid-free paper   21/3151/Di   5 4 3 2 1 0

Dedication

David S. Alberts
I would like to dedicate this book to my beautiful wife of 42 years, Heather, who has taught me to "walk the talk" of cancer prevention every day of my life, and to my magnificent grandchildren, Sammy, Sophie, Sydney and Emma, who I am certain will carry the banner of health promotion to the mid-century for a much healthier American society.

Lisa M. Hess
I would like to dedicate this book to my precious daughter Rachael, who every moment teaches me the value of health and the beauty of life.

Preface

Each year, more than 550,000 deaths result from invasive cancer in the United States alone. This is greater than the deaths that would be caused by two Boeing 747 airplane crashes every day, 365 days per year. The number of deaths in this one country alone is enough to make the mind grow numb. Recently, the American Cancer Society documented that for those under the age of 85, cancer deaths outnumber heart disease deaths and cancer is the leading cause of death among both men and women (Jemal, et al. *CA Cancer J Clin* 2005; 55:10–30).

Cancer death rates from the most common solid tumors, such as breast cancer, colon cancer and prostate cancer, are declining at a relatively slow rate despite recent advances in screening technologies, methods of early detection, and improved cytotoxic and biologic therapy.

If we are to see a major reduction in cancer mortality, especially for those patients under the age of 65 years, a great deal more emphasis and research funding must be placed on cancer prevention and early detection. Furthermore, efforts must be made to educate primary care physicians and caregivers, who are the first line of defense against cancer. Until physicians, nurse practitioners and physician assistants are empowered to see each patient in their practices as a target for cancer prevention interventions, we may never make a dramatic impact on cancer death rates.

Fundamentals of Cancer Prevention is a text specifically for primary healthcare providers written by the Cancer Prevention and Control Program faculty of the Arizona Cancer Center and collaborators. This first edition has attempted to provide a comprehensive educational experience for primary healthcare providers. We believe that only through the dissemination of information to those individuals who see patients before cancer begins will major strides be made to see a reduction in the burden of cancer worldwide. We look forward to working with this extremely important segment of our healthcare network to conquer the ever-increasing problem of cancer mortality and morbidity.

Tuscon, February 2005

David S. Alberts
Lisa M. Hess

Contents

List of Contributors

Mailing address of all authors (except K. Hunt, H. Greenlee, N. Aziz, and R. Lutz)
Arizona Cancer Center
Cancer Prevention and Control
1515 N. Campbell Avenue
PO Box 245 024
Tuscon, AZ 85724
USA

Ahmann, Frederick
Alberts, David
Baldwin, Susie
Chen, Zhao
Coe, Kathryn
Coons, Stephen Joel
Craig, Benjamin
Garcia, Francisco
Garland, Linda
Gerner, Eugene
Hakim, Iman
Hess, Lisa
Ismail, Ayaaz
Jacobson, Elaine
Jacobson, Myron
Kim, Hyuntae

Kim, Moonsun
Krouse, Robert
Lance, Peter
Larkey, Linda
Lluria-Prevatt, Maria
Lopez, Ana Maria
McKenzie, Naja
Mehl-Madrona, Lewis
Newton, J.
Palmer, Craig
Stopeck, Alison
Stratton, Suzanne
Thomson, Cynthia
Thompson, Patricia
Wondrak, Georg

Aziz, Noreen
Office of Cancer Survivorship
DCCPS, NCI 6130 EPN, Room 4090
Bethesda, MD 20892
USA

Lutz, Robert
Empire Health Systems
Spokane, WA 99210
USA

Hunt, Katherine
Mayo Clinic
13400 E. Shea Blvd.
Desk CR
Scottsdale, AZ 85259, USA

Greenlee, Heather
Columbia University
Mailman School of Public Health
722 West 168th Street
New York, NY 10032, USA

Introduction to Cancer Prevention

David S. Alberts and Lisa M. Hess

College of Medicine, University of Arizona, Tucson AZ 85724

The goals of cancer prevention are to reduce the incidence, morbidity and mortality due to cancer through the identification and elimination of precancerous lesions (termed intraepithelial neoplasias or IENs) and/or the early detection of minimally invasive cancers. Cancer is a global term for a variety of diseases that are characterized by uncontrolled cellular growth. The site of origin of the disease is used to define general categories of cancer (e.g. breast cancer, skin cancer). Worldwide, the incidence and mortality from cancer has been increasing, despite recent advances in the understanding and treatment of many diseases. This emphasizes the need to define the etiology and molecular basis of cancer and to prevent that cancer from developing. The concept of cancer prevention is changing gradually as we gain a greater understanding of the genetic and molecular basis of carcinogenesis. Certainly, it is understood that the cancer patient is not well one day and the next day diagnosed with cancer. It is estimated that there is an average lag of at least 20 years between the development of the first cancer cell and the onset of metastatic disease for a broad range of solid tumors. In that there were an estimated 563,700 cancer deaths in the U.S. in 2004, and given the 20+ year lag time, more than ten million "healthy" Americans harbor ultimately deadly cancers.

It is increasingly apparent that virtually all cancers proceed from the first initiated tumor cell (e.g. mutated DNA) to mild, moderate and severe dysplasia, invasive carcinoma (invasion of cells through the basement membrane) and metastatic disease (Fig. 1). Dysplasias are represented by small, intermediate and advanced adenomatous polyps in the colon, atypical hyperplasia and ductile carcinoma in situ in the breast and simple hyperplasia, atypical hyperplasia and carcinoma in situ in the endometrium. These precancerous lesions IENs can be identified both histologically and by molecular signatures, using a variety of anlytical methods (e.g. cDNA microarray) (O'Shaughnessy, Kelloff et al. 2002).

Many researchers worldwide have focused their life's work to identify ways to prevent cancer. This book provides an overview on the science and practice of cancer prevention for primary caregivers and the research community. The first section of this book (Chapters 1 through 8) provides information on economic issues in cancer prevention, dietary and environmental risk, cultural considerations in cancer prevention and issues related to drug development. The second section of the book (Chapters 9 through 16) focuses on the prevention of specific disease sites and provides the reader with a discussion of the epide-

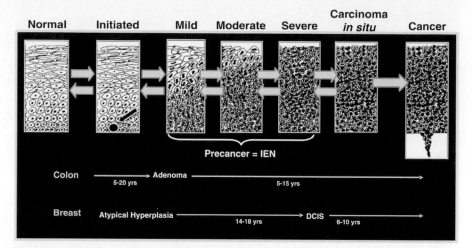

Fig. 1. Progression of precancer to cancer in humans is a multi-year process, adapted from O'Shaughnessy et al. (O'Shaughnessy, Kelloff et al. 2002)

miology, screening, and prevention of each disease, including both practice guidelines as well as theories and future research directions.

Overview of Cancer Prevention

It is estimated that there are over 8.1 million cases of cancer diagnosed per year worldwide (Parkin, Pisani et al. 1999). The five most common worldwide cancers, excluding non-melanoma skin cancer, include lung, stomach, breast, colorectal and liver cancer (Table 1). There are gender and regional differences in worldwide cancer diagnoses. Most lung cancers (about 58%) occur in developed countries. China accounts for 38% of all stomach cancers and 53.9% of all liver cancers diagnosed worldwide. Liver cancer is primarily diagnosed (81% of all cancers worldwide) in developing nations (e.g., Sub-Saharan Africa, Asia). Thirty-four percent of all colorectal cancer cases are diagnosed in developed nations. Among women, breast cancer accounts for 21% of all cancers and is the most common cancer in developed countries. Cervical cancer is the third most common cancer among women; 30% of all cases are diagnosed in south-central Asia. Prostate cancer is the fourth most common cancer among men worldwide, but is the most common cancer diagosed among men in North America. Prostate cancer incidence in North America is more than 80-fold the incidence rate in China.

In the United States (U.S.), there were 1,368,030 cancers diagnosed in 2004, excluding non-melanoma skin cancer, and cancer accounted for 563,700 deaths (Jemal, Tiwari et al. 2004). Cancer is a major health burden in the U.S., accounting for one of every four deaths. The most common cancers diagnosed in the U.S. are presented in Table 2. The three most common cancers account for a similar number of diagnoses among men and women. Among men, prostate, lung and colorectal cancer account for 396,840 diagnoses in 2004. Among women, breast, lung and colorectal cancer together accounted for 369,970 diagnoses.

Number (in thousands)	
Both sexes	
Lung	1036.9
Stomach	798.3
Breast	795.6
Colon/rectum	782.8
Liver	437.4
Prostate	396.1
Cervix	371.2
Males	
Lung	771.8
Stomach	511.0
Colon/rectum	401.9
Prostate	396.1
Liver	316.3
Esophagus	212.6
Bladder	202.5
Females	
Breast	795.6
Colon/rectum	381.0
Cervix	371.2
Stomach	287.2
Lung	265.1
Ovary	165.5
Endometrium	142.4

Table 1. Worldwide annual cancer incidence of the most common cancers (Parkin, Pisani et al. 1999)

Number	
Both sexes	
Prostate	230,110
Breast	217,440
Lung/bronchus	173,770
Colon/rectum	146,940
Melanoma	55,100
Males	
Prostate	230,110
Lung/bronchus	93,110
Colon/rectum	73,620
Bladder	60,240
Melanoma	29,900
Females	
Breast	215,990
Lung/bronchus	80,660
Colon/rectum	73,320
Endometrium	40,320
Ovary	25,580

Table 2. Annual cancer incidence of the most common cancers in the U.S. (Jemal, Tiwari et al. 2004)

Table 3. Factors associated with Cancer Risk, adapted from Giovannucci (Giovannucci 1999)

Factor	Association to Cancer Risk
Height	Increases prostate, colon and breast cancer risk
Obesity	Increases colon, breast, kidney, endometrial and gallbladder cancer risk; may increase ovarian cancer risk
Physical inactivity	Increases colon cancer risk; may increase breast and prostate cancer risk

The goal of cancer prevention is to reduce the morbidity and mortality from cancer by reducing the incidence of cancer. The development of effective cancer prevention strategies has the potential to impact more than eight million cancer diagnoses and to prevent more than 5.2 million cancer-related deaths each year worldwide (Parkin, Pisani et al. 1999; Pisani, Parkin et al. 1999). More than half of all cancer incidence and 2.8 million deaths occur in developed countries. Even with the current knowledge available, it is estimated that 60,000 cancer deaths could be prevented each year in the U.S. alone (Curry 2003). According to the Director of the National Cancer Institute, Andrew C. Von Eschenbach, M.D., one of the primary reasons why current knowledge and information about cancer and its prevention is not applied to the general public is due to an overload of complicated information. The dissemination of complicated information is problematic, but is essential to reduce the burden of cancer.

There are many factors known to reduce overall cancer incidence, such as minimizing exposure to carcinogens (e.g. avoiding tobacco), dietary modification, reducing body weight, increasing physical activity, or through medical intervention (surgery and/or chemoprevention). Current data, primarily obtained from epidemiologic research, suggests that there are a combination of factors involved in the development of cancer. As shown in Table 3, there is a critically important interaction of body height, presence of obesity, physical inactivity and cancer risk (Giovannucci 1999). Thus, it is important for primary caregivers as well as the research community to take a multidisciplinary approach to investigating and understanding cancer prevention.

There are three basic approaches to prevent cancer: primary, secondary and tertiary prevention. Primary prevention involves a reduction of the impact of carcinogens, such as through administration of a chemopreventive agent or the removal of environmental carcinogens. The goal of primary prevention is to prevent a cancer from beginning to develop by reducing individual risk. Current primary prevention methods include lifestyle modification or interventions that modify risk. Primary prevention methods are best suited for those cancers in which the causes are known. Worldwide, more than 1.3 million cancer cases are attributed to tobacco exposure (Parkin, Pisani et al. 1999). Modification of tobacco or other carcinogen exposure and other factors (i.e. dietary or environmental) could have a significant impact on worldwide health through primary prevention efforts. Many cancers are now known to be directly attributable to viral infections (e.g. human papillomavirus infection is a necessary factor in the development of cervical cancer; *Helicobacter pylori* is an initiator and promotor for gastric cancer). A number of primary prevention efforts are now being developed (e.g. cervical cancer vaccines; antibiotics and vaccines to eradicate

Helicobacter pylori) to prevent the development of these cancers via the prevention of viral infection.

Secondary prevention involves the concept of a precancerous lesion, or abnormal changes that precede the development of malignancy. Secondary prevention involves screening and early detection methods (e.g. mammogram, prostate-specific antigen test) that can identify abnormal changes before they become cancerous, thereby preventing the cancer before it fully develops. In some cases, secondary prevention can involve the treatment of precancerous lesions in an attempt to reverse carcinogenesis (e.g. cause the lesion to regress).

Tertiary prevention involves the care of established disease and the prevention of disease-related complications and often encompasses the treatment of patients at high risk of developing a second primary cancer. Tertiary prevention, often referred to as cancer control, involves a variety of aspects of patient care, such as quality of life, adjuvant therapies, surgical intervention and palliative care.

Multi-step Carcinogenesis Pathway

Prevention of cancer requires an understanding of the process of cancer initiation and the steps to progression of disease. This process is referred to as carcinogenesis, a process of genetic alterations that cause a normal cell to become malignant. Cancer prevention involves the identification and classification, as well as interventions for the regression or removal of precursor lesions, often referred to as intraepithelial neoplasia (IEN), before they can become cancerous. As shown earlier in Figure 1, the process of carcinogenesis may take many years. In the case of colorectal cancer, it may take up to 35 years from the first initiated colonic mucosal cell to an adenomatous polyp to develop invasive cancer. The same is true for prostate cancer, which progresses over as many as 40 to 50 years from mild to moderate, then severe intraepithelial neoplasia, to latent cancer (see Chapter 13).

The vast majority of current treatment modalities are used to treat far advanced and/or metastatic cancers; however, now that it is possible to identify IENs for virtually every solid tumor type, lifestyle changes, simple surgical procedures and che-

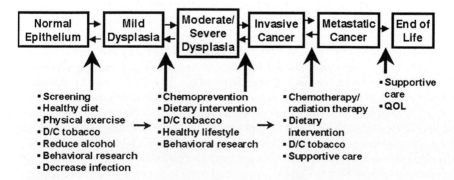

Fig. 2. Multi-step carcinogenesis pathway, adapted from Alberts, et al. (Alberts 1999)

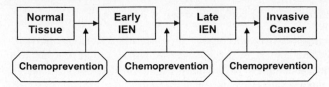

Fig. 3. Chemoprevention of intraepithelial neoplasia (IEN)

mopreventive agents can be used to impede the development of these potentially dangerous precancerous lesions (Fig. 2). For example, multiple lifestyle changes, taken together, could profoundly reduce the risk of the first initiated cell progressing to mild dysplasia. This would include reducing dietary fat intake, increasing the number of servings of fruits and vegetables, minimizing alcohol intake, tobacco exposure cessation and markedly increasing physical activity. These changes may potentially reduce risk for several cancers by up to 60 to 80% (Doll and Peto 1981). Furthermore, the addition of an effective chemoprevention agent, such as tamoxifen for moderately or severely dysplastic intraepithelial neoplasia such as ductile carcinoma in situ, can reduce cancer risk by as much as 50% (Fisher, Costantino et al. 1998). Thus, the concept of cancer prevention is now evolving into the mainstream of cancer therapeutics.

The process of carcinogenesis involves multiple molecular events over many years to evolve to the earliest dysplastic lesion or IEN. This multi-year process provides numerous opportunities to intervene with screening, early detection, surgical procedures, and chemoprevention (i.e. the use of specific nutrients and/or chemicals to treat IENs and/or delay their development) (Sporn 1976). Figure 3 presents the concept that an effective chemopreventive agent could prevent IEN growth, progression or, ultimately, invasion through the tissue basement membrane.

Cancer Prevention Research

The importance of conducting and participating in clinical trials cannot be understated. Every person is at risk of genetic mutations that may lead to cancer. Due to both endogenous or exogenous factors, every human body has undergone genetic alterations. For many individuals, these initiating factors are the early steps to the development of IEN or cancer. The time period from the first initiated cell to the time of cancer is estimated to be approximately 20 years. In 2004, there were an estimated 563,700 deaths due to cancer in the U.S. This would translate to more than 11,000,000 individuals in the U.S. alone who are currently in some phase of cancer progression that will ultimately result in death (Wattenberg 1993).

Cancer prevention trials are research studies designed to evaluate the safety and effectiveness of new methods of cancer prevention or screening. They are key to understanding the appropriate use of chemoprevention agents or screening tools. The focus of cancer prevention research can involve chemoprevention (including vaccination), screening, genetics, and/or lifestyle changes (e.g. diet, exercise). Cancer chemoprevention research differs from treatment research in several important ways as shown in Table 4. Cancer chemoprevention trials generally are performed in relatively healthy

Table 4. Cancer chemoprevention versus cancer treatment phase III trials, adapted from Alberts, et al. (Alberts 2004)

Characteristic	Cancer Chemoprevention Trials	Cancer Treatment Trials
Participants	Relatively healthy volunteers with IENs or at moderate/high risk	Patients diagnosed with invasive cancer
Trial design	Commonly double-blind, placebo controlled	Unblinded to both patient and investigator
Dosage	Minimize dose, emphasize safety	Maximize dose, emphasize efficacy
Toxicity	Dosage changes with any toxicity, concern for long-term use of agent	Moderate toxicity acceptable, less concern with toxicity due to severity of disease
Adherence	Concern for "drop ins" due to media or hype	Concern for "drop outs" due to toxicity
End point	Surrogate biomarkers; cancer incidence	Mortality
Sample size	A few thousand to several thousand participants	A few hundred to a thousand participants
Trial duration	Often 5–10 years	Several months to several years

volunteers who have well-documented IENs (e.g. colorectal adenomas, bladder papillomas, ductal carcinoma in situ, actinic keratosis in the skin) or at increased risk due to genetic or other factors. These trials are usually double-blind (i.e. both physician and participant do not know the assigned treatment), placebo-controlled and involve a few thousand to several thousand randomized participants. As opposed to cancer treatment phase III trials, that rarely extend beyond five years in duration, cancer chemoprevention trials often take 5 to 10 years to complete.

The phases of investigation in cancer prevention research trials (phase I through IV trials) are described in more detail in Chapter 7. Briefly, phase I trials take place after an agent has demonstrated activity with low toxicity in preclinical models. Phase I trials are brief (several weeks), preliminary research studies in humans to determine safety of an agent. Phase II trials are longer in duration (several weeks to months) to determine the activity of an agent and to further evaluate safety. Phase III trials are large, randomized trials to evaluate the effectiveness and safety of an agent in a sample of the target population. For a chemopreventive agent to be used in a phase III research setting, it must meet several criteria. The agent must have strong data supporting its mechanistic activity and there must be preclinical efficacy data from appropriate models. If the chemopreventive agent is a nutritient, there must be strong epidemiologic data supporting its potential effectiveness and it must have demonstrated safety and activity in phase II trials. Finally, phase III trials of a novel chemopreventive agent should not be performed in the absence of a fundamental understanding of its mechanism of action.

When the mechanism of activity of a putative chemoprevention agent has not been explored in the setting of broad populations, the results of phase III trials can be alarming. Two examples of this include the results of the Finnish Alpha-Tocopherol, Beta-Carotene (ATCB) Trial and the University of Washington Carotene and Efficacy

Trial (CARET). Both of these phase III trials used relatively high doses of beta-carotene as compared to placebo in heavy smokers to reduce the incidence of and mortality from lung cancer (1994; Omenn, Goodman et al. 1996). Unfortunately, both trials found that the beta-carotene intervention was asociated with a 18 to 28% increase in lung cancer incidence and an associated increase in mortality. Perhaps the reason for these unexpected and extremely unfortunate results relates to the fact that at high beta-carotene concentrations in the setting of high partial pressures of oxygen (e.g. as achieved in the lung) and in the presence of heat (e.g. as achieved in the lung with cigarette smoking), beta-carotene can become an autocatalytic pro-oxidant (versus its usual role as an anti-oxidant) (Burton and Ingold 1984).

The design of chemoprevention phase III trials must be founded on a hypothesis that is soundly based on the mechanism of action of the agent, epidemiologic data and its preclinical efficacy. The population to be enrolled to a phase III prevention trial must be relatively high risk, to assure that there will be a sufficient number of events (e.g. precancers or cancers) to compare the treatment to the control. Phase III prevention trials should include both intermediate (e.g. IEN) and long-term (e.g. cancer) endpoint evaluations. Most importantly, the endpoint analyses should be planned in advance, including well-defined and well-powered primary and secondary analyses.

One example of a potentially high-impact phase III chemoprevention trial is the Breast Cancer Prevention Trial with Tamoxifen (BCPT) (Fisher, Costantino et al. 1998). Healthy women at increased risk of breast cancer were randomized to either tamoxifen (20 mg per day) or placebo for up to five years. Tamoxifen was selected for this trial because of its well-documented mechanism of action (i.e. binding to the estrogen receptor to prevent estrogen's effect on tumor cell proliferation), its strong safety profile in the setting of adjuvant breast cancer therapy, and its extreme activity in the prevention of contralateral breast cancer in patients with stage I/II breast cancer. After 69 months of follow up, tamoxifen was found to be associated with an overall 49% reduction in the risk of invasive breast cancer (Fisher, Costantino et al. 1998). The benefit of breast cancer risk must be balanced with its toxicities, which include a

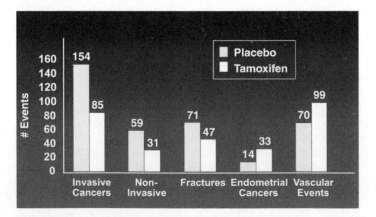

Fig. 4. Events in the Breast Cancer Prevention Trial

greater than two-fold increase in early stage endometrial cancer and an increased incidence of deep vein thrombosis and pulmonary embolism (Fig. 4). Since the publication of these results, much discussion has led to the identification of women who would most benefit from treatment with tamoxifen. Certainly, women who are at increased breast cancer risk, have already undergone a hysterectomy, and who at lower risk for thrombophlebitis (e.g. due to higher levels of physical activity, lack of obesity) would be good candidates for this intervention. Tamoxifen is a relatively expensive drug, but it is now approved by the U.S. Food and Drug Administration for the reduction of breast cancer risk among women at high risk. Nevertheless, without adequate health insurance coverage, there is very limited access to this prevention treatment among underserved populations.

The translation of research findings to the clinic is the ultimate goal of cancer prevention research. Chemoprevention agents or screening modalities must be acceptable to the target population that would benefit from such interventions. For example, the ideal chemoprevention agent would have a known mechanism of action and would have no or minimal toxicity, high efficacy, be available orally or topically, have an acceptable treatment regimen, and would be inexpensive. Similarly, screening or early detection modalities should be minimally invasive, have high sensitivity and specificity, and be acceptable to the target population. Interventions that fail to maintain adequate adherence or that have high attrition rates during phase III trials will likely also not be acceptable to the patient in clinical practice.

References

Alberts, D.S., R.R. Barakat, et al. (1994). "The effect of vitamin E and beta carotene on the incidence of lung cancer and other cancers in male smokers. The Alpha-Tocopherol, Beta Carotene Cancer Prevention Study Group." N Engl J Med **330**(15): 1029–1035.

Alberts, D.S., R.R. Barakat, et al. (2004). Prevention of gynecologic malignances. Gynecologic Cancer: Controversies in Management. D.M. Gershenson, W.P. McGuire, M. Gore, M.A. Quinn, G. Thomas (Eds.), Philadelphia, El Sevier Ltd.

Burton, G.W. and K.U. Ingold (1984). "Beta-Carotene: an unusual type of lipid antioxidant." Science **224**(4649): 569–573.

Curry, S.J., T. Byers, M. Hewitt (2003). Fulfilling the Potential for Cancer Prevention and Early Detection. Washington DC, National Academies Press, National Cancer Policy Board, Institute of Medicine.

Doll, R. and R. Peto (1981). "The causes of cancer: quantitative estimates of avoidable risks of cancer in the United States today." J Natl Cancer Inst **66**(6): 1191–1308.

Fisher, B., J.P. Costantino, et al. (1998). "Tamoxifen for prevention of breast cancer: report of the National Surgical Adjuvant Breast and Bowel Project P-1 Study." J Natl Cancer Inst **90**(18): 1371–1388.

Giovannucci, E. (1999). The epidemiologic basis for nutritional influences on the cancer cell. Nutritional Oncology. D. Heber, Blackburn, G.L., Go, V.L.W. San Diego, Academic Press.

Jemal, A., R.C. Tiwari, et al. (2004). "Cancer statistics, 2004." CA Cancer J Clin **54**(1): 8–29.

Omenn, G.S., G.E. Goodman, et al. (1996). "Risk factors for lung cancer and for intervention effects in CARET, the Beta-Carotene and Retinol Efficacy Trial." J Natl Cancer Inst **88**(21): 1550–1559.

O'Shaughnessy, J.A., G.J. Kelloff, et al. (2002). "Treatment and prevention of intraepithelial neoplasia: an important target for accelerated new agent development." Clin Cancer Res **8**(2): 314–346.

Parkin, D.M., P. Pisani, et al. (1999). "Estimates of the worldwide incidence of 25 major cancers in 1990." Int J Cancer **80**(6): 827–841.

Pisani, P., D.M. Parkin, et al. (1999). "Estimates of the worldwide mortality from 25 cancers in 1990." *Int J Cancer* **83**(1): 18–29.

Sporn, M.B. (1976). "Approaches to prevention of epithelial cancer during the preneoplastic period." *Cancer Res* **36**(7 PT 2):2699–2702.

Wattenberg, L.W. (1993). "Prevention–therapy–basic science and the resolution of the cancer problem." *Cancer Res* **53**(24): 5890–5896.

Assessing Human and Economic Benefits of Cancer Prevention

Stephen Joel Coons and Benjamin M. Craig

College of Pharmacy, University of Arizona, Tucson AZ 85721

It is critically important to discuss and attempt to quantify the human and economic value of cancer prevention. The purpose of this chapter is to provide an overview of the ways in which this value can be defined and assessed.

As will be described in much more detail in subsequent chapters, cancer prevention takes many forms. Virtually all prevention activities involve: (1) engaging in particular behaviors (e.g., routinely participating in recommended screenings, taking tamoxifen for secondary prevention of breast cancer); (2) avoiding particular behaviors (e.g., sunbathing, smoking); or (3) changing particular behaviors once they have become habitual or routine (e.g., quitting smoking, lowering dietary fat). Each of these prevention behaviors, or the lack of them, can have short- and long-term health, quality of life, and/or economic consequences.

Outcomes Assessment

In order to discuss the impact of cancer and, hence, the substantial benefits of preventing it, it is necessary to define *outcomes*. A conceptual framework articulated by Kozma et al. places outcomes into three categories: economic, clinical, and humanistic (Kozma, Reeder et al. 1993). Economic outcomes are changes in the consumption and production of resources caused by disease or intervention, such as cancer prevention. The changes may be direct (e.g., cost of a medication) or indirect (e.g., early retirement due to reduced productivity). Clinical outcomes are the medical events that occur as a result of the condition or its treatment as measured in the clinical setting. Humanistic, or patient-reported, outcomes include condition or treatment-related symptoms and side effects, satisfaction, and self-assessed function and well-being, or health-related quality of life.

The major cancer clinical trial cooperative groups in North America and Europe have recognized the importance of this outcomes triad in evaluating and improving the net benefit of cancer therapy (Bruner, Movsas et al. 2004). Humanistic and economic outcomes, which are the focus of this chapter, are increasingly being incorporated into clinical trials (Lipscomb, Donaldson et al. 2004). In addition, the importance of outcomes assessment in cancer was reinforced with the establishment of the National Cancer Institute's (NCI) Outcomes Research Branch in 1999 (Lipscomb and Snyder 2002). According to the NCI, "outcomes research describes, interprets, and predicts the impact of various influences, especially (but not exclusively) interventions on 'final' endpoints that matter to decision makers: patients, providers, private payers, government agencies, accrediting organizations, or society at large" (Lipscomb and Snyder 2002).

Humanistic Outcomes

Quality of life is a commonly used term that usually conveys a general feeling rather than a specific state of mind. A person's quality of life, or subjective well-being, is based on personal experience and expectations, that affect and can be influenced by many factors, including standard of living, family life, friendships, and job satisfaction. Although health can impact these factors, health care is not directly aimed at enhancing them. Studies of health outcomes use the term *health-related quality of life* to distinguish health effects from the effects of other important personal and environmental factors. There is growing awareness that in certain diseases, such as cancer, or at particular stages of disease, health-related quality of life may be the most important health outcome to consider in assessing treatment (Staquet, Aaronson et al. 1992).

In much of the empirical literature, explicit definitions of quality of life are rare; readers must deduce its implicit definition from the manner in which it is operationalized and measured. However, some authors have provided definitions of health-related quality of life that can guide its measurement. For example, Schron and Shumaker define it as "a multidimensional concept referring to a person's total well-being, including his or her psychological, social, and physical health status" (Schron and Shumaker 1992). Till et al. (Till 1984) state that health-related quality of life "includes psychologic and social functioning as well as physical functioning and incorporates positive aspects of well-being as well as negative aspects of disease or infirmity". These two definitions differ in certain respects, but an important conceptual characteristic they share is multidimensionality. Although the terminology may vary, commonly measured dimensions of health-related quality of life include the following:

▪ Physical health and functioning
▪ Psychological health and functioning
▪ Social and role functioning
▪ Perceptions of general well-being

An example of operationally defined health-related quality of life is provided in the National Surgical Adjuvant Breast and Bowel Project P-1 Study (Day, Ganz et al. 1999). The investigators measured health-related quality of life (HRQL) by administering the P-1 HRQL Questionnaire. This 104-item questionnaire included the Center for Epidemiological Studies Depression Scale (CES-D), the Medical Outcomes Study (MOS) 36-Item Short-Form Health Survey (SF-36), the MOS sexual functioning scale, and a symptom checklist. This battery of multiple instruments and scales enabled the investigators to assess dimensions of functioning and well-being they felt were most relevant in the target population.

Measuring Health-Related Quality of Life

Although health-related quality of life is subjective, when operationally defined (as with the P-1 HRQL Questionnaire), it can be validly and reliably measured. Cullen et al., in their review of the short-term quality of life impact of cancer prevention and screening activities, addressed other ways in which it has been operationalized through the use of new and existing measurement tools (Cullen, Schwartz et al. 2004).

There are hundreds of health-related quality of life instruments available (McDowell 1996; Bowling 1997), some of which have been developed specifically for use in people with cancer (Bowling 2001; Donaldson 2004). A primary distinction among the instruments is whether they are specific or generic.

Specific instruments are intended to provide greater detail concerning particular outcomes, in terms of functioning and well-being, uniquely associated with a condition and/or its treatment. Disease- or condition-specific instruments may be more sensitive than a generic measure to particular changes in health-related quality of life secondary to the disease or its treatment. For example, the Functional Assessment of Cancer Therapy (FACT) subscales, such as the neurotoxicity subscale (FACT-NTX,) address specific concerns (e.g., finger numbness, difficulty buttoning), which would not be addressed in a generic instrument. In addition, specific measures may appear to be more clinically relevant to patients and health care providers since the instruments address issues directly related to the disease (Guyatt, Feeny et al. 1993). However, a concern regarding the use of only specific instruments is that by focusing on the specific impact of a disease or its treatment, the general or overall impact on functioning and well-being may be overlooked. Therefore, the use of both a generic and a specific instrument may be the best approach to evaluating HRQL. This was the approach taken by the developers of the UCLA Prostate Cancer Index, which covers both general and disease-specific (e.g., sexual, urinary and bowel function) concerns (Litwin, Hays et al. 1998).

Patient-Reported Instruments. The pioneering work of Karnofsky and Burchenal in the 1940s that produced the Karnofsky Performance Scale recognized the need to assess the patient's functional status in the context of cancer chemotherapy (Karnofsky 1949). This tool, which was designed for clinician assessment of observable physical functioning, is still used today. It was one of the first steps in the development of patient-centered and, ultimately, patient-reported outcome measures. Since then, a considerable amount of time and effort has been invested in the development of cancer-specific instruments for use in clinical trials and routine patient monitoring. Another of these instruments is the Q-TWiST (Quality-Adjusted Time Without Symptoms and Toxicity), which addressed both quality and quantity of time following cancer treatment (Gelber, Goldhirsch et al. 1993). Other examples are the EORTC QLQ-C30 and the Functional Assessment of Cancer Therapy-General (FACT-G) (Aaronson, Ahmedzai et al. 1993; Cella, Tulsky et al. 1993). The European Organization for Research and Treatment of Cancer (EORTC) has worked extensively in the area of instrument development (www.eortc.be/home/qol). In addition, the developers of the FACT-G have a

Table 1. Domains/dimensions addressed by the FACT-G and EORTC QLQ-C30

EORTC QLQ-C30	FACT-G
Physical functioning	Physical well-being
Role functioning	Social/Family well-being
Cognitive functioning	Emotional well-being
Emotional functioning	Functional well-being
Social functioning	
Global quality of life	
Fatigue	
Nausea and vomiting	
Pain	

broad array of cancer-specific instruments available (www.facit.org). Table 1 lists the dimensions covered by the EORTC QLQ-C30 and the FACT-G. Each of these instruments was designed to be supplemented with additional modules or scales aimed at specific cancer patient subgroups.

Since primary cancer prevention involves avoiding the occurrence of disease, general measures may be more applicable in that context. Generic, or general, instruments are designed to be applicable across a wide variety of populations, across all diseases or conditions, and across different medical interventions (Patrick and Deyo 1989). The two main types of generic instruments are health profiles and preference-based measures.

Health Profiles. Health profiles provide multiple outcome scores representing individual dimensions of health-related quality of life. An advantage of a health profile is that it enables clinicians and/or researchers to measure the differential effects of a disease state or its treatment on particular dimensions. The most commonly used generic instrument in the world today is the SF-36 (www.sf36.org), which was used as a component of the P-1 HRQL Questionnaire discussed above. The SF-36 includes eight multi-item scales (Table 2) which address a wide array of dimensions (Ware and Sherbourne 1992). Each of the scale scores can range from 0 to 100, with higher scores representing better functioning or well-being. It is brief (it takes about 10 minutes to complete) and its reliability and validity have been documented in many clinical situations and disease states. A means of aggregating the items into physical and mental component summary scores is available (Ware 1994). However, the SF-36 does not provide an overall summary or index score, which distinguishes it from the preference-based measures.

Preference-Based Measures. For health-related quality of life scores to be most useful as an outcome in economic analysis, they need to be on a scale anchored by 0.0 (i.e., death) and 1.0 (i.e., perfect health). The values for the health states represented on the scale reflect the relative desirability or preference level for individual health states as judged by population- or patient-based samples. Although one can undertake direct preference measurement, a number of preference-based instruments are already available for which the health state preferences have been derived empirically through population studies. Examples include the Quality of Well-Being Scale (QWB) (www.medicine.ucsd.edu/fpm/hoap/qwb.htm), the Health Utilities Index (HUI) (www.healthutilities.com), the EuroQol Group's EQ-5D (www.euroqol.org), and the SF-6D (www.sf36.org). The SF-6D was developed to provide an overall summary or index score for data collected with the SF-36 (Brazier, Roberts et al. 2002). The domains addressed by each of these instruments are listed in Table 2.

Quality-Adjusted Life Years (QALYs). The instruments described above are administered to measure respondents' health status, which is then mapped onto the instrument's multiattribute health status classification system producing a health-related quality of life score on the 0.0 to 1.0 scale. Scores on this scale, which may represent the health-related consequences of disease or its treatment, can be used to adjust length of life for its quality resulting in an estimate of *quality-adjusted life years* (QALYs). QALYs integrate in a single outcome measure the net health gains or losses,

Table 2. Domains included in selected generic instruments

SF-36
Physical functioning
Role limitations due to physical problems
Bodily pain
General health perceptions
Vitality
Social functioning
Role limitations due to emotional problems
Mental health

Quality of Well-Being Scale (QWB)
Mobility
Physical activity
Social activity
Symptoms/Problems

Health Utilities Index (HUI)	
HUI2	**HUI3**
Sensation	Vision
Mobility	Hearing
Emotion	Speech
Cognition	Ambulation
Self-care	Dexterity
Pain	Emotion
Fertility	Cognition
	Pain

EQ-5D
Mobility
Self-care
Usual activity
Pain/discomfort
Anxiety/depression

SF-6D
Physical functioning
Role limitation
Social functioning
Mental health
Bodily pain
Vitality

in terms of both quantity and quality of life. The metric of life-years saved (LYS) is not sufficient since death is not the only outcome of concern; health-related quality of life changes can occur with or without changes in life years. The QALY approach assumes that one year in full health is scored 1.0 and death is 0.0. Years of life in less than full health are scored as less than 1.0 QALY. For example, based on a review by

Tengs and Wallace, a year of life with small-cell lung cancer after the disease has progressed is equal to 0.15 QALY (Tengs and Wallace 2000).

QALYs can be a key outcome measure, especially in diseases such as cancer, where the treatment itself can have a major impact on patient functioning and well-being. Although the QALY is the most commonly used health outcome summary measure, it is not the only one. Other conceptually equivalent outcomes include *years of healthy life* (YHL), *well years* (WYs), *health-adjusted person years* (HAPYs), and *health-adjusted life expectancy* (HALE). As observed by Ubel, without an outcome measure such as QALYs, it would be impossible to compare the relative cost-effectiveness of life-prolonging versus life-enhancing interventions, much less interventions that do both (Ubel 2001). The remainder of this chapter discusses the economic issues and methodologies relevant to cancer prevention.

Economic Outcomes and Cancer

Prevention of cancer renders an economic benefit for society by reducing the amount of resources necessary for the treatment of cancer. The NCI reports that cancer treatment accounted for $41 billion in 1995, just under 5 percent of total U.S. spending for medical treatments (NCI 2004). By investing in cost-saving cancer prevention modalities, more resources may be available for the overall health care system. Johnson and colleagues estimate that 53% and 13% of the medical expenditures for persons with lung cancer and chronic obstructive pulmonary disease are attributable to smoking, respectively (Johnson, Dominici et al. 2003). Substantial medical resources would become available, if smoking were reduced.

Economic benefits rendered by improving health go beyond the costs associated with medical treatments. The economic benefits of cancer prevention include decreases in the frequency of health-related disruptions in productive activity, such as lost work days. By promoting health, cancer prevention reduces the need for assistance with personal care services and allows greater intangible benefits, like dignity, autonomy, and individuality. Simply put, prevention is better than cure because, as stated by Thomas Adams, a 17th century physician, it saves the labor of being sick.

Although the economic benefits of cancer prevention are widely acknowledged, especially by NCI, there is a paucity of evidence regarding these benefits. The information regarding economic outcomes that is available is rarely translated for and applied to evidence-based medical decision making. As a result, cancer prevention is often inefficiently utilized. Researchers who study the economic outcomes of cancer prevention provide valuable information to individuals and institutions, who may fail to consider the full scope of the economic benefits (Fryback and Craig 2004). For example, some managed care organizations have responded to the increasing cost of medical care by increasing the cost borne by patients, and these higher copayments may deter the use of cancer prevention strategies. Individuals and institutions may observe short-run reductions in costs, but this shortsightedness can lead to greater long-run costs.

Decision makers at the individual, institutional, or governmental levels require evidence on economic outcomes of cancer prevention to improve their ability to make informed choices with regard to prevention activities, thereby maximizing limited resources. In this section, we describe core concepts in economic outcomes research and provide examples to illustrate their importance.

Defining and Measuring Economic Outcomes

Every cancer prevention strategy entails a change in the use of scarce resources, also known as an economic outcome. If we were to list the resources necessary to produce an intervention and the resources saved due to the intervention, we would have a description of the net bundle of resources attributable to the intervention. This bundle is known as the intervention's *opportunity cost*. Once the intervention is undertaken, the opportunity to use these resources differently is lost. Consideration of the economic outcomes associated with interventions is important for individuals and institutions that practice evidence-based medicine.

Economic outcomes, changes in resources due to an intervention, may be categorized by system, path, and flow. Resources from the medical system, such as physician time, medications, and hospital beds, are distinguished from non-medical resources, such as community, familial, and personal goods. For example, fuel consumption by an ambulance is a medical outcome, whereas fuel for personal transportation to a clinic is a non-medical outcome. Medical and non-medical resources are differentiated, because each system faces different budgetary constraints.

Economic outcomes are also separated by their path, whether they are directly related to an intervention or indirectly related through a change in health caused by the intervention. For example, a nicotine patch may be consumed as part of a smoking cessation intervention, therefore a direct economic outcome of the intervention. The patch may change smoking-related behaviors, such as smoking breaks at work. Changes in productivity are indirect economic outcomes of the intervention. The direct and indirect outcomes are components of the smoking cessation program's opportunity cost. The concept of indirect and direct economic outcomes is unrelated to the accounting term "indirect costs" referring to overhead or fixed costs.

Economic outcomes represent an inflow of resources through consumption or an outflow of resources through production. Patients directly consume medical resources over the course of an intervention, but patients are also producers of resources. Smoking cessation programs change the consumption of resources, such as cigarettes, nicotine replacement medications, and counseling. These programs may also affect the productivity of individuals, either by making their lives more productive, or by extending their productive lives. When considering the economic benefits of cancer prevention, the effect on the consumption of current resources may be small compared to the benefits in terms of productive activities. Economic outcomes can be characterized as medical or non-medical, direct or indirect, and an inflow or outflow of resources.

Unit of Economic Outcomes. Economic outcomes are best measured in natural units. Natural units often appear in the form of number of hours, quantities of a specific medication, or distance traveled. Natural units describe the changes in the inflow and outflow of resources related to the intervention. Clinical-economic trials, which are randomized controlled trials that prospectively collect economic endpoint data, provide the strongest evidence on economic outcomes, because these trials randomly assign alternatives to participants to identify causality. In a prospective substudy of a randomized clinical trial, Sculpher and colleagues (Sculpher, Palmer et al. 2000) evaluated alternative drug therapies, reltitrexed and fluorouracil with folinic acid, for advanced colorectal cancer based on the number of trips made to and from the hospital and the time lost from usual activity over the therapy period. In their study, they examined medical records for medical resource consumption data and self-report data to assess travel mode, distance, and time. This is an excellent example of a clinical-economic trial that collected economic endpoint data in natural units. These natural units can be translated into monetary values according to the perspective of the decision maker.

In economics, price is cost plus marginal profit, but outside of economics, price is often confused with cost and charges. Price represents the market value of a good, if sold. If the objective of the study is to predict revenue (or expenditure), natural units are to be translated using market values (i.e., prices). Market values fluctuate over time or region, according to market forces. If the objective is to predict cost of an intervention, natural units are to be translated according to the cost of producing those resources. The cost of producing resources may also depend upon market price of the inputs necessary for resource production. For example, a mammogram may cost a provider organization $50 to produce, but they set a price of $75, because that is what the market will bear. The difference between price and cost, $25, is the marginal profit for the health organization. The inclusion and extent of marginal profit in the translation of natural units into monetary values depends on the perspective of the decision maker. The reasonable amount of profit on a mammogram for a clinic is up for interpretation.

A charge is a payment of a claim, the rightful reimbursement for the provision of goods and services according to a contract. It is neither a price nor a cost, because of its dependence on the contractual relationship between institutions. For example, managed care organizations often shift funds between services, overcharging for specialist visits to subsidize mammography under the same contract. Unlike prices, the charge for one resource may depend on the charges for other resources under the same contract. This dependent relationship makes it difficult to interpret endpoints measured through charges. However, it is well-documented that charges exceed cost in most circumstances. The economic outcomes may be represented in monetary terms, such as costs, prices, and charges, depending on perspective. However, it is important the perspective of the translation (i.e., unit of analysis) match the perspective of the decision maker, so that they may practice evidence-based medicine.

Perspective of Economic Outcomes. The monetary value of an economic outcome depends on the perspective of the decision maker (e.g., individual, institutional, societal). Individuals face different prices (or costs) than institutions, so they translate natural units into monetary values differently. The societal perspective considers the economic outcome borne by all individuals, and uses market value to translate natural units into monetary values. For example, the monetary value of an hour of a physician's time may be equal to a copayment from a patient's perspective, an institution-specific wage from a managed care organization's perspective, or a market wage from the societal perspective.

Differing perspectives may lead decision makers to disagree on policies regarding cancer prevention. Smoking cessation programs have medical and non-medical economic outcomes. Medical outcomes attributable to certain programs may entail a monetary loss from the perspective of a managed care organization. After incorporating the non-medical outcomes, the programs may appear to save resources from the societal perspective. Disagreement between governmental and institutional decision makers over the economic consequences of smoking cessation programs are related to the translation of natural units into monetary values. Furthermore, societal and institutional perspectives often disagree about the inclusion of institutional profit in the translation.

Evaluative and Descriptive Analyses in Cancer Prevention

The economic benefits of cancer prevention are commonly described as a matter of investment in health (Wagner 1997). By investing medical resources in cancer prevention today, substantial economic benefits may accrue in the future. The purpose of evaluative analyses in cancer prevention is to examine the economic and health outcomes of alternative interventions, so that decision makers may better understand the potential impact of cancer prevention. There are four forms for economic evaluation: cost-minimization, cost-effectiveness, cost-utility, and cost-benefit. In addition, there are also descriptive studies that present economic outcomes of alternative interventions and disease, but do not directly compare health and economic outcomes. Descriptive analyses include cost-of-illness, cost identification, and cost-consequence studies. In this section, examples of evaluative and descriptive analyses in cancer prevention are provided.

Economic Evaluations. To promote evidence-based medical decision making, economic evaluations present the economic and health outcomes of alternative interventions. If an intervention costs more and is less effective than another intervention, the choice between the two interventions is clear. However, in many cases, the dominance of one intervention over another may depend on the relative importance of economic and health outcomes. For example, an intervention may cost more and be more effective or cost less and be less effective relative to another intervention. Economic evaluations verbally or quantitatively summarize the evidence to inform such difficult decisions.

The four types of economic evaluations (cost-minimization, cost-effectiveness, cost-utility, and cost-benefit) measure economic outcomes in monetary units, but each handles health outcomes in different ways. In cost-minimization studies, health outcomes are not measured, but assumed. For example, if two prevention interventions are known to have equivalent health outcomes, a study may examine which use the least amount of medical resources to minimize the cost to the health care system. Cost-effectiveness, cost-utility, and cost-benefit evaluations measure health outcomes, but using different units. Health outcomes in cost-effectiveness analyses are measured in natural units, such as number of life years saved. Cost-utility analyses use QALYs and cost-benefit analyses use monetary units, such as dollars. It can be difficult to translate health outcomes into QALYs or monetary units, so the typical form of economic evaluation is a cost-effectiveness analysis.

To summarize the evidence, cost-effectiveness and cost-utility analyses separate out the difference in cost and effectiveness between interventions and examine their ratio, known as an incremental cost-effectiveness ratio (ICER). This ratio measures the amount of resources required for each unit of health outcome (i.e., the amount of dollars required to increase life expectancy by one day). The ratios can be difficult to interpret because a positive value may signify an increase in cost and an increase in effectiveness, or a decrease in cost and a decrease in effectiveness. An intervention that saves money may have the same ratio as one that requires additional resources, so it is important to look at both the ratio and budgetary implications of the choice.

Cost-effectiveness analyses of cancer screening are commonplace, particularly in the cervical cancer literature (Eddy 1990; Kulasingam and Myers 2003; Goldie, Kohli et al. 2004). Brown and Garber examined three cervical screening technologies (Thin-Prep, AutoPap, and Papnet) among a cohort of 20-to 65-year-old women from the societal perspective (Brown and Garber 1999). Outcomes of interest, including life expectancy and lifetime direct medical cost, were compared among the three technologies and between each technology and conventional Pap at various intervals. The authors found that, depending on the technology and frequency of screening, these technologies increased life expectancy by 5 hours to 1.6 days and increased cost by $30 to $257 (1996 U.S. dollars) relative to conventional Pap. In this case, small increases in life expectancy are related to small increases in cost. When used with triennial screening, each technology produced more life years at a lower cost relative to conventional Pap used with biennial screening. In other words, conventional Pap used with biennial screening is dominated by each technology used with triennial screening. Among the new technologies, AutoPap dominated ThinPrep, but Papnet cost $43 more and produced 0.11 additional days of life expectancy. The incremental cost-effectiveness ratio, $391 ($43/0.11) per day of life saved, suggests that if society values a day of life more than $391 then Papnet may be preferred over AutoPap. The analysis does not account for nonmedical or indirect costs and examines only life expectancy, excluding the potential burden of cancer in terms of quality of life.

Compared to cost-effectiveness analyses, cost-utility analyses have the advantage of being able to combine multiple health and clinical outcomes into QALYs. Two cost-utility analyses of cervical cancer screening have estimated health outcomes in terms of QALYs (Goldie, Weinstein et al. 1999; Mandelblatt, Lawrence et al. 2002). Goldie and colleagues assess alternative screening strategies in HIV-infected women and Mandelblatt and colleagues examine combinations of conventional Pap and HPV testing at various intervals among a longitudinal cohort of women beginning at age 20 and continuing until age 65, 75 or death.

Evidence on economic outcomes is not meant to dictate the choice among alternative interventions. It is only one consideration among many possible considerations. Economic evaluations are conducted to assist policy makers in their deliberation over access to cost-effective cancer prevention strategies by providing evidence on the potential impact of the alternative strategies. In the absence of evidence-based policy, cancer prevention resources may not be allocated efficiently according to the perspectives of the decision makers.

Descriptive Studies. Cost-of-illness studies compare economic outcomes by disease and cost-identification studies examine the difference in economic outcomes across alternative interventions. Taplin and colleagues (Taplin, Barlow et al. 1995) conducted a cost-of-illness study and evaluated the direct cost of treating colon, prostate, and breast cancer. Their results suggest that the direct cost of cancer treatment increases with stage of diagnosis. Tsao and colleagues estimated that the cost of treating a patient with stage III or stage IV cutaneous melanoma is roughly 40 times the cost of treating a stage I patient (Tsao, Rogers et al. 1998). Although increasing medical cost by stage may not be surprising, Ramsey and colleagues found that even after controlling for stage, direct costs were lower among persons with screen-detected versus symptom-detected colorectal cancer in the 12 months following diagnosis (Ramsey, Mandelson et al. 2003). The findings of these cost-of-illness studies supports the premise that primary and secondary cancer prevention may result in substantial economic benefits, potentially saving economic resources from the managed care perspective.

Cost-identification studies can improve medical decision making by dispelling perceptions of cost savings. Esser and Brunner reviewed 33 studies that examine economic outcomes of granulocyte colony-stimulating factor (G-CSF) in the prevention and treatment of chemotherapy-induced neutropenia (Esser and Brunner 2003). Contrary to conventional opinion, they found little evidence that G-CSF is cost saving as primary or secondary prophylaxis, and only minor cost savings in patients undergoing bone marrow transplant. This tertiary prevention review is particularly notable because of reports that G-CSF expenses amount to 10% of the total budget of US hospital pharmacies with limited observed clinical benefits.

Evidence from cost-identification studies may also emphasize the importance of cancer prevention as a cost containment strategy. Loeve and colleagues conducted a cost-identification study for endoscopic colorectal cancer screening and found that endoscopic colorectal cancer screening has the potential to be cost saving (Loeve, Brown et al. 2000). They stated that similar analyses of screening programs for breast and cervical cancer have not demonstrated potential cost savings under any reasonable assumptions.

Some cost-identification studies have focused on the travel and time costs of cancer prevention. O'Brien and colleagues estimated direct health service costs and the indirect cost of time off work among chemotherapy patients using patient and nurse survey data as well as administrative data from 107 participants (O'Brien, Rusthoven et al. 1993). Houts and colleagues asked 139 patients receiving outpatient chemotherapy to keep diaries of nonmedical expenses resulting from their disease and its treatment, and documented the economic experiences of these patients (Houts, Lipton et al. 1984). These small, local cost-identification studies reveal a need to better understand the nonmedical economic outcomes using a patient-centered approach. Information on out-of-pocket savings in the long-run due to cancer prevention might be useful to motivate individuals at risk, and lead them to make more informed decisions regarding their health behaviors and use of medical services.

Cost-consequence studies entail a simple tabulation of health and economic outcomes of interventions. This rare and informal type of economic analysis is like a cost-identification analysis except that it includes health outcome information. The findings of a cost-consequence study are presented without summary statements about cost-effectiveness, which distinguishes it from economic evaluations.

Conclusion

The purpose of this chapter was to introduce the reader to ways of quantifying the human and economic value of cancer prevention activities. The human and economic costs of cancer to individuals, families, communities, and society are substantial (Brown, Lipscomb et al. 2001). It is imperative that personal and financial investments in cancer prevention be made; however, since healthcare resources are limited, those available must be used efficiently and equitably. To justify investments in cancer prevention, it is essential to have data about the relative costs and outcomes of prevention activities. Resources should be used for programs that produce the greatest benefit for the greatest number of people. The lack of good information about input–output relationships in health care has led to enormous variations in costs and practice patterns. The creation of more useful data and the more informed use of data currently available can enhance the public's health, patient care, and the quality of health care resource allocation decisions at many levels (e.g., individual, health plan, society).

References

Aaronson, N.K., S. Ahmedzai, et al. (1993). "The European Organization for Research and Treatment of Cancer QLQ-C30: a quality-of-life instrument for use in international clinical trials in oncology." *J Natl Cancer Inst* **85**(5): 365-376.

Bowling, A. (1997). *Measuring Health: A Review of Quality of Life Measurement Scales.* Philadelphia, Open University Press.

Bowling, A. (2001). *Measuring Disease: A Review of Disease-Specific Quality of Life Measurement Scales.* Philadelphia, Open University Press.

Brazier, J., J. Roberts, et al. (2002). "The estimation of a preference-based measure of health from the SF-36." *J Health Econ* **21**(2): 271–292.

Brown, A.D. and A.M. Garber (1999). "Cost-effectiveness of 3 methods to enhance the sensitivity of Papanicolaou testing." *JAMA* **281**(4): 347–353.

Brown, M.L., J. Lipscomb, et al. (2001). "The burden of illness of cancer: economic cost and quality of life." *Annu Rev Public Health* **22**: 91–113.

Bruner, D.W., B. Movsas, et al. (2004). "Outcomes research in cancer clinical trial cooperative groups: the RTOG model." *Qual Life Res* **13**(6): 1025–1041.

Cella, D.F., D.S. Tulsky, et al. (1993). "The Functional Assessment of Cancer Therapy scale: development and validation of the general measure." *J Clin Oncol* **11**(3): 570–579.

Cullen, J., M.D. Schwartz, et al. (2004). "Short-term impact of cancer prevention and screening activities on quality of life." *J Clin Oncol* **22**(5): 943–952.

Day, R., P.A. Ganz, et al. (1999). "Health-related quality of life and tamoxifen in breast cancer prevention: a report from the National Surgical Adjuvant Breast and Bowel Project P-1 Study." *J Clin Oncol* **17**(9): 2659–2669.

Donaldson, M.S. (2004). "Taking stock of health-related quality-of-life measurement in oncology practice in the United States." *J Natl Cancer Inst Monogr* (33): 155–167.

Eddy, D.M. (1990). "Screening for cervical cancer." *Ann Intern Med* **113**(3): 214–226.

Esser, M. and H. Brunner (2003). "Economic evaluations of granulocyte colony-stimulating factor: in the prevention and treatment of chemotherapy-induced neutropenia." *Pharmacoeconomics* **21**(18): 1295–1313.

Fryback, D.G. and B.M. Craig (2004). "Measuring economic outcomes of cancer." *J Natl Cancer Inst Monogr* (33): 134–141.

Gelber, R.D., A. Goldhirsch, et al. (1993). "Evaluation of effectiveness: Q-TWiST. The International Breast Cancer Study Group." *Cancer Treat Rev* **19** Suppl A: 73–84.

Goldie, S.J., M. Kohli, et al. (2004). "Projected clinical benefits and cost-effectiveness of a human papillomavirus 16/18 vaccine." *J Natl Cancer Inst* **96**(8): 604–615.

Goldie, S.J., M.C. Weinstein, et al. (1999). "The costs, clinical benefits, and cost-effectiveness of screening for cervical cancer in HIV-infected women." *Ann Intern Med* **130**(2): 97–107.

Guyatt, G.H., D.H. Feeny, et al. (1993). "Measuring health-related quality of life." *Ann Intern Med* **118**(8): 622–629.

Houts, P.S., A. Lipton, et al. (1984). "Nonmedical costs to patients and their families associated with outpatient chemotherapy." *Cancer* **53**(11): 2388–2392.

Johnson, E., F. Dominici, M. Griswold, S.L. Zeger (2003). "Disease cases and their medical costs attributable to smoking: an analysis of the national medical expenditure survey." *Journal of Econometrics* **112**(1): 135–151.

Karnofsky, D., J. Burchenal (1949). The clinical evaluation of chemotherapeutic agents in cancer. *Evaluation of Chemotherapeutic Agents*. C. Macleod. New York, Columbia University Press.

Kozma, C.M., C.E. Reeder, et al. (1993). "Economic, clinical, and humanistic outcomes: a planning model for pharmacoeconomic research." *Clin Ther* **15**(6): 1121–1132; discussion 1120.

Kulasingam, S.L. and E.R. Myers (2003). "Potential health and economic impact of adding a human papillomavirus vaccine to screening programs." *Jama* **290**(6): 781–789.

Lipscomb, J., M.S. Donaldson, et al. (2004). "Cancer outcomes research and the arenas of application." *J Natl Cancer Inst Monogr*(33): 1–7.

Lipscomb, J. and C.F. Snyder (2002). "The Outcomes of Cancer Outcomes Research: focusing on the National Cancer Institute's quality-of-care initiative." *Med Care* **40**(6 Suppl): III3–10.

Litwin, M. S., R.D. Hays, et al. (1998). "The UCLA Prostate Cancer Index: development, reliability, and validity of a health-related quality of life measure." *Med Care* **36**(7): 1002–1012.

Loeve, F., M. L. Brown, et al. (2000). "Endoscopic colorectal cancer screening: a cost-saving analysis." *J Natl Cancer Inst* **92**(7): 557–563.

Mandelblatt, J.S., W.F. Lawrence, et al. (2002). "Benefits and costs of using HPV testing to screen for cervical cancer." *JAMA* **287**(18): 2372–2381.

McDowell, I., C. Newell (1996). *Measuring Health: A Guide to Rating Scales and Questionnaires*. Philadelphia, Oxford University Press.

NCI (2004). *Cancer Progress Report – 2003 Update*. Rockville, National Cancer Institute.

O'Brien, B.J., J. Rusthoven, et al. (1993). "Impact of chemotherapy-associated nausea and vomiting on patients' functional status and on costs: survey of five Canadian centres." *CMAJ* **149**(3): 296–302.

Patrick, D.L. and R.A. Deyo (1989). "Generic and disease-specific measures in assessing health status and quality of life." *Med Care* **27**(3 Suppl): S217–232.

Ramsey, S.D., M.T. Mandelson, et al. (2003). "Cancer-attributable costs of diagnosis and care for persons with screen-detected versus symptom-detected colorectal cancer." *Gastroenterology* **125**(6): 1645–1650.

Schron, E.B. and S.A. Shumaker (1992). "The integration of health quality of life in clinical research: experiences from cardiovascular clinical trials." *Prog Cardiovasc Nurs* **7**(1): 21–28.

Sculpher, M., M.K. Palmer, et al. (2000). "Costs incurred by patients undergoing advanced colorectal cancer therapy. A comparison of raltitrexed and fluorouracil plus folinic acid." *Pharmacoeconomics* **17**(4): 361–370.

Staquet, M., N. Aaronson, et al. (1992). "Health-related quality of life research." *Qual Life Res* **1**: 3.

Taplin, S.H., W. Barlow, et al. (1995). "Stage, age, comorbidity, and direct costs of colon, prostate, and breast cancer care." *J Natl Cancer Inst* **87**(6): 417–426.

Tengs, T.O. and A. Wallace (2000). "One thousand health-related quality-of-life estimates." *Med Care* **38**(6): 583–637.

Till, J.E., McNeil, B.J., Bush, R.S. (1984). "Measurement of multiple components of quality of life." *Cancer Treatment Symposia* **1**: 177–181.

Tsao, H., G.S. Rogers, et al. (1998). "An estimate of the annual direct cost of treating cutaneous melanoma." *J Am Acad Dermatol* **38**(5 Pt 1): 669–680.

Ubel, P. (2001). *Pricing Life: Why it's Time for Health Care Rationing*. Cambridge, MIT Press.

Wagner, J.L. (1997). "Cost-effectiveness of screening for common cancers." *Cancer Metastasis Rev* **16**(3-4): 281–294.

Ware, J., M. Kosinski, S. Keller (1994). *SF-36 Physical and Mental Health Summary Scales: A User's Manual*. Boston, The Health Institute.

Ware, J.E., Jr. and C.D. Sherbourne (1992). "The MOS 36-item short-form health survey (SF-36). I. Conceptual framework and item selection." *Med Care* **30**(6): 473–483.

The Role of Diet, Physical Activity and Body Composition in Cancer Prevention

Cynthia A. Thomson[1], Zhao Chen[1], and Robert B. Lutz[2]

[1] College of Agriculture and Life Sciences and College of Public Health, University of Arizona, Tucson, AZ 85724
[2] Empire Health Systems, Spokane, WA 99210

"Let food be thy medicine and medicine be thy food." These words were spoken by Hippocrates in 440 BC, yet today they have as much application to health and the diet-cancer link as ever. To expand on this notion, Hippocrates also stated that, *"All parts of the body that have a function, if used in moderation, and exercised in labors to which each is accustomed, become healthy and well developed and age slowly; but if unused and left idle, they become liable to disease, defective in growth and age quickly."* Epidemiological evidence gathered over the past 50 years continues to support the belief that between 30 and 50% of all cancers could be prevented through optimal dietary selections and a physically active lifestyle (Doll and Peto 1981). Yet over this same time span we have continued to make poor food choices, reduce our level of physical activity and experience a continuing rise in the rates of overweight and obesity to the extent that obesity has become an epidemic in the U.S. Not surprisingly, these trends have undermined efforts to reduce cancer incidence.

This chapter will address the role of diet, physical activity and body composition in cancer prevention. In addition to summarizing the current evidence regarding associations between diet, physical activity and cancer prevention, the content will discuss the mechanistic underpinnings by which diet and physical activity can modulate the cancer process, review current guidelines as well as propose new guidelines for reducing cancer risk through lifestyle modification, and provide tools to support the integration of cancer preventive diets and activity patterns into clinical practice.

Primary Prevention

The association between diet, physical activity and cancer has been well described in the scientific literature. In terms of primary prevention, current data support the need for improved food choices and increased physical activity to prevent several of the leading cancers diagnosed in the U.S.

In reviewing the evidence for a preventive role for diet (Table 1), it is apparent that the majority of research indicating a protective effect is related to intake of vegetables, and to some, but much lesser extent, fruit (Riboli and Norat 2003). Evidence for other dietary components such as fiber, fat, and alcohol is less consistent, but generally indicates a probable relationship (WCRF; Key, Schatzkin et al. 2004). The protective role of constituents of select vegetables, such as folate, monounsaturated fat, and dietary phytochemicals, further supports the role of vegetables in chemoprevention (Steinmetz and Potter 1996; La Vecchia 2001).

Table 1. Relationship between diet and cancer, adapted (WCRF; Riboli and Norat 2003)

Cancer Site	Diet Component	Degree of Evidence
Oral		
Decrease Risk	Vegetables	++
	Fruit	++
Increased Risk	Alcohol	++
Esophagus		
Decreased Risk	Vegetables	++
	Fruit	++
Increased Risk	Alcohol	++
Stomach		
Decreased Risk	Vegetables	++
	Fruit	++
	Grains	±
Increased Risk	Alcohol	+
Pancreas		
Decreased Risk	Vegetables	+
	Fruit	+
	Fiber	±
Increased Risk	Meat	±
	Cholesterol	±
Colorectal		
Decreased Risk	Vegetables	+
	Fruit	NA
	Fiber	±
Increased Risk	Alcohol	+
	Meat	+
	Saturated Fat	±
	Dairy	NA
Breast		
Decreased Risk	Vegetables	++
	Fruit	++
	Fiber	±
Increased Risk	Alcohol	+
	Red meat	±
	Dairy	NA
Ovary		
Decreased Risk	Vegetables	±
	Fruit	±
Increased Risk	Animal fat	NA
	Vegetable fiber	NA
	Dairy	NA
Cervix		
Decreased Risk	Vegetables	±
	Fruit	±
Prostate		
Decreased Risk	Vegetables	±
	Fruit	NA
Increased Risk	Alcohol	NA
	Red meat	±
	Dietary fat	±
	Dairy	±

Table 1 (continued)

Cancer Site	Diet Component	Degree of Evidence
Bladder		
Decreased Risk	Vegetables	++
	Fruit	++
Increased Risk	Alcohol	NA
	Dietary fat	NA

NA Not available; ++ Convincing/consistent; + Weak but probable; ± Inconsistent evidence

One of the more controversial areas of diet cancer research is the potential protective role of fiber in reducing the recurrence of adenomas of the colon. Two key studies published in 2000 indicated that both daily consumption of a high fiber, wheat-bran cereal and daily intake of a high vegetable, fruit and fiber diet were not associated with a reduction in polyp recurrence (Alberts, Martinez et al. 2000; Schatzkin, Lanza et al. 2000). Although these trials were well designed, researchers continue to speculate that either the dose of fiber was insufficient or that once a premalignant lesion is identified and the gastrointestinal tissue is "initiated," an increase in daily fiber intake will not reduce the risk for polyp recurrence. More recent European data, where fiber intakes are greater then in the United States, suggest that fiber may be protective against colorectal cancer (Bingham, Day et al. 2003).

In addition, the evidence is predominantly associated with protection against the development of solid, organ-specific tumors. Of interest, several of the most significant associations are shown for hormone-related cancers such as breast, prostate and ovarian cancer, or for cancers of the gastrointestinal tract where direct contact between food constituents and the damaged tissue is possible, including oral, esophageal, gastric and colorectal cancers.

A review of the available epidemiological evidence supporting a relationship between physical activity and cancer (Table 2) finds the first suggestion dating to the early 1920s when association between occupational physical activity and cancer prevention was noted (Siverston and Dahlstrom 1922). Since that time, a fairly robust and yet fairly recent literature has developed that has further explored and defined this relationship. Findings have consistently demonstrated an association between physical activity and chronic diseases, such as cardiovascular disease and type 2 diabetes (USDHHS 1996). This prompted the American Cancer Society to publish guidelines for physical activity and cancer prevention (Byers, Nestle et al. 2002). Americans were encouraged to "adopt a physically active lifestyle" that was defined as:

■ Adults: Engaging in at least moderate activity for ≥30 minutes ≥5 days of the week; ≥45 minutes of moderate-to-vigorous physical activity (MVPA) ≥5 days per week (may further enhance reductions in the risk of breast and colon cancer).
■ Children and adolescents: Engaging in at least 60 minutes per day of MVPA at least 5 days per week.

These recommendations could be met in a variety of ways other than sports, to include leisure time physical activity (e.g. walking/hiking, swimming, resistance train-

Table 2. Association between physical activity and cancer risk-cohort studies, adapted (Thune and Furberg 2001)

Study Population	Sample size (M-male; F-female)	Cancer Site	RR[1] (95% CI[2]) Highest vs. Lowest LPA[3] Levels
Texas Cooper Clinic (Kampert, Blair et al. 1996)	25,341 (M) 7,080 (F)	Overall	0.2 (0.1–1.1) 0.4 (0.2–0.6)
Whitehall Study (Smith, Shipley et al. 2000)	6,702 (M)	Overall	0.8 (0.6–0.9)
Health Professionals' Follow-up (Giovannucci, Ascherio et al. 1995)	47,273 (M)	Colon	0.5 (0.3–0.9)
Nurses' Health Study (Martinez, Giovannucci et al. 1997)	52,875 (F)	Colon	0.5 (0.3–0.9)
Harvard Alumni (Lee, Paffenbarger et al. 1991)	17,148 (M)	Rectum	1.7 (0.4–7.7)
College Alumni (Sesso, Paffenbarger et al. 1998)	1,566	Breast	Total 0.7 (0.5–1.4) Pre[4] 1.8 (0.8–4.3) Post[5] 0.5 (0.3–0.9)
Nurses' Health Study (Rockhill, Willett et al. 1999)	121,701	Breast	0.8 (0.7–0.9)
Population-health screening (Thune, Brenn et al. 1997)	25,624	Breast	Total 0.6 (0.4–1.0) Pre[4] 0.5 (0.3–1.1) Post[5] 0.7 (0.4–1.1)
Swedish Twin Registry (Terry, Baron et al. 1999)	11,659	Endometrium	0.2 (0.3–0.8)
Iowa Women's Health Study (Mink, Folsom et al. 1996)	31,396	Ovary	2.1 (1.2–3.4)
Harvard Alumni (Lee and Paffenbarger 1994)	17,607	Prostate	0.6 (0.2–1.4)
Physicians' Health Study (Liu, Lee et al. 2000)	22,071	Prostate	1.1 (0.9–1.4)
NHANES I (Clarke and Whittemore 2000)	5,377	Prostate	C[6] 1.7 (0.8–2.3) AA[7] 3.7 (1.7–8.4)
Norway General Population (Thune and Lund 1994)	53,242	Testicle	2.0 (0.6–6.9)
Harvard Alumni (Lee, Sesso et al. 1999)	13,905	Lung	0.4 (0.4–1.0)

[1] RR – Relative risk; [2] CI – Confidence Interval; [3] LPA – Leisure time physical activity; [4] Pre – Premenopausal; [5] Post – Postmenopausal; [6] C – Caucasian; [7] AA – African American

ing); occupational physical activity (e.g. walking and lifting, manual labor) and home activities (e.g. lawn and house work).

Despite the supportive evidence, much remains unknown. This includes:
- Identification of the appropriate "dose" of physical activity
- Identification of the optimal time of life for intervention
- Determination of the "optimal" type of physical activity
- Mechanisms of action

It is probable that as cancer is a multifactorial disease, there will be no "one size fits all" explanation and that to some degree variations in providing physical activity prevention recommendations will exist. Nonetheless, the above-stated guidelines are a good starting point in moving individuals to a more active health-promoting lifestyle.

Note that the associations identified in large epidemiological trials account for only small reductions in risk; however, the potential additive effects of several lifestyle modifications could be considerable. In addition, these are modifications that are achievable, cost-effective and have no or minimal side effects. Thus, pursuit of such changes in lifestyle is an appropriate strategy to reduce cancer risk (Sass 2002).

Body Weight and Body Composition

Importantly, body weight and composition have also been identified as modifiable risk factors for cancer. Table 3 below outlines the current associations between overweight/ obese status and cancer risk.

Thus, primary prevention of undesirable body weight status should be considered in the first line of defense against the development of cancer. In fact, there are known periods in the lifecycle when undesirable weight gain is more common. These include:
- Adolescence/pre-pubertal
- Entry into the work force
- College entry
- Marriage
- Childbirth
- Menopause
- Retirement
- Stressful life events, such as death of a significant other, divorce, illness
- Activity-limiting illness
- Select medication use (i.e., oral contraceptives, postmenopausal hormone therapy, anti-depressants, insulin, etc.)

Not only should research focus on these vulnerable populations or time periods in life, clinicians should also be acutely aware of circumstantial changes in their patients' lives placing them at risk for undesirable weight gain. To this end, clinicians should not limit assessment to monitoring for changes in body weight over time, but should also proactively instruct patients regarding weight gain-prevention during these vulnerable life circumstances.

Table 3. Role of body weight and body composition in cancer prevention, adapted from IARC/WHO (IARC 2002)

Cancer Site	Percentage of Cancers Associated with Obese Status
Breast (post-menopausal)	9%
Colorectal	11%
Endometrial	39%
Esophagus	12%
Kidney	25%
TOTAL	5%

Survivorship

As survival rates for cancer have steadily increased (five-year survival for all cancers and stages is 62; 90% for the most common cancers with early detection) (ACS 2003), there is increasing interest in the role of lifestyle modification in preventing cancer recurrence and enhancing the quality of life (QOL) for people with cancer, both during and after treatment (Courneya 2003). The American Cancer Society has recently released its recommendations on lifestyle approaches for individuals during the various stages of cancer treatment (Brown, Byers et al. 2003).

A new focus in cancer prevention research is related to preventing recurrence of cancer in people previously treated for cancer. Historically, clinicians and researchers have relied on the primary prevention model to direct patients regarding optimal diet and physical activity patterns to reduce cancer recurrence risk. Unfortunately, there are currently a paucity of available data.

The magnitude and direction of this association varies depending on the type of cancer. For example, increased body weight and body fat negatively affect the prognosis of breast cancer, while survivorship in lung cancer patients is improved among those with stable weight or even weight gain. Weight gain is a common problem among breast cancer patients who receive adjuvant chemotherapy (Dixon, Moritz et al. 1978; Heasman, Sutherland et al. 1985; Ganz, Schag et al. 1987; Demark-Wahnefried, Winer et al. 1993; Demark-Wahnefried, Rimer et al. 1997; Goodwin, Ennis et al. 1999). This change in weight associated with breast cancer treatment not only generates psychosocial stress in women but also affects long-term cancer prognosis and survivorship, particularly among older breast cancer patients.

There are inconsistent results regarding the relationship between weight and fat distribution in breast cancer patients and their cancer prognosis and survivorship. A study in the Netherlands found no significant differences in survival time between heavier (for height) (body mass index, BMI, of 26 or greater) and lighter patients (BMI less than 26). There was also no association between central fat distribution, measured by the ratio of subscapular and triceps skinfold thickness, and survival time in breast cancer patients, after stratification by axillary node status, estrogen receptor status, and method of detection (den Tonkelaar, de Waard et al. 1995). However, in the Iowa Women's Health Study (698 postmenopausal patients with unilateral breast cancer), after adjusting for age, women in the highest tertile of BMI had a 1.9-fold higher risk (95% CI = 1.0–3.7) of dying after breast cancer than those in the lowest tertile, adjusted for other prognostic variables (age, smoking, education level, extent of breast cancer, and tumor size) (Zhang, Folsom et al. 1995). Kumar and colleagues suggested that among breast carcinoma patients, android body fat distribution, as indicated by a higher suprailiac to thigh ratio, was a statistically significant (p <0.0001) predictor of poorer 10-year survivorship (Kumar, Cantor et al. 2000). In contrast, Schapira and colleagues reported that perimenopausal and postmenopausal women with upper body fat distribution appeared to be a subset of women with a more favorable prognosis, as measured by less lymph node involvement, smaller tumors, and higher levels of ER in their tumors (Schapira, Kumar et al. 1991). Clearly, more studies are needed to understand the impact of weight, and fat distribution on cancer prognosis among breast cancer survivors. Even more importantly, this warrants further investigation in other tumor types, particularly hormone-related cancers, such as ovarian, endometrial and prostate.

The role of physical activity in reducing the risk for cancer recurrence has received minimal scientific attention to date. However, with increasing survival, this is a fast growing research area. A recent review of the literature identified 43 studies – 21 randomized controlled trials and 22 quasi-experimental studies (Irwin and Ainsworth 2004). The majority were feasibility studies that looked primarily at psychosocial outcomes rather than physiological measures. Overall, evidence suggests that among patients currently undergoing therapy and/or previously treated for cancer, increased energy expenditure in the form of regular physical activity provides benefits in biopsychocial and physiological measures. These factors have been most studied in women with breast cancer, and to a lesser degree in other cancers (Irwin and Ainsworth 2004).

In another review of this literature, 19 intervention trials and 9 observational studies have been reviewed in women either undergoing treatment for breast cancer or post-therapy. Statistically significant results have been demonstrated in a number of objective and subjective outcome measures (Courneya 2003). These have included exercise and functional capacity, body weight and composition, flexibility, nausea, physical well-being, functional well-being, mood states, anxiety and depression, satisfaction with life, and overall quality of life. These trials, as reviewed by Courneya et al. (Courneya 2003), have used a variety of exercise interventions (e.g. self-directed or home-based versus supervised exercise) for variable study lengths. Many have made use of the traditional "exercise prescription" guidelines with respect to frequency, intensity, type and tempo with only a few studies looking at resistance training. Whereas methodologies have often differed, sample sizes have been small, and research vigor has been variable, thereby limiting interpretation of findings, the cumulative evidence supports the safety and benefits of physical activity for women who have breast cancer.

Similarly, 19 studies have been reviewed in non-breast cancer patients (Courneya 2003). A number of physiological and psychological variables have been measured. Again, variable study designs and small populations have been noted. These studies have likewise generally supported a recommendation for physical activity in individuals undergoing treatment or in recovery from cancer.

Cardiovascular fitness and QOL were assessed in 53 postmenopausal women who had received treatment for breast cancer. They were randomly assigned to an exercise group or control. The intervention consisted of training on a bicycle ergometer 3 times/week for 15 weeks. Primary outcome measures included changes in VO_{2max} and QOL, as measured by the Functional Assessment of Cancer Therapy-Breast subscale. Peak oxygen consumption increased by 0.24 L/min in the exercise group, whereas it decreased by 0.05 L/min in the control group (mean difference, 0.29 L/min; 95% confidence interval [CI], 0.18 to 0.40; $p < 0.001$). Overall QOL increased by 9.1 points in the exercise group compared with 0.3 points in the control group (mean difference, 8.8 points; 95% CI, 3.6 to 14.0; $p = 0.001$). Pearson correlations indicated that change in peak oxygen consumption correlated with change in overall QOL (r = 0.45; $p < 0.01$). The researchers concluded that this exercise intervention positively affected cardiovascular fitness and QOL in postmenopausal women who had undergone treatment for breast cancer (Courneya 2003).

A recent trial evaluated the effects of structured exercise on physical functioning and other dimensions of health-related QOL in women with stages I and II breast cancer (Segal, Evans et al. 2001). One hundred twenty-three women with stage I or II breast cancer were randomly allocated to one of three intervention groups: usual care (control group), self-directed exercise, or supervised exercise. Quality of life, aerobic capacity, and body weight measures were repeated at 26 weeks. The primary outcome measure was the change in the Short Form-36 physical functioning scale between baseline and 26 weeks. Findings demonstrated a decrease in physical functioning in the control group by 4.1 points, whereas it increased by 5.7 points and 2.2 points in the self-directed and supervised exercise groups, respectively ($p=0.04$). Post hoc analysis demonstrated a significant and clinically important difference between the self-directed and control groups (9.8 points; $p=0.01$) and a more modest difference between the supervised and control groups (6.3 points; $p=0.09$). No significant differences between groups were observed for changes in quality of life scores. In a secondary analysis of participants stratified by type of adjuvant therapy, supervised exercise improved aerobic capacity ($+3.5$ mL/kg/min; $p=0.01$) and reduced body weight (-4.8 kg; $p<0.05$) compared with usual care only in participants not receiving chemotherapy. The researchers concluded that exercise can lessen some of the negative side effects of breast cancer treatment. Self-directed exercise was seen as an effective method to improve physical functioning as compared to usual care. In participants not receiving chemotherapy, supervised exercise could increase aerobic capacity and reduce body weight compared with usual care.

Researchers have also looked at physical activity in men undergoing androgen deprivation therapy for prostate cancer (Segal, Reid et al. 2003). This treatment often causes fatigue, functional decline, increased body fatness, and loss of lean body tissue, side-effects that may negatively affect health-related quality of life. They hypothesized that resistance exercise would counter some of these side-effects by reducing fatigue, elevating mood, building muscle mass, and reducing body fat. They recruited 155 men with prostate cancer scheduled to receive androgen deprivation therapy for at least 3 months after recruitment. Volunteers were randomly assigned to an intervention group that participated in a resistance exercise program 3 times/week for 12 weeks (82 men) or to a waiting list control group (73 men). The primary outcome measures were fatigue and disease-specific quality of life as assessed by self-reported questionnaires; secondary outcome measures were muscular fitness and body composition. Men assigned to resistance exercise had less interference from fatigue on activities of daily living ($p=0.002$) and higher quality of life ($p=0.001$) than men in the control group. Men in the intervention group demonstrated higher levels of upper body ($p=0.009$) and lower body ($p<0.001$) muscular fitness than men in the control group. The 12-week resistance exercise intervention did not improve body composition as measured by changes in body weight, body mass index, waist circumference, or subcutaneous skinfolds. They concluded that resistance training could decrease fatigue, improve QOL, and enhance musculoskeletal fitness in men with prostate cancer receiving androgen deprivation therapy (Segal, Reid et al. 2003).

One hundred and two survivors of colorectal cancer were randomly assigned to an exercise group versus control in another research trial (Courneya 2003). The exercise group was asked to perform moderate intensity exercise 3-5 times/week for 20–30 minutes for 16 weeks. The control group was instructed not to enroll in a structured exercise program. The primary outcome measure was change in QOL as measured by the Functional Assessment of Cancer Therapy-Colorectal (FACT-C) scale. Although adherence in the exercise group was good (75.8%) significant contamination in the control group occurred (51.6%). Intention-to-treat analysis revealed no significant differences between groups for change in the FACT-C (mean difference −1.3; 95% CI: −7.8 to 5.1; $p = 0.679$). In an 'on-treatment' ancillary analysis, comparison was performed of participants who decreased versus increased their cardiovascular fitness. This analysis revealed significant differences in favor of the increased fitness group for the FACT-C (mean difference 6.5; 95% CI: 0.4–12.6; $p = 0.038$). The researchers concluded that increased cardiovascular fitness was associated with improvements in QOL in colorectal cancer survivors (Courneya 2003).

It is important to recognize that during the various phases of cancer treatment and post-treatment, people often experience significant limitations in their functional capacity. Fatigue, diminished exercise capacity, and decreased strength often exist. The decision how best to incorporate physical activity necessarily requires individualization based upon pre-existing exercise levels, current physical status, and goals and expectations. For those with low pre-existing physical activity levels, simple stretching or a few minutes of walking performed regularly may be all that is tolerated. For those with more active backgrounds, maintenance of levels may be desirable. Physical activity levels may be increased as physical abilities are enhanced. With the paucity of available data, it is probable that the guidelines published by the American Cancer Society for prevention are appropriate for prevention of recurrence (Byers, Nestle et al. 2002).

Clinical Trials of Lifestyle Modification

The large and growing number of cancer survivors has led to new research in the area of diet and cancer recurrence. Below is a summary of current trials and primary outcomes to be assessed (Table 4).

Although the results of these intervention trials are pending, there is theoretical and mechanistic support that modification in diet and physical activity toward a more plant-based, energy-controlled diet combined with greater levels of physical activity that would result in optimal body composition and body weight will reduce recurrence rates. To date, none of the large intervention trials include such a multi-pronged approach nor do the trials seek to reduce or even control body weight (Pierce, Faerber et al. 2002). A differential response was demonstrated in the Women's Intervention Nutrition Study. On average, women on the low-fat diet lost body weight, while those following their usual diets gained body weight, although the mean difference was less than 10 pounds (Pierce, Faerber et al. 2002). Thus, although the efficacy of current interventions will increase our understanding and potentially provide a foundation for clinical recommendations related to diet and the prevention of breast cancer recurrence, further research is warranted to definitively test the role of weight control in recurrence of several cancers. For example, previous studies have demonstrated exercise training effects on reproductive function (i.e., menstrual study length, suppression of ovulation, estrogen and progesterone levels) that would be pertinent to the etiology of breast and endometrial cancer (Williams, Bullen et al. 1999). Insulin, as a biomarker for diabetes, cardiovascular disease, and overweight and metabolic syndrome, has been assessed with respect to exercise effects (Boule, Haddad et al. 2001).

Table 4. Ongoing clinical trials evaluating the role of diet or physical activity in reducing cancer recurrence

Trial Name	Target Population	Sample Size	Intervention	Primary Outcome
Women's Healthy Eating and Living Study	Breast cancer survivors within 4 years of treatment for stage I, II or IIIa disease	3109	Diet: High vegetable, fruit and fiber, low fat, plant-based	Breast cancer recurrence
Women's Intervention Nutrition Study	Breast cancer survivors within 1 year of treatment, stage I or II, standardized chemotherapies	2500	Diet: Low fat: 15 to 20% total energy	Breast cancer recurrence
CAN-HOPE Trial (Courneya 2003)	Post-surgical colorectal cancer survivors	102	Ex ercise: self-directed 16-wk MPA*	Physical fitness; QOL*
Resistance Exercise & Prostate Cancer Trial (Segal, Reid et al. 2003)	Prostate cancer survivors on androgen deprivation	155	Resistance exercise, 12-wk	Fatigue; QOL*
(Courneya, Mackey et al. 2003)	Stage 1 & 2 breast cancer survivors receiving treatment	123	Home-based at 50% VO_{2max},* 5 days/wk vs. 3 days/wk monitored & 2 days/wk self-monitored	QOL*; Fitness; Body weight
Rehabilitation Exercise for Health After Breast Cancer (REHAB) (Segal, Evans et al. 2001)	Postmenopausal breast cancer survivors following therapy ± hormone therapy	53	Bicycle ergometer 3 times/wk, 15 weeks	VO_{2max}; QOL*; biological outcomes

* MPA-moderate physical activity; QOL-quality of life; VO_{2max}-maximum oxygen consumption

Optimizing Bone Health

Bone metabolism can be disrupted by metastatic bone disease that often develops as a result of many interactions between tumor cells and bone cells. Cancer patients with bone metastases may experience bone pain, fractures, hypercalcemia and spinal cord compression. Given the long survival time after bone metastasis in certain types of cancer, these skeletal complications may have profound adverse effects on cancer survivors' quality of life. There is some evidence that bisphosphonates that are used to promote bone integrity clinically may not only reduce the symptoms and complications of cancer-related bone metastases, but may also inhibit the development of bone metastases (Coleman 2001).

Low bone density, deterioration of bone microstructure, and increased risk of fracture are characteristics of osteoporosis. Poor nutrition, reduced sex hormones levels, prolonged pharmacological intervention, disease, and low physical activity level or decreased mobility are all risk factors for osteoporosis. As a result of cancer prognosis and treatment, patients with cancer are often predisposed to low bone mineral density (BMD) and increased risk for osteoporotic fractures in later life. Cancer treatments may increase the risk for developing osteoporosis through a variety of biological mechanisms, including treatment-induced hypogonadism, disturbances of thyroid and growth hormones, hormone-independent effects of chemotherapy on bone cells, and nutrient malabsorption after gastrectomy (Pfeilschifter and Diel 2000).

Studies have shown that young women who experience premature menopause following chemotherapy for breast cancer demonstrate excess bone loss and a higher risk for early development of osteoporosis (Headley, Theriault et al. 1998; Shapiro, Manola et al. 2001; Vehmanen, Saarto et al. 2001). The rate of bone loss among postmenopausal breast cancer patients is less well characterized. However, a recent study found that regardless of whether the breast cancer diagnosis is before or after menopause, women with a history of breast cancer often have an increased risk for bone fractures after age 50 (Chen, Maricic et al. in press, 2005).

Anti-resorptive agents may reduce the bone loss associated with chemotherapy-induced ovarian failure in premenopausal women (Saarto, Blomqvist et al. 1997). It has been reported that adjuvant clodronate treatment significantly reduced chemotherapy-induced bone loss (Vehmanen, Saarto et al. 2001). However, clodronate may have limited effects in preventing bone loss among postmenopausal breast cancer patients after the termination of hormone replacement therapy (HRT). In a randomized control trial among postmenopausal breast cancer patients, women who had recently discontinued HRT experienced more rapid bone loss than HRT non-users. Neither three-year antiestrogen therapy alone nor antiestrogen together with clodronate could totally prevent the bone loss related to HRT withdrawal, even though clodronate seemed to retard it (Saarto, Blomqvist et al. 1997).

Prostate cancer is the most common malignancy among American men. Since prostate cancer is testosterone dependent, androgen deprivation therapy (ADT) with GnRH agonists (GnRH-a) is often used in treating prostate cancer, which renders these men hypogonadal. Testosterone plays an important role in maintaining bone as well as skeletal muscle mass; ADT-induced hypogonadism potentially has a significant impact on body composition. Recently, Smith reviewed studies on bone loss and osteoporosis-associated ADT among men with prostate cancer (Smith 2002). The cumulative evidence indicates that prostate cancer patients without apparent bone metastases are at increased risks of osteoporosis and obesity, as well as low lean and soft tissue mass, after ADT (Stoch, Parker et al. 2001; Basaria, Lieb et al. 2002; Berruti, Dogliotti et al. 2002; Chen, Maricic et al. 2002). Bisphosphonates reduce the loss of bone density among prostate cancer patients after ADT (Smith, McGovern et al. 2001). More research is needed to investigate bone loss among other prostate cancer populations.

The increasing incidence of childhood cancers and the improved treatment for childhood malignancies have resulted in a growing number of childhood cancer survivors in the U.S. The improved survival of children with malignant diseases is in part due to the application of intensive, multi-modality therapies that include radiotherapy, surgery, glucocorticoids, and cytotoxic agents. However, such interventions have the potential to induce complex hormonal, metabolic, and nutritional effects that may interfere with longitudinal bone growth and skeletal mass acquisition during the critical growth phases of childhood and adolescence. Recently, in a review paper, van Leeuwen and colleagues (van Leeuwen, Kamps et al. 2000) concluded that many factors might simultaneously or independently affect final height and BMD in adults who survived childhood cancers. Multi-agent chemotherapy, corticosteroids, malignancy itself, cranial radiotherapy, and physical inactivity may reduce long bone growth resulting in short body height. These factors may also cause low peak bone mass, which may lead to long-term consequences including increased risk for bone fractures in later life.

Total and near-total thyroidectomy, with or without radioiodine ablative therapy, are in the mainstay of current treatments for well-differentiated thyroid cancer. Supraphysiologic amounts of oral thyroxine are also administered to suppress serum thyroid stimulating hormone (TSH) to below detectable levels. It is well known that overt clinical hyperthyroidism may increase bone turnover and decrease BMD, but the effect of suppressive thyroxine treatment on BMD is less well known. After reviewing current evidence on bone density among thyroid cancer patients who were treated with suppressive thyroxine, Quan and colleagues (Quan, Pasieka et al. 2002) concluded that there is no significant change in BMD for premenopausal women or in men after diagnosis and treatment for thyroid cancer; however, the findings for postmenopausal women are controversial and remain unclear.

Gastric cancer is one of the most common causes of cancer death. The only treatment that leads to cures in some patients is surgery. Liedman has reviewed the impact of gastrectomy on food intake, body composition, and bone metabolism (Liedman 1999). Previous studies have suggested that substantial weight loss, amounting to about 10% of preoperative weight, occurred during the early postoperative period, including a decrease in lean soft tissue. To study the changes in body composition and BMD after gastrectomy, Liedman and colleagues (Liedman, Henningsson et al. 2000) conducted a small longitudinal study among 22 gastric cancer patients who were long-term survivors after total gastrectomy (mean of eight years). Whole body dual x-ray absorptiometry (DXA) scans were performed at a mean of five and eight years after the operation. The results showed that patients lost an average of 3.2 kg of body weight ($p < 0.006$) with a corresponding loss of lean body mass ($p < 0.0001$). However, there was no difference in bone density from values seen in age- and sex-matched controls. There was a slight elevation of osteocalcin levels and a minor increase in parathyroid hormone levels. The impact of total gastrectomy on calcium homeostasis and BMD seems to be marginal in this study. However, the authors argued that the observed close relationship between BMD and body weight suggested the pivotal importance of maintaining body weight after gastrectomy.

There is very limited information on bone density among cervical cancer and ovarian cancer patients. A small case-control study in 40 cervical cancer patients treated with radiotherapy and 40 matched controls found no significant difference in the BMD between the two groups and no significant change in BMD one to seven years after the therapy in the patient group (Chen, Lee et al. 2002). In another small study, fifteen women (mean age 38.2 ± 7.8 years; range 30 to 46 years) with ovarian cancer who had been treated with chemotherapy for six cycles every four weeks following surgical cytoreduction were measured for bone loss. A significant bone loss was observed ($p < 0.001$), and baseline lean mass predicted bone loss with anticancer chemotherapy (Douchi, Kosha et al. 1997).

It is fundamental that health professionals and cancer patients learn about the risk of osteoporosis associated with both cancer prognosis and treatment and to take an active role in preventing, treating and managing osteoporosis. Preventive measures should be recommended to all patients. Risk assessments, including (BMD) testing for osteoporosis, should be performed, and treatments should be initiated for people with low bone density or at high risk of bone fracture. Although specific guidelines and consensus on the treatment and prevention of osteoporosis among cancer survivors are lacking, research evidence suggests that both non-pharmacologic approaches and some pharmacologic approaches to prevent and treat osteoporosis among the general population may be applicable to cancer populations (Mincey, Moraghan et al. 2000; Pfeilschifter and Diel 2000).

Pharmacologic approaches include anti-resorptive therapy and anabolic therapy. Most of the bone-active agents currently available in the U.S. act by inhibiting bone resorption. Estrogens, selective estrogen receptor modulators (SERMs), bisphosphonates, calcitonin, calcium and vitamin D all have anti-resorptive properties. However, estrogen therapy is neither an option for cancer survivors nor recommended for prevention or treatment of osteoporosis for women without vasomotor symptoms. There are several anabolic agents that have the ability to increase bone formation. These include parathyroid hormone, fluoride, growth hormone, insulin-like growth factor-1, androgens, tibolone, strontium and statins. Since many of these agents may increase the risk of malignancy, they are not good candidates for osteoporosis therapy among cancer patients.

Falls are responsible for 90% of hip fractures. Nutrition, exercise and fall prevention are important non-pharmacologic approaches for fracture risk reduction. Adequate calcium and vitamin D intake are necessary for bone health. Vitamin K, caffeine, soy, and high protein and sodium diet may also affect bone density, but their relationship to osteoporosis has not been well established. Exercise provides an approximate two-fold benefit for osteoporosis risk reduction, including a significant improvement or maintenance of bone density as well as a reduced risk of falls. In a 2004 report on osteoporosis by the U.S. Surgeon General, lifestyle approaches to promote bone health are supported by a rich body of research evidence (DHHS 2004).

Mechanisms of Carcinogenesis

Although there are literally dozens of biological mechanisms by which diet and physical activity protect against the development of cancer, a few have been of particular biological relevance. These include insulin resistance, modulation of immunity, including the inflammatory response, and DNA damage-repair. Each of these are described and discussed in more detail below.

Insulin Resistance. Insulin resistance has been described as the dysregulation of insulin response to elevations in blood glucose levels. Among individuals demonstrating insulin resistance, even moderate intake of low fiber, high carbohydrate food items (high glycemic foods) can result in significant elevations of plasma insulin levels. Insulin is well known to be growth promoting, and thus, increased plasma insulin levels in the presence of pre-cancerous or cancer cells are thought to provide the necessary microenvironmental stimulus for cancer development and growth. In other words, hyperinsulinemia is a

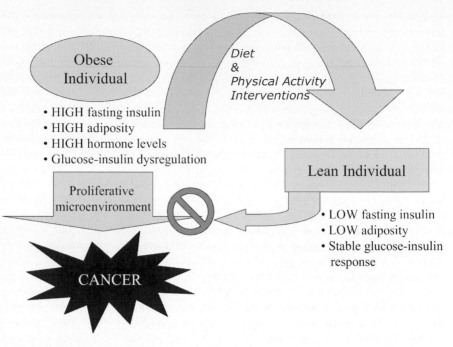

Fig. 1. Insulin resistance, obesity and carcinogenesis.

compensatory response to control blood glucose levels within the normal range in people who demonstrate a blunted response to insulin. Evidence suggests that hyperglycemia and, in some cases, the corresponding insulinemia, are associated with increased risk of several cancer types including colorectal, breast and prostate cancers. Elevations in triglycerides, C-peptide (a marker of pancreatic insulin secretion) and insulin-like growth factor 1, and reductions in select insulin binding proteins, have also been associated with increased cancer risk in both animal models and human trials, thus further supporting the insulin resistance theory of carcinogenesis (Fig. 1).

In turn, dietary selections and eating patterns further augment this cancer-promoting process. It has been shown that diets high in refined sugars and carbohydrates elevate blood glucose levels and insulin response more so than diets high in complex or high fiber foods. Intake of protein- or fat-containing food items along with refined carbohydrates will reduce the maximal height on the insulin response curve as measured in peripheral blood over time, but will not prevent the rise all together. In addition, the normal biological control of blood glucose and insulin response is significantly reduced in the presence of adiposity with aging. Certain populations, such as the Pima Indians, may have a genetic predisposition toward insulin resistance. Cell culture studies using a wide variety of cancer cell lines exposed to exogenous insulin and/or simple sugars, such as sucrose and high fructose corn syrup, also indicate that carcinogenesis is promoted in such an environment.

Both optimal dietary selections and increased physical activity can modulate both the potential for developing insulin resistance as well as reverse the process in those previously demonstrated to have insulin resistance. Weight loss is pivotal to these protective effects. Significant reductions in energy intake (10 to 20% of energy requirements) should be prescribed for weight loss of one kilogram weekly until weight is within normal acceptable limits. Concurrent with energy restriction, emphasis should be placed on increasing energy expenditure, starting with a goal expenditure of 1000 kcal per week and increasing to 2500 to 3000 kcal/week. Weight loss is the single most effective intervention to prevent or reverse insulin resistance. Although the evidence does not currently exist regarding the specific macronutrient composition of the diet to prevent or control insulin resistance, the biologic and pathophysiologic features of the insulin resistance syndrome indicate that a diet restricted in simple sugars, including high fructose corn syrup and refined carbohydrates, is warranted. Efforts to increase high-fiber foods, which are low in sugars, and to consume a protein or fat food source, along with any carbohydrate-rich food, may also be of benefit. It is important to note that there are circumstances when a person of seemingly normal body weight may demonstrate increased adiposity and thus be prone to insulin resistance syndrome. In these cases, dietary modification as described above should be considered; however, optimizing physical activity levels will be central to reversing the adverse effects of hyperinsulinemia.

Immune Modulation. Cancer is thought to be a disease of the immune system. Theoretically, if the immune system is functioning optimally, cancer should not occur. To this end, research has focused both on understanding the role of the immune system in cancer prevention as well as how lifestyle behaviors can modulate immune response. Several nutrients have been shown to play a role in immune function ranging from protein, the building block of immune cells, to numerous micronutrients, such as vitamins A, C, E, and zinc and copper. The role of select nutrients in immune modulation is summarized in Table 5. The appropriate level of nutrient intake for promoting optimal immune response has not been clearly established. For some nutrients it appears that there is a window; intake below or above this range may have immunosuppressive effects (e.g. zinc). For other nutrients, levels must be significantly depressed before immune suppression is shown (e.g. vitamin A). What is clear is that among immunosuppressed populations (such as HIV-infected individuals), the risk for cancer is increased. In addition, these same populations generally demonstrate improved immunity in response to nutrient-dense diets or supplementation. However, if the provision of nutrients to these high-risk individuals also reduces cancer occurrence has yet to be established.

In general, it is important to assess the adequacy of the diet in terms of the immune-modulating nutrients. Particularly for individuals at increased genetic risk for cancer, optimizing micronutrient intake is a feasible and potentially health promoting approach to reducing cancer risk. Although the risk may remain, dietary modification to promote intake of a nutrient-dense diet can delay disease onset or reduce disease severity. In fact, a recent study of lifestyle behaviors among women with BRCA1 and BRCA2 genes demonstrated a 10- to 13-year delay in onset of breast cancer among women with a healthy body weight and particularly among those who reported regular physical activity (King, Marks et al. 2003).

As discussed earlier, obesity is a contributing factor in the development of several cancers. It has been demonstrated that obese individuals have suppressed immune re-

Table 5. Role of nutrients in enhancing immunity

Nutrient	Food Sources	Demonstrated Effects on Immune Response
Vitamins		
Vitamin A	Fortified dairy, yellow-orange vegetables	Improve mucosal integrity, increase T cell function, increase antigen (Ag)-specific immunoglobin-G response
Vitamin C	Citrus, peppers, broccoli	Increase T cell response, increase phagocytosis, increase epithelial integrity
Vitamin E	Seeds, almonds, oils, Raisin Bran	Increase cytokine production, increase B cell function, increase T cell cytotoxicity, increase phagocytosis
Minerals		
Copper	Beef liver, cashews, molasses	Increase B cell function, increase T cell response, increase phagocytic function
Iron	Fortified cereals, liver, clams	Increase B cells, increase Ab production, increase lymphoid tissue
Magnesium		Increase cytotoxic cells, increase cytokine production
Zinc	Oysters, wheat germ, dark meat, poultry	Increase B cell function, increase cytokine production, increase cell mediated immunity
Other Nutrients		
Omega-3 fatty acids	Salmon, cold water fish, flax	Decrease inflammatory response
Protein	Lean meat, low-fat dairy, egg white	Increase total lymphocyte count/response to Ag, increase epithelial integrity

sponse. Not only are the numbers of CD4- and CD8-positive T cells reduced, macrophage response is delayed in obese subjects as is natural killer cell cytotoxicity. It therefore appears that one plausible mechanism by which cancer risk is elevated in obese individuals may be related to the resultant immunosuppression, the onset of which is related to an accumulation of adipose tissue.

Inflammatory Response. One factor relevant to immune response and cancer risk theoretically identifies cancer as an inflammatory disease. In fact, inflammatory biomarkers have been shown to be elevated in a variety of cancer patients before, during and after cancer therapy. Inflammation results in cellular damage and thus is thought to be a contributory factor in the multi-step pathway to carcinogenesis. Inflammation is also characterized by an accumulation of macrophages that in turn release reactive oxygen species, another contributing factor in cancer development. This biological response may be of particular importance to the obese patient who not only demonstrates reduced macrophage-related response to antigens, but also accumulates macrophages locally in adipose tissue thus elevating the level of localized oxidative damage in these cells.

There are several naturally-occurring inflammatory response modifiers in the human diet. Of particular interest are the omega-3 fatty acids. Fatty acids have demonstrated effects on membrane fluidity and eicosanoid production that in turn alters signal-transduction pathways, membrane-bound receptors and enzyme activity. The end

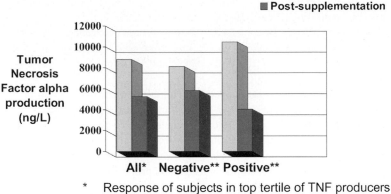

■ Pre-supplementation
■ Post-supplementation

*   Response of subjects in top tertile of TNF producers
**   Response of subjects in the top tertile of TNF production who
      tested as shown for TNFA (-308) allele 2

Fig. 2. Genetic polymorphisms and anti-inflammatory response to omega-3 fatty acid supplementation (Kornman, Martha et al. 2004)

result of these biological effects is an alteration in cytokine release and inflammatory response. Increasing omega-3 fatty acid intake results in a reduction in omega-6 fatty acid and in particular arachidonic acid, a pro-inflammatory compound. Fish oil, an abundant source of omega-3 fatty acids, when supplemented in the diet, results in a significant decrease in the omega-6 to omega-3 fatty acid ratio. Omega-3 fatty acids and foods high in omega-3 fatty acids, including alpha linolenic acid, are considered anti-inflammatory and thus may play a role similar to prescribed cyclooxygenase inhibitors in reducing cancer risk. Recent evidence also suggests that responsiveness to omega-3 fatty acid supplementation may be modulated by genetic background (Fig. 2).

Oxidative Damage. Related to the inflammatory response is the role of oxidative DNA damage in cancer development and progression. All living organisms consuming oxygen experience oxidative damage to tissue on an ongoing basis. In turn, within the human, adaptive mechanisms exist to either reverse the oxidative damage inherent to our biological processes or minimize the effects by clearing byproducts of oxidative damage from the body, thus reducing cancer risk. The role of antioxidants in reducing oxidative damage and promoting repair has been well described in the literature (Ames 1983; Halliwell 2002). Many clinicians fail to recognize that beyond the more well-known antioxidants (e.g. vitamins C and E and selenium) are several naturally-occurring phytochemicals that also have significant antioxidant properties. These include carotenoids found in vegetables and fruits, polyphenols found in teas, resveratrol found in grapes, limonene from citrus peel, or isoflavones found in soy foods. The cancer preventive role of vegetables and fruits likely stems in part from the high antioxidant content.

Several studies have been published over the past five to ten years demonstrating the potential for vegetables and fruit to reduce oxidative damage. In a study by Thompson and colleagues (Thompson, Heimendinger et al. 1999), a controlled feeding of vegetable (carrot) juice resulted in a significant reduction in oxidative damage biomarkers among healthy individuals. Another study showed a similar response using a high vegetable and fruit diet (Djuric, Heilbrun et al. 1991). Similar results have been shown while feeding a variety of foods rich in antioxidant properties, not only to healthy individuals but also to smokers, people diagnosed with cancer and long-term cancer survivors (Djuric, Depper et al. 1998; van Zeeland, de Groot et al. 1999; Collins and Harrington 2002).

Reduction in oxidative damage through dietary modification seems an appropriate approach to reducing cancer risk. However, there is no direct evidence that such an approach will result in reduced cancer rates. A prudent diet should include a wide variety of vegetables and fruits with attention to a broad range of food colors. The diet should also include additional food selections that promote greater intake of dietary constituents that have demonstrated antioxidant properties such as green tea, citrus peel, onion, garlic, and soy foods.

Biological Mechanisms of Physical Activity

Whereas the exact biological mechanisms defining the relationship between physical activity and cancer remain unknown, many plausible explanations have been identified. It is likely that multiple mechanisms exist that demonstrate individual variability, based upon genetics, environment, cancer type and stage, and the form of physical activity performed.

Insulin, Glucose and Insulin-Like Growth Factor. Elevations in insulin and insulin-like growth factor-1 (IGF-1) have been associated with increased rates of many cancers (LeRoith, Baserga et al. 1995). IGF-1 is down regulated by increased synthesis of a binding protein (IGFBP-3) which is enhanced by physical activity. Decreased IGF-1 may also lead to increases in sex hormone binding globulin (SHBG), thereby leading to decreases in unbound sex steroids. Finally, a strong relationship exists between physical activity and circulating levels of insulin and insulin sensitivity. This relationship may also be mediated through adiposity.

Body Composition and Obesity. Obesity and fat distribution have been associated with increased rates of many cancers. Abdominal fat, specifically visceral or intra-abdominal fat, is the most metabolically active fat store. This relationship is mediated through variations in hormone levels, to include sex steroid hormones, insulin and IGF-1. Physically active individuals are generally neither obese nor demonstrate central distribution of body fat (Westerlind 2003). Visceral fat is preferentially affected by aerobic exercise (Schwartz, Shuman et al. 1991). Calorie restriction has been demonstrated to have a protective effect (Kritchevsky 1999) and although compensatory mechanisms often exist for calorie expenditure from exercise, it is plausible that this relationship may exist to a degree in individuals who are physically active.

Immune Function. The effects of physical activity on the immune system have often been held as a primary link between physical activity and cancer, although it is believed that the majority of cancers are nonimmunogenic (Westerlind 2003). Regular, moderate exercise and physical activity have been noted to affect a number of immune parameters, both numerically and functionally, to include: macrophages, natural killer cells (NK), cytotoxic T lymphocytes, and lymphokine-activated killer cells (LAK) (Newsholme 1994). Aging-associated decreases in immune function (immune senescence) have been suggested as a possible explanation for the increased rates of cancer seen with aging. Conversely, regular physical activity has been noted to enhance T-cell function of elderly men and women (Mazzeo 1994). Therefore, overall immune enhancement and slowing of immune senescence may represent the physical activity-immunity relationship.

Oxidative Damage. Physical activity and exercise demonstrate varying degrees of oxidative damage and generation of free radicals. Whereas moderate activity causes no to minimal damage in young and/or trained athletes (Margaritis, Tessier et al. 1997), strenuous exercise may increase rates of oxidative stress (Poulsen, Loft et al. 1996). Free radicals may adversely affect DNA and may stimulate mutagenesis and tumor proliferation (Dreher and Junod 1996). Moderate physical activity and training effects may enhance the body's innate antioxidant system and scavenging of free radicals. Conversely, intense exercise may overwhelm the body's ability to manage oxidative stress, leading to increased oxidative damage.

Steroid Sex Hormones. Steroid sex hormones are associated with the development of reproductive cancers in both women and men. The varied effects of exercise on these hormones is believed to be responsible for this protective relationship.

Epidemiologic evidence generally supports an inverse relationship between physical activity and the incidence of prostate cancer (Oliveria and Lee 1997), although it has been noted that there is an inverse relationship between upper body mass and prostate cancer, possibly due to higher testosterone levels from increased muscularity (Severson, Grove et al. 1988). It has been identified that chronic endurance activities may decrease levels of testosterone, although this effect has not been reported consistently (Lucia, Chicharro et al. 1996; Hackney, Fahrner et al. 1998). A relationship has been identified between sedentary occupations and increased risk of testicular cancer (Coggon, Pannett et al. 1986), whereas 15 or more hours of vigorous physical activity per week has been noted to decrease the risk of this cancer (1994). Concentrations of SHBG may be increased, thereby leading to depressed levels of free circulating testosterone.

Likewise in women, SHBG levels may demonstrate a similar response to exercise. Additional mechanisms may lead to decreases of both estrogen and progesterone, in premenopausal women, causing increased menstrual irregularities, a shortened luteal phase, and increased anovulatory cycles (Westerlind 2003). Decreased hormone levels have also been identified in postmenopausal women that appear to be unrelated to body fat (Nelson, Meredith et al. 1988).

It is generally noted that physical activity decreases bowel transit time, possibly mediated by increased vagal tone and increased peristalsis. This may lead to decreased exposure time of toxins with the bowel mucosa and inhibit promotion of carcinogenesis.

Diet-gene Interactions. Briefly, it is important to mention the role genetics is likely to play in the future of cancer-preventive diets and lifestyle interventions for individuals and sub-groups at risk. A person's reponsiveness to dietary intervention is increasingly being identified as being affected by the complexity of an individual's genotype and genetic polymorphisms. It is likely that many of the inconsistencies demonstrated

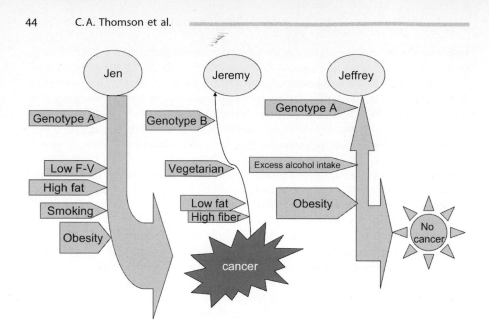

Fig. 3. Diet, genetics and the potential to develop cancer

in the epidemiological assessment of relationships between dietary constituents and specific cancer endpoints may be explained by genetic variability. In a given population, the interplay between an individual's genotype and dietary exposures throughout the lifespan may significantly influence whether or not that individual is diagnosed with cancer (Fig. 3). Understanding this relationship, future dietary interventions can be targeted to those at risk and can be adapted for individual likelihood of response.

Guidelines for Cancer Preventive Lifestyle

Several organizations have provided guidance in terms of dietary recommendations to reduce cancer risk. Generally, the recommendations are similar across organizational groups, such as the American Cancer Society, World Cancer Research Fund, and the Committee on Medical Aspects of Food and Nutrition Policy of the United Kingdom. The recommendations are largely based on epidemiological evidence, much of which has been supported by plausible mechanisms of biological action. In forming such policy and recommendations, these organizations often give consideration to the plausibility that individuals or populations will be able to effectively achieve and maintain the dietary pattern described. To this end, to some extent the recommended intakes may not be consistent with published literature, but instead reflect a positive change in intake toward an optimal level. While much of the evidence remains insufficient and further research is warranted, providing dietary guidelines is prudent in that there is a consistency in the evidence collected that supports dietary change in the American population. These same dietary guidelines, in a majority of the cases, may also result in reduced rates of other chronic diseases.

Currently, the guidelines provided by the American Cancer Society for primary cancer prevention and recurrence should serve as the foundation of any recommendations provided to individuals (Byers, Nestle et al. 2002; Brown, Byers et al. 2003). Individualization is essential, based upon the person's physical status, prior physical activity and exercise history, and goals and expectations.

The following is a summary of dietary and physical activity recommendations developed in the context of this chapter that should be considered in providing lifestyle advice to people seeking to reduce their cancer risk. These recommendations should be considered for all adults and efforts should be made to integrate these same recommendations in youth prior to puberty.

- Achieve and maintain a healthy body weight and body composition
  - Be aware of small, incremental changes that over time result in excess adiposity
  - Restrict energy intake
  - Increase energy expenditure
  - Perform both aerobic and weight-bearing activities daily
- Eat at least five servings of vegetables daily
  - Include a dark green leafy vegetable daily
  - Include a dark orange-yellow vegetable daily
- Eat at least three servings of fruit daily
  - Consume fresh or dried fruit
  - Include one serving of citrus daily
- Eat at least 30 grams of fiber daily
  - Select both soluble and insoluble fiber sources
  - Select only whole grain breads and cereals
- Reduce intake or avoid processed or refined carbohydrates
  - Select whole grain breads
  - Read labels and avoid foods with greater than 10 grams of sugar per serving
  - Avoid foods and beverages containing high fructose corn syrup
  - Prepare food at home more; reduce meals from fast food restaurants
- Include foods rich in antioxidants
  - Vegetables and fruits
  - Teas
- Include omega-3 rich foods daily
  - Cold-water fish
  - Flax seed
  - Omega-3 oils
- Adopt a physically active lifestyle
  - Adults: Engage in at least moderate aerobic physical activity for at least 30 minutes on most, preferably all, days of the week. Recognition of the exercise continuum indicating that health and fitness gains are enhanced by greater volumes of activity should serve as a goal to achieve at least 20 to 60 minutes of continuous or intermittent (minimum of 10 minute bouts accumulated throughout the day) moderate to vigorous aerobic physical activity regularly (Pollock, Gaesser et al. 1998, UDHHS 1996).
  - Adults: Engage in resistance training 2–3 days per week. A minimum of 8 to 10 exercises involving the major muscle groups should be performed that incorporate a minimum of one set of 8 to 15 repetitions.

▪ Youth: Accumulate at least 60 minutes, and up to several hours, of age-appropriate moderate-to-vigorous physical activity on most, preferably all, days of the week (NASPE 2004).

▪ All individuals should incorporate more physical activity into their daily lives. Simple measures such as the following can enhance regular activity and improve health:

- Take the stairs rather than the elevator or escalator
- "Actively commute" by walking or bicycling where and when appropriate
- Schedule active family outings and vacations
- Engage in moderate housework and yardwork where and when available
- Take 10-minute minimum walk breaks at work
- Wear a pedometer to gauge daily activity level
- Get together regularly with friends and/or family members for hikes or walks
- Walk the dog
- Take the first available parking space and walk to the store entrance
- Carry bags of groceries in from the car one at a time

The American Cancer Society identifies specific issues for survivors of cancer that may preclude their participation in physical activity (Brown, Byers et al. 2003).

▪ Individuals with anemia should refrain from activity, other than that of daily living, until anemia improves.

▪ Individuals with compromised immune systems should avoid public gyms and other public venues; survivors post bone marrow transplantation should avoid these spaces for one year following transplant.

▪ Persons experiencing significant fatigue should listen to their bodies and do as much as they feel able to do and are encouraged to do 10 minutes of stretching daily.

▪ Individuals should avoid chlorinated pools if undergoing radiation therapy.

▪ Persons with indwelling catheters should avoid water or other microbial exposures that may result in infections. They should also avoid resistance training that may cause dislodgement of the catheter.

▪ Persons who are experiencing significant peripheral neuropathy that may impede their ability to perform exercises and activities that make use of the affected limbs may consider using a recumbent bicycle or similar exercise equipment in controlled settings rather than performing activities outdoors.

As previously mentioned, it is important for clinicians to individualize physical activity and exercise recommendations as determined by the unique situation of the patient. An emphasis should be placed upon getting all individuals to limit their sedentary behavior and increase their activity as tolerated.

Tools for Research and Clinical Practice

Researchers and clinicians can benefit from having the appropriate tools necessary to integrate diet and nutrition as well as physical activity and body composition assessment and behavior change instruments available. The remainder of this chapter focuses on key issues in measurement, assessment and implementation of behavior change in this context. Some will have greater application to the researcher, while others will be most appropriately applied in clinical practice.

Measuring Diet

Dietary measurement is among the most challenging issues facing researchers and clinicians alike. Current dietary measurement tools rely heavily on self report. It has been demonstrated that people have difficulty accurately recalling dietary intake and due to social desirability may have significant discomfort in reporting intake even when accurately recalled. This is particularly true for overweight persons, and has been primarily described among women.

There are three major approaches to measuring diet reported in the scientific literature. These include: the Food Frequency Questionnaire (FFQ), where individuals recall intake of a specific list of foods (80 to 250 items), frequency of intake, and approximate serving sizes; dietary recalls, where individuals report their intake in terms of food items, amounts and preparation methods for one or more 24-hour periods; and the dietary record, where individuals record all food consumed, amounts, brands and preparation methods for a pre-defined period of time. Each approach has both strengths and weaknesses. Correlations between these approaches generally range between 30 and 60% supporting the concern for significant reporting error when it comes to dietary measurement. However, until more accurate approaches are developed, these approaches remain the basis for much of the dietary measurement reported in the literature.

To best assess intake, researchers recommend that more than one approach be used and when possible, biological markers of intake also be measured. Presented in Table 6 are several biomarkers of dietary intake that can be employed in an effort to validate self-reported intake.

In addition, investigators have developed several focused food frequency questionnaires to more accurately capture intake of select foods that have been recognized for their chemopreventive properties. These include the Citrus Intake Questionnaire, the

Table 6. Biological markers (assays) used to validate self-reported dietary intake

Dietary Constituent of Interest	Biomarker/Functional Biomarker
Fiber	Fecal hemicellulose; fecal weight, short-chain fatty acids
Folate	Plasma folate; red blood cell folate; plasma homocysteine
Vitamin B12	Plasma B12
Vitamin C	Plasma vitamin C; urine deoxypyridinoline
Vitamin E	Plasma tocopherols; LDL oxidation
Calcium	Bone density; serum osteocalcin
Selenium	Plasma or whole blood selenium; toenail selenium; plasma GSH peroxidase activity
Carotenoids	Plasma levels (alpha- and beta-carotene; lutein; lycopene
Cruciferous vegetables/isothiocyanates	Urinary dithiocarbamates
Citrus/limonene	Urinary perillylic acid
Tea polyphenols	Urinary polyphenols

Table 7. Dietary Measurement Websites

Organization	Website address	Components
Arizona Cancer Center Diet and Behavioral Measurement Service	http://www.azdiet-behavior.azcc.arizona.edu	Food Frequency Questionnaires including FFQs for Tea, Citrus and Cruciferous Vegetables
Block, Gladys-Investigator	http://www.nutritionquest.com/fat_screener.html	Fat Screener
National Cancer Institute	http://riskfactor.cancer.gov/diet/screeners/fruitveg/	Fruit and Vegetable Screener
U.S. Department of Agriculture	http://www.usda.gov/cnpp/healthyeating.html	Healthy Eating Index

Arizona Tea Questionnaire, the Soy Foods Questionnaire and most recently the Cruciferous Vegetable Questionnaire. These focused instruments allow for more complete and valid assessment of intake of the designated foods, thus supporting more reliable assessment of the association between these foods and cancer risk reduction. Several of these instruments are available through the Dietary and Behavioral Measurements Service at the University of Arizona.

Other clinical and research tools are available online. These include the National Cancer Institute FFQ, Block Fat Screener, and the NCI Fruit and Vegetable Screener. The U.S. Department of Agriculture also has an online Healthy Eating Index; individuals can enter daily dietary intake and can receive an immediate assessment of specific macro and micronutrients, a graphic comparison of how their intake compares to the Food Guide Pyramid, and a summary of individual intake versus national dietary goals. The Healthy Eating Index also affords the individual an opportunity to track progress over time as new dietary behaviors are adapted. A summary of diet evaluation resources is listed in Table 7.

Assessment of Physical Activity and Energy Expenditure

Researchers should be familiar with the various methods of assessing physical activity and energy expenditure. The former term is broadly defined as any bodily movement that is produced by the contraction of skeletal muscle and that substantially increases energy expenditure. The latter specifically addresses the energetic cost associated with a specific physical activity and is dependent upon the numerous processes and personal characteristics (e.g., age, body mass, fitness level) associated with that activity (Montoye, Kemper et al. 1996).

Physical Activity Questionnaires. Physical activity questionnaires are simple and inexpensive methods of obtaining data from participants. As they are dependent upon individual self report, they are subject to recall and social bias. They are nonetheless useful and are often used in conjunction with more objective measures.

Global short surveys (1 to 5 questions) that focus upon general aspects of physical activity provide limited information and lack specificity, but provide an overview of physical activity patterns that may provide background information for more focused studies. Recall, or longer surveys (10 to 20 questions), are often used to obtain baseline data for comparison with post-intervention data. These instruments provide more detailed information about specific aspects of physical activity (e.g. frequency, amount) over a defined period of time (e.g. days, weeks, months). Quantitative history tools generally have more questions (greater than 20) and provide very detailed information about physical activity patterns over longer periods of time (e.g. past year, period in lifetime, entire lifetime). These instruments address the volume of activity and allow for the determination of dose-response effects on outcome measures of interest (e.g. kcal/week).

Physical Activity Logs, Records and Recalls. Physical activity records provide an on-going account of an individual's physical activity during a defined period of time in an attempt to capture all forms of activity. Physical activity logs are often used to determine adherence to specific protocols. They call for identifying specific aspects of physical activity over determined intervals (e.g. every 15 minutes). Physical activity recall is usually performed by telephone or personal interviews and attempt to catalogue an individual's physical activity patterns over a defined period of time (e.g. day, week).

Indirect Measures of Energy Expenditure. There are a wide variety of tools and methods that can be applied in either laboratory or field situations. They provide reliable and valid measures of free living situations but vary in their logistical burden of performance. Doubly labeled water (DLW) provides an accurate assessment of energy expenditure based upon the volume of carbon dioxide (VCO_2) produced and oxygen uptake volume (VO_2). Stable isotopes of water are consumed, and then fractional excretion is calculated through urinary measures. Energy expenditure is calculated from determination of VCO_2 and VO_2. Although an accurate measure, it cannot provide specific information about the characteristics of physical activity that have contributed to the energy expenditure, such as intensity, frequency or duration. VO_2 estimates energy intake based upon equations that provide a relationship between oxygen utilization by tissues and caloric utilization by activity (one liter O_2 approximately equals 5 kcal). These estimates are commonly determined by a treadmill or bicycle ergometer and are often used to provide an individual with an exercise prescription that defines the volume and intensity of activity to be performed (e.g. 60 to 90% of maximum heart rate, or 50 to 85% of VO_{2max}).

Heart rate is a commonly used measure that provides an indirect estimate of workload or energy expenditure. It is based upon a linear relationship that may exist between heart rate and VO_2, but as it is significantly affected by a number of parameters, its accuracy is less than other measures. It nonetheless is easily measured and is a useful measure in interventions that provide an exercise prescription to participants.

Motion detectors are mechanical instruments that are worn to quantify a measure of physical activity. These instruments are based upon the premise that motion is related to energy expenditure. Accelerometers have commonly been utilized and provide researchers with an accurate assessment of activity intensity and volume over a determined time interval. Limitations, such as the inability to measure activities that may not cause trunk movement (e.g. resistance training), prevent them from accurately providing a measure of the wearer's total energy expenditure.

Pedometers are simple devices that have become increasingly popular for physical activity assessment. They measure the number of steps that are taken while worn, but cannot differentiate characteristics of step-based activities, nor can they measure other forms of activity accurately (e.g., bicycling). Pedometers are inexpensive and have been associated with an increase in motivation toward behavior change, thus making them popular for clinical practice and research. In general, research studies are more likely to rely on accelerometers to measure physical activity because they have a higher correlation with actual energy expenditure [$r = 0.34$–0.49 (Freedson and Miller 2000) versus $r = 0.66$–0.96 (Sherman, Morris et al. 1998)].

Measurement of Body Composition

Anthropometric Measurements. Anthropometry has been used to predict body composition in laboratory and field situations. Some examples of anthropometric variables relevant to body composition are weight, trunk depth, stature, arm span, knee height, breadth of biacromial, bi-iliac, knee, ankle, elbow and wrist, circumference of waist, hip, thigh, calf, arm and wrist, and skinfold thickness at the subscapular, midaxillary, suprailia, triceps and biceps. These variables can be used to predict percent body fat, body density, fat-free mass, total body muscle mass, and total body bone mineral content. A number of body composition predictive models with anthropometric variables have been developed and cross-calibrated. Because anthropometric procedures are non-invasive and the instruments used for anthropometric measurements are portable and relatively inexpensive, anthropometry tends to be used for large population-based studies. However, in comparison to other laboratory techniques for body composition measurements, anthropometric measurements may be less accurate.

Bioelectric Impedance Analysis (BIA). BIA is often a substitute or supplement to conventional anthropometry in field research or epidemiologic studies on body composition. Impedance is the frequency-dependent opposition of a conductor to the flow of an alternating electric current and reflects both resistance and reactance. The use of BIA to estimate body composition is based on the assumption that different body tissue components have different conductive and dielectric properties at different frequencies of current. The conductive and dielectric properties can be measured through impedance. All BIA devices are composed of three essential parts: alternating electrical current sources; cables and electrodes to introduce the current into the body and to send the voltage drop due to impedance; and a system for measuring impedance. BIA is portable and easy to use. Predictive equations of impedance can be developed and calibrated for estimating total and regional body composition, including fat and fat-free mass. However, the general applicability of BIA is often limited by the availability of appropriately calibrated and cross-validated predictive equations in different populations who have different hydration status and thickness of subcutaneous fat. These factors may significantly affect the precision of BIA assessments. Although limited evidence suggests a significant correlation between changes in total body water assessed from BIA and deuterium dilution among some cancer patients (Simons, Schols et al. 1999), BIA does not provide reliable measurements of body composition for cancer patients with ascites (Sarhill, Walsh et al. 2000). Until more research has been conducted, caution should be taken when applying general BIA predictive equations for body composition estimations among cancer patients.

Dual-energy X-ray Absorptiometry (DXA). A new generation of bone densitometry not only measures bone density, but also measures soft tissue mass. Body soft tissue measurements by DXA are derived from the assumed constant attenuation of pure fat and of bone-free lean tissue. The advantages of DXA in measuring body composition include its qualities as a noninvasive, highly precise and accurate instrument, and that it emits very low radiation (less than a standard x-ray). DXA scans may provide total body and regional measurements of bone mineral content, bone mineral density, soft tissue mass, lean soft tissue mass, and fat tissue mass as well as percent fat tissue mass. Hydration levels and body thickness have very small effects on the precision of DXA-derived body composition assessments. Hence, DXA can be used in both general and patient populations. With new developments in DXA hardware and software, the total body scan time has been significantly shortened, and body composition analyses can be conducted for any defined regions by the investigator. However, the high cost of DXA units and the need of special radiologic training for DXA operators limit the application of DXA for body composition measurements in standard research and clinical practice. Nevertheless, given the growing numbers of DXA instruments, and especially DXA-mobile units, the utility of DXA in field and epidemiologic and clincal studies of body composition will increase. Body composition measurement will likely have an increasing role in the supportive care of the patient, specifically to evaluate nutritional status and treatment effects on health.

Other Techniques. Hydrodensitometry, hydrometry, whole-body counting, neutron activation analysis, ultrasound, and imaging techniques, such as computed tomography (CT) and magnetic resonance imaging (MRI), are other techniques for body composition assessments. The hydrodensitometry method, which measures percent body fat, requires that the subject completely submerge in water and assumes consistent densities of the constituents of the body from person to person. The hydrometry method measures total body water, as well as intracellular and extracellular water, based on the distribution of isotopic tracers in different water compartments. Whole-body counting and neutron activation analysis can be used to measure skeletal muscle mass and other body composition through assessing natural potassium concentration, or assessing selectively activated atoms in the body. Ultrasound has been used to measure regional body composition for over 30 years. However, the precisions of ultrasound-derived body composition measurements are less satisfactory in comparison with DXA measurements.

Most previous studies have used body mass index or weight and waist-to-hip ratio as proxies for obesity and fat distribution. Measurement errors due to improper anatomical placement of the measuring tape and other technician operation errors, particularly with repeated measures, may limit the ability to detect an association of obesity or fat distribution with cancer.

Measurement of Bone Health

The World Health Organization (WHO) criteria for the diagnosis of osteoporosis are based on DXA measurements of BMD of the hip and spine for postmenopausal women. The criteria are T-scores that indicate the number of standard deviations below or above the average peak bone mass in young adults of the same sex (Table 8).

Table 8. World Health Organization (WHO) criteria for diagnosis of bone status

T-score	Classification
–1 or higher	Normal
–1 to –2.5	Osteopenia (or low bone density)
–2.5 or lower	Osteoporosis
–2.5 or lower + facture	Severe osteoporosis

The National Osteoporosis Foundation (NOF) Guidelines suggest that all women age 65 years or more, postmenopausal women with fractures, and younger postmenopausal women with one or more risk factors have a bone density test. The NOF suggests initiating therapy for women who have a T-score below –2.0 by central DXA and no additional risk factors, a T-score below –1.5 by central DXA with one or more additional risk factors, or for women with prior vertebral or hip fractures (Wei, Jackson et al. 2003). According to the International Society for Clinical Densitometry (ISCD), the WHO criteria should neither be applied to healthy premenopausal women nor applied in its entirety to men. The ISCD recommends using Z-scores, rather than T-scores, for osteoporosis diagnosis in premenopausal women. Z-scores indicate the number of standard deviations below or above the average population bone mass, determined by age and gender. The diagnosis of osteoporosis in premenopausal women should not be made on the basis of densitometric criteria alone. Osteoporosis may be diagnosed for premenopausal women with low BMD and secondary causes (e.g. glucocorticoid therapy, hypogonadism, hyperparathyroidism) or risk factors for fracture. The criteria for osteoporosis diagnosis among men may differ by age: in men age 65 and older, T-scores should be used and osteoporosis diagnosed if the T-score is at or below –2.5; between age 50 and 65, T-scores may be used and osteoporosis diagnosed if both the T-score is at or below –2.5 and other risk factors for fracture are identified; and for men under age 50, diagnosis should not be made on densitometric criteria alone. Men at any age with secondary causes of low BMD (e.g., glucocorticoid therapy, hypogonadism, hyperparathyroidism) may be diagnosed clinically with osteoporosis supported by findings of low BMD. For young adults and children (age 20 or under) the value of BMD in predicting fractures is not clearly determined. Z-scores may be used and the diagnosis should not be made on the basis of densitometric criteria alone. Low bone density for chronological age may be stated if Z-score is below -2.0 (2004).

There are many different techniques, including DXA, ultrasound devices, and quantitative CT (Maricic and Chen 2000) for central or peripheral BMD measurements. Both the NOF and the ISCD recommend using central DXA scans for osteoporosis diagnosis so as to be in agreement with the WHO criteria. Forearm (33% radius) BMD should be measured for osteoporosis diagnosis under the following circumstances: hip and or spine cannot be measured or interpreted; hyperparathyroidism; and very obese patients (over the weight limit for DXA tables) (ICSD 2004).

Biomarkers for Bone Metabolism. Biochemical bone markers reflect bone metabolism or bone turnover. There are two types of bone biomarkers — markers of bone formation and markers of bone absorption (Table 9).

Table 9. Biochemical markers of bone health

Markers of Bone Formation	Osteoblast-derived enzymes ▦ Total alkaline phosphatase ▦ Bone-specific alkaline phosphatase Bone matrix formation products ▦ Osteocalcin ▦ Type 1 collage propeptides
Markers of Bone Resorption	Osteoclast-derived enzymes ▦ Acid phosphatase ▦ Tartrate-resistant acid phosphatase Bone matrix degradation products ▦ Collagen cross-links (pyridinoline, deoxypyridinoline, N-telopeptide, C-telopeptide) ▦ Hydroxyproline

When used in conjunction with BMD measurements, the measurement of bone biomarkers may assist clinical decision making regarding the initiation and maintenance of therapy. However, the clinical use of bone biomarkers is complicated by multiple sources of variability related to biological factors and to the assay itself. Some examples of biological factors that may influence these markers include age, sex, ethnicity, physical activity, diet, drug therapy, medical conditions, and time of specimen collection. Assay variability can arise from variations in specimen processing, assay precision and accuracy, standardization, cross-reaction with other organ markers, nongaussian distribution, and interlaboratory variation. Therefore, bone biomarkers are poorly accepted by clinicians (Stepan 2003) and should be used only as secondary or experimental measures of bone density. The value of using biomarkers in aiding treatment decision for osteoporosis or monitoring treatment effects for osteoporosis among cancer patients have yet to be investigated.

Success usually comes when behavior change is made using small, incremental steps. Food and other lifestyle choices are influenced by several factors including perceived risk, cost, convenience, taste (e.g. food), social support, self-efficacy, and environment. Table 10 provides examples of behavior strategies or 'prescriptions' that can be employed to promote behavior change and, as a result, achieve the desired health outcome.

Conclusion

The role of diet, physical activity and body composition continues to be an area of active research both in terms of primary prevention and in terms of reducing morbidity and mortality among those previously treated for cancer. Evidence to date supports efforts to improve dietary selections toward a more plant-based, low fat, complex carbohydrate-rich diet along with daily, regular and varied physical activity. Maintenance of a healthy body weight throughout life is strongly recommended to reduce cancer risk. Measuring diet, physical activity and body composition is both plausible and challenging. Practitioners should develop strategies to routinely evaluate the diet, physical activity and body composition of each patient to promote early and effective behavior change to reduce cancer risk.

Table 10. Desired health outcome and possible behavioral strategies

Health or behavioral outcome sought	Behavioral strategy
Weight loss	■ Cut all portions in half ■ Use a salad plate to serve food ■ Restrict fast food restaurant visits to once/week ■ Record intake ■ Substitute calcium chews for dessert
Increased fruit and vegetable intake	■ Select a new fruit or vegetable from the produce department each week ■ Purchase a 5-a-day cookbook and try 3 new recipes each week ■ Keep a fruit bowl readily available at work and home ■ Select at least five different colors of produce at the marker each week ■ Visit the Farmer's market weekly – bring a friend ■ Add fresh fruit to cereal ■ Have a fruit smoothie for breakfast ■ Put blended vegetables into your pasta sauce ■ Make salads a meal
Increased fiber intake	■ Select and eat cereal with at least 6 grams of fiber per serving ■ Try oatmeal again ■ Purchase the heaviest bread on the shelves ■ Eat five to nine servings of vegetables and fruits daily ■ Add seeds to cereal, salads, etc ■ Snack on air-popped popcorn
Normal glucose-insulin levels	■ Avoid any food with greater than 10 grams sugar/serving ■ Switch from soda to fresh lemonade or tea with no added sugar ■ Consume protein-carbohydrate combined meals ■ Replace white bread with whole grain; replace white rice with brown; replace white potato with sweet potato
Daily physical activity	■ Wake up 30 minutes early and walk ■ Find a friend to walk with ■ Jump rope during television commercials ■ Garden ■ Ride a bike to work or on errands ■ Try a new sport ■ Join a team ■ Train for a charity walk/run ■ Keep an activity log – reward yourself when goals are met

References

(1994). "Aetiology of testicular cancer: association with congenital abnormalities, age at puberty, infertility, and exercise. United Kingdom Testicular Cancer Study Group." *Bmj* **308**(6941): 1393–1399.

(2004). "Diagnosis of osteoporosis in men, premenopausal women, and children." *J Clin Densitom* **7**(1): 17–26.

ACS (2003). Cancer Facts and Figures, 2003. Atlanta, American Cancer Society.

Alberts, D.S., M.E. Martinez, et al. (2000). "Lack of effect of a high-fiber cereal supplement on the recurrence of colorectal adenomas. Phoenix Colon Cancer Prevention Physicians' Network." *N Engl J Med* **342**(16): 1156–1162.

Ames, B.N. (1983). "Dietary carcinogens and anticarcinogens. Oxygen radicals and degenerative diseases." *Science* **221**(4617): 1256–1264.

Basaria, S., J. Lieb, 2nd, et al. (2002). "Long-term effects of androgen deprivation therapy in prostate cancer patients." *Clin Endocrinol (Oxf)* **56**(6): 779–786.

Berruti, A., L. Dogliotti, et al. (2002). "Changes in bone mineral density, lean body mass and fat content as measured by dual energy x-ray absorptiometry in patients with prostate cancer without apparent bone metastases given androgen deprivation therapy." *J Urol* **167**(6): 2361–2367; discussion 2367.

Bingham, S.A., N.E. Day, et al. (2003). "Dietary fibre in food and protection against colorectal cancer in the European Prospective Investigation into Cancer and Nutrition (EPIC): an observational study." *Lancet* **361**(9368): 1496–1501.

Boule, N.G., E. Haddad, et al. (2001). "Effects of exercise on glycemic control and body mass in type 2 diabetes mellitus: a meta-analysis of controlled clinical trials." *Jama* **286**(10): 1218–1227.

Brown, J.K., T. Byers, et al. (2003). "Nutrition and physical activity during and after cancer treatment: an American Cancer Society guide for informed choices." *CA Cancer J Clin* **53**(5): 268–291.

Byers, T., M. Nestle, et al. (2002). "American Cancer Society guidelines on nutrition and physical activity for cancer prevention: Reducing the risk of cancer with healthy food choices and physical activity." *CA Cancer J Clin* **52**(2): 92–119.

Chen, H.H., B.F. Lee, et al. (2002). "Changes in bone mineral density of lumbar spine after pelvic radiotherapy." *Radiother Oncol* **62**(2): 239–242.

Chen, Z., M. Maricic, et al. (2002). "Low bone density and high percentage of body fat among men who were treated with androgen deprivation therapy for prostate carcinoma." *Cancer* **95**(10): 2136–2144.

Chen, Z., M. Maricic, et al. (in press, 2005). "Fracture risk among breast cancer survivors: results from the Women's Health Initiative observational study." *Arch Int Med*.

Clarke, G. and A.S. Whittemore (2000). "Prostate cancer risk in relation to anthropometry and physical activity: the National Health and Nutrition Examination Survey I Epidemiological Follow-Up Study." *Cancer Epidemiol Biomarkers Prev* **9**(9): 875–881.

Coggon, D., B. Pannett, et al. (1986). "A survey of cancer and occupation in young and middle aged men. II. Non-respiratory cancers." *Br J Ind Med* **43**(6): 381–386.

Coleman, R.E. (2001). "Metastatic bone disease: clinical features, pathophysiology and treatment strategies." *Cancer Treat Rev* **27**(3): 165–176.

Collins, A. and V. Harrington (2002). "Repair of oxidative DNA damage: assessing its contribution to cancer prevention." *Mutagenesis* **17**(6): 489–493.

Courneya, K.S. (2003). "Exercise in cancer survivors: an overview of research." *Med Sci Sports Exerc* **35**(11): 1846–1852.

Courneya, K.S., J.R. Mackey, et al. (2003). "Randomized controlled trial of exercise training in postmenopausal breast cancer survivors: cardiopulmonary and quality of life outcomes." *J Clin Oncol* **21**(9): 1660–1668.

Demark-Wahnefried, W., B.K. Rimer, et al. (1997). "Weight gain in women diagnosed with breast cancer." *J Am Diet Assoc* **97**(5): 519–526, 529; quiz 527–528.

Demark-Wahnefried, W., E.P. Winer, et al. (1993). "Why women gain weight with adjuvant chemotherapy for breast cancer." *J Clin Oncol* **11**(7): 1418–1429.

den Tonkelaar, I., F. de Waard, et al. (1995). "Obesity and subcutaneous fat patterning in relation to survival of postmenopausal breast cancer patients participating in the DOM-project." *Breast Cancer Res Treat* **34**(2): 129–137.

DHHS (2004). Bone Health and Osteoporosis: A Report of the Surgeon General. Rockville, U.S. Department of Health and Human Services, Office of the Surgeon General.

Dixon, J.K., D.A. Moritz, et al. (1978). "Breast cancer and weight gain: an unexpected finding." *Oncol Nurs Forum* **5**(3): 5–7.

Djuric, Z., J.B. Depper, et al. (1998). "Oxidative DNA damage levels in blood from women at high risk for breast cancer are associated with dietary intakes of meats, vegetables, and fruits." *J Am Diet Assoc* **98**(5): 524–528.

Djuric, Z., L.K. Heilbrun, et al. (1991). "Effects of a low-fat diet on levels of oxidative damage to DNA to human peripheral nucleated blood cells." *J Natl Cancer Inst* **83**(11): 766–769.

Doll, R. and R. Peto (1981). "The causes of cancer: quantitative estimates of avoidable risks of cancer in the United States today." *J Natl Cancer Inst* **66**(6): 1191–1308.

Douchi, T., S. Kosha, et al. (1997). "Predictors of bone mineral loss in patients with ovarian cancer treated with anticancer agents." *Obstet Gynecol* **90**(1): 12–15.

Dreher, D. and A.F. Junod (1996). "Role of oxygen free radicals in cancer development." *Eur J Cancer* **32A**(1): 30–38.

Freedson, P.S. and K. Miller (2000). "Objective monitoring of physical activity using motion sensors and heart rate." *Res Q Exerc Sport* **71**(2 Suppl): S21–29.

Ganz, P.A., C.C. Schag, et al. (1987). "Rehabilitation needs and breast cancer: the first month after primary therapy." *Breast Cancer Res Treat* **10**(3): 243–253.

Giovannucci, E., A. Ascherio, et al. (1995). "Physical activity, obesity, and risk for colon cancer and adenoma in men." *Ann Intern Med* **122**(5): 327–334.

Goodwin, P.J., M. Ennis, et al. (1999). "Adjuvant treatment and onset of menopause predict weight gain after breast cancer diagnosis." *J Clin Oncol* **17**(1): 120–129.

Hackney, A.C., C.L. Fahrner, et al. (1998). "Basal reproductive hormonal profiles are altered in endurance trained men." *J Sports Med Phys Fitness* **38**(2): 138–141.

Halliwell, B. (2002). "Effect of diet on cancer development: is oxidative DNA damage a biomarker?" *Free Radic Biol Med* **32**(10): 968–974.

Headley, J.A., R.L. Theriault, et al. (1998). "Pilot study of bone mineral density in breast cancer patients treated with adjuvant chemotherapy." *Cancer Invest* **16**(1): 6–11.

Heasman, K.Z., H.J. Sutherland, et al. (1985). "Weight gain during adjuvant chemotherapy for breast cancer." *Breast Cancer Res Treat* **5**(2): 195–200.

IARC (2002). Overweight and lack of exercise. *International Agency for Research on Cancer Handbook of Cancer Prevention*.

ICSD (2004). "Technical standardization for dual-energy x-ray absorptiometry." *J Clin Densitom* **7**(1): 27–36.

Irwin, M.L. and B.E. Ainsworth (2004). "Physical activity interventions following cancer diagnosis: methodologic challenges to delivery and assessment." *Cancer Invest* **22**(1): 30–50.

Kampert, J.B., S.N. Blair, et al. (1996). "Physical activity, physical fitness, and all-cause and cancer mortality: a prospective study of men and women." *Ann Epidemiol* **6**(5): 452–457.

Key, T.J., A. Schatzkin, et al. (2004). "Diet, nutrition and the prevention of cancer." *Public Health Nutr* **7**(1A): 187–200.

King, M.C., J.H. Marks, et al. (2003). "Breast and ovarian cancer risks due to inherited mutations in BRCA1 and BRCA2." *Science* **302**(5645): 643–646.

Kritchevsky, D. (1999). "Caloric restriction and experimental carcinogenesis." *Toxicol Sci* **52**(2 Suppl): 13–16.

Kumar, N.B., A. Cantor, et al. (2000). "Android obesity at diagnosis and breast carcinoma survival: Evaluation of the effects of anthropometric variables at diagnosis, including body composition and body fat distribution and weight gain during life span, and survival from breast carcinoma." *Cancer* **88**(12): 2751–2757.

La Vecchia, C. (2001). "Diet and human cancer: a review." *Eur J Cancer Prev* **10**(2): 177–181.

Lee, I.M. and R.S. Paffenbarger, Jr. (1994). "Physical activity and its relation to cancer risk: a prospective study of college alumni." *Med Sci Sports Exerc* **26**(7): 831–837.

Lee, I.M., R.S. Paffenbarger, Jr., et al. (1991). "Physical activity and risk of developing color-ectal cancer among college alumni." *J Natl Cancer Inst* **83**(18): 1324–1329.

Lee, I.M., H.D. Sesso, et al. (1999). "Physical activity and risk of lung cancer." *Int J Epidemiol* **28**(4): 620–625.

LeRoith, D., R. Baserga, et al. (1995). "Insulin-like growth factors and cancer." *Ann Intern Med* **122**(1): 54–59.

Liedman, B. (1999). "Symptoms after total gastrectomy on food intake, body composition, bone metabolism, and quality of life in gastric cancer patients – is reconstruction with a reservoir worthwhile?" *Nutrition* **15**(9): 677–682.

Liedman, B., A. Henningsson, et al. (2000). "Changes in bone metabolism and body compo-sition after total gastrectomy: results of a longitudinal study." *Dig Dis Sci* **45**(4): 819–824.

Liu, S., I.M. Lee, et al. (2000). "A prospective study of physical activity and risk of prostate cancer in US physicians." *Int J Epidemiol* **29**(1): 29–35.

Lucia, A., J.L. Chicharro, et al. (1996). "Reproductive function in male endurance athletes: sperm analysis and hormonal profile." *J Appl Physiol* **81**(6): 2627–2636.

Margaritis, I., F. Tessier, et al. (1997). "No evidence of oxidative stress after a triathlon race in highly trained competitors." *Int J Sports Med* **18**(3): 186–190.

Maricic, M. and Z. Chen (2000). "Bone densitometry." *Clin Lab Med* **20**(3): 469–488.

Martinez, M.E., E. Giovannucci, et al. (1997). "Leisure-time physical activity, body size, and colon cancer in women. Nurses' Health Study Research Group." *J Natl Cancer Inst* **89**(13): 948–955.

Mazzeo, R.S. (1994). "The influence of exercise and aging on immune function." *Med Sci Sports Exerc* **26**(5): 586–592.

Mincey, B.A., T.J. Moraghan, et al. (2000). "Prevention and treatment of osteoporosis in wo-men with breast cancer." *Mayo Clin Proc* **75**(8): 821–829.

Mink, P.J., A.R. Folsom, et al. (1996). "Physical activity, waist-to-hip ratio, and other risk fac-tors for ovarian cancer: a follow-up study of older women." *Epidemiology* **7**(1): 38–45.

Montoye, H.J., H.C.G. Kemper, et al. (1996). *Measuring Physical Activity and Energy Expendi-ture*. Champaign, Human Kinetics.

NASPE (2004). *Physical Activity for Children: A Statement of Guidelines for Children Ages 5–12*. Reston, NASPE Publications.

Nelson, M.E., C.N. Meredith, et al. (1988). "Hormone and bone mineral status in endurance-trained and sedentary postmenopausal women." *J Clin Endocrinol Metab* **66**(5): 927–933.

Newsholme, E.A., Parry-Billings, M. (1994). Effects of exercise on the immune system. *Physi-cal Activity, Fitness and Health: International Proceedings Consensus Statement*. C. Bou-chard, Shephard, R.J., Stephens, T. Champaign, Human Kinetics.

Oliveria, S.A. and I.M. Lee (1997). "Is exercise beneficial in the prevention of prostate can-cer?" *Sports Med* **23**(5): 271–278.

Pfeilschifter, J. and I.J. Diel (2000). "Osteoporosis due to cancer treatment: pathogenesis and management." *J Clin Oncol* **18**(7): 1570–1593.

Pierce, J.P., S. Faerber, et al. (2002). "A randomized trial of the effect of a plant-based diet-ary pattern on additional breast cancer events and survival: the Women's Healthy Eating and Living (WHEL) Study." *Control Clin Trials* **23**(6): 728–756.

Pollock, M.L., G.A. Gaesser, et al. (1998). "American College of Sports Medicine Position Stand. The recommended quantity and quality of exercise for developing and maintain-ing cardiorespiratory and muscular fitness, and flexibility in healthy adults." *Med Sci Sports Exerc* **30**(6): 975–991.

Poulsen, H.E., S. Loft, et al. (1996). "Extreme exercise and oxidative DNA modification." *J Sports Sci* **14**(4): 343–346.

Quan, M.L., J.L. Pasieka, et al. (2002). "Bone mineral density in well-differentiated thyroid cancer patients treated with suppressive thyroxine: a systematic overview of the litera-ture." *J Surg Oncol* **79**(1): 62–69; discussion 69–70.

Riboli, E. and T. Norat (2003). "Epidemiologic evidence of the protective effect of fruit and vegetables on cancer risk." *Am J Clin Nutr* **78**(3 Suppl): 559S–569S.

Rockhill, B., W.C. Willett, et al. (1999). "A prospective study of recreational physical activity and breast cancer risk." *Arch Intern Med* **159**(19): 2290–2296.

Saarto, T., C. Blomqvist, et al. (1997). "Clodronate improves bone mineral density in post-menopausal breast cancer patients treated with adjuvant antioestrogens." *Br J Cancer* **75**(4): 602–605.

Sarhill, N., D. Walsh, et al. (2000). "Bioelectrical impedance, cancer nutritional assessment, and ascites." *Support Care Cancer* **8**(4): 341–343.

Sass, J. (2002). "Lead IARC towards compliance with WHO/IARC Declarations of Interests (DOI) policy." *Int J Occup Environ Health* **8**(3): 277–278.

Schapira, D.V., N.B. Kumar, et al. (1991). "Obesity and body fat distribution and breast cancer prognosis." *Cancer* **67**(2): 523–528.

Schatzkin, A., E. Lanza, et al. (2000). "Lack of effect of a low-fat, high-fiber diet on the recurrence of colorectal adenomas. Polyp Prevention Trial Study Group." *N Engl J Med* **342**(16): 1149–1155.

Schwartz, R.S., W.P. Shuman, et al. (1991). "The effect of intensive endurance exercise training on body fat distribution in young and older men." *Metabolism* **40**(5): 545–551.

Segal, R., W. Evans, et al. (2001). "Structured exercise improves physical functioning in women with stages I and II breast cancer: results of a randomized controlled trial." *J Clin Oncol* **19**(3): 657–665.

Segal, R.J., R.D. Reid, et al. (2003). "Resistance exercise in men receiving androgen deprivation therapy for prostate cancer." *J Clin Oncol* **21**(9): 1653–1659.

Sesso, H.D., R.S. Paffenbarger, Jr., et al. (1998). "Physical activity and breast cancer risk in the College Alumni Health Study (United States)." *Cancer Causes Control* **9**(4): 433–439.

Severson, R.K., J.S. Grove, et al. (1988). "Body mass and prostatic cancer: a prospective study." *Bmj* **297**(6650): 713–715.

Shapiro, C.L., J. Manola, et al. (2001). "Ovarian failure after adjuvant chemotherapy is associated with rapid bone loss in women with early-stage breast cancer." *J Clin Oncol* **19**(14): 3306–33011.

Sherman, W.M., D.M. Morris, et al. (1998). "Evaluation of a commercial accelerometer (Tritrac-R3 D) to measure energy expenditure during ambulation." *Int J Sports Med* **19**(1): 43–47.

Simons, J.P., A.M. Schols, et al. (1999). "Weight loss and low body cell mass in males with lung cancer: relationship with systemic inflammation, acute-phase response, resting energy expenditure, and catabolic and anabolic hormones." *Clin Sci (Lond)* **97**(2): 215–223.

Siverston, I., Dahlstrom, A.W. (1922). "The relation of muscular activity to carcinoma: a preliminary report." *J Cancer Research* **6**: 365–378.

Smith, G.D., M.J. Shipley, et al. (2000). "Physical activity and cause-specific mortality in the Whitehall study." *Public Health* **114**: 1–8.

Smith, M.R. (2002). "Osteoporosis during androgen deprivation therapy for prostate cancer." *Urology* **60**(3 Suppl 1): 79–85; discussion 86.

Smith, M.R., F.J. McGovern, et al. (2001). "Pamidronate to prevent bone loss during androgen-deprivation therapy for prostate cancer." *N Engl J Med* **345**(13): 948–955.

Steinmetz, K.A. and J.D. Potter (1996). "Vegetables, fruit, and cancer prevention: a review." *J Am Diet Assoc* **96**(10): 1027–1039.

Stepan, J.J. (2003). "Clinical utility of bone markers in the evaluation and follow-up of osteoporotic patients: why are the markers poorly accepted by clinicians?" *J Endocrinol Invest* **26**(5): 458–463.

Stoch, S.A., R.A. Parker, et al. (2001). "Bone loss in men with prostate cancer treated with gonadotropin-releasing hormone agonists." *J Clin Endocrinol Metab* **86**(6): 2787–2791.

Terry, P., J.A. Baron, et al. (1999). "Lifestyle and endometrial cancer risk: a cohort study from the Swedish Twin Registry." *Int J Cancer* **82**(1): 38–42.

Thompson, H.J., J. Heimendinger, et al. (1999). "Effect of increased vegetable and fruit consumption on markers of oxidative cellular damage." *Carcinogenesis* **20**(12): 2261–2266.

Thune, I., T. Brenn, et al. (1997). "Physical activity and the risk of breast cancer." *N Engl J Med* **336**(18): 1269–1275.

Thune, I. and A.S. Furberg (2001). "Physical activity and cancer risk: dose-response and cancer, all sites and site-specific." *Med Sci Sports Exerc* **33**(6 Suppl): S530–50; discussion S609–610.

Thune, I. and E. Lund (1994). "Physical activity and the risk of prostate and testicular cancer: a cohort study of 53,000 Norwegian men." *Cancer Causes Control* **5**(6): 549–556.

USDHHS (1996). Physical Activity and Health: A Report of the Surgeon General. Atlanta, US Dept of Health and Human Services, Centers for Disease Control, National Center for Chronic Disease Prevention and Health Promotion.

van Leeuwen, B.L., W.A. Kamps, et al. (2000). "The effect of chemotherapy on the growing skeleton." *Cancer Treat Rev* **26**(5): 363–376.

van Zeeland, A.A., A.J. de Groot, et al. (1999). "8-Hydroxydeoxyguanosine in DNA from leukocytes of healthy adults: relationship with cigarette smoking, environmental tobacco smoke, alcohol and coffee consumption." *Mutat Res* **439**(2): 249–257.

Vehmanen, L., T. Saarto, et al. (2001). "Long-term impact of chemotherapy-induced ovarian failure on bone mineral density (BMD) in premenopausal breast cancer patients. The effect of adjuvant clodronate treatment." *Eur J Cancer* **37**(18): 2373–2378.

WCRF *Food, Nutrition, and the Prevention of Cancer: A Global Perspective*, World Cancer Research Fund.

Wei, G.S., J.L. Jackson, et al. (2003). "Osteoporosis management in the new millennium." *Prim Care* **30**(4): 711–741, vi–vii.

Westerlind, K.C. (2003). "Physical activity and cancer prevention–mechanisms." *Med Sci Sports Exerc* **35**(11): 1834–1840.

Williams, N.I., B.A. Bullen, et al. (1999). "Effects of short-term strenuous endurance exercise upon corpus luteum function." *Med Sci Sports Exerc* **31**(7): 949–958.

Zhang, S., A.R. Folsom, et al. (1995). "Better breast cancer survival for postmenopausal women who are less overweight and eat less fat. The Iowa Women's Health Study." *Cancer* **76**(2): 275–283.

Hereditary Risk for Cancer

Katherine S. Hunt

Mayo Clinic-Scottsdale, Scottsdale, AZ 58259

Understanding the role of heredity in cancer is a key component of cancer prevention. Individuals at a high risk for cancer due to hereditary predisposition can now be identified through a comprehensive cancer risk assessment evaluation and/or cancer genetic testing. Identification of individual's positive for mutations or those at high risk prior to cancer occurrence provides an opportunity to intervene with prevention and screening strategies documented to reduce cancer incidence or the mortality from cancer occurrence. Currently, there are over 200 hereditary cancer syndromes described in the literature (Schneider 2001). The scope of this chapter is not to describe all hereditary cancer syndromes, but to provide the tools to identify a hereditary cancer syndrome in a family and describe the process individuals and families undergo to determine a hereditary susceptibility towards cancer. The more common hereditary breast, ovarian and colon cancer syndromes will be described along with recommended screening and surveillance, prophylactic and chemoprevention options currently available to those at increased risk.

Cancer as a Genetic Disorder

Cancer is the outcome of an evolution of genetic mutations and epigenetic effects on our DNA over time. Therefore, cancer is a genetic disease however, not all cancer is hereditary. To understand the hereditary predisposition to cancer, it is first important to provide a basic review of the molecular genetics involved in cancer progression.

Molecular Genetics

A gene is the basic unit of heredity, encoded in the deoxyribonucleic acid (DNA) that make up our 46 chromosomes found in the nucleus of our cells. Our chromosomes travel in pairs. The first 22 pairs are the autosomes. Genes located on an autosomal chromosome are present in both males and females and are therefore inherited in an autosomal inheritance pattern. The 23rd chromosome pair make up the sex chromosomes. Males have an X and a Y chromosome. Females carry two X chromosomes. Genes located on the X and the Y chromosomes are sex-linked and not identified in hereditary cancer.

Genetic information is inherited from parents through the chromosomes. Half of the total genetic information comes from each parent's chromosomes (23 from each parent). The germline cells found in ovum and sperm are the only cells that do not return to the original total number of 46 following mitosis.

Mutations can be classified in three groups: *genome mutations* are those that change the total number of chromosomes in the cell, *chromosomal mutations* change the structure of the individual chromosomes and *genetic mutations* change our genetic sequence (Nussbaum 2001). For the purpose of this discussion on hereditary cancer, the focus will be only on genetic mutations as they apply to hereditary cancer syndromes.

Mutations can occur in the germline cells and in somatic cells. The germline mutations are the only mutations passed from generation to generation and are therefore responsible for hereditary predisposition to cancer.

Tumor Suppressor Genes

The majority of hereditary cancer syndromes are caused by mutations in the tumor suppressor genes in the germline cells (Schneider 2001). The function of the proteins expressed from tumor suppressor genes is to negatively regulate cellular growth, especially in damaged cells (Schneider 2001). Tumor suppressor genes are inherited dominantly in hereditary cancer syndromes, but behave recessively on the cellular level (Franks 1997). When an individual inherits a mutation on one copy of a tumor suppressor gene, the protein produced from the working gene will maintain cell growth and suppress cancer (Schneider 2001). If this individual were to loose the working copy of the same gene, tumor growth can occur in the target cell. Mutations in tumor suppressor genes do not always begin with a germline mutation followed by a somatic mutation. Cancer may also result from two somatic mutations. This form of cancer initiation is thought to represent the majority of sporadic cancer occurrences (Schneider 2001).

Alfred Knudson advanced the understanding of cancer as a hereditary disease with his model of retinoblastoma. This model explained cancer as a two-hit progression of cancer. He compared the inherited form of retinoblastoma, occurring in nine out of every ten children with an inherited mutation, to the sporadic form that occurrs in one of every 20,000 children in the U.S. (Knudson 1971). The children with the inherited mutation were much more likely to be affected with cancer because they were born with "one hit" or germline mutation versus the sporadic cases requiring two acquired mutations in the somatic cells.

Vogelstein furthered the two-hit theory with his model of carcinogenesis first described in 1990 (Fearon and Vogelstein 1990). Vogelstein's model described multiple hits occurring in normal colon cells causing increasingly more mutations and resulting in carcinoma.

His model was based on the adenomatous polyposis coli (APC) tumor suppressor gene which is mutated in the germ-line cells in inherited cases of familial adenomatous polyposis (FAP). The first mutation in the APC gene, whether it be somatic or hereditary, can be thought of as "the gate-keeper" gene (Schneider 2001). A mutation in the gate-keeper gene allows for additional gene mutations, such as activation of the K-RAS oncogene and loss of other tumor suppressor genes to occur more readily. The succession of genetic mutations and the order in which these mutations occur is important in determining stages of development of adenomas.

Understanding changes in the gene on the molecular level will eventually lead to better treatment protocols and prevention recommendations tailored to an individual's genetic changes (Schneider 2001).

Oncogenes

There are relatively few hereditary cancer syndromes which occur as a result of oncogenes (Schneider 2001). Oncogenes arise from proto-oncogenes which are responsible for regulating the cell's signaling pathway. A mutation in the proto-oncogene activates the oncogene causing either increased expression of the proto-oncogene protein or a change in the structure and function of the proto-oncogene's protein (Schneider 2001). Most mutations occur on the somatic level and behave dominantly, requiring only one mutation to cause abnormal cell growth. As is described in Vogelstein's cancer progression model, more than one activated oncogene in a target cell or cells is necessary for cancer to occur.

DNA Repair Genes

The purpose of DNA repair genes is to identify and repair DNA errors made in the nucleotide sequence during replication. DNA repair involves several steps, including identifying the error in the DNA strand, gathering necessary proteins for repair, incision of the DNA and excision of the nucleotide sequence that is erroneous, new synthesis of the correct nucleotides and reattachment of the correct sequence (Schneider 2001). Mutations in the genes involved in the repair process can lead to accumulations of DNA errors within a cell. A defective DNA repair gene has a secondary effect on cancer progression, whereas mutations in oncogenes and tumor suppressor genes cause a primary effect (Schneider 2001).

Several DNA repair genes, called mismatch repair genes (MMR) have been implicated in hereditary nonpolyposis colorectal cancer syndrome (HNPCC), which is described later. MMR genes work in the cell to repair errors that occur during replication. In cells with mutated mismatch repair genes, a phenomenon called microsatellite instability (MSI) occurs. MSI refers to the instability of the microsatellite sequences, short repeats of six or less base pairs, causing long strings of the same repeated sequence. The presence of MSI results in the progression of more somatic mutations in the cell (Offit 1997).

Epigenetic Mechanisms

Epigenetic effects imply a non-genetic influence on the DNA that changes gene expression through the activation or silencing of growth regulatory genes. Genomic imprinting and methylation are two examples of epigenetic mechanisms causing gene silencing. When growth regulation genes are silenced by this mechanism, cells may receive a potential hit (Schneider 2001). Epigenetic effects are important because these changes may be the most common alteration seen in human cancer. Because epigenetic mechanisms are not thought to be the result of DNA changes, the process may be reversible, leading to better targeted treatment options for patients in the future (Schneider 2001).

Cancer occurs as a multi-step model in which a succession of events, genetic mutations, environmental agents, epigenic agents, lead to cancer progression. Learning the molecular changes in cells and following the sequential progression of cancer may allow the development of effective interventions that will stop cancer progression on the molecular level.

Cancer as a Hereditary Disease

The majority of the 200 hereditary cancer syndromes described in the literature are rare and account for between 5% and 10% of all cancers. Identifying a sporadic occurrence of cancer versus a familial or hereditary form is the first step in locating patients at higher cancer risk, and thus providing appropriate screening and prevention recommendations. Differentiation between sporadic and hereditary cancer is often obvious while elucidating a hereditary versus familial form of cancer can be subtle. The latter requires familiarity with the hereditary cancer syndromes in addition to obtaining a well documented and detailed family history from the patient.

A sporadic cancer family can be described by a single occurrence of cancer, typically at a later age of onset. For example, the proband (the affected family member from which the family is ascertained) is a 70 year old woman recently diagnosed with breast cancer. There are no other incidences of cancer in first degree relatives (mother and father, sisters and brothers) or second degree relatives (grandparents, aunts and uncles). Family history is also negative for cancer in the third degree relatives (cousins and great aunts and uncles). The cancer described in this family would be classified as a sporadic incidence of cancer with no concern of inherited susceptibility.

Familial cancer syndromes are more difficult to differentiate from hereditary cancer due in large part to the variability in gene expression exhibited by hereditary cancer syndromes. The typical family history reported for a potential familial form of cancer is described with at least two relatives who are affected with similar cancers or two relatives with distinct cancers. The ages of onset in familial cancer tend to occur at a later age. For example, the proband is diagnosed with breast cancer at age 68. The proband's mother has never been affected with cancer, but a maternal aunt was diagnosed at a later age, early 80s, also with breast cancer. This family history is not as compelling for hereditary cancer because the ages of onset are closer to expected age of diagnosis for sporadic cancers. In addition, and more importantly, the cancer occurrences do not follow an autosomal dominant inheritance pattern. Another example of possible familial cancer is the following: a proband is diagnosed with prostate cancer at age 75 and reports a maternal grandfather affected with colon cancer at age 72. Despite two cancer occurrence in this family, the ages of onset are later and autosomal dominant inheritance is not demonstrated.

Two hallmarks of hereditary cancer are early ages of onset and occurrence in at least two successive generations. Hereditary cancer may occur up to 20 years younger than the expected age for the specified cancer. Individuals who carry an autosomal dominant mutation for hereditary breast and ovarian cancer are at an increased risk for bilateral cancers, as well as for a second occurrence of cancer. Most hereditary cancer syndromes are also associated with increased risk for multiple primary cancers. These factors contribute to the importance of identifying at-risk individuals so that recommendations can be given to prevent cancer from occurring or to reduce morbidity and mortality from cancer. Perhaps the most important characteristic of hereditary cancer syndromes is the potential for increased risk to the relatives of the affected individual who is found to carry a hereditary predisposition gene.

Because the hereditary cancer genes are located on the autosomal chromosomes, both males and females may inherit these cancer susceptibility genes. Expression of disease after inheriting the gene will differ between men and women depending on the types of cancer exhibited in the hereditary cancer syndrome as well as the type of mutation inherited. For an autosomal dominantly inherited hereditary cancer syndrome, there is a 50% risk of passing down a genetic mutation from the carrier to an offspring. In a typical family history with a hereditary cancer gene mutation there tends to be at least one affected relative in each generation. However, this is not consistently demonstrated. There are many families in which an individual carries one of the gene mutations for an autosomal dominant cancer syndrome, yet they do not express the phenotype of the mutation and are not affected with cancer. This phenomenon is observed because hereditary cancer syndromes demonstrate variable expression of the disease phenotype. Another example of variable expressivity is seen with the lack of similarity among the ages of diagnosis between relatives with the same cancer. In addition, most hereditary cancer genes exhibit incomplete penetrance. Penetrance describes an all or none effect of gene expression. Individuals will either have signs and symptoms of the disease or they will not.

There are only a few hereditary cancer syndromes inherited in an autosomal recessive manner. Autosomal recessive disorders occur when an individual inherits the same genetic mutation on each chromosome. A carrier for an autosomal recessive gene is not affected with the disease. When parents carry the same autosomal recessive gene mutation, the risk to have an affected child is one in four or 25%.

Common Hereditary Cancer Syndromes

Hereditary Breast and Ovarian Cancer. Genetic predisposition provides one of the most significant risk factors for women to develop either breast or ovarian cancer or both cancers. Of all the genetic predisposition genes, the breast and ovarian cancer genes provide one of the highest risks for increased cancer susceptibility. Genetic testing became available for the breast and ovarian cancer syndrome in the mid 1990s. Currently, there are two genes described for the hereditary breast and ovarian cancer syndrome. The first gene described, BRCA1, located on chromosome 17q21 was identified in 1989 and sequenced in 1994 (Hall, Lee et al. 1990; Miki 1994). The second gene, BRCA2, located on chromosome 13q12 was sequenced in 1995 (Wooster, Bignell et al. 1995).

The BRCA1 and BRCA2 genes are thought to account for approximately 80%–90% of all hereditary breast and ovarian cancers (Thull and Vogel 2004). Similar to other hereditary cancers, between 5% and 10% of all breast cancer and 10% of all ovarian cancer (Malander, Ridderheim et al. 2004) is thought to be due to inherited susceptibility.

The incidence of a BRCA1 or BRCA2 gene mutation in individuals of Northern European descent is between one in 800 to one in 2,500 (Schneider 2001). Several founder mutations specific to geographically isolated populations have been identified in hereditary breast and ovarian cancer. The most well described founder mutation is found in the Ashkenazi Jewish population in which the carrier frequency for a BRCA1 or BRCA2 gene mutation is one in 40 or approximately 2.5% (Tonin, Weber et al. 1996). Other founder mutations have been identified in the Dutch and Icelandic populations (Johannesdottir, Gudmundsson et al. 1996; Tonin, Weber et al. 1996; Peelen, vanVliet et al. 1997; Petrij-Bosch, Peelen et al. 1997).

The BRCA1 gene is large, with 24 exons, encoding a protein of 1863 amino acids and works as a tumor suppressor gene (Miki 1994). The protein function of a normal

BRCA1 gene is to recognize DNA damage (Couch, Weber et al. 1996). Referring back to the model of carcinogenesis, the inherited mutation of one BRCA1 gene leads to increased susceptibility to mutations in the remaining somatic copy of the BRCA1 gene beginning the pathway to carcinogenesis.

The 800 hereditary mutations identified on the BRCA1 gene are found throughout the gene sequence. The majority of these mutations lead to premature protein termination and are frameshift or nonsense mutations (Barnes-Kedar and Plon 2002). Testing for a BRCA1 gene mutation is complex. This complexity is due in part to the fact that the majority of gene mutations described to date have been identified as private mutations which are unique to each family undergoing testing (Tirkkonen, Johannsson et al. 1997). An exception to these private mutations is seen with the founder mutations. The BRCA1 contains two of the three founder mutations for the Ashkenazi Jewish population. Approximately 1% of the Ashkenazi Jewish population carry the mutation, 185delAG, and 0.1% of the Ashkenazi population carry the founder mutation, 5382insC (Peelen, vanVliet et al. 1997).

The BRCA2 gene is even larger than the BRCA1 gene with 27 exons, encoding a protein of 3418 amino acids (Tirkkonen, Johannsson et al. 1997). The BRCA2 gene, like BRCA1 is also a tumor suppressor gene with protein product is also involved in DNA repair (Couch, Weber et al. 1996). There have been approximately 100 mutations reported in the BRCA2 gene and these mutations also play a role in premature chain termination (Tirkkonen, Johannsson et al. 1997). Unique to the BRCA2 gene is a region identified as the ovarian cancer cluster region (OCCR). Mutations found in this region confer lower risks for women to develop breast cancer and increased risks for developing ovarian cancer (Thompson, Easton et al. 2001). There is one Ashkenazi Jewish founder mutation on BRCA2, 6174delT. This mutation is seen in approximately 1% of individuals of Ashkenazi Jewish descent (Peelen, vanVliet et al. 1997). Interestingly, neither the BRCA1 or BRCA2 genes exhibit mutations in truly sporadic breast cancer.

In addition to increased susceptibility to breast and ovarian cancer, mutations in the BRCA1 and BRCA2 genes confer risks for other cancers as well. While this is still controversial, early studies report an increased risk for colon cancer in carriers of the BRCA1 gene mutations (Ford, Easton et al. 1994). Follow-up studies failed to duplicate these risks (Peelen, de Leeuw et al. 2000). Males who carry the BRCA1 gene mutation may also have an increased risk for prostate cancer (Liede, Karlan et al. 2004).

Male breast cancer has also been correlated with a BRCA2 gene mutation. There are a variety of other cancers also associated with the BRCA2 gene mutations, including prostate, pancreatic, gallbladder, bile duct, stomach and malignant melanoma (Risch, McLaughlin et al. 2001).

Current estimation of cancer risks for carriers of a BRCA1 or BRCA2 mutation indicate the lifetime risk for breast cancer is between 50% to 87%. The risks for ovarian cancer differ between the BRCA1 and the BRCA2 gene mutations.

The risks for ovarian cancer in women who carry a BRCA1 gene are estimated to be 15% to 40%. The risks for ovarian cancer in women who carry a BRCA2 gene are 14% to 27% (Struewing, Hartge et al. 1997; Risch, McLaughlin et al. 2001).

The risks for breast cancer in men who carry a BRCA2 mutation is between 2.8% to 6.3% (Thompson, Easton et al. 2001). The risks for prostate cancer in men who carry a BRCA1 gene mutation is between 8% and 16% based on one study (Ford, Easton et al. 1994). The risks for prostate cancer in men who carry the BRCA2 gene mutation is between 7% and 16% and had been estimated to be as high as 20% before age 80 with the relative risks greater for men younger than 65 (Struewing, Hartge et al. 1997, 1999).

The risks for colon cancer in men and women who carry a BRCA1 gene mutation is 6% based on data reported from the Breast Cancer Linkage Consortium. Pancreatic cancer was also found in studies to be increased in BRCA2 mutation carriers with a 2.1% cumulative risk by age 70 (1999).

The wide range of cancer risks described from mutations in the BRCA1 and BRCA2 genes can be explained by inadequate study designs with potential for biased ascertainment as well as variable expressivity of the gene, environmental factors and other gene modifiers. A recent report on risks for breast and ovarian cancer in Ashkenazi Jewish women with inherited BRCA1 and BRCA2 mutations identified physical exercise and lack of obesity in adolescent as modifiable risk factors, delaying the age of breast cancer onset (King, Marks et al. 2003). Further studies are underway to determine effects of environmental factors and other modifier genes on the expression of these gene mutations.

Cowden Syndrome. There are a handful of other hereditary cancer syndromes that increase susceptibility to breast cancer. These syndromes are typically much rarer in the general population and include an increased susceptibility to a variety of other cancers as well. Cowden syndrome, also called multiple hamartoma syndrome, accounts for less than 1% of hereditary breast and ovarian cancer. The incidence of Cowden syndrome is approximately one in every 200,000 to 250,000 individuals (Schneider 2001). The incidence of this syndrome is likely underreported given the variety of unusual findings. Cowden syndrome is inherited in an autosomal dominant pattern conferring a 50% risk to the offspring of an affected male or female. The gene for Cowden syndrome is located on chromosome 10q23 and penetrance of the gene may be as high as 100% (Nelen, Padberg et al. 1996). The gene mutated in Cowden syndrome, PTEN, is a tumor suppressor gene, only nine exons in length. The role of the protein product is to control cell cycle arrest and apoptosis (Schneider 2001). As many as 80% of individuals with clinic findings suggestive of Cowden syndrome will have gene mutation identified with clinical testing (Eng 2000).

The clinical features of Cowden syndrome are unique from hereditary breast and ovarian cancer due to the physical findings associated with this syndrome. The pathognomonic features of Cowden syndrome are facial trichilemmomas, acral keratoses, oral papillomatous papules and mucosal lesions (Eng 2000). Major criteria used to establish a clinical diagnosis include breast cancer, thyroid cancer, especially papillary carcinoma, macrocephaly, Lhermitte-Duclos disease or cerebral dysplastic gangliocytoma, and endometrial cancer. The minor criteria include other thyroid lesions, mental retardation, gastrointestinal hamartomas, fibrocystic breasts, lipomas or fibromas, genitourinary tumors (renal cell carcinoma, uterine fibroids) and genitourinary malformations. Diagnosis is confirmed clinically when the affected proband presents with either six facial papules listed in the pathognomonic criteria, two major criteria that must include macrocephaly or Lhermitte-Duclos disease, one major criteria and three minor criteria, or four minor criteria (Eng 2000).

The lifetime risk for breast cancer in women who are identified with Cowden syndrome is between 25% to 50%, and at least 75% of women with Cowden syndrome have benign breast disease (fibroadenoma and fibrocystic breasts) (Brownstein, Wolf et al. 1978). Male breast cancer has also been identified in men who carry a PTEN mutation, but the specific risks are not documented (Fackenthal, Marsh et al. 2001). Endometrial cancer is also considered in Cowden syndrome with risks reported between 5% and 10% (Eng 2000).

Li Fraumeni syndrome. Li Fraumeni syndrome (LFS) is another rare syndrome conferring increased risk for breast cancer in affected women. The incidence of LFS is unknown. LFS accounts for less than 1% of hereditary breast cancer. The inheritance of LFS, similar to the other hereditary breast cancer syndromes, is autosomal dominant. The gene is located on chromosomes 17p13.1 (Levine 1997). Individuals who meet diagnostic criteria for LFS could elect to undergo genetic testing. The majority of families who meet diagnosed criteria for LFS are found to carry an identifiable genetic mutation. The gene for LFS, p53, is also a tumor suppressor gene and is involved in cell repair, the apoptosis pathway and maintaining genomic stability (Schneider 2001). A mutation in the hCHK2 gene has been identified in some families with LFS (Barnes-Kedar and Plon 2002).

The clinical characteristics of LFS include early onset of breast cancer (before the fortieth decade of life), soft tissue sarcomas, primary brain tumors, adrenocortical carcinomas and acute leukemias (Malkin, Li et al. 1990). Other cancers associated with LFS include malignancies in the stomach, colon and lung as well as childhood neuroblastomas and increased risk of melanoma (Schneider 2001). Clinical diagnosis is considered when the proband reports being diagnosed with an isolated sarcoma before age 40. In addition to reporting one first degree relative and another first or second degree relative affected with associated LFS tumors, clinical diagnosis of LFS is considered when cancer is diagnosed before age 45 or a sarcoma is diagnosed at any age (Garber, Goldstein et al. 1991).

The risk of all cancers in individuals with LFS is estimated to be 50% by age 30 and 90% by age 70. Mutations in the LFS also place a carrier at a 50% risk of a second primary tumor (Schneider 2001; Thull and Vogel 2004).

Ataxia-Telangiectasis. Ataxia-Telangiectasis (A-T) is one of the few hereditary cancer syndromes inherited in an autosomal recessive manner. This rare syndrome, affecting between one in 30,000 to one in 100,000 individuals, is characterized by cerebellar ataxia, immune defects, telangiectasias, radiosensitivity and predisposition to malignancies, especially leukemias and lymphomas (Izatt, Greenman et al. 1999; Schneider 2001). While the syndrome itself places the affected individuals at a substantial increased risk of dying from cancer, the carriers of the gene for A-T are also at an increased risk of breast cancer.

The gene for A-T, ATM, is located on chromosome 11q22.3. The penetrance of this gene is 100%. The ATM gene is found in every organ and is believed to be involved in maintaining genomic stability (Savitsky, Sfez et al. 1995). The increased risk of breast cancer in carriers of an ATM mutation is not well established. Earlier data indicated that a carrier female could have a five to seven-fold increased relative risk of breast cancer (Schneider 2001). Breast cancer caused by mutations in the ATM gene account for approximately 8% of all breast cancer cases (Swift, Morrell et al. 1991).

Hereditary Nonpolyposis Colorectal Cancer. Hereditary forms of colorectal cancer (CRC) account for between 10% and 20% of the total number of colorectal cancer.

The most common form of inherited colorectal cancer is hereditary nonpolyposis colorectal cancer (HNPCC), also called Lynch syndrome. HNPCC has an interesting history, dating back to 1895. Aldred Warthin, a well-known pathologist, published the first report on HNPCC documenting the kindred of his seamstress who died of endometrial cancer at a young age. Before genetic susceptibility testing was available, Warthin's seamstress predicted her early demise based on the fact her relatives all died of colorectal, gastric or endometrial cancer (Lynch and Lynch 2000). Many years later, international recognition of other similar families led to the official recognition of hereditary nonpolyposis colorectal cancer (Lynch and Lynch 1998).

The incidence of HNPCC is one in 200 to one in 1,000 and accounts for approximately 1 to 6% of colon cancers (Hampel and Peltomaki 2000). HNPCC is inherited in an autosomal dominant pattern. The penetrance of the gene is as high as 90% (Lynch and Lynch 1998).

The genes implicated in HNPCC are numerous and complex. The HNPCC genes are DNA repair genes involved in mismatch repair. As a result of mutations in the MMR genes, MSI is a characteristic of HNPCC tumors. Ninety-five percent of the tumors in individuals with HNPCC exhibit MSI (Hampel and Peltomaki 2000). There are five genes responsible for the mismatch repair pathway associated with HNPCC (Wooster, Bignell et al. 1995). The first gene, MLH1, is located on chromosome 3p21.3. The second gene, MSH2, is located on 2p22-p21. These two genes represent the majority of families with an identifiable mutation (Peltomaki and Vasen 1997). The third gene, MSH6, is located on 2p16 and the fourth and fifth genes, PMS2 and MLH3, are still undergoing validation studies to determine their role in colon cancer and MSI. There have been over 400 different mutations reported in these genes, with MLH1 accounting for 50% of the mutations and MSH2 accounting for 40% (Umar, Boland et al. 2004).

Individuals with HNPCC have up to an 80% lifetime risk of colorectal cancer. Colorectal cancer typically occurs at a younger age with mean age of 44 years, and a 60 to 70% likelihood for tumors to be located in the proximal colon. It has also been associated with an increased risk of synchronous or metachronous colon cancer (Hampel and Peltomaki 2000). The colonic adenomas in HNPCC occur with the same frequency and in the same location within the colon as in the general population; however, the adenomas are larger, occur earlier in life, and have a higher grade of dysplasia and villous features. The characteristics of carcinomas of the colon include poor differentiation, tumor infiltrating lymphocytes, mucin and signet ring histology (Lynch and Lynch 2000).

While the average age of cancer diagnosis is 44 years, patients with HNPCC are reported to have a better survival than age and stage matched sporadic patients (Lynch and Lynch 1998). Studies have suggested this survival difference can be explained by the response to chemotherapy in HNPCC as compared to sporadic tumors (Watanabe, Wu et al. 2001). Gender differences are a possible factor in HNPCC tumor expression; the male risk of colon cancer is reported to be 91% and female risk is 69% (Dunlop, Farrington et al. 1997). Women affected with HNPCC have up to a 60% lifetime risk to be affected with endometrial cancer, with the average age at diagnosis of 46 years (Aarnio, Sankila et al. 1999). Improved survival in women affected with HNPCC type endometrial cancer versus sporadic occurrence is also observed (Solomon 2004).

Stomach or gastric cancers were described historically, but perhaps because of changes in Western diets and gene modifying events, the incidence of stomach cancer in HNPCC has declined. The risk of stomach cancer is reported to be as high as 13% with the average age at diagnosis being 56 years. Women are also at 12% increased risk of ovarian cancer, with the mean age at onset of 42.5 (Solomon 2004).

The International Collaborative Group on Hereditary Nonpolyposis Colorectal Cancer (ICG-HNPCC) created the Amsterdam Criteria in an attempt to standardize the diagnostic criteria for families suspected of having HNPCC. Subsequently, Amsterdam Criteria II was proposed by the ICG-HNPCC to include additional colon cancers (Thull and Vogel 2004). In 1996, the National Cancer Institute developed the Bethesda Guidelines that described criteria for identifying colorectal tumors that should be tested for MSI. These guidelines were revised in 2002 in an attempt to increase sensitivity in identifying HNPCC MSI tumors (Umar, Boland et al. 2004). The updated Bethesda guidelines are outlined below under genetic testing for HNPCC. It is important to realize that families who do not meet Amsterdam Criteria I or II are not to be excluded from a diagnosis of HNPCC.

Familial Adenomatous Polyposis. Although familial adenomatous polyposis (FAP) is responsible for only about 1% of all hereditary colorectal cancers, it has played a large role in understanding the multiple gene model of cancer progression. The incidence of FAP is one in 6,000 to one in 13,000 individuals. Similar to HNPCC, FAP is inherited in an autosomal dominant manner with 75 to 80% of individuals reporting an affected parent. The remaining one-fourth to one-third of cases result from *de novo* mutations (Amos 2004). The penetrance of the gene is close to 100% (Schneider 2001). The gene, located on chromosome 5q21 is called adenomatous polyposis coli protein (APC). The APC gene is a tumor suppressor and works to maintain apoptosis and decrease cell proliferation in addition to participating in many other important cellular functions. As with HNPCC, BRCA1 and BRCA2 genes, mutations in the APC gene result in truncated protein products.

Unlike HNPCC, FAP is characterized by hundreds to thousands of precancerous colon polyps that begin to develop at a mean age of 16 years (range of 7 to 36 years) (Solomon 2004). By age 35, 95% of individuals with FAP have colorectal polyps. Colon cancer risk is 100% by the mean age of 40 without intervention (Hampel and Peltomaki 2000). Clinical diagnosis of FAP is made in an individual with more than 100 colorectal adenomatous polyps or in any individual with less than 100 adenomatous polyps who had one relative affected with FAP (Solomon 2004).

Associated extracolonic cancers include polyps of the upper gastrointestinal tract, osteomas, dental anomalies, congenital hypertrophy of the retina pigment epithelium (CHRPE), congenital hypertrophy of the retinal pigment epithelium, soft tissue tumors, desmoid tumors, and brain cancer. Increased risks for papillary thyroid carcinoma in younger women and hepatoblastoma in affected children have also been documented (Hampel and Peltomaki 2000). Variability in clinical symptoms is quite extensive between affected family members. Gardner syndrome, a variant of FAP, is also associated with extracolonic features, osteomas, dental abnormalities, desmoid tumors and sebaceous cysts (Hampel and Peltomaki 2000).

Attenuated Familial Adenomatous Polyposis. Attenuated FAP (AFAP) is described as a form of FAP with fewer colorectal polyps, between 50 to 100 with average number of 30, occurring at a later age and found more proximally in the colon than classic

FAP (Lynch and Lynch 1998). AFAP is more likely to be confused with HNPCC than classic FAP for this reason. The colon polyps take on a polypoid shape in AFAP (Hampel and Peltomaki 2000). The average age for colon cancer in individuals with AFAP is 50 to 55 years (Solomon 2004). Multiple extracolonic polyps, such as fundus gland polyps and duodenal polyps, are detected but individuals with AFAP do not typically exhibit CHRPE characteristics. AFAP is inherited autosomally dominant and the mutations for AFAP are also located on the APC gene. Mutations are characteristically located on either the extreme 5′ region of the first four exons or the 3′ region of the APC gene (Hampel and Peltomaki 2000).

MYH Associated Polyposis (MYH) is a newly described autosomal recessive hereditary cancer syndrome associated with multiple adenomas and a phenotype similar to AFAP.

Peutz-Jeghers Syndrome. Another rare colorectal cancer syndrome characterized by polyposis is Peutz-Jeghers Syndrome (PJS). This syndrome occurs in one of every 120,000 and has distinct clinical features. PJS exhibits an autosomal dominant inheritance pattern with the gene, STK11, located on 19p13.3 (Hemminki, Markie et al. 1998). The gene product of the PJS gene is involved in a signaling pathway for cellular apoptosis (Amos 2004). Because only 50% of individuals affected with PJS test positive for a mutation in the STK11 gene, other genes are believed to be responsible for the disease (Ylikorkala, Avizienyte et al. 1999).

PJS is clinically diagnosed in an individual with pathognomonic hyperpigmented macules on the lips and buccal mucosa. These macules also occur on the eyes, genitalia, anus, hands and feet (Hampel and Peltomaki 2000). Individuals affected with PJS are at increased risk of multiple hamartomous polyps in the small bowel, stomach, colon and rectum, causing intussusception and obstruction (Hemminki 1999). Individuals affected are 10 to 18 times more likely to be diagnosed with intestinal and other cancers during their lifetime. Breast and cervical cancers are also described in individuals with PJS (Boardman, Thibodeau et al. 1998).

Genetic Counseling

Given the complexities involved in genetic testing and the clinical diagnosis of hereditary cancer syndromes described above, the clinician must be prepared to understand basic Mendelian inheritance as it is applied to hereditary cancer in the family, explain the hereditary components of a cancer syndrome, and understand the complexities of genetic testing. An increase in the number of syndromes identifiable through mutational analysis coupled with the complexities inherent in testing and the potential psychological impact on affected individuals has created the need for specialized cancer genetics and high-risk clinics.

In order to accurately address patient concerns related to cancer risk, the American Society of Clinical Oncology (ASCO 2003), the American Society of Human Genetics (ASHG 1994), and the American College of Obstetricians and Gynecologists (ACOG 1997) have issued the recommendation of pre- and post-testing counseling by appropriately trained individuals with knowledge of the complex genetic issues related to hereditary cancer syndromes (ACOG 1997).

In order to meet this recommendation, genetic counseling is now offered in cancer centers and other institutions throughout the country. Genetic counseling is defined as a communication process that deals with the human problems associated with the occurrence, or risk of occurrence, of a genetic disorder in a family (1975). Genetic counseling is offered by individuals with a M.D., Ph.D, or M.S. who are certified by either the American Board of Medical Genetics or the American Board of Genetic Counseling (Peters and Stopfer 1996). Genetic counselors trained at the Master's degree level attend an accredited genetic counseling training program. A national list of genetic counselors is available through the National Society of Genetic Counselors website (NSGC 2004).

The compilation of a comprehensive family history is the first step in identifying possible hereditary cancer families. As Aldred Warthin discovered upon learning about the extensive family cancer history of his seamstress, paying attention to what has happened in a family can serve to benefit future generations. A pedigree analysis is perhaps the most critical tool for defining a high-risk candidate and the need for further evaluation in a cancer genetics or high-risk clinic. The family history of cancer is often the strongest epidemiological risk factor that can be identified (Vogelstein 2002). Once completed, a pedigree analysis includes identifying patterns of clinical clues, based on the phenotypic expression of cancer, and matching these clues with a hereditary cancer syndrome diagnosis. Documentation of cancers, when possible, through medical records and pathology reports are necessary for the most accurate risk assessment and identification of a potential hereditary cancer syndrome.

Given the time consuming nature of taking such a thorough family history, most individuals can be screened with a family history questionnaire that can be completed by a patient either during or prior to their visit with the clinician. At the very minimum, a screening questionnaire should ask the patient to report all first and second degree relatives, the types of cancers they were affected with, ages at diagnosis, and should include both the maternal and paternal family histories. Other useful screening questions include the patient's ethnicity, primary cancers versus metastatic cancers and the presence of colon polyps in family histories of colon cancer.

Cancer Risk Assessment Models. After a family history has been evaluated thoroughly, the patient may be provided with a risk assessment for either being affected with cancer or if they have already been diagnosed with a cancer, for carrying a germ line mutation for a hereditary cancer syndrome. This discussion will focus on the cancer risk assessment models that may be utilized during this portion of the evaluation.

Epidemiologic Models of Breast Cancer Risk. There are two well known models used to predict breast cancer risk in women: the Gail model and the Claus model. The Gail model is the only statistically validated model.

The Gail model was developed using risk factors for breast cancer identified in the Breast Cancer Detection Demonstration Project (Baker 1982). The model asks women to report age at menarche, age at first live birth, number of previous breast biopsies, number of first degree relatives with breast cancer, and current age. Any atypical hyperplasia diagnosed from biopsies is also evaluated at this time. Using this data, the Gail model provides women with both five-year and lifetime risk of developing breast cancer. An updated version of the Gail model can be downloaded from the National Cancer Institute website (NCI 2004). The updated version provides risks for invasive breast cancer only, derives baseline incidence rates from SEER data, and includes a separate baseline incidence for black women (NCI 1998).

The Gail model was developed prior to the discovery of the BRCA1 and BRCA2 genes and therefore only limited family history is included. This leads to underestimation of cancer risks in women with a more extensive family history of early-onset breast cancer, ovarian cancer, male breast cancer or paternal relatives with breast cancer. Therefore, the Gail model is not recommended for use in high-risk families (Barnes-Kedar and Plon 2002).

The Claus model consists of published tables to estimate risk of breast cancer over time. This model requires family history information, including paternal history and occurrences of ovarian cancer to calculate cancer risk (Domchek, Eisen et al. 2003). Individuals receiving risk values from this model are encouraged to remember that the model can be imprecise since it does not account for subtle features of hereditary cancer. Like the Gail model, Claus should also be avoided in individuals with a strong family history of cancer. New models are under development that will incorporate both family history and individual risk factors (Tyrer, Duffy et al. 2004).

Genetic Testing Models. The patient is offered an estimation of the prior probability of an individual to carry a gene mutation in one of the hereditary cancer susceptibility genes. Prior probabilities models are available for hereditary breast and ovarian cancer and for HNPCC.

Models for predicting breast cancer mutation probability include the Couch, Shattuck-Eidens, Frank and the Berry-Parmigiani-Aguilar or BRCAPRO models (Claus, Risch et al. 1994; Shattuck-Eidens, Oliphant et al. 1997; Frank, Manley et al. 1998; Parmigiani, Berry et al. 1998). In addition, a computer program has been developed (CA-Gene) that calculates risk by incorporating the Couch, Shattuck-Eidens and BRCAPRO models. It also provides mutation prevalence estimates from Myriad Genetic Laboratories. This program is offered as a free service on the internet (Parmigiani 2004). For a more extensive review of each of these models, see Domchek et al. (Domchek, Eisen et al. 2003).

There is a colorectal cancer model available (the Wijnen model) to predict an individual's probability for testing positive for a gene mutation for HNPCC. The Wijnen model predicts prior probability for a muation in either the MLH1 or the MSH2 genes. The average age of diagnosis of colorectal cancer, presence of endometrial cancer in the family, and the Amsterdam criteria are entered into the program to calculate prior probability risk. If an individual's prior probability for carrying a mutation on one of these two genes is calculated to be equal to or greater than 20%, Wijnen suggests clinicians first offer germ line testing without MSI testing (Wijnen, Vasen et al. 1998).

Informed Consent Prior to Genetic Testing. The availability of the models described above to predict prior probability of a germ-line mutation will likely result in more individuals and families requesting genetic testing. The issues surrounding genetic testing for hereditary cancer syndromes have been debated extensively. The conclusion of these debates is that the decision to undergo genetic testing should remain a personal choice. Therefore, proper informed consent requires a thorough discussion with the patient prior to genetic testing. A comprehensive informed consent has been documented and includes a discussion of, but is not limited to: the purpose of the test (including testing which is part of a research protocol, costs, turnaround time, and documentation of results), the predictive value of a positive, negative or indeterminate result, and corresponding cancer risk information. It should also include options for cancer risk management if the test is positive, negative or indeterminate, the possible psychological implications of testing, individualized assessment of insurance, employment discrimination risks, and alternatives to genetic testing, such as the possible delay of decision making to a future date (Geller, Botkin et al. 1997).

The importance of adhering to this informed consent process was demonstrated in a study that examined the use and interpretation of genetic testing for mutations on the APC gene. The study found that 20% of physicians ordered testing erroneously for FAP, only 18.6% of individuals in this study received genetic counseling before the test and in 31.6% of the cases the physicians misinterpreted the results (Giardiello, Brensinger et al. 1997).

In direct response to the complexity of genetic testing issues, as well as in an attempt to define those who would most benefit from genetic testing, the American Society of Clinical Oncology (ASCO) recommends genetic testing be offered when personal or family history is representative of a possible hereditary cancer syndrome, the test is able to be adequately interpreted, and the results from the genetic test will assist with medical management decision for the individual and their family. ASCO guidelines go on to state that clinicians offering genetic testing must include pre- and post-test genetic counseling, documentation of a family history of cancer, and must provide a risk assessment as well as discuss options for prevention and early detection (ASCO 2003).

Genetic Testing

Genetic Testing for Hereditary Breast and Ovarian Cancer. Although there is no recommended numerical "prior probability" to indicate when to offer gene testing for the BRCA1 and BRCA2 genes, responsibility of when to offer genetic testing is based on the judgement of the clinician. Once an individual has undergone a family history evaluation, provided with risk assessments, demonstrated to meet the criteria outlined by ASCO guidelines, genetic testing is typically offered. Eighty to 90% of the time, hereditary breast and ovarian cancer is caused by BRCA1 and BRCA2 mutations. A recent study from Sweden reported one in 10 ovarian cancer patients carry a BRCA1 or BRCA2 mutation (Malander, Ridderheim et al. 2004). Genetic testing for the BRCA1 and BRCA2 genes is one of the most requested genetic tests for hereditary cancer.

The standard protocol for initiating genetic testing is to test for the BRCA1 and BRCA2 genes on the affected individual in a family before offering testing to the at-risk relatives. Given the high incidence of "private mutations", and the likelihood of other hereditary breast cancer genes yet to be discovered, the results will be most definitive in an individual already affected with cancer. If no living affected relatives are available, it is feasible to begin testing close family members.

Genetic analysis of the BRCA1 and BRCA2 genes include complete sequencing with results available in four to five weeks. In 2004, the price of this test was approximately $3,000 (U.S. dollars). Most insurance companies will cover at least a portion of the cost of this test. Individuals of Ashkenazi Jewish descent can elect to undergo the ethnicity panel, screening for the three common founder mutations. The cost of this test in the U.S. was approximately $400 in 2004. Issues related to health insurance discrimination are becoming less common. Most states currently have legislation to prohibit health insurers from using the results from a genetic test to deny coverage, set premiums or drop coverage. Additionally, there is pending federal legislation to provide a more comprehensive law to prohibit health insurance and job descrimination.

A positive result from a BRCA1 or BRCA2 genetic test identifies a deleterious mutation in the individual tested. Relatives of the BRCA positive individual can then be offered testing for the same mutation, which is called a single-site analysis. The siblings and offspring of a carrier proband are at a 50% risk to inherit the same mutation. In 2004, the cost for the single-site analysis was $325 in U.S. dollars. In some families, more than one deleterious mutation is identified, complicating the testing protocol. In these situations, it is recommended that all at risk relatives undergo genetic counseling prior to undergoing genetic testing.

A negative result indicates no deleterious mutations were identified in the examined gene. Negative results are considered either a true negative or uninformative. A true negative occurs when a mutation has already been identified in an affected family member. Therefore, the individual who tested negative did not inherit the mutation in their family history. The absence of a germline mutation indicates this individual is not at an increased risk of breast, ovarian and possible other cancers, but they will still face the general population risk of breast, ovarian and other cancers as well.

A result is uninformative when an individual who tested negative was diagnosed with cancer and their family history is indicative of the breast and ovarian syndrome. In families in which a true autosomal dominant cancer syndrome is present, but no mutation has been located, either the family carries a different susceptibility gene or there is a mutation on the BRCA1 or BRCA2 gene that is not detectable by current testing methods. In families for which no mutation is identified, yet there is a pedigree suggestive of hereditary cancer, risk assessment for cancer must be based on the family history.

A negative test result in an individual not affected with cancer may also be uninformative when they are tested before an affected relative. Until the affected relative is tested, it is impossible to know whether the results were negative because they did not inherit the cancer susceptibility gene or because there is no such mutation in the family. If affected relatives are unavailable to clarify the results, risk assessment should again be based on the family history of cancer.

The final possible result for individuals undergoing BRCA1 and BRCA2 analysis is a variant of uncertain significance. Variants occur in 10% of the samples that are analyzed at Myriad Genetics, Inc. (Salt Lake City, UT) (Frank, Manley et al. 1998). This result is most commonly reported when a missense mutation is identified. Missense mutations may or may not affect the protein function of the gene product.

Until a protein assay is developed to determine the effect on protein expression, interpretation of this result is based on clinical observation. All affected relatives in a family are offered testing to determine if the variant tracks with cancer. Receiving a result of a variant of unknown significance leaves the clinician with limited information about cancer risks. Medical management decisions can not be made from this result.

Genetic Testing for Hereditary Nonpolyposis Colon Cancer. Given that 95% of tumors in individuals with HNPCC are MSI positive, testing the tumor for MSI is recommended prior to genetic testing (Hampel and Peltomaki 2000). The Bethesda guidelines have been developed to identify individuals affected with colon cancer who would be appropriate candidates for MSI testing. The revised Bethesda Guidelines recommend testing tumors for MSI in individuals who meet one or more of the following criteria:

1. Colorectal cancer diagnosed before age 50;
2. Presence of synchronous, metachronous colorectal or the HNPCC associated tumor irrespective of age at diagnosis;
3. Colorectal cancer with microsatellite instability and the presence of tumor infiltrating lymphocytes, Crohn's-like lymphocytic reaction, mucinous/signet-ring differentiation or medullary growth pattern;
4. Colorectal cancer diagnosed in one or more first degree relatives with an HNPCC-related tumor, and one cancer diagnosed less than 50 years old; or
5. Colorectal cancer diagnosed in two or more first or second degree relatives with HNPCC-related tumors, irrespective of age at diagnosis (Umar, Boland et al. 2004).

If the tumor is MSI positive, germline testing is offered. The probability of detecting a germline mutation when an individual meets Amsterdam Criteria I is 40 to 80%. When the Bethesda Guidelines are met and a tumor is MSI positive, the probability of detecting a mutation nears 50% (Kohlman 2004). Since 5% of tumors from verified HNPCC cases do not exhibit MSI, screening negative for this feature does not rule out the diagnosis of HNPCC. In addition, many individuals with colon cancer have MSI but do not have HNPCC.

Genetic Testing for Familial Adenomatous Polyposis. Germline testing in individuals with a clinical diagnosis of FAP is typically preformed to identify a mutation in the family so that at-risk relatives can undergo genetic testing. As with hereditary breast and ovarian cancer syndromes and testing for the BRCA1 and BRCA2 genes, it is emphasized in testing individuals for the APC gene mutations, that a clinical diagnosed individual be tested prior to the at-risk relatives. Molecular testing is also offered to confirm the clinical diagnosis in patients with FAP who may have less than 100 adenomatous polyps. Full gene sequencing will detect up to 90% of mutations on the APC gene. A protein truncation test, when performed alone will be positive in about 80% of individuals affected with FAP. If there are at least two affected individuals available for testing, linkage analysis can also be attempted and is informative in 95% of families tested (Solomon 2004).

Because screening for FAP begins as young as ten years old and children who carry an APC gene mutation are at risk for hepatoblastoma, molecular genetic testing is offered to at-risk children under the age of eight. While there is no evidence of psychological problems when testing is performed this early, some recommend that long-term psychological counseling be provided to these individuals (Solomon 2004).

Genotype-phenotype correlations are predicted to be available in the future allowing for individualized preventative screening and medical management recommendations.

Genetic Testing for Attenuated FAP. Because the APC gene is responsible for both FAP and AFAP, the recommendation for genetic testing is the same. The mutations for attenuated FAP are located on the far ends, the 3' or 5' ends of the gene. Since AFAP and HNPCC can present in a similar manner, molecular testing may be used to confirm or rule out a diagnosis. Molecular testing is offered to individuals 18 and older for AFAP given the later age of onset of symptoms (Solomon 2004). Genetic testing is also available for MYH-associated polyposis with both common mutations and founder mutations already described.

Cancer Screening, Surveillance and Prophylactic Management for Hereditary Cancer Syndromes

The purpose of offering a risk assessment evaluation and genetic testing is to identify individuals at increased risks for cancer prior to cancer initiation so that screening and prevention strategies can be implemented. Medical management guidelines have already been published for hereditary breast and ovarian cancer as well as hereditary colorectal cancer syndromes. The major components of these guidelines will be described.

Prevention Strategies for Hereditary Breast/Ovarian Cancer. The manner in which individuals incorporate positive genetic test results for a BRCA1 or BRCA2 mutation is the initial step in understanding the effect genetic testing has on screening and surveillance and other prophylactic options. Behavioral modification, when necessary, is the first line of defense towards this effort. Currently several studies are working to identify the long-term effects of learning genetic predisposition to cancer prior to a cancer diagnosis (Risch, McLaughlin et al. 2001). Early results indicate that fewer women than expected opted for prophylactic surgery after testing positive for a BRCA1 or BRCA2 gene (Lerman, Hughes et al. 2000). More research is necessary to understand the psychological effects of identifying a positive mutation. The findings of these studies will aid in developing behavioral interventions to increase understanding of, and adherence to, available options for this at-risk population.

The options available to women who are at an increased risk of breast and ovarian cancer can be divided into three categories: screening and surveillance; prophylactic surgery; and chemoprevention. Screening recommendations for women positive for a BRCA1 or BRCA2 mutation were written by a NIH consensus panel and published in 1997 (Burke, Daly et al. 1997) and are summarized below.

- Breast cancer screening: Clinical breast exam every six months, mammograms every six to 12 months beginning at age 25, and education regarding monthly self-examination.
- Ovarian cancer screening: Annual transvaginal ultrasounds, serum CA-125 levels and biannual pelvic exams. This information is based on expert opinion with no data indicating that these screening methods will reduce mortality from ovarian cancer in women who test positive for a BRCA1 or BRCA2 mutations (Risch, McLaughlin et al. 2001).
- Colon cancer screening: Male and female carriers of the BRCA1 and BRCA2 are informed of the possible increased risk of colorectal cancer and advised to follow the guidelines for screening published for the general population (Liede, Karlan et al. 2004).

The recommendations above have not been studied to prove benefit of surveillance on cancer-related mortality in women who are BRCA1 or BRCA2 mutation carriers. These recommendations are therefore based on expert opinion only. New studies have recently been published indicating an increased sensitivity of detection of breast cancer by magnetic resonance imaging (MRI) compared to standard mammography (Kriege, Brekelmans et al. 2004; Warner, Plewes et al. 2004). While MRI has shown to be more sensitive than mammography, the specificity is lower for MRI versus mammography (Kriege, Brekelmans et al. 2004; Warner, Plewes et al. 2004). In addition, these studies still have not proven benefit of MRI surveillance on cancer-related mortality in women who carry a BRCA1 or BRCA2 mutation.

Male carriers of mutations in BRCA1 or BRCA2 should also be offered appropriate screening and surveillance. Currently there is no standard recommendation for breast cancer screening in male carriers. Men can be advised to perform breast self-examination and contact their physician if any changes are detected. Screening with mammography is not typically recommended for males. Prostate cancer screening includes an annual prostate specific antigen (PSA) test and a digital rectal examination for men over the age of 40 (Liede, Karlan et al. 2004).

Prevention Strategies for Hereditary Colorectal Cancer Syndromes. Two groups have published screening guidelines for individuals with HNPCC. The ICG-HNPCC first published their guidelines in 1996, which were reviewed by a task force from The Cancer Genetics Studies Consortium in 1997 (Weber 1996; Burke, Daly et al. 1997). In general, both groups recommended colonoscopy every one to three years, starting at age 20 to 25, for all at-risk relatives.

Initial recommendations for endometrial cancer screening were changed by the task force in 1997. Currently, screening for endometrial cancer is recommended beginning from age 25 to 35. Screening methods include either annual endometrial aspirate (in premenopausal women) or transvaginal ultrasound with biopsies of suspicious areas. Screening for gastic cancers or urinary tract cancers are only recommended if these cancers occurred in other family members. Due to lack of sufficient data proving efficacy, serum CA-125 screening for ovarian cancer has not been recommended. Several studies have reported on the efficacy of such screening strategies in HNPCC families and conclude a decrease in incidence and mortality from colorectal cancer (Vasen, van Ballegooijen et al. 1998).

Guidelines for individuals with FAP have been updated and published by the Mayo Clinic. Screening for FAP begins as early as age ten, with prophylactic colectomy recommended between the age 17 to 20. An individual who does not undergo a proctocolectomy will require surveillance of the rectal stump every six months. Individuals with FAP are also encouraged to undergo baseline endoscopic screening for adenomas in the stomach and duodenum and a follow-up every three to five years after colectomy (Hampel and Peltomaki 2000). Surveillance for colon cancer in individuals with AFAP is similar, but typically begins at age 20 with annual colonoscopy.

To screen for other cancers, sonography and palpation is recommended in young women with FAP. Liver palpation, serum alpha-fetoprotein measurement and ultrasound are recommended for at-risk children until age six (Hampel and Peltomaki 2000).

Prophylactic Surgery. Early studies have indicated a risk reduction of 90% in breast cancer incidence and mortality after prophylactic mastectomy in high-risk women (Hartmann, Sellers et al. 1999). A recent study reported a 95% reduction in breast cancer in BRCA1 and BRCA2 mutation carriers after prophylactic mastectomy with prior or concurrent bilateral prophylactic oophorectomy (Rebbeck, Friebel et al. 2004). Bilateral prophylactic oophorectomy (BPO) is offered for women at increased risks for ovarian and breast cancer. Rebbeck et al. studied effects of BPO in carriers of a BRCA1 mutation and reported a 50% reduction in risk of breast cancer (Rebbeck, Friebel et al. 2004). Early studies have suggested increased life expectancy in BRCA1 and BRCA2 carriers who undergo prophylactic mastectomy and oophorectomy (Schrag, Kuntz et al. 1997).

Prophylactic surgery has not been proven to be effective in individuals affected with HNPCC, but the option for either subtotal colectomy (or proctocolectomy) with ileorectal anastomosis should be given to the patient after the first colon cancer diagnosis is made or when adenomas are diagnosed. In addition, women should be offered total abdominal hysterectomy and bilateral salphingooophorectomy (King, Dozois et al. 2000).

Chemoprevention. Because tamoxifen has been proven at reducing contralateral breast cancer in women with a history of breast cancer, studies are ongoing to test the risk reduction in women who carry a BRCA1 or BRCA2 mutation. One case-control study reported tamoxifen is protective from contralateral breast cancer in women with a BRCA1 or BRCA2 conferring more protection to the BRCA1 carriers (Risch, McLaughlin et al. 2001). Investigators are also exploring the possible prevention effects of oral contraceptive use in women who carry a BRCA1 or BRCA2 mutation. Initial studies have suggested a reduction in the risk of ovarian cancer in BRCA1 or BRCA2 carriers after oral contraceptive use for an average of four years (Narod, Risch et al. 1998). Several chemoprevention trials are underway to test sulindac and other non-steroidal anti-inflammatory drugs to prevent the development and advancement of polyps in FAP individuals (Hampel and Peltomaki 2000).

Conclusion

Cancer genetics and hereditary cancer syndromes are opening up an entirely new arena for cancer prevention. Education is the first step in the process of cancer prevention for hereditary cancer syndromes.

Compiling a detailed three generation family history is perhaps the single most important preventative action clinicians can do for their patients. Understanding the concepts of cancer genetics and inheritance of hereditary cancer allows the clinician to properly identify those at increased risk.

Educating the general population on the importance of maintaining accurate family records, especially of diagnosis and ages of onset is also necessary. Educating individuals and families and helping them appreciate the role of heredity in cancer, will empower patients to learn more about their family history.

Understanding the genetic risks conferred to patients who carry hereditary cancer gene mutations allows for more personalized medical management strategies. Information provided through the genetic test results may serve to increase an individual's lifespan and/or prevent cancer occurrence.

Our continued understanding of the molecular genetics of cancer at the cellular level is leading to better targeted therapies and chemoprevention options. Learning how the environment can effect a gene's function will allow individuals to modify lifestyle choices and play a part in their own cancer prevention.

References

(1975). "Genetic counseling." *Am J Hum Genet* **27**(2): 240–242.

(1999). "Cancer risks in BRCA2 mutation carriers. The Breast Cancer Linkage Consortium." *J Natl Cancer Inst* **91**(15): 1310–1316.

Aarnio, M., R. Sankila, et al. (1999). "Cancer risk in mutation carriers of DNA-mismatch-repair genes." *Int J Cancer* **81**(2): 214–218.

ACOG (1997). "ACOG committee opinion. Breast–ovarian cancer screening. Number 176, October 1996. Committee on Genetics. The American College of Obstetricians and Gynecologists." *Int J Gynaecol Obstet* **56**(1): 82–83.

Amos, C., M. Frazie, T. McGarrity (2004). Peutz-Jeghers Syndrome. In GeneReviews. *www.genetests.org*, University of Washington, Accessed April 2, 2004.

ASCO (2003). "American Society of Clinical Oncology policy statement update: genetic testing for cancer susceptibility." *J Clin Oncol* **21**(12): 2397–2406.

ASHG (1994). "Statement of the American Society of Human Genetics on genetic testing for breast and ovarian cancer predisposition." *Am J Hum Genet* **55**(5): i–iv.

Baker, L.H. (1982). "Breast Cancer Detection Demonstration Project: five-year summary report." *CA Cancer J Clin* **32**(4): 194–225.

Barnes-Kedar, I.M. and S.E. Plon (2002). "Counseling the at risk patient in the BRCA1 and BRCA2 Era." *Obstet Gynecol Clin North Am* **29**(2): 341–366, vii.

Boardman, L.A., S.N. Thibodeau, et al. (1998). "Increased risk for cancer in patients with the Peutz-Jeghers syndrome." *Ann Intern Med* **128**(11): 896–899.

Brownstein, M.H., M. Wolf, et al. (1978). "Cowden's disease: a cutaneous marker of breast cancer." *Cancer* **41**(6): 2393–2398.

Burke, W., M. Daly, et al. (1997). "Recommendations for follow-up care of individuals with an inherited predisposition to cancer. II. BRCA1 and BRCA2. Cancer Genetics Studies Consortium." *JAMA* **277**(12): 997–1003.

Claus, E.B., N. Risch, et al. (1994). "Autosomal dominant inheritance of early-onset breast cancer. Implications for risk prediction." *Cancer* **73**(3): 643–651.

Couch, F.J., B.L. Weber, et al. (1996). "Mutations and polymorphisms in the familial early-onset breast cancer (BRCA1) gene." *Human Mutation* **8**(1): 8–18.

Domchek, S.M., A. Eisen, et al. (2003). "Application of breast cancer risk prediction models in clinical practice." *J Clin Oncol* **21**(4): 593–601.

Dunlop, M.G., S.M. Farrington, et al. (1997). "Cancer risk associated with germline DNA mismatch repair gene mutations." *Hum Mol Genet* **6**(1): 105–110.

Eng, C. (2000). "Will the real Cowden syndrome please stand up: revised diagnostic criteria." *J Med Genet* **37**(11): 828–830.

Fackenthal, J.D., D.J. Marsh, et al. (2001). "Male breast cancer in Cowden syndrome patients with germline PTEN mutations." *J Med Genet* **38**(3): 159–164.

Fearon, E.R., B. Vogelstein (1990). "A genetic model for colorectal tumorigenesis." *Cell* **61**(5): 759–767.

Ford, D., D.F. Easton, et al. (1994). "Risks of cancer in BRCA1-mutation carriers." *Lancet* **343**(8899): 692–695.

Frank, T.S., S.A. Manley, et al. (1998). "Sequence analysis of BRCA1 and BRCA2: correlation of mutations with family history and ovarian cancer risk." *J Clin Oncol* **16**(7): 2417–2425.

Franks, L.M., Teich, N.M. (1997). *Introduction to the Cellular and Molecular Biology of Cancer.* London, Oxford University Press.

Garber, J.E., A.M. Goldstein, et al. (1991). "Follow-up study of twenty-four families with Li-Fraumeni syndrome." *Cancer Res* **51**(22): 6094–6097.

Geller, G., J.R. Botkin, et al. (1997). "Genetic testing for susceptibility to adult-onset cancer. The process and content of informed consent." *Jama* **277**(18): 1467–1474.

Giardiello, F.M., J.D. Brensinger, et al. (1997). "The use and interpretation of commercial APC gene testing for familial adenomatous polyposis." *N Engl J Med* **336**(12): 823–827.

Hall, J.M., M.K. Lee, et al. (1990). "Linkage of early-onset familial breast cancer to chromosome-17q21." *Science* **250**(4988): 1684–1689.

Hampel, H. and P. Peltomaki (2000). "Hereditary colorectal cancer: risk assessment and management." *Clin Genet* **58**(2): 89–97.

Hartmann, L.C., T.A. Sellers, et al. (1999). "Clinical options for women at high risk for breast cancer." *Surg Clin North Am* **79**(5): 1189–1206.

Hemminki, A. (1999). "The molecular basis and clinical aspects of Peutz-Jeghers syndrome." *Cell Mol Life Sci* **55**(5): 735–750.

Hemminki, A., D. Markie, et al. (1998). "A serine/threonine kinase gene defective in Peutz-Jeghers syndrome." *Nature* **391**(6663): 184–187.

Izatt, L., J. Greenman, et al. (1999). "Identification of germline missense mutations and rare allelic variants in the ATM gene in early-onset breast cancer." *Genes Chromosomes Cancer* **26**(4): 286–294.

Johannesdottir, G., J. Gudmundsson, et al. (1996). "High prevalence of the 999del5 mutation in icelandic breast and ovarian cancer patients." *Cancer Res* **56**(16): 3663–3665.

King, J.E., R.R. Dozois, et al. (2000). "Care of patients and their families with familial adenomatous polyposis." *Mayo Clin Proc* **75**(1): 57–67.

King, M.C., J.H. Marks, et al. (2003). "Breast and ovarian cancer risks due to inherited mutations in BRCA1 and BRCA2." *Science* **302**(5645): 643–646.

Knudson, A.G. (1971). "Mutation and cancer – statistical study of retinoblastoma." *Proceedings of the National Academy of Sciences of the United States of America* **68**(4): 820–823.

Kohlman, W., Gruber, S.B. (2004). Hereditary Non-Polyposis Colon Cancer. In GeneReviews, *www.genetests.org*, accessed November 10, 2004.

Kriege, M., C.T. Brekelmans, et al. (2004). "Efficacy of MRI and mammography for breast-cancer screening in women with a familial or genetic predisposition." *N Engl J Med* **351**(5): 427–437.

Lerman, C., C. Hughes, et al. (2000). "Prophylactic surgery decisions and surveillance practices one year following BRCA1/2 testing." *Prev Med* **31**(1): 75–80.

Levine, A.J. (1997). "p53, the cellular gatekeeper for growth and division." *Cell* **88**(3): 323–331.

Liede, A., B.Y. Karlan, et al. (2004). "Cancer risks for male carriers of germline mutations in BRCA1 or BRCA2: a review of the literature." *J Clin Oncol* **22**(4): 735–742.

Lynch, H.T. and J.F. Lynch (1998). "Genetics of colonic cancer." *Digestion* **59**(5): 481–492.

Lynch, H.T. and J.F. Lynch (2000). "Hereditary nonpolyposis colorectal cancer." *Semin Surg Oncol* **18**(4): 305–313.

Malander, S., M. Ridderheim, et al. (2004). "One in 10 ovarian cancer patients carry germ line BRCA1 or BRCA2 mutations: results of a prospective study in Southern Sweden." *European Journal of Cancer* **40**(3): 422–428.

Malkin, D., F.P. Li, et al. (1990). "Germ line p53 mutations in a familial syndrome of breast cancer, sarcomas, and other neoplasms." *Science* **250**(4985): 1233–1238.

Miki, Y., J. Swensen, et al. (1994). "Isolation of BRCA1, the 17q-linked breast and ovarian cancer susceptibility gene." *Science* **266**: 61–71.

Narod, S.A., H. Risch, et al. (1998). "Oral contraceptives and the risk of hereditary ovarian cancer. Hereditary Ovarian Cancer Clinical Study Group." *N Engl J Med* **339**(7): 424–428.

NCI (1998). Breast Cancer Risk Assessment Tool for Health Care Providers. N. C. I. Office of Cancer Communication, Bethesda.

NCI (2004). Breast Cancer Risk Assessment Tool. *http://bcra.nci.nih.gov/brc/*, Accessed November 10, 2004.

Nelen, M.R., G.W. Padberg, et al. (1996). "Localization of the gene for Cowden disease to chromosome 10q22-23." *Nat Genet* **13**(1): 114–116.

NSGC (2004). National Society of Genetic Counselors Home Page. *www.nsgc.org*, Accessed November 10, 2004.

Nussbaum, R.L., McInnes, R.R., Willard, H.F. (2001). *Thompson and Thompson Genetics in Medicine*. Philadelphia, W.B. Saunders Company.

Offit, K. (1997). *Clinical Cancer Genetics: Risk Counseling and Management*. New York, Wiley-Liss.

Parmigiani, G., D. Berry, et al. (1998). "Determining carrier probabilities for breast cancer-susceptibility genes BRCA1 and BRCA2." *Am J Hum Genet* **62**(1): 145–158.

Parmigiani, G., W. Wang (2004). BRCAPRO. B. Lab, *http://astor.som.jhmi.edu/BayesMendel/brcapro.html*, accessed November 10, 2004.

Peelen, T., W. de Leeuw, et al. (2000). "Genetic analysis of a breast-ovarian cancer family, with 7 cases of colorectal cancer linked to BRCA1, fails to support a role for BRCA1 in colorectal tumorigenesis." *Int J Cancer* **88**(5): 778–782.

Peelen, T., M. vanVliet, et al. (1997). "A high proportion of novel mutations in BRCA1 with strong founder effects among Dutch and Belgian hereditary breast and ovarian cancer families." *American Journal of Human Genetics* **60**(5): 1041–1049.

Peltomaki, P. and H.F. Vasen (1997). "Mutations predisposing to hereditary nonpolyposis colorectal cancer: database and results of a collaborative study. The International Collaborative Group on Hereditary Nonpolyposis Colorectal Cancer." *Gastroenterology* **113**(4): 1146–1158.

Peters, J.A. and J.E. Stopfer (1996). "Role of the genetic counselor in familial cancer." *Oncology (Huntingt)* **10**(2): 159–166.

Petrij-Bosch, A., T. Peelen, et al. (1997). "BRCA1 genomic deletions are major founder mutations in Dutch breast cancer patients." *Nat Genet* **17**(3): 341–345.

Rebbeck, T.R., T. Friebel, et al. (2004). "Bilateral prophylactic mastectomy reduces breast cancer risk in BRCA1 and BRCA2 mutation carriers: the PROSE Study Group." *J Clin Oncol* **22**(6): 1055–1062.

Risch, H.A., J.R. McLaughlin, et al. (2001). "Prevalence and penetrance of germline BRCA1 and BRCA2 mutations in a population series of 649 women with ovarian cancer." *Am J Hum Genet* **68**(3): 700–710.

Savitsky, K., S. Sfez, et al. (1995). "The complete sequence of the coding region of the ATM gene reveals similarity to cell cycle regulators in different species." *Hum Mol Genet* **4**(11): 2025–2032.

Schneider, K. (2001). *Counseling About Cancer: Strategies for Genetic Counseling*. New York, Wiley-Liss.

Schrag, D., K.M. Kuntz, et al. (1997). "Decision analysis – effects of prophylactic mastectomy and oophorectomy on life expectancy among women with BRCA1 or BRCA2 mutations." *N Engl J Med* **336**(20): 1465–1471.

Shattuck-Eidens, D., A. Oliphant, et al. (1997). "BRCA1 sequence analysis in women at high risk for susceptibility mutations. Risk factor analysis and implications for genetic testing." *JAMA* **278**(15): 1242–1250.

Solomon, C., Burt, R.W. (2004). Familial adenomatous polyposis. In GeneReviews. *www.genetests.org*, University of Washington, Accessed April 2, 2004.

Struewing, J.P., P. Hartge, et al. (1997). "The risk of cancer associated with specific mutations of BRCA1 and BRCA2 among Ashkenazi Jews." *N Engl J Med* **336**(20): 1401–1408.

Swift, M., D. Morrell, et al. (1991). "Incidence of cancer in 161 families affected by ataxia-telangiectasia." *N Engl J Med* **325**(26): 1831–1836.

Thompson, D., D. Easton, et al. (2001). "Variation in cancer risks, by mutation position, in BRCA2 mutation carriers." *American Journal of Human Genetics* **68**(2): 410–419.

Thull, D.L. and V.G. Vogel (2004). "Recognition and management of hereditary breast cancer syndromes." *Oncologist* **9**(1): 13–24.

Tirkkonen, M., O. Johannsson, et al. (1997). "Distinct somatic genetic changes associated with tumor progression in carriers of BRCA1 and BRCA2 germ-line mutations." *Cancer Research* **57**(7): 1222–1227.

Tonin, P., B. Weber, et al. (1996). "Frequency of recurrent BRCA1 and BRCA2 mutations in Ashkenazi Jewish breast cancer families." *Nature Medicine* **2**(11): 1179–1183.

Tyrer, J., S.W. Duffy, et al. (2004). "A breast cancer prediction model incorporating familial and personal risk factors." *Stat Med* **23**(7): 1111–1130.

Umar, A., C.R. Boland, et al. (2004). "Revised Bethesda Guidelines for hereditary nonpolyposis colorectal cancer (Lynch syndrome) and microsatellite instability." *J Natl Cancer Inst* **96**(4): 261–268.

Vasen, H.F., M. van Ballegooijen, et al. (1998). "A cost-effectiveness analysis of colorectal screening of hereditary nonpolyposis colorectal carcinoma gene carriers." *Cancer* **82**(9): 1632–1637.

Vogelstein, B., Kinzler, K.W. (2002). *The Genetic Basis of Human Cancer.* New York, McGraw-Hill Professional.

Warner, E., D.B. Plewes, et al. (2004). "Surveillance of BRCA1 and BRCA2 mutation carriers with magnetic resonance imaging, ultrasound, mammography, and clinical breast examination." *JAMA* **292**(11): 1317–1325.

Watanabe, T., T.T. Wu, et al. (2001). "Molecular predictors of survival after adjuvant chemotherapy for colon cancer." *N Engl J Med* **344**(16): 1196–1206.

Weber, T. (1996). "Clinical surveillance recommendations adopted for HNPCC." *Lancet* **348**: 465.

Wijnen, J.T., H.F. Vasen, et al. (1998). "Clinical findings with implications for genetic testing in families with clustering of colorectal cancer." *N Engl J Med* **339**(8): 511–518.

Wooster, R., G. Bignell, et al. (1995). "Identification of the Breast-Cancer Susceptibility Gene Brca2." *Nature* **378**(6559): 789–792.

Ylikorkala, A., E. Avizienyte, et al. (1999). "Mutations and impaired function of LKB1 in familial and non-familial Peutz-Jeghers syndrome and a sporadic testicular cancer." *Hum Mol Genet* **8**(1): 45–51.

Human Categories and Health:
The Power of the Concept of Ethnicity

Kathryn Coe[1] and Craig T. Palmer[2]

[1] Mel and Enid Zuckerman College of Public Health, University of Arizona, Tucson, AZ 85724
[2] Department of Anthropology, University of Missouri-Columbia, Columbia, MO 65211

The inclusion of ethnic minorities in cancer prevention studies is a scientific, logistic, cultural, and ethical issue. A great deal has yet to be learned about cancer in these populations. Many questions remain unanswered, such as why some ethnic minorities are more likely to get certain cancers, be diagnosed at later stages, and die of their disease. Further, there is a great need to be more successful in the recruitment of ethnic minorities to cancer prevention research trials. It is unclear why their participation in many clinical studies remains low. The answer to these questions, we argue, lies in an a deeper understanding of the meaning of ethnicity. Definitions of ethnicity are inconsistent and unclear; researchers employ the concept to measure every important indicator associated with inequality or difference: socioeconomic status, cultural lifestyles and values, and genetic predispositions are all being measured by the ethnicity variable. A discussion of the multifactorial elements, implicit or explicit, in the use of the terms race, ethnicity, and culture can be used to point out the elements that are fundamental to these terms and that may influence health behaviors and outcomes. The concept of ethnicity is more useful for understanding health than are the concepts of race or culture because it has, since the origins of the term, focused on the role of traditions while acknowledging that genetics are involved. Ethnicity is best understood when we adopt the interactionist view that specifies that both genes and environmental factors interact in human development and play a role in health and illness. By taking an interactionist view, more successful cancer prevention interventions and research trials can be developed.

For a number of reasons, the inclusion of ethnic minorities in cancer research trials is an important concern for researchers. There are a growing number of reports of robust relationships between ethnic group or ethnicity (the characteristics that make that group distinctive) and health outcomes (Kato 1996; Patrinos 2004). Ethnic minorities experience significant health disparities.

Certain cancers, for example, are more common in ethnic minorities than in other populations. Even among those populations in which cancers incidence rates are lower, the mortality may be higher. Today, Hispanic/Latino women who live in the United States, when compared to non-Hispanic white women, have twice the incidence rate of and 1.4 times the mortality from cervical cancer (Reynolds 2004). Relative to non-Hispanic whites, a greater proportion of African American, American Indian, Hawaiian, and Hispanic patients are diagnosed with testis cancer at later stages (Lou Biggs and Schwartz 2004). American Indian women, when compared to their white counterparts, have a significantly lower five-year cancer survival rate (Samet, Key et al. 1987).

In addition, the cancer rates in ethnic populations are rising; during the last century, cancer was a disease so seldom diagnosed among American Indians that anthropologists were led to argue that they were immune to cancer or had some natural protection from the disease (Hrdlicka 1905; Leven 1910). Among the First Nations people of Canada, cancer incidence rates increased significantly between 1968 through 1975 and from 1984 to 1991 for all cancers and for the major cancers (e.g., breast, lung, prostate and colorectal) (Marrett and Chaudhry 2003). Further, there are regional differences in the types of cancers diagnosed. For example, American Indians in New Mexico are at higher risk of gestational trophoblastic neoplasia (Smith, Qualls et al. 2004).

Despite increasing cancer mortality and morbidity, cancer screening rates are lower in ethnic minority populations than in whites (Walsh, Kaplan et al. 2004). Substantial subgroups of American women, specifically those of ethnic minorities, have not been screened for cervical cancer nor are they screened at regular intervals. Hispanic women are less likely to receive screening mammograms than are white or African American women (Bazargan, Bazargan et al. 2004), even though breast cancer is the leading cause of cancer-related deaths in the Hispanic population (Darling, Nelson et al. 2004). There are also disparities related to treatment; in a recent study of prostate cancer, racial/ethnic minorities were found to be less likely to receive definitive therapy for the treatment of disease (Underwood, De Monner et al. 2004).

While these problems are significant, it is not clear why these disparities exist. The factors contributing to these disparities, such as the increased likelihood of ethnic minorities to get certain cancers, to die of certain cancers, to be diagnosed at a late stage in the disease progression, and the decreased likelihood to be screened for cancer or to receive the best treatment, remain elusive.

One problem with research in ethnicity and health is that researchers employ the term to measure every important indicator associated with inequality or difference: socioeconomic status, cultural lifestyles and values, and genetic predispositions are all being measured by the ethnicity variable. The independent importance of this variable, however, is evident in the fact that even if we control for other factors, race and ethnicity are predictors of disparities (Palacio, Kahn et al. 2002; Cohen 2003; Opolka, Rascati et al. 2003; Guller, Jain et al. 2004).

To begin to investigate these issues, it is important to understand not only what ethnicity is, but why it might impact health. Only then can we use this knowledge to develop an effective and fruitful approach to health disparities research (Ashing-Giwa, Padilla et al. 2004). Due to the scientifically verifiable robust relationships that exist between ethnic groups and health outcomes (Kato 1996; Patrinos 2004), the term 'ethnicity' is increasingly being used as categorical variables in social research related to cancer and its prevention. While an association between ethnicity and health outcomes does exist,

> ... the use of ethnicity as a grouping variable in health research is disturbing to scientists. It is poorly defined, is not objectively measured, and cannot be studied in a true experiment. Thus, scientific conclusions about the causal relationship between ethnicity and health are difficult to make (Kato 1996).

The failure of scholars to agree on the traits necessary or sufficient for ethnic membership has led to controversy, with some researchers dismissing the term as a political category that is otherwise meaningless. The strong association between ethnicity and health indicates that we should not consider abandoning the term, but rather suggests that it deserves careful study (Kato 1996). This is true not only for the study of health and ethnicity, but for the study of ethnicity in general because "the academic specialty usually called 'race and ethnic relations' is rich in literature but poor in theory" (Van den Berghe 1981).

The Failure of Attempts to Define Ethnicity

Much of the confusion related to the term ethnicity is the result of attempts to equate ethnicity with either the biological or genetic concept of race or the environmental concept of culture. These attempts have failed because ethnicity incorporates both genetic and environmental factors.

Race originally was a taxonomic term coined by biologists to refer to a subspecies. For example, Kroeber wrote that a race "is a group united by heredity, a breed or genetic strain or subspecies" (Kroeber 1923). It corresponded, he continued, "to a breed in domestic animals" (Kroeber 1923, p. 75). Hoebel was yet more explicit. "A race is a biologically inbred group possessing a distinctive combination of physical traits that tend to breed true from generation to generation" (p. 69). The assumption that race was defined by genetic differences between races, often *mislabled* as biologic differences, is illustrated by the fact that such a grouping is at times called a Mendelian population (Zuckerman 1990). The genetic differences responsible for the physical and behavioral similarities (e.g., phenotypes) found among individuals in Mendelian populations occur because all individuals in this small population share relatively recent common ancestry.

It seemed obvious to early explorers that geographically isolated human populations also seemed to be distinguishable in terms of phenotypic characteristics. Among the earliest published human racial classifications was Francois Bernier's *Nouvelle division de la terre par les différents espèces ou races qui l'habitent* ("New division of Earth by the different species or races which inhabit it") (Bernier 1684). In the 19th century, race continued to be identified based on similarity in appearance and was generally measured by skin color and other obvious morphologic characteristics. As Kroeber recognized, in gross physiology, all human races were much alike (Kroeber 1923). However, it was also true that a great many distinct characteristics distinguished different categories of humans (e.g., skin and hair color, stature, cephalic index, nasal index, texture of the hair, hairiness of the body, prognathism). It was not clear which of these markers might be the most important in classifying races. While heredity was involved (in that children resembled their parents), these physical similarities were related to a common geographic place of origin: the white race, with its origin in the Caucasus; the yellow race, with its origin in Mongolia; the black race, with its origin in Ethiopia or Africa (Cuvier 1848; Gould 1981). Racial categories were seen as typologies; one of such types (black) differed from another (white, yellow, or red) (Crews and Bindon 1991). Early discussions of the meaning of race focused solely on physical chararacteristics; culture was ignored.

By the 20th century, the conditions once considered to be necessary or sufficient for membership in a particular human race were beginning to be problematic. Although the characteristics that determined racial membership were due to genetic similarities resulting from common ancestry and reproductive isolation, these characteristics were beginning to appear to be arbitrary. Researchers began to argue that the term race might not be an appropriate term for human groups. In fact, a long tradition of scholarly research has argued that race is an arbitrary system of visual classification that fails to and, indeed cannot, "demarcate distinct subspecies of the human population" (Fullilove 1998).

Similarity in physical and behavioral features may be a product of genetic admixture brought about by the migrations that began to occur early in human prehistory or may be due to convergent evolution, with similar environmental pressures selecting for similar responses, including both physical and behavioral characteristics. People in Africa and in India, while perhaps sharing a dark skin, are not closely related; their dark skin may be an adaptation to particular environmental pressures. Among humans, as among other species, physical appearance is neither a reliable nor a valid indicator of relatedness or shared descent. "We are genetically far more nuanced and variable than is reflected in just skin coloration" (Patrinos 2004).

While some of the debate was related to the central concept of humans as animals, there was ample reason to reject the idea of race. While subspecies and Mendelian populations are usually small, races are often large. In addition, as races were identified by ideal type, intermediate types that failed to match the ideal, such as brown as opposed to black, led to the breakdown of the typology. These variants could neither be forced into one of the ideal types nor ignored (Crews and Bindon 1991).

Particular mate choices, including a long history of arranged marriages and tribal endogamy can lead to rapid selection for certain morphological characteristics. "Cultural restrictions for mate selection based on external morphological characteristics may lead to rapid differentiation of skin, eye, or hair color between populations while leaving aspects of basic biology and energy metabolism relatively unaffected" (Crews and Bindon 1991). Visual differences are superficial and, in fact, the racial categories being promoted did not typically reflect the factors important for human classification. Most importantly, studies of actual genetic clinal distributions found that the vast majority of genetic differences occur within any given racial category, with only a very small percentage of the variation occurring between racial classifications (Lewontin 1972). As early as 1923, Kroeber argued that "variations between individuals of the same race are often greater than differences between the races" (Kroeber 1923, p. 126). These studies led to the realization that phenotypic differences do not necessary indicate that there are dramatic genotypic differences. In addition, there was the real fear that a clear designation of racial categories would contribute to racism. Thus, the concept of race fell into disfavor.

The rejection of the concept of race led to the popularity of ethnicity as a replacement in both scientific and nonscientific research (Bhopal and Donaldson 1998). The roots of the term *ethnic* are Greek (as well as Latin *ethnicus*, German *ethnikos* and French *ethnique*), meaning a nation or people and its cultural practices. By 1957, ethnicity was a term most commonly used to refer to nations or groups that were neither Christian nor Jewish, but heathen (1957). Ethnicity was used to distinguish "them" from "us," with us being the explorers and scholars writing about exotic peoples. The second meaning of ethnic referred to "any of the basic divisions or groups of mankind, as distinguished by customs, characteristics, (or) language" (1957). Ethnic groups were identifiable and distinguishable on the basis of cultural traits, which included not only the shared language and cultural practices, but also the knowledge, attitudes, and beliefs shared by members of a cultural group.

At its origin, ethnicity was used to distinguish cultural homogeneity (ethnic group) from biological homogeneity (race) (Damon 1969). The use of the term "ethnic group" was promoted, based at least partially on the idea that it would stimulate discussion as to its meaning and thus clarify the meaning of race (Montagu 1962). Attempts to replace the term race with the term ethnicity, and thus shift from genetic racial categories to cultural ethnic categories, have not proven to be successful (Crews and Bindon 1991).

Ethnicity is not simply a synonym for culture. Although researchers often deny that there is a genetic component to ethnicity (Amick 1995), ethnicity does in fact have a genetic aspect. While ethnicity has been tied to cultural behavior since its origin, there is an association with other traits that are not necessarily cultural. The realization that ethnicity is not just cultural has lead to the persistence of attempts to equate ethnicity with race. For example, the terms race and ethnicity are still often found together, and at least implicitly are often used as synonyms (Bulmer 1999; Kromkrowski 2002; Scupin 2003).

Ethnic groups are also often described as being sub-groups of races, and to the extent that ethnicity is seen as a sub-grouping of race, it has an implied genetic component (Miranda 1997). While physical appearance may be due to convergent evolution, it can be related to genetic differences (Crews and Bindon 1991). Looking like the other members of your ethnic group was important (Westermarck 1921). Non-cultural phenotypes are the most reliable markers of ethnicity (Van den Berghe 1981). For example, an individual who looks Asian is classified as Asian, even if he or she follows no Asian cultural practices (Kato 1996). Despite attempts to define ethnicity in purely cultural terms, ethnicity is popularly seen as biological, as related to ancestry and genetics (Nagel 1996). The failure of the term ethnicity to completely replace race indicates that there is a clear sense that something important would be lost by a complete shift from a biological or genetic to a cultural definition.

There are contradictions encountered when ethnicity is used interchangeably with race. It is recognized that racial categories "are not co-extensive with any existing ethnic group" (Crews and Bindon 1991). The Serbians and Croatians are classified as white; however, few would argue that they represent a single ethnic group (Crews and Bindon 1991). As a result, many researchers have returned to using the term race, but have redefined it in an attempt to make it more applicable to human categories (Bhopal 1999). Some researchers use the term race, but assert that there are no identifiable innate genetic differences between races that can explain disparities in health (Fullilove 1998). If no innate genetic differences exist, it is unclear why race should be used at all instead of simply using cultural differences for these categorizations. Despite all of the problems with the term race, it has neither been abandoned nor replaced with culture because of the view that ignoring race in health statistics could lead us to ignore the disparities these statistics bring to light (Buehler 1999).

Instead of attempting to redefine race, the best solution may be to more clearly define ethnicity. The inability to define ethnicity in exclusively genetic or cultural terms implies that both factors need to be incorporated. Ethnicity must be understood within the context of the interactive view of human development.

The Interactive View of Human Development

An accurate understanding of the relationships among race, ethnicity, and culture requires an understanding of the interactive theory of human development (Alcock 2001). According to the interactive theory, the development of humans and all living organisms involves an incredibly complex interaction of both genetic and environmental factors. This requires an understanding of the terms biologic, genetic, environmental, innate, learned, culture, and tradition as well as an understanding of their interactions.

Biologic, Genetic and Environmental. Much of the confusion over the meaning of ethnicity stems from the meaning of biological difference. This can be avoided by simply remembering that biology is the study of life (Thornhill 2000). Hence, to describe something as biological is simply declaring it living. Often, biological is incorrectly interchanged with the term genetic. These terms are not interchangeable; the traits of living, biological things (e.g. organs, limbs, skin, eye color, behaviors) are all phenotypes. In contrast, the genes within any individual organism are merely its genotype. Phenotypes are not the same as genotypes. Any part of an organism's phenotype is the result of an interaction between genes and environmental factors.

To understand this point it is crucial to recognize that environmental factors include more than just those things normally associated with the environment. To a biologist, the environment includes all exogenetic factors, that is, everything that the genes of an organism interact with during the development of an organism, both before and after birth. Such factors include not only the air, water, nutrients, and other chemicals the organism consumes, but the other living things, including humans, the organism encounters. Further, the environment includes not only things external to the organism, but also chemicals within the organism that interact with genes. Hence, everything biologic is the product of both genes and environmental factors. Even an individual cell, the most fundamental building block of any larger organism, is a product of genes and certain aspects of the environment. The constant intertwining of genetic and environmental factors continues throughout the life of the organism. This is true even for behavior, the muscular-induced movements of organisms.

Learned and Innate. Because behavior is part of the phenotype of an organism, it is a product of the interaction of both genetic and environmental factors. This fact makes the distinction between learned and innate behaviors untenable. A behavior is learned when a specific environmental factor has been identified as necessary for the behavior's occurrence. For example, when it is identified that a person must get on a bicycle and fall off several times before they are able to ride successfully, riding a bicycle is claimed to be a learned behavior. However, focusing on only this particular necessary environmental factor causes people to overlook all of the other factors that are also necessary for a human to ride a bicycle. These include all kinds of other environmental factors during the development of the child such as oxygen, water, and nutrients, as well as certain genes that enable physical functioning to interact with environmental factors. Remove any of these necessary environmental or genetic factors and bicycle riding will never occur. All behaviors that we call learned are the result of many environmental factors and genes.

A behavior is innate when certain environmental factors are identified that are *not* necessary for a behavior to occur. For example, the sucking behavior of infants occurs before the infant ever sees another infant making the motion or is even exposed to a nipple. This is claimed to be an innate behavior. However, it is important that not only the unnecessary environmental factors be considered. There are many other factors that occur during development that are necessary if an infant is to perform the sucking motion. These include not only certain genes, but the interaction of those genes with such environmental factors in utero, including maternal nutrition. All behaviors that we call innate are also the result of many environmental factors and genes.

Since all behavior, whether it is claimed to be learned or innate, is the result of an interaction between genes and numerous environmental factors, the distinction between learned and innate behavior has no meaning. The debate between whether a behavior is learned or innate should be replaced with attempts to identify what genes and what environmental factors are necessary to produce a given behavior or for that matter, disease.

Heritability and Inheritable. It is crucial to understand the term heritability and how it differs from the term inherited. Heritability is the degree to which differences between individuals are due to differences in genes. Heritability is expressed as the proportion of the variation among individuals with regard to a certain trait that is attributable to genetic rather than environmental variation (Falconer 1981). For example, differences between individual humans in height has a heritability index as high as 0.9 in some human populations (Bodmer 1976). This means that about 90 percent of the difference in height between individuals is due to genetic differences, and about 10 percent to differences in environment (e.g., nutrition, disease). However, this does not mean than any given individual's height is 90% genetic. The height of any individual is the result of an inseparable interaction of genes and environmental factors (Alcock 2001).

The difference between heritability and inheritable is crucial because a trait can be inherited regardless of its heritability. Highly heritable traits may be inherited; for example, a tall parent can have a tall offspring. However, a highly heritable trait may not be inherited. The offspring of a tall parent may be short because of the environment in which the offspring develops (e.g., an environment lacking nutrition or containing disease). On the other hand, inheritance often occurs in the absence of heritability. Although two hands are normally inherited from one's parents, hand number is not a heritable trait – that is, there is essentially no genetic variance underlying hand number. In times past, hand number in humans was under strong selection, and that greatly reduced variation affecting the development of this trait.

Cultural. Although culture often is asserted to involve mental states, and sometimes to involve only mental states, culture becomes important in scientific studies when certain kinds of behavior or their consequences are observed. Most social scientists refer to culture when describing socially learned behavior (Flinn 1997), but what may appear to be essential to culture is not just that it is learned and shared, but that it is acquired from another individual and potentially transmittable to a third (Palmer 1997; Thornhill 2000; Coe 2003). To say that culture is socially learned behavior means only that the developmental causes of the behavior include, not that they are limited to, learning experiences involving other human beings. Speaking a language, for example, is clearly a cultural behavior, because the environmental influences leading to its occurrence include social learning. But the presence of another person is far from sufficient. Speaking a language only occurs when certain necessary genes have interacted with numerous environmental factors in addition to other people speaking the language.

If cultural is a term used to refer to socially learned and transmitted behaviors, then a culture would include a set of people who share a vast amount of socially learned behaviors. That is, the members of a culture share more socially learned behaviors with other members of that culture than they do with members of other cultures. If two cultures are geographically isolated, the cultural behaviors tend to be fairly distinct. However, in most cases, human cultures have been in contact and cultural behaviors are exchanged. Today it is probably more often likely to be true that the boundaries between cultures are at least somewhat arbitrary because of cultural behaviors being shared between what are designated as distinct cultures. The term sub-culture is often used because within a culture some sets of individuals share more cultural behaviors with each other than they do with other individuals in their culture.

Traditional. Traditional refers to only those behaviors that are socially learned from a parent or other ancestor. Thus traditional behavior is a subset of cultural behavior and occurs when genes interact with many environmental factors, including a parent or other ancestor engaged in the behavior. Speaking a language for example is always cultural, but it may or may not be traditional. An individual may have learned French at school, not from parents or grandparents. Speaking a language learned from someone other than an ancestor is not traditional; learning a language from an ancestor is traditional. Until recently, not only language, but nearly all other cultural behaviors were traditional.

Until recently, most shared socially learned behaviors, which were seen as characteristic of and as distinguishing a particular culture, were a consequence of social learning from common ancestors. The shared socially-learned behaviors defining a culture were traditional behaviors, and the members of the culture tended to be co-descendants, all of whom inherited culture from a common ancestor through grandparents and parents. While this continues to be the case in many parts of the world in what we have come to call ethnic groups, the shared socially learned behaviors in other areas, such as in much of the U.S., are primarily due to social learning from people other than ancestors. In such areas, the shared socially learned behaviors defining a culture are often not traditional.

The Interactive View of Development and Health

The view that race correlates with health assumes that genes alone produce aspects of a phenotype that is correlated in some way with health. Race may be useful in studying health issues occurring in environments in which the health issues are highly heritable as well as inheritable, but only to the extent that the racial categories used correlate with the particular genetic differences related to the health issue. The fact that such correlation is often absent, because most genetic variation is found within a given racial category instead of between racial categories, weakens the relation between race and health. This approach is further weakened by the fact that genes alone do not create aspects of a phenotype that affect health. Even if certain genes are found to correlate with a racial category and the racial category correlates with a health issue, the health issue may not be causally related to those genes. The health issue may actually be related to some aspect of the environment (e.g., diet or exposure to pollutants) that also correlates with the racial category in that particular setting. These factors severely weaken the use of race as a variable in health research.

The typical view of culture is also limited because of its focus in the development of cultural behavior. By focusing only on the necessity of interaction with other people, the other factors, including genes, tend to be ignored. These other factors may also be necessary for the development of cultural behaviors and that might be related to health conditions. A focus on only cultural variables limits our ability to explain highly heritable health conditions. For example, without an understanding of the heritability of a health condition, merely detecting a correlation between a certain cultural practice and a health issue would not indicate whether or not the health issue was likely to be inherited. This is because the inheritance of the health condition by offspring might depend on inheriting both certain genetic factors and certain environmental factors (e.g., diet) from the parents. To provide a clear example, a study conducted in Brazil of Leber's hereditary optic neuropathy (LHON) began by identifying four index cases from a remote area. Molecular analysis of blood showed that they were LHON, homoplasmic 11778, J-haplogroup. As these four individuals had an extensive family living in that rural area, 273 of the 295 family members were investigated (Sadun, Carelli et al. 2002). The team conducted epidemiological interviews attempting to identify possible environmental risk factors and conducted comprehensive neuro-ophthalmological examinations, psychophysical tests, Humphrey visual field studies, fundus photography, and blood testing for both mitochondrial genetic analysis and nuclear gene linkage analysis. They found that the individuals were all descendants of an immigrant from Verona, Italy and that subsequent generations of his descendants demonstrated penetrance rates of 71, 60, 34, 15, and 9%. Age at onset ranged from 10 to 64 years of age. Current visual acuities varied from light perception to 20/400. The team was left unable to answer the question of why only some of the genetically affected individuals manifested the disease (Sadun, Carelli et al. 2002). The obvious answer is that the expression of a disease is a consequence not only of the genes but of complex environmental factors.

Ethnicity is better able to explain health issues than are either race or culture because it incorporates both genetic and environmental (including cultural) factors. This is because ethnicity is defined by descent from common ancestors and involves the inheritance of both genes and culture. This is also why attempts to equate ethnicity with either genetic race or environmental culture have failed.

"(T)he notion that ethnicity has something to do with kinship or 'blood' is not new. Indeed descent seems to be, implicitly and very often explicitly, the essential element of the definition of those groups of 'significant others' that go under a wide variety of labels: tribe, band, horde, deme, ethnic group, race, nation, and nationality" (Van den Berghe 1981).

Ethnicity, when defined by descent, incorporates both genetic and cultural factors, including those factors related to health. The key to such an understanding is an appreciation of the importance of cultural traditions and an understanding of how they are inherited. Inheritance occurs "when and only when both genetic and environmental influences are repeated between generations" (Thornhill 2000). Traditions are a form of culture that is transmitted vertically, across generations from ancestors to descendants, parent to child. Traditions make up a significant amount of human behavior and distinguish the sets of co-descendants referred to as ethnic groups. Ethnic groups are distinguished by both genetic and environmental factors because traditions are inherited from one's ancestors when both the necessary genes and environmental factors are present.

In contrast to a race, an ethnic group is a set of co-descendants that cannot be identified solely by non-cultural phenotypes. Ethnicity is a category of co-descendants often identifiable only through particular traditional cultural traits. Typically these include language, clothing, tattooing, hair styles, dance, art, and other traits. In contrast to a race, an ethnic group is a set of people perceived to be co-descendants of a recent common ancestor (i.e., members share a more recent common ancestor with other members of the ethnic group than with nonmembers). An ethnic group is perceived to be identifiable through traditional cultural markers.

The realization that ethnicity is a combination of genetic and cultural factors does not simplify the concept of ethnicity. Although ethnicity incorporates both genetic and cultural factors, it does not perfectly correlate with either. Descent from a common ancestor predicts that members of an ethnic group may be more likely to have a certain gene, but a correlation between genes and ethnicity is far from perfect. Each child inherits only 50% of our genes. While traditional behaviors identify one's ethnicity, not all members of an ethnic group will share all traditional behaviors. The amount of correlation between ethnic groups and both genes and traditions is also likely to vary from one ethnic group to another.

In the 21st century, we are less likely to find individuals who share genes due to common ancestry and who have maintained ancestral traditions. However, in the past, traditions remained unchanged for centuries or even millennia (Coe 2003). Although all forms of culture imply social interaction, traditions imply enduring social interactions between individuals sharing ancestry. The transmission of a tradition, such as learning how to make pottery, can require decades of social interaction during which strong social ties were formed and the history of the people was learned (Coe 2003). It is for this reason that anthropologists have seen traditions as embedded in social support (Corin 1995), as identifiers of group membership, and as very difficult to change without damaging important social ties (Coe 2003). Ethnicity is often communicated by using such things as distinctive cuisine and body decoration. Many ethnic groups have had explicit rules specifying that clan or tribal "brothers" or "sisters" were to be treated as if they were real brothers and sisters. "Siblings" were to be treated preferentially; outsiders (e.g., those of another clan or tribe) were not to be given the same consideration. One function of ethnic costumes and outfits seems to have been to identify, continuously and unambiguously, cooperative units – the ethnic groups. For much of human history, it would have been important to identify one's affiliation with certain others and dangerous to point out one's distinctiveness, or lack of membership. Farley recognized this separation when he wrote, "we are all ethnics; we represent some groupings of people who are or have been separate or different from other groupings of people" (Farley 1988, p. 2). Others have emphasized the importance of the we-they component of ethnicity when describing the "...unity that characterizes all ethnic groups... Despite differences, there is an overarching sense of 'we' (and of 'they') that emerges when collective fates and interests are at stake and when the larger group confronts outsiders" (Nagel 1996).

The failure to understand the vertical nature of culture led many sociologists to see culture as a product of horizontal social conformity acquired through proximity and readily subject to change. For this reason, sociologists predicted, especially in the decades after World War II, the demise of ethnicity. They felt that the horizontal social conformity they thought essential to ethnic identification would break down in industrialized, urban societies such as the United States (Park 1950; Wilson 1967; Bonacich 1980; Keefe, Padilla et al. 1987). It was believed that ethnic groups would eventually disappear because technology is associated with urbanism that is, in turn, associated with mobility and the loss of community. Individualism (refusing to conform to others around you) and growing alienation (implied by this lack of conformity) would thus result in the loss of ethnicity.

While many of the traditional behaviors associated with ethnic groups have disappeared, it is important to recognize that identification with ethnic groups has not. A number of studies conducted in the second half of the 20th century have shown maintenance of or increase in ethnic identification despite a historical loss of traditions and weakening of mechanisms that protected ethnic boundaries (e.g., rules of endogamy; loss of ancestral language) (Scupin 2003). For example, American individuals of Irish descent continue to identify with their ancestry despite the fact the family may have been in America for generations and the descendants have never traveled to Ireland. While many traditional behaviors that once distinguished ethnic groups have disappeared, the ethnic wars now occurring around the world demonstrate that ethnicity, including the strong passions associated with in-group membership and the antagonism directed against outsiders, remains (Coe 2003; Scupin 2003).

Ethnicity is further complicated by the fact that there are nearly an infinite number of common ancestors that could be used to delineate an ethnic group. A focus on more distant common ancestors identifies a larger ethnic group because it implies a larger set of co-descendants, while a focus on a more recent common ancestor identifies a smaller ethnic group (Palmer 1997). All mammals, for example, share a common ancestor, although that ancestor is quite distant. All humans share a closer common ancestor with each other than with other mammals. A Hopi shares a more recent common ancestor with other Hopi than with members of other Pueblo tribes. However, a Hopi shares a more recent common ancestor with members of other Pueblo tribes than with members of Athabascan tribes, such as the Navajo and Apache. A Hopi may share a more recent common ancestor with other American Indians, including the Athabascans, than with those of European descent (Dillehay 2001). Humans routinely expand or contract their ethnic category by focusing on more distant or nearer common ancestors in different situations. For example, a person may be a Lakota in one situation and a Native American in another.

The use of cultural behaviors and their products to identify ethnicity also complicates the concept of ethnicity. Individuals can manipulate their ethnicity by manipulating their cultural behaviors. Sociologists have noted that the ethnicity claimed by an individual could change depending on the social situation (Nagata 1974; Cohen 1978; Okamura 1981; Nagel 1996). Individuals, particularly given the mixed ancestry of most Americans, can identify with different ethnic groups at different times, there are limitations. As van den Berghe points out, "the fiction of kinship, even in modern indus-trial societies, has to be sufficiently credible for ethnic solidarity to be effective. One cannot create an instant [ethnic group] by creating a myth. The myth has to be rooted in historical reality to be accepted. Ethnicity can be *manipulated* but not *manufac-tured*" (Van den Berghe 1981). The tie of ethnicity to at least a plausible approxima-tion of ancestry is what makes ethnicity a more powerful concept than culture.

The importance of the interactive view of development when applied to health is il-lustrated by Alcock, who writes:

"... every visible attribute of every organism is the product of a marvelously complex and all-pervasive interaction between genes and environment. The evidence for the interactive theory of development is overwhelming, but a nice illustration of the point comes from work showing that persons with different genes can develop similar traits given the appropriate environments. A famous example of this sort comes from studies of a human gene we will label PAH. ... [I]ndividuals with certain alleles of the PAH gene make forms of phenylalanine hydroxylase that may fail to do their job properly. Persons carrying these variant genes are generally unable to convert phe-nylalanine to tyrosine and therefore phenylalanine typically builds up in their cells. The extra phenylalanine [results] in the formation of considerable amounts of... [phenylpyruvic acid], which happens to be developmentally damaging in large quan-tities... [with] the sad result [being]... a child who suffers from severe mental retar-dation" (Alcock 2001).

Because this form of mental retardation is influenced by a particular gene, individuals unaware of the interactive view of development tend to only focus on this particular factor, calling it a genetic disease that is innate in those who have it. This view is in-accurate because it ignores the other factors involved in the development of the mental retardation.

Because of our recently acquired understanding of the interactive view of develop-ment,

"today any newborn testing positive for phenylketonuria is immediately placed on a highly restrictive diet very low in phenylalanine. This intervention does not change the genes of the babies, but it does change the chemical environment of the brain cells, and thereby helps prevent the buildup of phenylalanine and its devastating by-product, phenylpyruvic acid. As a result, brain cell development usually proceeds more or less normally, as does intellectual development. Thus, having certain alleles of the PAH gene does not condemn one to be mentally retarded. The disease is not genetically determined..." (Alcock 2001).

Identifying Ethnicity Using Proxy Measures

Another advantage to a clear understanding of ethnicity is that it reveals limitations to some of the various ways that are currently used to identify a person's ethnicity. Based on the assumption that culture is acquired horizontally, general geographic ori-gin (e.g., Cuban American, Asian American) was assumed to be a good proxy measure for ethnicity (Ortiz and Arce 1984; Kato 1996). We often continue to see geography as-sociated with ethnicity and race. Patrinos wrote in a recent edition of *Nature Genetics*:

"With very rare exceptions, all of us in the U.S. are immigrants. We bring with us a subset of genes from our homelands, and for many Americans, often first-generation but more commonly second-generation, the plural noun 'homelands' is appropriate" (Patrinos 2004). However, a general geographic place, such as a country, often contains numerous ethnic groups with distinct traditions. For example, the category of Native American contains hundreds of distinct tribes. Limiting geographic origin to a smaller area is helpful, although it does not solve the problem in the case of multiple ethnic groups who inhabit a geographic area.

Other proxy measures for ethnicity are language and surname, but these are also problematic. In the 1930s, the U.S. Census Bureau began to look at Hispanics, persons of Spanish/Hispanic origin, as a separate group (Miranda 1997). An early policy in the southwestern states was to group together individuals with Spanish surnames. This practice was abandoned when a study conducted by the U.S. Census Bureau indicated that about one third of those who claimed Spanish descent did not have Spanish surnames, and around a third of those with Spanish surnames did not claim Spanish descent (United States. Bureau of the Census. 1973). While in the U.S. individuals frequently inherit the last name of their fathers, those individuals may be likely to identify with maternal traditions and ethnic identity. Some surnames are shared with other ethnic groups, such as the Spanish surname Miranda, which is shared by Italians, Portuguese, Filipinos, and Brazilians (Miranda 1997). Language as a proxy measure for ethnicity would lead us to omit individuals who do not speak the language of their ethnic group. For example, a Hispanic individual may or may not speak Spanish. Many entire ethnic groups in the U.S. have lost their traditional language, but continue to identify with the ethnic group.

Failure to define the term ethnicity explicitly and empirically has led to an inability to identify why and how ethnicity might be related to differential health outcomes, and even to the argument that ethnicity may not be an important variable in health research. It is crucial to remember that ethnicity is based on ancestry, and that any number of traditional cultural behaviors may be used to identify a person with that ancestry. This approach facilitates the identification of correlations between ethnicity and health as it focuses attention on any number of possible traditions that might influence health.

Ethnicity and Health

The realization that ethnicity is a combination of genetic and cultural factors does not simplify the relationship between ethnicity and health. It does, however, direct research toward better ways to deal with the complexities of this relationship due to the focus on the inheritance of both genes and traditions that occur in the development of offspring. This makes the concept of ethnicity extremely powerful in sorting out the various genetic and environmental factors that influence individuals and their health. Consider a population where there is a correlation between a health issue and ethnicity. An understanding of what ethnicity is, and of the interactive theory of human development, allows an efficient approach to identifying the genetic and environmental factors involved in the health condition.

If there is a correlation between ethnicity and the health condition, that could mean that the condition is more common within the ethnic group for a number of reasons. The correlation could be due to genes inherited by the recent common ancestry of the ethnic group, the cultural traditions inherited by the recent common ancestry of the ethnic group, or due to some other variable that just happens to correlate with the ethnic group (e.g., residence near a toxic waste dump, socioeconomic class). Differences in health outcomes and in the behaviors that influence those outcomes may be artifacts of the tendency for certain ethnic groups to share a common socioeconomic status (Landry 1987). This realization directs investigators towards the tests needed to determine exactly which factors are related. In addition to genetic testing, variation in traditions within the ethnic group could be examined to determine which factors may be causal.

A number of anthropologists have identified traditions that are important to the persistence and well-being of groups, and hence, likely to be related to some aspect of health.

"Cultural influences on health and medical care involve such basic aspects of human behavior and belief systems as religious practices, language, folk medicine, diet, dress, norms and values, and help seeking behavior. These cultural practices in turn have an impact on perceptions of symptoms, definitions of illness, delivery of health services, disease prevention, health promotion, medical practice and patient adherence" (King and Williams 1995).

Health outcomes are not only influenced by culture, but also by discrimination by the dominant culture, self-imposed isolation, physical environment, resources available, socioeconomic and political factors, limitations of health care (including provider ignorance of the sociocultural determinants of health and disease), or genetic factors (Farley 1988).

People of persistence are those ethnic groups around the world that maintain a unique group identity despite intense contact with other cultures. Anthropologists have argued that the cultural features crucial to persistence include common "language, style of dress and adornment, religion, patterns of social interaction, and food habits" (Crews and Bindon 1991), as well as the close kinship ties that are necessary for and resulting from the transmission of traditions (Coe 2003). Ethnic clothing often functions to continuously and unambiguously identify ethnic or ancestral groups. We know that a member of the Tsachilai tribe is a Tsachila by the manner of their dress, body paint, and even their hair arrangement (Coe 2003). This body decoration is inherited from one's ancestors, identifies one as a descendant of that ancestor, and identifies others who share that ancestry and with whom each must cooperate. Even today in the U.S., individuals who cooperate (e.g., sorority sisters, gang members) tend to dress similarly and often claim metaphorical ancestry. Dietary traditions have been promoted as an important tradition that persists long after other aspects of culture are no longer evident (Van den Berghe 1981). Food-sharing rituals persist because they involve family and reinforce the important kinship ties that form the basis of social support (Van den Berghe 1981).

The importance of tradition is evident in the American Indian populations of the United States. American Indian tribes, as members of unique and diverse ethnic groups, tend to each have rules encouraging respect for elders (e.g., honor your elders who are the bearers of traditions) and ancestors, who are the creators of tradition. Such respect may be necessary for the successful transmission of tradition, including those related to health, and for building strong social relationships. Mothers are important in Native American societies, as families and extended families revolve around them and their children (Coe 2003). "So important are mothers that even very ferocious people...would never hurt a mother because the mother is considered the fountain of kinship" (Briffault 1931).

Religion, which in the past was often inherited from one's ancestors through one's grandparents and parents, is also often associated with rules specifying appropriate kinship behavior. Of importance to the field of cancer prevention, religion and beliefs "are at the core of preventive and curative health practices" (Airhihenbuwa 1995). Healthful behaviors are learned from ancestors via close kin and result in an obligation owed to one's ancestors. Religions around the world promote kinship behaviors that make the transmission of traditions possible. Christians, as one example, encourage individuals to honor their parents and care for their children. This rule, however, is not unique to Christianity. Kinship is the informal hierarchy used for teaching the young and reminding adults of culturally appropriate behavior. Storytelling, along with modeling and guided learning, is the method most often used to teach traditions. Humans respond to stories and they influence behavior (Coe 2003).

Some of the evidence of the relationship between traditions and health are the consequences of losing these traditions. Rapid loss of cultural traditions, whatever the cause, can leave populations vulnerable to certain health problems (Swedlund and Armelagos 1990; Corin 1995; Coe 2003). A loss of traditions, particularly those encouraging kinship behavior, may be associated with an increase in high-risk behaviors, including substance abuse and failure of a pregnant woman to protect her health and the fetus (Coonrod, Bay et al. 2004).

Applications to Disparity Research

Cancer health disparities in ethnic minorities are a serious problem in the United States. If we recognize that ethnicity is inherited and refers to categories of individuals who are co-descendants of a common ancestor, we may begin to understand its importance and the role it may play in both health and research. Ancestors are a key to understanding ethnicity, yet it is important to determine the breadth of how ancestry is defined. The guidelines of the 1990 census recognize the importance of ancestry and inheritance of ethnicity. "A person is of Spanish/Hispanic origin if the person's origin (ancestry) is Mexican, Mexican-American, Chicano, Puerto Rican, Cuban, Argentinean, Colombian, Costa Rican, Dominican, Ecuadorian, Guatemalan, Honduran, Nicaraguan, Peruvian, Salvadorian, from other Spanish-speaking countries of the Caribbean or Central or South America, or from Spain" (United States. Bureau of the Census. 1990).

Although ancestry is included in this definition, the term Hispanic refers to a very heterogeneous population. Hispanics share only a very distant ancestors, perhaps one that lived tens of thousand of years ago, because the ancestors of Hispanics came from indigenous populations spread across the Americas, as well as from populations living in Europe, Asia, and Africa. Some Hispanic ancestors, like those of American Indians, came hundreds or even thousands of years ago from different and diverse ecological habitats. These ancestors brought distinct cultural behaviors that underwent unique adaptations in response to the environment encountered in the New World. These practices were blended with older ones to produce a rich and highly diverse cultural fabric. Today, through the process of acculturation to a more western lifestyle, many of these traditions are rapidly disappearing. Hispanic is an extremely complex term that has historical, social, cultural, legal and political connotations and ramifications.

It is not clear how much of the variance in health outcomes can be explained by unique genetics and cultural practices attributed to such a diverse ethnic category. There are regional patterns and socioeconomic patterns to disease incidence that may or may not be associated with ethnicity. Not unrelated is the fact that in general, ethnic minorities face greater barriers obtaining access to medical care (De la Cancela 1992; Hale 1992). Lack of access to health care providers means not only that diagnoses are underreported, but also that diseases are diagnosed at later and more serious stages. Nevertheless, by recognizing that ethnicity is related to descent, we gain a great deal of understanding. The proper focus on individuals sharing common descent has a genetic component (genes are inherited from ancestors) as well as cultural components (traditions are inherited from ancestors).

Many of the problems currently faced in health research disparities are related to our current inability to understand ethnicity and its importance. Researchers have often used the wrong frame of reference. In so doing, researchers have placed themselves in the position of trying to understand ethnicity from the standpoint of a period of time in which intermarriage, migration, and westernization have led to ethnic groups in which the members have few, if any, cultural traits in common.

For this reason that Fullilove criticized health research for focusing on "small periods of time...[e]ven longitudinal studies are limited to 40 or 50 years. The evolution of human behavior and ecosystems within which it is located must be understood from the perspective of much longer time frames" (Fullilove 1998). Ethnicity, as van den Berge explains, has to be validated by several generations of common historical experience (Van den Berghe 1981, p. 16).

By focusing on ethnicity as a descent category that develops over time we can turn this complex concept into a powerful means of identifying both the genetic and environmental (including cultural) factors influencing health. However, this will only be possible if political agendas are kept separate from the scientific study of ethnicity and health. This represents a considerable challenge because as ethnicity is associated with in-group and out-group identity, it has always been political, associated with judgments of good and bad, appropriate and inappropriate. In 1923, Kroeber cautioned anthropologists, warning them that discussions of race were very likely to be guided by "feeling, usually of considerable strength, which tends to vitiate objective approach" (Kroeber 1923, p. 205). For some researchers and many lay people, ethnicity is pejorative, a name given to minority populations by a "dominant" society. For these individuals, the established race and ethnic classifications or taxonomies in American societies evolved from systems of stratification, power, and ideology (Amick 1995). In this setting, certain populations are seen as marginal, dismissed as "ethnics" because they lack political power and have a low social status (Amick 1995). For others, ethnicity is a positive, "Diversity and ethnicity are basic to our species. Many of us want to be different in belief, looks and actions from others..." (Farley 1988, p. 1). The positive nature of ethnicity may be implied in the way people continue to identify with ethnic groups, long after identifying features have been lost and boundaries erased and even when faced with prejudice for such an identification.

Both of these positions, however, may be guilty of the naturalistic fallacy. From a scientific point of view, ethnicity is neither good nor bad, it just is. Cross-cultural judgments that conclude that some ethnic groups are somehow less or better than others, are simply judgments. To the extent that such judgments affect health and access to health services they are examples of racism or ethnocentrism. Clearly, while this political aspect of ethnicity should be the focus of study, we should recognize that if we are to understand the fundamental meaning of ethnicity, we have to appreciate that there are, inherently, no differential values related to ethnic group membership. All of our ancestors, evolutionarily speaking, were equally successful. They all left behind them a line of descendants that began with the origins of life on earth and continues until today. Ethnicity and race as a political category have unfortunately led to claims that current racial and ethnic designations have little relevance to science and are essentially pragmatic or politically expedient categories (Weissman 1990; Hahn 1992; Hahn, Mulinare et al. 1992). Ethnicity, however, is much more.

Conclusion

Ethnicity cannot be understood as a term useful in scientific study until its necessary elements (genes, environment, heritability, inheritability, culture and traditions) are understood. Once we understand that all these elements play a role in the disease process, we can begin to move forward in the study of the relationship between ethnicity and disease. Both the genetic and environmental background are important. The field of genomics now makes it possible to study the underlying mechanisms of human health in relation to diet and other environmental factors (Desiere 2004). However, the environment is more than drugs and toxic pollutants; it is complex and involves social relationships and traditional behaviors.

Traditions do not only serve as in-group and out-group identification. The process of transmitting a tradition from one generation to the next builds the social relationships that are crucial to health. Health behaviors, today as in the past, are by and large taught in families. Family members are present to reinforce these behaviors. Kinship is centered on a maternal-child relationship that is characterized by the responsibilities the one at the top of the hierarchy, the mother, has to those beneath. Lay health worker programs, which appear to be effective in promoting health, are built on this basic maternal-child, duty-responsiveness model (Staten, Gregory-Mercado et al. 2004). However, more than a benevolent hierarchy is implicated in promoting health behaviors. We ignore families in our health promotion efforts at our peril because families reinforce behaviors in a myriad of ways.

Finally, programs that interest ethnic minorities and non-minorities should be developed based on the methods used in traditional societies to educate the young and to reinforce beliefs among adults. Cultures are holistic; education takes place during all activities of daily living. Learning incorporates the humanities, the spiritual and the pragmatics of subsistence strategies for procuring food. Those from whom we learn are those we trust. Learning traditionally has not been done in a classroom setting but involves modeling and guided practice. A lecture approach to health will never be attractive to most people who have been raised in a rich cultural environment.

References

(1957). *Webster's New World Dictionary of the American Language*. Cleveland, World Publishing.

Airhihenbuwa, C.O. (1995). *Health and culture: beyond the Western paradigm*. Thousand Oaks, Calif., Sage Publishers.

Alcock, J. (2001). *The Triumph of Sociobiology*. New York, Oxford University Press.

Amick, B. C. (1995). *Society and health*. New York, Oxford University Press.

Ashing-Giwa, K.T., G.V. Padilla, et al. (2004). "Breast cancer survivorship in a multiethnic sample: challenges in recruitment and measurement." *Cancer* **101**(3): 450–465.

Bazargan, M., S. H. Bazargan, et al. (2004). "Correlates of cervical cancer screening among underserved Hispanic and African-American women." *Prev Med* **39**(3): 465–473.

Bernier, F. (1684). "A New Division of the Earth, according to the Different Species or Races of Men who Inhabit It." *Journal de Scavans* (April 24).

Bhopal, R. (1999). "Bhopal Responds to Rabin and Buehler." *American Journal of Public Health* **89**(5): 784.

Bhopal, R. and L. Donaldson (1998). "White, European, Western, Caucasian, or what? Inappropriate labeling in research on race, ethnicity, and health." *Am J Public Health* **88**(9): 1303–1307.

Bodmer, W.F. and L. Cavalli-Sforza (1976). *Genetics, Evolution and Man*. San Francisco, W.H. Freeman and Company.

Bonacich, E. (1980). "Class approaches to ethnicity and race." *Insurgent Sociologist* **X**(2): 9–24.

Briffault, R. (1931). *The mothers, the matriarchical theory of social origins*. New York, Macmillan Co.

Buehler, J. W. (1999). "Abandoning race as a variable in public health research." *Am J Public Health* **89**(5): 783; author reply 784.

Bulmer, M. and J. Solomos (1999). *Ethnic and Racial Studies Today*. London, Routledge.

Coe, K. (2003). *The Ancesstress Hypothesis*. Newark, Rutgers University Press.

Cohen, J.J. (2003). "Disparities in health care: an overview." *Acad Emerg Med* **10**(11): 1155–1160.

Cohen, R. (1978). "Ethnicity: Problem and Focus in Anthropology." *Annual Review of Anthropology* **7**: 379–403.

Coonrod, D.V., R.C. Bay, et al. (2004). "Ethnicity, acculturation and obstetric outcomes. Different risk factor profiles in low- and high-acculturation Hispanics and in white non-Hispanics." *J Reprod Med* **49**(1): 17–22.

Corin, E. (1995). The cultural frame: Context and meaning in the construction of health. *Society and health*. B.C. Amick, S. Levine, A. Tarlov and D.C. Walsh. New York, Oxford University Press.

Crews, D.E. and J.R. Bindon (1991). "Ethnicity as a taxonomic tool in biomedical and biosocial research." *Ethn Dis* **1**(1): 42–49.

Cuvier, G., Pritchard, J.C., Agassiz, J., Pickering, C. (1848). *Races of Man and Their Geographical Distribution*.

Damon, A. (1969). "Race, ethnic group, and disease." *Soc Biol* **16**(2): 69–80.

Darling, C.M., C.P. Nelson, et al. (2004). "Improving breast health education for Hispanic women." *J Am Med Womens Assoc* **59**(3): 171, 228–229.

De la Cancela, V. (1992). "Keeping African American and Latino males alive: Policy and program initiatives in health." *Journal of Multi-Cultural Community Health* **2**: 331–339.

Desiere, F. (2004). "Towards a systems biology understanding of human health: Interplay between genotype, environment and nutrition." *Biotechnol Annu Rev* **10**: 51–84.

Dillehay, T. (2001). *The Settlement of the Americas*. New York, Basic Books.

Falconer, D. (1981). *Introduction to Quantitative Genetics*. New York, Longman.

Farley, E. (1988). Cultural diversity in health care: The education of future practitioners. *Ethnicity and Health*. W. Van Horne and T. Tonnesen. Milwaukee, University of Wisconsin, Institute on Race and Ethnicity.

Flinn, M. (1997). "Culture and the evolution of human learning." *Evolution and Human Behavior* **18**: 23–67.

Fullilove, M. T. (1998). "Comment: abandoning "race" as a variable in public health research – an idea whose time has come." Am J Public Health 88(9): 1297–1298.

Gould, S.J. (1981). The Mismeasure of Man. New York, W.W. Norton and Company, Inc.

Guller, U., N. Jain, et al. (2004). "Insurance status and race represent independent predictors of undergoing laparoscopic surgery for appendicitis: secondary data analysis of 145, 546 patients." J Am Coll Surg 199(4): 567–575; discussion 575–577.

Hahn, R.A. (1992). "The state of federal health statistics on racial and ethnic groups." JAMA 267(2): 268–271.

Hahn, R.A., J. Mulinare, et al. (1992). "Inconsistencies in coding of race and ethnicity between birth and death in US infants. A new look at infant mortality, 1983 through 1985." JAMA 267(2): 259–263.

Hale, C. (1992). A demographic profile of African Americans. Health Issues in the Black Community. R.L. Braithwaite and S.E. Taylor. San Francisco, Jossey-Bass: xxix, 371.

Hrdlicka, A. (1905). "Disease of the Indians, more especially of the southwest United States and northern Mexico." Washington Medical Annals 6(3): 72–94.

Kato, P.M. (1996). On nothing and everything: The relationship between ethnicity and health. In: Handbook of Diversity Issues in Health Psychology. P.M. Kato and T. Mann. New York, Plenum Press: xxviii, 439.

Keefe, S.E., A.M. Padilla, et al. (1987). Chicano Ethnicity. Albuquerque, N.M., University of New Mexico Press.

King, G. and D. Williams (1995). Race and Health: A Multidimensional Approach to African-American Health. In: Society and Health. B.C. Amick, S. Levine, A. Tarlov and D.C. Walsh. New York, Oxford University Press: 93–130.

Kroeber, A.L. (1923). Anthropology: Race, Language, Culture, Psychology, Prehistory. New York, Harcourt, Brace and Company.

Kromkrowski, J.A. (2002). Annual Editions: Racae and Ethnic Relations. Guilford, McGraw-Hill.

Landry, B. (1987). The New Black Middle Class. Berkeley, University of California Press.

Leven, I. (1910). "Cancer among the American Indians and its bearing upon the ethnological distribution of the disease." Zeitschrift Krebsforsch 9: 423–425.

Lewontin, R. (1972). "The appointment of human diversity." Evolutionary Biology 6: 381–398.

Lou Biggs, M. and S.M. Schwartz (2004). "Differences in testis cancer survival by race and ethnicity: a population-based study, 1973–1999 (United States)." Cancer Causes Control 15(5): 437–444.

Marrett, L.D. and M. Chaudhry (2003). "Cancer incidence and mortality in Ontario First Nations, 1968–1991 (Canada)." Cancer Causes Control 14(3): 259–268.

Miranda, M. L. (1997). A History of Hispanics in Southern Nevada. Reno, Nev., University of Nevada Press.

Montagu, A. (1962). "The Concept of Race." American Anthropologist 64(5, Part 1): 919–928.

Nagata, J. A. (1974). "What Is a Malay? Situational Selection of Ethnic Identity in a Plural Society." American Ethnologist 1(2): 331–350.

Nagel, J. (1996). American Indian Ethnic Renewal: Red power and the Resurgence of Identity and Culture. New York, Oxford University Press.

Okamura, J. (1981). "Situational ethnicity." Ethnic and Racial Studies 4: 452–465.

Opolka, J.L., K.L. Rascati, et al. (2003). "Role of ethnicity in predicting antipsychotic medication adherence." Ann Pharmacother 37(5): 625–630.

Ortiz, V. and C. Arce (1984). "Language orientation and mental health status among persons of Mexican descent." Hispanic Journal of Behavioral Sciences 6: 127–143.

Palacio, H., J. G. Kahn, et al. (2002). "Effect of race and/or ethnicity in use of antiretrovirals and prophylaxis for opportunistic infection: a review of the literature." Public Health Rep 117(3): 233-51; discussion 231–232.

Palmer, C. and L. Steadman (1997). "Human kinship as a descendant-leaving strategy: a solution to an evolutionary puzzle." Journal of Social and Evolutionary Systems 20(1): 39–52.

Park, R.E. (1950). Race and Culture. Glencoe, Ill., Free Press.

Patrinos, A. (2004). "'Race' and the human genome." Nat Genet 36 (Suppl 1): S1–2.

Reynolds, D. (2004). "Cervical cancer in Hispanic/Latino women." *Clin J Oncol Nurs* **8**(2): 146–150.

Sadun, A.A., V. Carelli, et al. (2002). "A very large Brazilian pedigree with 11778 Leber's hereditary optic neuropathy." *Trans Am Ophthalmol Soc* **100**: 169-178; discussion 178–179.

Samet, J.M., C.R. Key, et al. (1987). "Survival of American Indian and Hispanic cancer patients in New Mexico and Arizona, 1969–1982." *J Natl Cancer Inst* **79**(3): 457–463.

Scupin, R. (2003). *Race and Ethnicity: An Anthropological Focus on the United States and the World*. Upple Saddle River, Prentice Hall.

Smith, H.O., C.R. Qualls, et al. (2004). "Gestational trophoblastic neoplasia in American Indians." *J Reprod Med* **49**(7): 535–544.

Staten, L.K., K.Y. Gregory-Mercado, et al. (2004). "Provider counseling, health education, and community health workers: the Arizona WISEWOMAN project." *J Womens Health (Larchmt)* **13**(5): 547–556.

Swedlund, A.C. and G.J. Armelagos (1990). *Disease in Populations in Transition: Anthropological and Epidemiological Perspectives*. New York, Bergin and Garvey.

Thornhill, R., Palmer, C. (2000). *A Natural History of Rape: Biological Bases of Sexual Coercion*. Cambridge, MIT Press.

Underwood, W., S. De Monner, et al. (2004). "Racial/ethnic disparities in the treatment of localized/regional prostate cancer." *J Urol* **171**(4): 1504–1507.

United States. Bureau of the Census. (1973). *Persons of Spanish origin in the United States, March 1971*. Washington D.C., U.S. Dept. of Commerce Social and Economic Statistics Administration Bureau of the Census: for sale by the Supt. of Docs. U.S. Govt. Print. Off.

United States. Bureau of the Census. (1990). *Your Guide for the 1990 U.S. Census Form*. Washington D.C., U.S. Dept. of Commerce.

Van den Berghe, P. (1981). *The Ethnic Phenomenon*. New York, NY, Elsevier.

Walsh, J.M., C.P. Kaplan, et al. (2004). "Barriers to colorectal cancer screening in Latino and Vietnamese Americans. Compared with non-Latino white Americans." *J Gen Intern Med* **19**(2): 156–166.

Weissman, A. (1990). "'Race-ethnicity': a dubious scientific concept." *Public Health Rep* **105**(1): 102–103.

Westermarck, E. (1921). *The History of Human Marriage*. London, Macmillan.

Wilson, W. (1967). *The Declining Significance of Race*. Chicago, University of Illinois.

Zuckerman, M. (1990). "Some dubious premises in research and theory on racial differences. Scientific, social, and ethical issues." *Am Psychol* **45**(12): 1297–1303.

Complementary and Alternative Approaches to Cancer Prevention

Linda K. Larkey[1], Heather Greenlee[2], and Lewis E. Mehl-Madrona[1]

[1] College of Medicine, University of Arizona, Tucson, AZ 85724
[2] Mailman School of Public Health, Columbia University, New York, NY 10032

Complementary and alternative medicine (CAM) includes a variety of therapeutic approaches not typically taught in conventional medical schools or used by the majority of conventionally trained physicians (Gordon and Curtin 2000). Complementary refers to modalities used to complement, that is, used in addition to conventional medicine, while alternative is usually used to describe treatments intended to replace conventional treatment (Murphy, Morris et al. 1997). Some such practices enjoy a history of research to support claims of efficacy but have not gained popularity among the majority of medical practitioners (e.g., use of acupuncture to reduce chemotherapy-induced nausea) (Dibble, Chapman et al. 2000; Mayer 2000; Shen, Wenger et al. 2000); others either lack or have unsupporting research to back claims of safety or efficacy (e.g., use of milk thistle to protect liver function during chemotherapy) (Ladas and Kelly 2003). Even so, the labeling of which modalities are complementary or alternative may shift over time as research and practice move some into conventional use and disprove others. Some practices less amenable to our current research epistemology may never move out of CAM nomenclature or perceptions (such as multi-modality system approaches, and perhaps, spirituality).

Currently, CAM broadly encompasses a range of substances, practices, practitioners, and belief systems that fall outside of the conventional medical model. CAM substances include botanicals (also known as herbs), vitamins, minerals, specific nutrients, enzymes, foods, and homeopathy. CAM practices include yoga, Qigong, meditation, dietary modifications such as macrobiotic or raw food, and numerous culturally-based interventions focusing on various combinations of body, mind or spiritual interventions. CAM practitioners use therapeutics with varying level of training, with great variation in licensing laws and insurance reimbursement depending on state (United States), province (Canada) or country (Cherkin, Deyo et al. 2002; Eisenberg, Cohen et al. 2002). These practitioners include, but are not limited to, naturopathic physicians, chiropractors, acupuncturists, herbalists (both Western and Chinese), massage therapists, Ayurvedic practitioners, Native American healers, Tibetan physicians, Reiki practitioners, Healing Touch practitioners, and spiritual healers. Although conventional in many cultures, belief systems or perceptions of health, healing and the body that are considered to be CAM by conventional medical practitioners in the United States (U.S.) include Traditional Chinese Medicine (TCM), Ayurvedic medicine, Tibetan medicine, and Native American medicine. These substances, practitioners, practices, and belief systems have undergone varying levels of scientific scrutiny, with the current emphasis in US research focusing on elucidating their biological mechanisms of action.

This chapter first addresses a variety of CAM modalities related to food, spices and botanicals. The research on these modalities most resembles conventional research on mechanisms of action, such as chemoprevention or dietary interventions that effect biochemical changes. This chapter also includes topics that are less well matched to the medical model of biochemical responses, including: (a) approaches based on the mind-body relationship; (b) traditional systems of healing founded in ancient wisdom and practice; and (c) the more esoteric areas of spirituality and energy medicine.

CAM and Cancer Prevention Research

Although there are no proven methods to definitively prevent cancer in either conventional medicine or complementary and alternative medicine (CAM), many of the cancer prevention approaches under investigation focus on dietary changes, nutritional supplements, lifestyle modifications (e.g., exercise), and decreasing environmental exposures, much of which falls into the field of CAM research.

Although the field of research on CAM in treatment of diseases, including cancer, has exploded in the past few years, there is a notable lag in the development of research protocols in the area of cancer prevention. Research on treating disease generally progresses through systematic phases of theory development, lab and animal testing, then small pilot trials to large population studies. However, prevention research may follow a less convenient trajectory. Theories of cancer prevention often originate from correlational, longitudinal databases or observations of populations, national or cultural patterns of diet or lifestyle that might impact cancer rates (Krishnaswamy 1996). Following epidemiologic investigation, potential mechanisms for affecting the precursors or biomarkers of cancer development (and those associated with prevention of recurrence when applicable) are studied. Trials to investigate the effects of actually manipulating such variables and eventually measuring cancer outcomes in CAM have yet to take a prominent role in the U.S. We are only just beginning to see the results of large-scale national trials in conventional chemoprevention (e.g., BCPT, The Breast Cancer Prevention Trial) (Fisher, Costantino et al. 1998) and in nutritional interventions (CARET, Carotene and Retinol Efficacy Trial) (Omenn, Goodman et al. 1996). It will require funding opportunities for preliminary research to investigate CAM to demonstrate its effects on biomarkers before such large investments will be made for research in CAM in cancer prevention in the U.S.

Cancer patients and survivors have increasingly turned to CAM approaches for treatment and alleviating side-effects of treatment, making it more important for researchers to test safety and effectiveness of these alternatives (Bernstein and Grasso 1983; Cassileth and Deng 2004). Since CAM approaches are typically less targeted towards killing cancer cells and more focused on supporting the immune system and strengthen the capacity for self-healing (Gordon and Curtin 2000), such treatment modalities may also serve at-risk or healthy populations for prevention purposes.

The use of CAM in cancer prevention has not been thoroughly evaluated despite growing evidence that the public is utilizing a wide range of practices and products with that intent. In 1990 it was estimated that 425 million visits to CAM providers were made in the U.S. (as compared to 388 million visits to conventional caregivers), and that CAM expenditures for that year in the U.S. amounted to approximately $13.7 billion (Eisenberg, Kessler et al. 1993). Estimates for out-of-pocket expenses rose to $27 to 34 billion by 1997 with a "staggering 629 million visits to alternative practitioners" (Neal 2001). Specific to cancer prevention, a recent study showed that 55% of sampled men with a family member diagnosed with prostate cancer were using some form of CAM and 30% were using supplements specifically purported to be prostate-specific cancer prevention agents (Beebe-Dimmer, Wood et al. 2004).

Foods, Spices, and Herbs

CAM cancer prevention strategies that employ foods, spices, botanicals, and specific nutrients are directed towards specific physiological pathways. Certain agents have a number of possible chemopreventive effects including antioxidant, immune modulating, hormone modulating, anti-angiogenic, apoptotic, and anti-metastatic properties. These have been described elsewhere (Boik 2001; Park and Pezzuto 2002). Some of the most promising candidates for further exploration, according to the existing literature, are summarized here.

The definitive line between a food, a spice and a botanical is easily blurred depending on how substances are prepared or formulated. For example, garlic may be considered a food, a flavoring, or extracted for botanical supplementation. In general, a food is considered something that is eaten as a primary source of nutrition. Much of the food chemoprevention literature focuses on fruits, vegetables and whole foods (i.e. foods that have not been commercially processed) (Vainio and Bianchini 2003). Cruciferous vegetables, fiber and soy are currently under investigation for activity in cancer prevention. These are addressed in this book's chapter on "Body Composition, Diet and Physical Activity." Other research efforts in cancer prevention are focused on the benefits of a specific diet, such as a macrobiotic diet (Kushi, Cunningham et al. 2001).

Spices are the aromatic parts of plants that are used as seasonings, rather than for nutrition. Some spices, as well as many foods, contain concentrated amounts of phytochemicals (naturally occurring biochemicals that give plants their color, flavor, smell, and texture) that may have preventive properties (Polk 1996; Nishino, Tokuda et al. 2000). Many of these properties have been demonstrated in *in vitro* and animal studies, with only limited data in humans (Lampe 2003). Antioxidants, which help prevent free radical formation and damage, are found in cloves, cinnamon, oregano, pepper, ginger, garlic, curcumin, coriander, and cardamom (Wu 2004). Biotransformation enzymes, which metabolize chemical carcinogens, are induced by coriander, curcumin, cinnamon, and *Wasabia japonica* (Japanese domestic horseradish). Garlic, cloves, cinnamon, chili, horseradish, cumin, tamarind, black cumin, pomegranate seeds, nutmeg, onion, and, celery have all demonstrated antibacterial activity. Ginger and curcumin have anti-inflammatory properties.

Botanicals, more commonly known as herbs, may be fresh, dried, freeze-dried, juiced, or extracted. Either the whole or specific parts of the plant are used, including the leaf, flower, stem or root. Much of the cancer-related research on botanicals to date focuses on the role of botanicals to treat cancer (e.g., mistletoe extract) (Zarkovic, Vukovic et al. 2001). However, most research in botanical chemoprevention has been limited to work *in vitro* (cell lines) and *in vivo* (biomarker evaluation).

The specific agents reviewed below provide examples of the various mechanisms being investigated in botanical chemoprevention research: curcumin for its antioxidant and anti-inflammatory properties; flaxseed for its hormone modulating effects; mushrooms for their immune modulating properties; and ginseng for its immune modulating and adaptogenic effects. It is imporant to note that these and other herbal agents have active substances that may interact with other herbs, supplements or medicines and that may have unexpected side effects. Herbal products that modulate certain enzymes or proteins may have adverse interactions with anti-cancer medications (e.g., ginko, echinacea, ginseng, St. Johns wort, kava) (Sparreboom, Cox et al. 2004). All foods, spices and herbs used for medicinal purposes should only be taken under the care and supervision of a practitioner highly trained in the area of botanical medicine.

Curcumin

Curcumin, an extract of tumeric, has attracted attention as a potent antioxidant with anti-inflammatory effects. It has demonstrated antitumorigenesis effects in experimental mouse models (Miquel, Bernd et al. 2002; Youssef, El-Sherbeny et al. 2004). It has also shown protective effects against DNA damage in human peripheral blood lymphocyte cells in both smokers and non-smokers. Recent studies of potential mechanisms of curcumin effects on invasive lung adenocarcinoma cells indicate that it may inhibit invasion via the regulation of selected gene expression (Chen, Yu et al. 2004). In colon cancer cells, curcumin has demonstrated the ability to induce apoptosis in cells expressing Cox-2 (Agarwal, Swaroop et al. 2003). Curcumin is a promising agent with a similar mechanism of action as other agents currently being investigated in the prevention of colon (Xu 2002), breast (Shen and Brown 2003), skin (Bachelor and Bowden 2004) and other cancers (Grossman 2003).

Flaxseed

Flaxseed is rich in lignans (a type of phytoestrogen) and fiber. Lignans are proposed to have chemoprotective properties in breast cancer due to their inhibition of estrogen production; they have been shown to inhibit growth of human mammary tumor cells (Hirano, Fukuoka et al. 1990), reduce mammary tumor initiation (Thompson, Seidl et al. 1996), stimulate sex hormone binding globulin which binds estrogens that increase cancer risk (Adlercreutz, Mousavi et al. 1992), and inhibit aromatase activity which then decreases endogenous estrogen level (Adlercreutz, Mousavi et al. 1992; Adlercreutz, Fotsis et al. 1994). More recent studies have focused on how flaxseed influences endogenous hormone concentration and urinary estrogen metabolites associated with increased cancer risk. Flaxseed in the diet has been shown to significantly reduce serum concentration of 17-beta-estradiol and estrone sulfate (Hutchins, Martini et al. 2001). Flaxseed supplementation significantly increased urinary 2-hydroxyestrone excretion and increased the 2:16 alpha-hydroxyestrone ratio in pre-menopausal (Haggans, Travelli et al. 2000) and post-menopausal women (Haggans, Hutchins et al. 1999). Flaxseed's influence on hormones (e.g., testosterone) and its high content of omega-3 fatty acids has led to initial research on its potential role in the prevention of prostate cancer (Demark-Wahnefried, Price et al. 2001).

Immune modulating mushrooms

Several mushrooms have been identified as having potential immune modulating effects (Pelley and Strickland 2000). Coriolus versicolor, historically used in Traditional Chinese Medicne (TCM), is often used in extract form. A protein-bound polysaccharide-K (PSK) and polysaccharide-P (PSP) from the mushroom is currently under investigation as a preventive and as an anti-cancer agent. Recent research has shown immune-stimulatory actions of these polysaccharides on T lymphocytes, B lymphocytes, monocytes/macrophages, bone marrow cells, natural killer cells, and lymphocyte-activated killer cells as well as promoting the proliferation and/or production of antibodies and various cytokines such as interleukin (IL)-2 and IL-6, interferons, and tumor necrotic factor (Chu, Ho et al. 2002; Fisher and Yang 2002). Maitake mushroom (*Grifola frondosa*) is an edible mushroom that is also under investigation for its anti-cancer properties. The most active ingredients in this mushroom appear to be polysaccharides 1,3 and 1,6 beta-glucan). These constituents are marketed in the form of proprietary D- or MD-fraction extracts. Maitake extracts have been shown to enhance bone marrow colony formation in vitro (Lin, She et al. 2004), induce apoptosis in prostate cancer cells (Fullerton, Samadi et al. 2000), and activate NK cells in cancer patients (Kodama, Komuta et al. 2003).

Ginseng

Several botanicals are purported to have adaptogenic effects that provide resistance to stress and fatigue. The most active components of *Panax ginseng* (Asian ginseng) are ginsenoside saponins (Tyler 1993). There are approximately 30 different saponins that have been isolated from Panax ginseng; a number of these have been evaluated for their potential use in the field of cancer prevention (e.g., ginsenoside Rg_3, Rg_5, Rh_1, and Rh_2) (Yun, Lee et al. 2001). The quantity of ginsenoside in roots vary by type and age of the plant. Ginsenosides have been shown to stimulate the immune system and inhibit cancer cell proliferation (Xiaoguang, Hongyan et al. 1998). Preliminary in vitro and epidemiologic evidence show non-specific preventive effects in multiple tumor sites (Shin, Kim et al. 2000; Yun 2001; Yun, Choi et al. 2001; Yun, Lee et al. 2001; Chang, Seo et al. 2003; Yun 2003).

While these and other botanicals show promise for a number of biological mechanisms related to cancer prevention, randomized controlled trials are needed in humans before they can be advocated as effective chemoprevention agents.

The Mind-Body Connection

Mind-body approaches to health are those practices that generate states of mental and physical relaxation (e.g., meditation), or those that strive to improve attitudes and emotions regarding health (e.g., psychotherapy and support groups). A long history of research has explicated numerous ways in which psychology interacts with physiology. Much of this work has been in the area of stress. The mechanisms of stress, and stress reduction through mind-body techniques, have been thoroughly described through more than five decades of research. Early work on stress and health focused on the correlates of risk and incidence of heart disease (Friedman and Rosenman 1974). In the 1980s, the emerging field of psychoneuroimmunology demonstrated the relationship between the hypothalamus, psychological states and immune function. This work began to extend the paradigm of the stress response to incorporate much more sophisticated models of the interactions between mind and body (Ader, Felten et al. 1991; Pert 1997; Zorrilla, Luborsky et al. 2001).

Much of the CAM literature written for cancer patients provides thorough reviews of mind-body options to consider and suggests the potential use of mind-body techniques for prevention of recurrence of disease (Lerner 1994; Gordon and Curtin 2000). Theories and research exploring the relationship between immune, nervous, and endocrine systems relate these factors directly to the development and progression of cancer. Current theories and ongoing research are contributing to our understanding of the effects of analogues of hypothalamic hormones on hormone-dependent cancer, the role of opioids and melatonin on cytokines, gene modulation, and the immune responses to psychotherapy in cancer patients (Temoshok 1987; Holland 1989; Schipper, Goh et al. 1995; Conti 2000; Elenkov and Chrousos 2002).

Stress and Immunity

Stress has a central role in health and well-being; the cascading effects of stress are known to have numerous consequences. Initially affecting the sympathetic nervous system with concomitant releases of epinephrine and norepinephrine, stress raises blood pressure and heart rate as a coping response. Activation of the hypothalamic-pituitary-adrenal (HPA) axis mediates the body's response to stress, exerting effects on the various peripheral target tissues through glucocorticoids. The acute stress response is associated with beneficial effects that help the individual survive a challenge by mobilizing fuels for energy, inhibiting reproductive behavior and increasing arousal and vigilance. However, when the body is chronically challenged, whether it is continuous or in intervals that are too frequent to allow for recovery and/or adaptation, these effects are detrimental and lead to an increased risk of disease (Raison and Miller 2001). Dysregulation of the sympathetic nervous system/HPA axis (due to increased exposure to cortisol), is hypothesized to contribute to the physiological decrements that accompany diseases associated with aging and suppressed immune function, factors implicated in cancer risk.

Interventions that use combinations of meditation, breathing, and movement indicate that responses to stress may be attenuated through such practice. Mind-body methods then emphasize breathing along with progressive muscle relaxation, meditation, yoga postures, or autogenic training (a technique that uses a combination of attention and somatic suggestion to assist relaxation) have been shown to help in reduction of hypertension (Astin, Shapiro et al. 2003), increased phagocytic activity (Peavey, Lawlis et al. 1985) and lowering of cortisol levels (Schmidt, Wijga et al. 1997; Kamei, Toriumi et al. 2000; Gaab, Blattler et al. 2003). Mindfulness meditation has become one of the more standardized and popular methods of meditation taught in the West. Studies show direct improvements of immune function among other health indicators in response to this form of meditation, which focuses on breathing, relaxation and a full consciousness of one's surroundings (Kabat-Zinn 1994; Williams, Kolar et al. 2001; Davidson, Kabat-Zinn et al. 2003). Popular among cancer patients since the late 1970s are the visualization techniques promoted by Carl Simonton (Simonton, Simonton et al. 1978). Preliminary studies of this technique have shown improvements in leucocyte and natural killer cell activity in response to imagery of healthy immune systems and retreating cancer cells (Achterberg and Lawlis 1984; Kiecolt-Glaser, Glaser et al. 1985; Gruber, Hall et al. 1988).

Qigong and tai chi exercises, ancient TCM practices that include breathing and movement, are often seen as mind-body approaches to health. Tai chi is one of the forms of qigong exercise that has become increasingly popular in the U.S.; qigong is gaining in use and popularity. The effects of qigong and tai chi are theoretically linked to the reduction of stress (Kerr 2002). These practices hold potential for affecting the immune system; there are reports of increased phagocytic activity, lymphocyte transformation, and improved cytokine profiles among those who practice qigong (Liu, Xu, Guomin et al. 1988; Chen and Yeung 2002) and similar results have been shown for tai chi practice (Wang, Collet and Lau 2004). One of the few studies of Qigong exercise effects on immunological function published in the U.S. showed a reduction in cortisol and an increase in the number of the cytokine-secreting cells (in particular, significant increases in the IFNgamma:IL10 ratio) (Jones 2001). Although much of the research on the mind-body connection has been done in the context of cancer patients, immune system responses may arguably translate to cancer prevention for those who utilize mind-body techniques in the context of wellness (Engelking 1994).

Psychological States, Interventions, and Cancer

Although theories have been proposed to associate certain predispositions of personality or psychological factors with the development of cancer, the research has been inconsistent making it difficult to summarize conclusions (Garssen and Goodkin 1999). Prospective studies have implicated a number of possible psychological risk factors for developing cancer, with the most consistent finding being repression of emotion or depression (Dattore, Shontz et al. 1980; Temoshok, Heller et al. 1985; Hislop, Waxler et al. 1987; Temoshok 1987; Kaasa, Mastekaasa et al. 1989) yet even these have been disputed (Hahn and Petitti 1988; Kreitler, Chaitchik et al. 1993). Preliminary understanding of these issues might best be studied in the context of survival, in that the factors influencing survival time may represent similar mechanisms that prevent recurrence.

Work with animal models has clearly shown a relationship between psychological determinants and tumor growth (LaBarba 1970; Sklar and Anisman 1981; Visintainer, Seligman et al. 1983), but in the human arena the relationship between psychology and the course of cancer progression is less clear. Factors shown to improve outcomes include social support (Ell, Nishimoto et al. 1989; Waxler-Morrison, Hislop et al. 1991), greater expression of distress, smaller numbers of severe or difficult life events (Ramirez, Craig et al. 1989), and "fighting spirit" (Pettingale, Morris et al. 1985). A discussion of the potential role of psychological variables moved to the forefront in 1989 with the publication of research that found a positive effect of a psychosocial intervention on breast cancer patients' survival time (a study that has since been called into question due to differences in baseline characteristics of patients and other study design issues) (Spiegel, Bloom et al. 1989). This study kicked off a series of similar research projects, but all trials specifically designed to test the impact of a psychological intervention on survival have so far given inconclusive results. Nevertheless, clinical experience points to the existence of a minority of cancer patients who make strong efforts to help themselves psychologically and appear to live longer than expected (Ikemi, Nakagawa et al. 1975; Achterberg, Mathews-Simonton et al. 1977; Roud 1986; Berland 1995).

Cunningham (Cunningham, Phillips et al. 2000; Cunningham, Phillips et al. 2002) conducted an exploratory study on metastatic cancer patients enrolled in a year-long psychospiritual intervention. Standard psychometric instruments did not predict length of survival in this study, but a subsequent analysis of qualitative interview data from 22 participants suggested that there may be a survival benefit among those who (a) believed that the group activity would help them, (b) invested a greater level of effort in the group activities, (c) engaged to a greater degree in personal and spiritual change, and (d) had improved perceptions of quality of life as compared to those who did not.

This finding may help explain the inconclusive results of previous studies that have randomized patients to intervention or control groups; those predisposed to involve themselves in psychological work may find opportunities in the context of an intervention or may seek such opportunities on their own. Furthermore, if only a small proportion of the patients in a therapy group become strongly involved in trying to help themselves psychologically, and theirs are the only lives substantially prolonged, this effect may be "diluted out" when group means are calculated. A randomized, controlled trial would thus need to be exceedingly large to produce a reliable treatment effect and would likely need to control for patients' expectations.

Given Cunningham's findings, there is reason to suspect that, although more challenging to design than originally thought, there is great potential for finding more robust relationships between the psychological, social, and even spiritual factors associated with patient involvement in their own healing. Preventing a recurrence of cancer may similarly be dependent upon a set of psychoneuroimmunological factors. Although developing a sense of purpose in life, having a supportive community, and having faith for healing may not manifest in the same way with healthy individuals as with those who have been challenged by a diagnosis of cancer, these factors are worth examining as reducing risk for disease as well as improving patient quality of life.

Social support and spirituality have been shown to be related to longevity and general health. Improved outcomes have been demonstrated in some studies of cancer patients who have strong social support (Worden and Weisman 1975; Funch and Marshall 1983); other studies have found no survival benefit (Goodwin, Leszcz et al. 2001). Investigations of the relationships between spirituality and cancer is based on the evidence that overall improved health has been shown to be related to spirituality, and healthy behaviors have been correlated with religious practice (Schiller and Levin 1988; Levin and Vanderpool 1991; Daaleman, Perera et al. 2004; Daniels, Merrill et al. 2004; Reindl Benjamins and Brown 2004). Continuing to explore social, psychological, and spiritual factors related to the mind-body connection may prove fruitful, but there remains a need for evidence regarding the specific mechanisms of these mind-body approaches that affect cancer outcomes.

Wellness

Much of the interest in CAM from the public and practitioners has been guided by and intrinsically linked to emerging views based on the concept of "wellness." The wellness concept became popular in the early 1970s, and out of that original thrust, many wellness centers began to emerge, some with a cancer focus, most without a particular disease focus. The term "wellness" has come to denote a way of thinking about health that goes beyond the simple absence of disease. In theory, wellness is not necessarily sought from a position of avoiding disease, but is holistic in the sense that it seeks to achieve greater balance and awareness in body, mind, and spirit, an evolution of one's whole being (Benson and Stuart 1993).

Several of the culturally-based systems of health, such as Traditional Chinese Medicine (TCM), Ayurvedic medicine, and practices associated with Native American healing, match the holistic precepts of wellness. Although there may be practitioners and patients with a single-minded focus on a particular modality, most proponents of CAM view health as multifaceted, promoting balance and wellness of body, mind, and spirit. Because the systems promoting wellness tend to be broad in focus, prevention of a specific disease such as cancer is not an exclusive goal. Nevertheless, the expected outcomes of improved wellness include enhanced immune function, stamina and overall well-being, factors that may reduce the risk of cancer as well as other diseases.

There is a particular challenge for drawing conclusions about the cancer preventive potential of wellness-focused systems. Most are promoted as an entire wellness package, where a set of principles guide lifestyle, such as diet, form of exercise, meditation or other mindful practices, spiritual views, and even botanicals, specifically chosen for balance based on the philosophy of that system. In the context of cancer treatment, several of these systems propose paradigms of etiology and progression, as well as healing, that are very different from the Western medical model, which focuses on the treatment of a specific diagnosis or symptom.

Researching non-Western systems is problematic. The multiple modalities usually prescribed for treatment are based on individual readings of the various levels of involvement in body, mind, social, environmental, and spiritual factors. Research methods are not designed to test non-Western systems that treat every individual differently according to particular needs. Because of the lack of accepted research methodology that is able to test this holistic approach to health, it is important that health care practitioners become aware of, and researchers to begin to solve the puzzles of, scientifically understanding these integrated systems.

CAM practitioners promote balance for healing or for overall well-being, but the goals of achieving wellness are put into the hands of the individual taking responsibility for her or his own health (Wong and McKeen 2001). The movement toward self-responsibility in health and examining life as a whole are principles that sprouted in Western culture. This movement took place concurrently with a rekindled interest in more natural forms of healing that included mind-body approaches, spirituality, and non-Western medical practices, and has been especially powerful among cancer patients (Tatsumura, Maskarinec et al. 2003).

An exemplar of this philosophy is the Wellness Community, an international network of non-profit centers "dedicated to providing free emotional support, education and hope for people with cancer and their loved ones" (Benjamin 1995; Penson, Talsania et al. 2004). Using a whole-person (holistic) approach, patients are encouraged to actively support each other "to regain control, reduce feelings of isolation and restore hope-regardless of the stage of disease" (Penson, Talsania et al. 2004). Varieties of meditation, Qigong, massage, yoga, Reiki, healing touch, and other such practices are common in these centers, which make available to cancer patients a supportive community as well as opportunities for spiritual, emotional and physical healing.

Popular writers such as Dr. Bernie Seigel (Seigel 1990) and Dr. Andrew Weil (Weil 1995) have intrigued the minds of readers with stories of healing as well as stories of profoundly changed lives. Many of these stories are recounted in books that catch the attention of the public, inspiring faith in the human ability to get well and stay well. For example, Dr. Caroline Myss, in her book about power and healing, suggests exploring symbolic meaning and balance, taking the reader through religious symbols, archetypal challenges, and stage-of-life passages to address life lessons and points of transition (Myss 1996). Moving through these lessons with conscious response is theorized to bring spiritual health cascading down through the psychological and physical systems. Even though Dr. Myss describes case histories of patients with cancer or precancerous conditions who get well, there is not sufficient documentation of measurable physiological outcomes over time, nor comparison to matched cases, to draw conclusions.

Research on spontaneous remission was more prevalent in the early 1900s; numerous examples defy our current understanding of the disease process (O'Regan and Hirshberg 1993). A common ingredient in these healing testimonies is spirituality (Hammerschlag 1988; Struve 2002). It is important for the reader to understand that these are testimonies, not scientific research. The role of spirituality in wellness, although only emerging in western societies over the past few decades, might be seen as a reclamation of ways of viewing health and life that have been prevalent in most cultures and societies worldwide.

Indigenous Cultural Systems of Healing

Many cultures throughout the world have produced comprehensive, sophisticated systems of describing disease states and methods of healing that are very different from the Western medical model. What characterizes many of the systems, and distinguishes them from western medicine, is the tendency to consider health to be a system of balance among body, mind and spirit-often including social and environmental factors as part of the whole in some systems, rather than a constellation of biochemical and hormonal balances identified at a microbiological level. From African healing arts to Samoan fofo; from Native American ceremony to Traditional Chinese Medicine, it appears that nearly all of the indigenous cultural systems view human health in the context of the natural world around us as well as the interaction of physical elements with mind and spirit (Kaptchuk 1983; Mehl-Madrona 2003; Mishra, Hess et al. 2003).

Each of these systems of healing typically has theories of how particular diseases develop, and consequently suggest tactics for prevention. Health and disease is understood in the context of a particular person's experience of life, family, dietary and environmental factors, social conditions, and spiritual responses. Ayurvedic medicine and Native American healing are given as two examples of systems of healing that promote living in harmony with nature, with one's given constitution, and connecting to spirit as ways to stay healthy.

Ayurveda

In Ayurvedic medicine, the build-up of toxic residues termed "ama" (more than physical substances in biomedical terms, but more subtle essences produced by imbalances in living, diet, and mental/emotional states) is believed to be one of the main causes of cancer. Recognizing one's primary "doshas," or essential natures, and living a lifestyle to manage and balance these elements alongside cleansing techniques designed to rid the body of ama, are considered to be the best approach to avoiding cancer from the Ayurvedic point of view (Chopra 2000; Herron and Fagan 2002). Ayurvedic medicine uses the terms "mind" and "consciousness" to refer to the origin of physical conditions. "When you look at Ayurveda's anatomical charts, you don't see the familiar organs pictured in Gray's Anatomy, but a hidden diagram of where the mind is flowing as it creates the body. This flow is what Ayurveda treats" (Chopra 1989).

Although the combination of these many lifestyle and mind-body approaches are seen as central to treating cancer, one agent Maharishi-4, an Ayurvedic food supplement, has been shown to regress mammary tumors in rats and has been evaluated for other anti-cancer effects due to its potent anti-oxidant properties (Fields 1990; Sharma, Dwivedi et al. 1990). Given that this is only one of the many modalities used in Ayurvedic medicine, and more emphasis is placed on building balance through assessment and lifestyle changes to support essential constitutions, much work must be done to test the potential for this system to affect cancer risk. Singh (Singh 2002). provides a much needed framework for presenting various aspects of Ayurvedic practice in cancer treatment, linking theoretical constructs of that system to potential explanations of medical biomarkers that could be explored to begin explicating mechanisms of action for treatment and prevention.

Deepak Chopra, M.D., has done much to promote the concept of mind-body healing and wellness through his center and his book entitled *Perfect Health; The Complete Mind-Body Guide*. This book repackaged Ayurvedic principles of healing into an approach more palatable to Western tastes. The details of the Ayurvedic system are generalized to principles that are recognizable in modern wellness teaching (Chopra 2000). Such programs continue to represent the basic tenets of wellness–balance in life and responsiveness to life's lessons. These basic tenets are hypothesized to bring optimum health, and hence may also prevent cancer.

Native American Healing Traditions

With so many tribes indigenous to the Americas, each with unique healing traditions, it becomes impossible to define a particular tradition as representative of Native American healing. There are, however, some themes that are common throughout the Americas. For example, Native American healers generally do not conceptualize a medicine-religion differentiation. Healing must acknowledge an Inner Healer. According to Dineh (Navajo) healer, Thomas Largewhiskers, this inner force explains why people get well or not, or how they stay healthy in the first place (Largewhiskers 2004). Many tribes and other indigenous cultures teach that spirit is indivisible from mind and body and that a healthy balance and connection with spirit is the path to prevention of disease.

An important source for connecting with spirit for healing and balance, for healthy and ill alike, is ceremony. Ceremony is not unique to Native American culture; it is often represented in one form or another in health systems that include a spiritual component (Hammerschlag and Silverman 1997). The importance of ceremony is consistent with the hypothesis that religiosity/spirituality may be associated with physiological processes – including cardiovascular, neuroendocrine, and immune function (Seeman, Dubin et al. 2003). Immune function is important in cancer and its prevention. Although the evidence has not demonstrated that spirituality slows the progression of cancer, studies conducted to date have been small and limited (Powell, Shahabi et al. 2003). In cultural systems that involve ceremony, prevention should address mind, body, and spirit.

Native American healing practices often hinge upon the skills of the medicine man who is able to intervene for the patient in the spirit world, and can "see" or listen to messages provided by Spirit to help the patient, including how to change aspects of the person's individual spirit or energy body through sound, touch, or prayer. This is a traditional way of viewing what is now often called "energy medicine," a field that combines technology, physics, and ancient wisdom for healing.

Energy Medicine

Energy medicine is often used to refer to practices that involve subtle or very low intensity nonmaterial stimuli for purposes of healing (Rubik 1995). These stimuli may be artificially generated electromagnetic fields (e.g., Pulsed Electromagnetic Field Therapy) or healing energies emitted by humans (e.g., Reiki, Healing Touch), and are theorized to work by causing a change in the human biomagnetic energy field and subsequently in biochemical responses.

Energy medicine includes a wide range of therapies. As noted above, many of the indigenous systems of healing acknowledge a life force such as Qi (the force that runs through meridians as defined in TCM), prana (in yoga practice and Ayruvedic medicine) or the fields of energy perceived and manipulated by those practicing any of the forms of energy healing (e.g., Healing Touch, Reiki, Therapeutic Touch). For purposes of this review, a broad definition will be used to encompass any modality designed to improve overall balance of the energy field either through internal intent or external application. The mechanisms by which energy healing may work to improve health are still being explicated. Without knowing yet whether there is one underlying principle or many ways in which nonmaterial stimuli might affect energy fields and, in turn, biological outcomes, these modalities will be considered as similar in this review.

The term "biomagnetic field" refers to the various electromagnetic fields that run through and around the body (Oschmann 2000). Electrical impulses generated in the heart and brain (as measured conventionally via electroencephalograph, or EEG, and electrocardiogram) are known to generate biomagnetic fields. Such fields have been detected by trained energy medicine practitioners as emanating from the whole body as well as specific parts, notably the hands.

The most controversial aspect of energy medicine is the assumption that biomagnetic fields are more than artifacts of electrical activity in the body and that they not only provide indicators of health, but that they can be altered to produce improved states of health. For example, TCM is based on the concept that there are flows of energy that can be mapped representationally across the surface of the skin (although they are believed to flow through and beyond the limits of the physical body). These flows have names that link them to organs of the body (e.g., liver meridian or kidney flow), but their function is seen as much broader, including emotional and symbolic as well as physiological functions.

Applications of electromagnetic fields within certain frequency ranges have been shown to have a number of biological consequences with potential application in medicine. Pain control using transcutaneous electrical nerve stimulation (TENS) is one of the more well-known developments in energy medicine. Tissue regeneration, bone repair (Sharrard 1990), improvements in osteoarthritis (Trock, Bollet et al. 1993), soft tissue wound healing (Becker 1990; O'Connor, Bentall et al. 1990), neuroendocrine modulations, and immune system stimulation (Cadossi, Emilia et al. 1988; Cadossi, Iverson et al. 1988; Cossarizza, Monti et al. 1989) have all been documented in response to various forms of electromagnetic stimuli. The usefulness for such externally, artificially applied therapies for cancer prevention have not been demonstrated; response to such therapies has only been documented in the context of disease.

The purpose for addressing the emerging field of energy medicine in the context of cancer prevention is twofold: 1) to explicate the non-Western theories underlying energy medicine approaches; and 2) to discuss the theory inherent in energy medicine-based systems that early correction of stagnation or imbalances in energy patterns may lead to the prevention of cancer. Non-Western theories are based on the concept that there are flows of energy or essence patterns in the body that are dynamically balanced and must not be blocked; the blockages of energy will allow the development of disease, including tumors and eventually cancer. Energy based medicine systems attempt to unblock these flows through various methods such as acupuncture treatments, specifically designed Qigong exercises, or externally applied biomagnetic emissions from the hands of a healer. Even more remarkable is the hypothesis that detection of neoplastic changes may be possible with methods that assess Qi imbalance.

One of the oldest documented forms of energy healing is the practice of qigong. An area of practice foreign to western medicine and philosophy, qigong is typically considered to be comprised of two forms, external and internal qigong. External qigong or external qi healing ("wai qi" or "wei qi") (Cohen 1997; Johnson 2000), an ancient Chinese method of healing touch, refers to the emission or direction of qi, theoretically similar to healing touch methods described above. It is administered by transfer from the hands of experienced qigong practitioners to other individuals for the purposes of healing or improving health. Trials of healer interventions have demonstrated a variety of healing effects on the human body (Benor 1993; Schwartz, Swanick et al. 2004).

The potential for Qigong exercises (i.e., internal qigong) designed to balance the meridians to have an effect on health indicators such as cytokine profiles has already been discussed in the section on mind-body interventions. Emitted qi also has been shown in numerous studies to have immune modulating effects, mostly reported from research conducted in China with incomplete information on study design (Liu). Preliminary evidence is good for demonstrating potential of qi emission to strengthen cellular immune function in animal models and humans.

More notable are the results that are beginning to be published in the U.S. on effects of qi emission (external qigong) on growth of induced lymphoma in mice. Although results seemed inconclusive relative to varying abilities of practitioners, one of the studies showed significant differences in tumor inhibition between intervention and control mice (Chen, Shiflett et al. 2002).

Beyond these claims, most of which focus either on healing for specific conditions, or improvement in immune status, there is much to be learned from the theories and practice of qigong. In this paradigm of health, the goal of balancing qi is woven through the practices. From the qi emission from the hands of a master practitioner who "sees" the blockages and areas of need in the biofield, to the exercises designed for movement of qi through specific meridians, to the herbal remedies that stimulate, calm or unblock meridian flow, each modality is intended to move one toward greater health. Validating through research a system so focused on prevention of disease, catching the imbalances in the energy field before illness manifests, seems unlikely.

Many people are familiar with the idea that TCM includes a range of modalities, such as acupuncture and herbal remedies. What is less well-understood is that these treatments are all designed to influence the energy map of the body; in TCM, a network of energy lines called meridians represent various organs and functions, physical and emotional, and the balance of these are purported to maintain health. The theory behind a particular remedy is not necessarily direct action upon an organ or a biochemical reaction (as is the case with Western views of herbs), but rather its effects on promoting, inhibiting, or balancing the targeted energy meridians (Kaptchuk 2002).

Explanations for what structures in the body might account for positional relationships to energy phenomena have more recently been proposed, most notably in the context of acupuncture. The clinical efficacy of acupuncture has been demonstrated in numerous studies, yet the theories of how it functions according to TCM are often not accepted even by physicians who practice this form of energy medicine (Kaptchuk 2002). Neurohumoral approaches in acupuncture research were instrumental in establishing the scientific validity of acupuncture. Recent advances in the morphogenetic singularity theory suggest that acupuncture points originate from the organizing centers in morphogenesis. Possible mechanisms of action are not necessarily dependent upon an association with nervous or lymphatic systems; acupuncture points and meridians have been shown to have high electric conductance that is related to high density of gap junctions in cellular structure (Shang 1993; Shang 2001).

There is evidence that acupuncture has immunomodulatory effects (Petti, Bangrazi et al. 1998; Kaptchuk 2002). For example, T cells and activity of NK cells in cancer patients treated with acupuncture have been shown to remain stable over the course of chemotherapy (Ye, Chen et al. 2002). In a group of relatively healthy young volunteers, acupuncture normalized leukocytes (Mori, Nishijo et al. 2002).

There are numerous modalities of healing that are theorized to involve the interaction of biomagnetic fields between two humans, one "sending" healing, the other "receiving". These include practices such as Reiki therapy, Johrei, Healing Touch, Therapeutic Touch, and laying on of hands in the context of prayer (Anderson 2001). Although practitioners from these various fields of practice may argue for marked differences in their intent and work, studies examining the biomagnetic fields emitted from the hands of healing practitioners across disciplines found similarity. Pulsing magnetic fields of extremely low frequency (ELF) emitted from the hands have been detected, the majority falling between 7–10 Hz with a range of 0.03 to 30 Hz (Zimmerman 1990; Seto, Kusaka et al. 1992). Similarly, healing practitioners using a variety of modalities also demonstrate similar EEG signatures while in the healing mode, altered state, or in prayerful focus (Beck 1986). Although healing effects of emissions in these studies were not tested, the frequencies measured all fell into the same range as those electromagnetic device therapies shown to have specific healing outcomes (e.g., 7 Hz for bone growth, 15–20 Hz for capillary formation and fibroblast proliferation) (Sisken and Walker 1995).

Speculations about how healing interventions may work vary. One explanation is that "intent" may have an effect through the mind on the frequencies emitted and received. Recent developments in the science of mind and experiments of consciousness are beginning to reveal effects for "intent" on physical matter, such as re-configuration of water molecules (Tiller 1997). Another theory suggests that physical resonance develops via "entrainment" (an accepted principle in physics whereby pulsing of waves or rhythms produced by pendulums in close proximity will entrain to the point of resonance) between the healer and target. Evidence of the potential for this explanation is provided in the work of Russek and Schwartz who show that even without intent for healing, two people sitting quietly with eyes closed in the same room will tend to couple both cardiac and brain wave rhythms (Russek and Schwartz 1994; Russek and Schwartz 1996).

The nature of human biofield-based energy healing has not been fully explained, but the effects have been well documented in randomized, controlled clinical trials on healing interventions such as Healing Touch, Therapeutic Touch and similar modalities. Despite continuing questions about exact modes of action, energy healing has been shown to significantly increase secretory immunoglobulin A (Wardell and Engebretson 2001; Wilkinson, Knox et al. 2002), enhance immune system response (Quinn and Strelkauskas 1993; Ryu, Jun et al. 1995; Kataoka, Sugiyama et al. 1997) and produce relaxation or stress-reduction effects in general (Wirth, Cram et al. 1997). Other research has shown consistent results for improving quality of life and reducing stress-related symptoms in cancer patients undergoing treatment (Post-White, Kinney et al. 2003; Cook, Guerrerio et al. 2004). Although the application of the findings from these studies and the potential for cancer prevention has not yet been investigated, the results of these studies should attract enough attention to begin investigations of effects on biomarkers related to cancer risk or protection.

Large, randomized clinical trials that also allow for individualized treatment and practice plans, as is common in many forms of complementary and alternative medicine, do not currently fit research design standards in the U.S. Until research is able to be designed to encompass such studies, only small parts of this puzzle may be examined to assess potential. One such puzzle piece may be the research that is beginning to emerge in the field of energy medicine through instruments designed to assess meridian flow.

Although the use of diagnostic methods such as "seeing" imbalances in the human energy field (the mark of a Qigong master being the ability to see or detect Qi imbalances without the need of questioning, blood tests, or even hands-on pulse readings) may seem foreign to the western medical mind, there are recent developments in measurement of biofield emissions that correlate with and validate these fields. For example, acupuncture meridians and stimulation/collection points are detectable via instruments such as the MSA-21 that assesses electrical impedance along the meridians (Roberts 2002).

Instruments are available to assess flow of electrical potential across entire meridians, such as the Gas Discharge Visualization device (GDV). The GDV captures the biofield emissions surrounding each of the 10 fingers resulting in the measurement of biophotonic discharge that is in direct proportion to the amount of energy flowing through the 14 main meridians. The coronal discharges measured by the GDV are detected as a result of the human bio-energy field interacting with the electrical field of the device. At the time of measurement, the emitted light from the interaction is captured by a video camera, and then the images are analyzed with sophisticated software using a mathematical tool known as fractal dimensionality. The data can be integrated over the whole body resulting in a quantifiable analysis of the energy flow and balance throughout the meridian system (Korotkov 2002).

Experiments with the GDV in Russia have suggested potential for the detection of breast cancer. A study of 194 women, 140 with breast cancer, was conducted to assess the diagnostic potential of the GDV to see how it may be used to reflect the patient's "energy state" in the process of chemotherapy, radiation therapy, and surgery. Statistically significant differences were found between the GDV parameters of the cancer patients when compared with a healthy control group. The patients with cancer had a wide range of stages and diagnoses (Korotkov 2002).

Despite growing evidence that biofields may be related to biological functions and may possibly precede material changes (Tiller, Dibble et al. 2001), it will take more rigorous research to define ways that protecting from assaults or correcting imbalances in those fields may affect health. There are experiments going on everyday through exposures and behaviors that we cannot fully understand the role of biofields in health until they are evaluated in randomized controlled trials.

Nevertheless, energy medicine practices are common throughout the world. In China, the largest population on earth practices Tai Chi daily to balance energy fields. Although no correlation has yet been established, cancer rates in China are generally low (except for cancers directly attributable to tobacco) (Yuan, Ross et al. 1996). In fact, reviewing cancer rates worldwide, one might want to consider moving to Qidong, China as a "best practice for preventing cancer"! Very controversial evidence continues to be wrestled with regarding exposure to electrical fields from power lines and cancer risk (Moulder and Foster 1995; Moulder and Foster 1999). The role of culture, health practices and spirituality, and many more suspects in the theatre of life exposures, need refined exploration. But until our understanding of mechanisms of energetic influences on the body and the biofield is understood in terms of the dominant microbiological paradigm, the research will neither be noticed nor applied to cancer prevention.

Conclusions

CAM is a continuously developing field, challenging researchers to find new epistemologies to match complex systems and competing evidence. For example despite a long history of holding certain hormones responsible for hormone-related cancers, new evidence is accumulating on the potential of endogenous and/or bioidentical supplemental progesterone to have protective effects against several cancers (Cowan, Gordis et al. 1981; Formby and Wiley 1998; Malet, Spritzer et al. 2000; Horita, Inase et al. 2001; Dai, Wolf et al. 2002). As findings emerge from the cancer treatment realm, its potential application to cancer prevention may be better understood. However, given the many systems approaches to healing that may never be fully defined or researched as a package, it may be important to find ways to investigate on a large scale what cultural lifestyles and accompanying methods of healing used in those cultures, may be associated with lower rates of cancer. It will be important to solve the problems of separating out cultural and genetic influences on racioethnic populations and ruling out spurious correlations from true effects and mediating factors in such observational studies. It may be necessary to develop an appropriate research paradigm to apply to trials on lifestyles that cannot be recreated or inhibited in real-life conditions, as is required in randomized controlled trials, before the potential for such systems is fully known.

In the meantime, smaller scale studies may begin to uncover select mechanisms of action of the elements of CAM. One of the primary funding agencies for examining alternative approaches to cancer treatment, control, and prevention of recurrence, the NCI's Office of Cancer Complementary and Alternative Medicine (NCCAM), has shifted many modalities previously considered CAM to conventional status. In particular, the NCCAM now suggests that many of the mind-body approaches for reducing stress and improving quality of life among patients with cancer or cancer survivors has become mainstream due to well documented theoretical foundation and scientific evidence (e.g., patient education, biofeedback, and cognitive-behavioral approaches). These mind-body approaches are now assigned to funding within the main body of NCI divisions unless the focus of research is more clearly placed on novel mechanisms of action for cancer that have yet to be investigated. Currently, both in the current research projects (NCI) and in the statements of the modalities suggested for investigation (e.g., phase I/II trials of CAM mechanisms of action), it is evident that in the future, CAM approaches will be sorted out into those that can be scientifically validated and those that have less support. This is good news; as the consumer continues to adjust lifestyle, seek wellness and attempt to prevent disease through conventional as well as alternative systems, knowledge that comes from well-designed research may guide this search toward more effective prevention strategies.

The creative search for alternative modes of treatment and supportive care for cancer patients may serve as a useful starting point to identify potential candidate agents and practices for research in prevention. In this light, some of the therapies gaining popularity for supportive care may gain attention in the future as more than simply positive experiences. For example, music, art therapy, and guided imagery all have a long tradition of use with cancer patients, and many oncologists encourage their patients to integrate such extra-medical practices into their treatment program. Often these are not seen as modalities that could affect the course of cancer, only to help the patients cope psychologically with their disease. However, as more evidence accumulates that such activities, even for healthy patients, might affect overall health and immunity, potentially even at the cellular level (Chopra 2000), these may also be explored as ways to improve one's chances of avoiding cancer. Until that day, one should consider adding flaxseed and curcumin to a diet rich in fruits and vegetables, engage in some form of daily meditation, practice yoga, tai chi or qigong to the point of obtaining a balanced GDV reading, and watch the research unfold over the next decade.

References

The Wellness Community (2004). Mission Statement.

Achterberg, J. and G. F. Lawlis (1984). *Imagery and Disease: Diagnostic Tools?* Champaign, Illinois, Institute for Personality and Ability Testing.

Achterberg, J., S. Mathews-Simonton, et al. (1977). "Psychology of the exceptional cancer patient: a description of patients who outlive predicted life expectancies." *Psychotherapy: Theory, Research, Practice, Training* **14**: 416–422.

Ader, R., D. L. Felten, et al., Eds. (1991). *Psychoneuroimmunology.* San Diego, Academic Press.

Adlercreutz, H., T. Fotsis, et al. (1994). "Determination of lignans and isoflavonoids in plasma by isotope dilution gas chromatography-mass spectrometry." *Cancer Detect Prev* **18**(4): 259–271.

Adlercreutz, H., Y. Mousavi, et al. (1992). "Dietary phytoestrogens and cancer: in vitro and in vivo studies." *J Steroid Biochem Mol Biol* **41**(3–8): 331–337.

Agarwal, B., P. Swaroop, et al. (2003). "Cox-2 is needed but not sufficient for apoptosis induced by Cox-2 selective inhibitors in colon cancer cells." *Apoptosis* **8**(6): 649–654.

Anderson, E.Z. (2001). "Energy therapies for physical and occupational therapists working with older adults." *Physical and Occupational Therapies in Geriatrics* **18**(4): 38–49.

Astin, J.A., S.L. Shapiro, et al. (2003). "Mind-body medicine: state of the science, implications for practice." *J Am Board Fam Pract* **16**(2): 131–147.

Bachelor, M.A. and G.T. Bowden (2004). "UVA-mediated activation of signaling pathways involved in skin tumor promotion and progression." *Semin Cancer Biol* **14**(2): 131–138.

Beck, R. (1986). "Mood modification with ELF magnetic fields: a preliminary exploration." *Archaeus* **4**: 48.

Becker, R.O. (1990). "A technique for producing regenerative healing in humans." *Frontier Perspectives* **1**(2): 1–2.

Beebe-Dimmer, J.L., J. Wood, P. David et al. (2004). "Use of complementary and alternative medicine in men with family history of prostate cancer: a pilot study." *Urology* **63**(2): 282–287.

Benjamin, H.H. (1995). *The Wellness Community Guide to Fighting Recovery from Cancer.* New York, Putnam.

Benor, D. (1993). *Healing research: Holistic Energy Medicine and Spiritual Healing.* Munich, Helix.

Benson, H. and E.M. Stuart (1993). *The Wellness Book: the Comprehensive Guide to Maintaining Health and Treating Stress-related Illness.* Secaucus, NJ, Carol Publishing Group.

Berland, W. (1995). Unexpected cancer recovery: Why patients believe they survive. *Advances: The Journal of Mind – Body Health*, Fetzer Institute. **11**: 5.

Bernstein, B.J. and T. Grasso (1983). "Prevalence of complementary and alternative medicine use in cancer patients." *Oncology (Huntington)* **15**(10): 1267–1272; discussion 1272–1278.

Boik, J. (2001). *Natural Compounds in Cancer Therapy.* Princeton, Minn., USA, Oregon Medical Press.

Cadossi, R., G. Emilia, et al. (1988). Lymphocytes and pulsing magnetic fields. In: *Modern Bioelectricity.* A.A. Marino. New York, Dekker: xviii, 1050.

Cadossi, R., R. Iverson, et al. (1988). "Effect of low-frequency low energy pulsing electromagnetic fields on mice undergoing bone marrow transplantation." *International Journal of Immunopathology and Pharmacology* **1**: 57–62.

Cassileth, B.R. and G. Deng (2004). "Complementary and Alternative Therapies for Cancer." *Oncologist* **9**(1): 80–89.

Chang, Y.S., E.K. Seo, et al. (2003). "Panax ginseng: a role in cancer therapy?" *Integr Cancer Ther* **2**(1): 13–33.

Chen, H.W., S.L. Yu, et al. (2004). "Anti-invasive gene expression profile of curcumin in lung adenocarcinoma based on a high throughput microarray analysis." *Mol Pharmacol* **65**(1): 99–110.

Chen, K. and R. Yeung (2002). "A review of qigong therapy for cancer treatment." *Journal of International Society of Life Information Science* **20**(2): 532–542.

Chen, K.W., S.C. Shiflett, et al. (2002). "A preliminary study of the effect of external qigong on lymphoma growth in mice." *J Altern Complement Med* **8**(5): 615–621.

Cherkin, D.C., R.A. Deyo, et al. (2002). "Characteristics of licensed acupuncturists, chiropractors, massage therapists, and naturopathic physicians." *J Am Board Fam Pract* **15**(5): 378–390.

Chopra, D. (1989). *Quantum Healing: Exploring the Frontiers of Mind/Body Medicine.* New York, Bantam Books.

Chopra, D. (2000). *Perfect Health: The Complete Mind-Body Guide.* New York Three Rivers Press.

Chu, K.K., S.S. Ho, et al. (2002). "Coriolus versicolor: a medicinal mushroom with promising immunotherapeutic values." *J Clin Pharmacol* **42**(9): 976–984.

Cohen, K. (1997). *The Way of Qigong = [Ch'i kung chi tao]: The Art and Science of Chinese Energy Healing*. New York, Ballantine Books.

Conti, A. (2000). "Oncology in neuroimmunomodulation. What progress has been made?" *Ann NY Acad Sci* **917**: 68–83.

Cook, C.A., J.F. Guerrerio, et al. (2004). "Healing touch and quality of life in women receiving radiation treatment for cancer: a randomized controlled trial." *Altern Ther Health Med* **10**(3): 34–41.

Cossarizza, A., D. Monti, et al. (1989). "Extremely low frequency pulsed electromagnetic fields increase interleukin-2 (IL-2) utilization and IL-2 receptor expression in mitogen-stimulated human lymphocytes from old subjects." *FEBS Lett* **248**(1–2): 141–144.

Cowan, L.D., L. Gordis, et al. (1981). "Breast cancer incidence in women with a history of progesterone deficiency." *Am J Epidemiol* **114**(2): 209–217.

Cunningham, A.J., C. Phillips, et al. (2000). "Association of involvement in psychological self-regulation with longer survival in patients with metastatic cancer: an exploratory study." *Adv Mind Body Med* **16**(4): 276–287.

Cunningham, A.J., C. Phillips, et al. (2002). "Fighting for life: a qualitative analysis of the process of psychotherapy-assisted self-help in patients with metastatic cancer." *Integr Cancer Ther* **1**(2): 146–161.

Daaleman, T.P., S. Perera, et al. (2004). "Religion, spirituality, and health status in geriatric outpatients." *Ann Fam Med* **2**(1): 49–53.

Dai, D., D.M. Wolf, et al. (2002). "Progesterone inhibits human endometrial cancer cell growth and invasiveness: down-regulation of cellular adhesion molecules through progesterone B receptors." *Cancer Res* **62**(3): 881–886.

Daniels, M., R.M. Merrill, et al. (2004). "Associations between breast cancer risk factors and religious practices in Utah." *Prev Med* **38**(1): 28–38.

Dattore, P.J., F.C. Shontz, et al. (1980). "Premorbid personality differentiation of cancer and noncancer groups: a test of the hypothesis of cancer proneness." *J Consult Clin Psychol* **48**(3): 388–394.

Davidson, R.J., J. Kabat-Zinn, et al. (2003). "Alterations in brain and immune function produced by mindfulness meditation." *Psychosom Med* **65**(4): 564–570.

Demark-Wahnefried, W., D.T. Price, et al. (2001). "Pilot study of dietary fat restriction and flaxseed supplementation in men with prostate cancer before surgery: exploring the effects on hormonal levels, prostate-specific antigen, and histopathologic features." *Urology* **58**(1): 47–52.

Dibble, S.L., J. Chapman, et al. (2000). "Acupressure for nausea: results of a pilot study." *Oncol Nurs Forum* **27**(1): 41–47.

Eisenberg, D.M., M.H. Cohen, et al. (2002). "Credentialing complementary and alternative medical providers." *Ann Intern Med* **137**(12): 965–973.

Eisenberg, D.M., R.C. Kessler, et al. (1993). "Unconventional medicine in the United States. Prevalence, costs, and patterns of use." *N Engl J Med* **328**(4): 246–252.

Elenkov, I.J. and G.P. Chrousos (2002). "Stress hormones, proinflammatory and antiinflammatory cytokines, and autoimmunity." *Ann NY Acad Sci* **966**: 290–303.

Ell, K., R. Nishimoto, et al. (1989). "A longitudinal analysis of psychological adaptation among survivors of cancer." *Cancer* **63**(2): 406–413.

Engelking, C. (1994). "New approaches: innovations in cancer prevention, diagnosis, treatment, and support." *Oncol Nurs Forum* **21**(1): 62–71.

Fields, J.Z., Rawal, P.A., Hagen, J.F., Ing, T., Wallace, R.K., Tomlinson, P.F., Schneider, R.H. (1990). "Oxygen free radical (OFR) scavenging effects of an anti-carcinogenic natural product, Maharishi Amrit Kalash." *The Pharmacologist* **32**(3): 155.

Fisher, B., J.P. Costantino, et al. (1998). "Tamoxifen for prevention of breast cancer: report of the National Surgical Adjuvant Breast and Bowel Project P-1 Study." *J Natl Cancer Inst* **90**(18): 1371–1388.

Fisher, M. and L.X. Yang (2002). "Anticancer effects and mechanisms of polysaccharide-K (PSK): implications of cancer immunotherapy." *Anticancer Res* **22**(3): 1737–1754.

Formby, B. and T.S. Wiley (1998). "Progesterone inhibits growth and induces apoptosis in breast cancer cells: inverse effects on Bcl-2 and p53." *Ann Clin Lab Sci* **28**(6): 360–369.

Friedman, M. and R.H. Rosenman (1974). *Type A Behavior and Your Heart*. New York, Knopf.

Fullerton, S.A., A.A. Samadi, et al. (2000). "Induction of apoptosis in human prostatic cancer cells with beta-glucan (Maitake mushroom polysaccharide)." *Mol Urol* **4**(1): 7–13.

Funch, D.P. and J. Marshall (1983). "The role of stress, social support and age in survival from breast cancer." *J Psychosom Res* **27**(1): 77–83.

Gaab, J., N. Blattler, et al. (2003). "Randomized controlled evaluation of the effects of cognitive-behavioral stress management on cortisol responses to acute stress in healthy subjects." *Psychoneuroendocrinology* **28**(6): 767–779.

Garssen, B. and K. Goodkin (1999). "On the role of immunological factors as mediators between psychosocial factors and cancer progression." *Psychiatry Res* **85**(1): 51–61.

Goodwin, P.J., M. Leszcz, et al. (2001). "The effect of group psychosocial support on survival in metastatic breast cancer." *N Engl J Med* **345**(24): 1719–1726.

Gordon, J.S. and S.R. Curtin (2000). *Comprehensive Cancer Care: Integrating Alternative, Complementary, and Conventional Therapies*. Cambridge, Mass., Perseus.

Grossman, H.B. (2003). "Selective COX-2 inhibitors as chemopreventive and therapeutic agents." *Drugs Today (Barc)* **39**(3): 203–212.

Gruber, B.L., N.R. Hall, et al. (1988). "Immune system and psychological changes in metastatic cancer patients using relaxation and guided imagery: a pilot study." *Scandinavian Journal of Behavior Therapy* **17**: 25–46.

Haggans, C.J., A.M. Hutchins, et al. (1999). "Effect of flaxseed consumption on urinary estrogen metabolites in postmenopausal women." *Nutrition & Cancer* **33**(2): 188–195.

Haggans, C.J., E.J. Travelli, et al. (2000). "The effect of flaxseed and wheat bran consumption on urinary estrogen metabolites in premenopausal women." *Cancer Epidemiol, Biomarkers Prev* **9**(7): 719–725.

Hahn, R.C. and D.B. Petitti (1988). "Minnesota Multiphasic Personality Inventory-rated depression and the incidence of breast cancer." *Cancer* **61**(4): 845–848.

Hammerschlag, C. and H. Silverman (1997). *Healing Ceremonies: Creating Personal Rituals for Spiritual, Emotion, Physical and Mental Health*. New York, Perigee.

Hammerschlag, C.A. (1988). *The Dancing Healers: A Doctor's Journey of Healing with Native Americans*. San Francisco, Harper & Row.

Herron, R.E. and J.B. Fagan (2002). "Lipophil-mediated reduction of toxicants in humans: an evaluation of an ayurvedic detoxification procedure." *Altern Ther Health Med* **8**(5): 40–51.

Hirano, T., K. Fukuoka, et al. (1990). "Antiproliferative activity of mammalian lignan derivatives against the human breast carcinoma cell line, ZR-75-1." *Cancer Invest* **8**(6): 595–602.

Hislop, T.G., N.E. Waxler, et al. (1987). "The prognostic significance of psychosocial factors in women with breast cancer." *J Chronic Dis* **40**(7): 729–735.

Holland, J.C. (1989). Behavioral and psychological risk factors in cancer: human studies. In: *Handbook of Psychooncology: Psychological Care of the Patient with Cancer*. J.C. Holland and J.H. Rowland. New York, Oxford University Press. xiv, 785.

Horita, K., N. Inase, et al. (2001). "Progesterone induces apoptosis in malignant mesothelioma cells." *Anticancer Res* **21**(6A): 3871–3874.

Hutchins, A.M., M.C. Martini, et al. (2001). "Flaxseed consumption influences endogenous hormone concentrations in postmenopausal women." *Nutrition & Cancer* **39**(1): 58–65.

Ikemi, Y., S. Nakagawa, et al. (1975). "Psychosomatic consideration of cancer patients who have made a narrow escape from death." *Dynamic Psychiatry* **8**: 77–91.

Johnson, J.A. (2000). *Chinese Medical Qigong Therapy: A Comprehensive Clinical Text*. Pacific Grove, CA, The International Institute of Medical Qigong.

Jones, B.M. (2001). "Changes in cytokine production in healthy subjects practicing Guolin Qigong: a pilot study." *BMC Complement Altern Med* **1**(1): 8.

Kaasa, S., A. Mastekaasa, et al. (1989). "Prognostic factors for patients with inoperable non-small cell lung cancer, limited disease. The importance of patients' subjective experience of disease and psychosocial well-being." *Radiother Oncol* **15**(3): 235–242.

Kabat-Zinn, J. (1994). *Wherever You Go, There You Are: Mindfulness Meditation in Everyday Life*. New York, Hyperion.

Kamei, T., Y. Toriumi, et al. (2000). "Decrease in serum cortisol during yoga exercise is correlated with alpha wave activation." *Percept Mot Skills* **90**(3 Pt 1): 1027–1032.

Kaptchuk, T.J. (1983). *The Web That Has No Weaver: Understanding Chinese Medicine*. New York, Congdon & Weed: Distributed by St. Martin's Press.

Kaptchuk, T.J. (2002). "Acupuncture: theory, efficacy, and practice." *Ann Intern Med* **136**(5): 374–383.

Kataoka, T., N. Sugiyama, et al. (1997). "Effects of qi-gong vital energy on human neutrophils." *Journal of International Society of Life Information Science* **15**: 129–134.

Kerr, C. (2002). "Translating "mind-in-body": two models of patient experience underlying a randomized controlled trial of qigong." *Cult Med Psychiatry* **26**(4): 419–447.

Kiecolt-Glaser, J.K., R. Glaser, et al. (1985). "Psychosocial enhancement of immunocompetence in a geriatric population." *Health Psychol* **4**(1): 25–41.

Kodama, N., K. Komuta, et al. (2003). "Effect of Maitake (Grifola frondosa) D-Fraction on the activation of NK cells in cancer patients." *J Med Food* **6**(4): 371–377.

Korotkov, K. (2002). *Human Energy Field: Study with GDV Bioelectrography*. Fair Lawn, NJ, Backbone Publishing Co.

Kreitler, S., S. Chaitchik, et al. (1993). "Repressiveness: cause or result of cancer?" *Psychooncology* **2**: 43–54.

Krishnaswamy, K. (1996). "Indian functional foods: role in prevention of cancer." *Nutrition Reviews* **54**(11 Pt 2): 127–131.

Kushi, L.H., J.E. Cunningham, et al. (2001). "The macrobiotic diet in cancer." *Journal of Nutrition* **131**(11 Suppl): 3056S–3064S.

LaBarba, R.C. (1970). "Experimental and environmental factors in cancer. A review of research with animals." *Psychosom Med* **32**(3): 259–276.

Ladas, E.J. and K.M. Kelly (2003). "Milk thistle: is there a role for its use as an adjunct therapy in patients with cancer?" *J Altern Complement Med* **9**(3): 411–416.

Lampe, J.W. (2003). "Spicing up a vegetarian diet: chemopreventive effects of phytochemicals." *Am J Clin Nutr* **78**(3 Suppl): 579S–583S.

Largewhiskers, T. (2004). Personal communication.

Lerner, M. (1994). *Choices in Healing: Integrating the Best of Conventional and Complementary Approaches to Cancer*. Cambridge, Mass., MIT Press.

Levin, J.S. and H.Y. Vanderpool (1991). "Religious factors in physical health and the prevention of illness." *Prev Hum Serv* **9**: 41–64.

Lin, H., Y.H. She, et al. (2004). "Maitake beta-glucan MD-fraction enhances bone marrow colony formation and reduces doxorubicin toxicity in vitro." *Int Immunopharmacol* **4**(1): 91–99.

Liu, H. (2004). Principles of prevention and treatment of cancers by qigong. In: *Summary of studies related to cancer executed and published in China*.

Malet, C., P. Spritzer, et al. (2000). "Progesterone effect on cell growth, ultrastructural aspect and estradiol receptors of normal human breast epithelial (HBE) cells in culture." *J Steroid Biochem Mol Biol* **73**(3–4): 171–181.

Mayer, D.J. (2000). "Acupuncture: an evidence-based review of the clinical literature." *Annu Rev Med* **51**: 49–63.

Mehl-Madrona, L. (2003). *Coyote healing: miracles of native America*. Rochester, VT, Inner Traditions/ Bear and Company.

Miquel, J., A. Bernd, et al. (2002). "The curcuma antioxidants: pharmacological effects and prospects for future clinical use. A review." *Arch Gerontol and Geriatr* **34**(1): 37–46.

Mishra, S.I., J. Hess, et al. (2003). "Predictors of indigenous healer use among Samoans." *Altern Ther Health Med* **9**(6): 64–69.

Mori, H., K. Nishijo, et al. (2002). "Unique immunomodulation by electro-acupuncture in humans possibly via stimulation of the autonomic nervous system." *Neurosci Lett* **320**(1–2): 21–24.

Moulder, J.E. and K.R. Foster (1995). "Biological effects of power-frequency fields as they relate to carcinogenesis." *Proc Soc Exp Biol Med* **209**(4): 309–324.

Moulder, J.E. and K.R. Foster (1999). "Is there a link between exposure to power-frequency electric fields and cancer?" *IEEE Eng Med Biol Mag* **18**(2): 109–116.

Murphy, G.P., L.B. Morris, et al. (1997). *Informed Decisions: The Complete Book of Cancer Diagnosis, Treatment, and Recovery*. New York, Viking.

Myss, C. (1996). *Anatomy of Spirit: The Seven Stages of Power and Healing*. New York, Three Rivers Press.

NCI Computer Retrieval of Information on Scientific Projects (CRISP) (2004). http://www.cit.nih.gov/ Accessed Feb 8, 2005.

Neal, R. (2001). "Report by David M. Eisenberg, M.D., on complementary and alternative medicine in the United States: overview and patterns of use." *J Altern Complement Med* **7 Suppl 1**: S19–21.

Nishino, H., H. Tokuda, et al. (2000). "Cancer chemoprevention by phytochemicals and their related compounds." *Asian Pac J Cancer Prev* **1**(1): 49–55.

O'Connor, M.E., R.H. Bentall, et al., Eds. (1990). *Emerging Electromagnetic Medicine Conference Proceedings*. New York, Springer.

Omenn, G.S., G.E. Goodman, et al. (1996). "Risk factors for lung cancer and for intervention effects in CARET, the Beta-Carotene and Retinol Efficacy Trial." *J Natl Cancer Inst* **88**(21): 1550–1559.

O'Regan, B. and C. Hirshberg (1993). *Spontaneous Remission: An Annotated Bibliography*. Sausalito, CA, Institute of Noetic Sciences.

Oschmann, J.L. (2000). *Energy, Medicine: The Scientific Basis*. Edinburgh, Churchill Livingston.

Park, E.J. and J.M. Pezzuto (2002). "Botanicals in cancer chemoprevention." *Cancer Metastasis Reviews* **21**(3–4): 231–255.

Peavey, B.S., G.F. Lawlis, et al. (1985). "Biofeedback-assisted relaxation: effects on phagocytic capacity." *Biofeedback Self Regul* **10**(1): 33–47.

Pelley, R.P. and F.M. Strickland (2000). "Plants, polysaccharides, and the treatment and prevention of neoplasia." *Critical Reviews in Oncogenesis* **11**(3–4): 189–225.

Penson, R.T., S.H. Talsania, et al. (2004). "Help me help you: support groups in cancer therapy." *Oncologist* **9**(2): 217–225.

Pert, C.B. (1997). *Molecules of Emotion: Why You Feel The Way You Feel*. New York, Scribner.

Petti, F., A. Bangrazi, et al. (1998). "Effects of acupuncture on immune response related to opioid-like peptides." *J Tradit Chin Med* **18**(1): 55–63.

Pettingale, K.W., T. Morris, et al. (1985). "Mental attitudes to cancer: an additional prognostic factor." *Lancet* **1**(8431): 750.

Polk, M. (1996). "Feast on phytochemicals." *AICR Newsletter* (51).

Post-White, J., M.E. Kinney, et al. (2003). "Therapeutic massage and healing touch improve symptoms in cancer." *Integr Cancer Ther* **2**(4): 332–344.

Powell, L.H., L. Shahabi, et al. (2003). "Religion and spirituality. Linkages to physical health." *Am Psychol* **58**(1): 36–52.

Quinn, J.F. and A.J. Strelkauskas (1993). "Psychoimmunologic effects of therapeutic touch on practitioners and recently bereaved recipients: a pilot study." *ANS Adv Nurs Sci* **15**(4): 13–26.

Raison, C.L. and A.H. Miller (2001). "The neuroimmunology of stress and depression." *Semin Clin Neuropsychiatry* **6**(4): 277–294.

Ramirez, A.J., T.K. Craig, et al. (1989). "Stress and relapse of breast cancer." *BMJ* **298**(6669): 291–293.

Reindl Benjamins, M. and C. Brown (2004). "Religion and preventative health care utilization among the elderly." *Soc Sci Med* **58**(1): 109–118.

Roberts, N., C.N. Shealy, et al. (2002). "Are there electrical devices that can measure the body's energy state change to an acupuncture treatment? Part I, The Meridian Stress Assessment (MSA-21) Device." *Subtle Energies and Energy Medicine Journal* **13**(3).

Roud, P.C. (1986). "Psychosocial variables associated with the exceptional survival of patients with advanced malignant disease." *Int J Psychiatry Med* **16**(2): 113–122.

Rubik, B. (1995). "Energy medicine and the unifying concept of information." *Altern Ther Health Med* **1**(1): 34–39.

Russek, L.G. and G.E. Schwartz (1994). "Interpersonal heart-brain registration and the perception of parental love: a 42 year follow-up of the Harvard Mastery of Stress Study." *Subtle Energies and Energy Medicine Journal* **5**(3): 195–208.

Russek, L.G. and G.E. Schwartz (1996). "Energy cardiology: a dynamical energy systems approach for integrating conventional and alternative medicine." *Advances: Journal of Mind-Body Health* **12**(4): 4–24.

Ryu, H., C.D. Jun, et al. (1995). "Effect of qigong training on proportions of T lymphocyte subsets in human peripheral blood." *Am J Chin Med* **23**(1): 27–36.

Schiller, P.L. and J.S. Levin (1988). "Is there a religious factor in health care utilization?: A review." *Soc Sci Med* **27**(12): 1369–1379.

Schipper, H., C.R. Goh, et al. (1995). "Shifting the cancer paradigm: must we kill to cure?" *J Clin Oncol* **13**(4): 801–807.

Schmidt, T., A. Wijga, et al. (1997). "Changes in cardiovascular risk factors and hormones during a comprehensive residential three month kriya yoga training and vegetarian nutrition." *Acta Physiol Scand Suppl* **640**: 158–162.

Schwartz, G.E., S. Swanick, et al. (2004). "Biofield detection: role of bioenergy awareness training and individual differences in absorption." *J Altern Complement Med* **10**(1): 167–169.

Seeman, T.E., L.F. Dubin, et al. (2003). "Religiosity/spirituality and health. A critical review of the evidence for biological pathways." *Am Psychol* **58**(1): 53–63.

Seigel, B.S. (1990). *Love, Medicine and Miracles: Lessons Learned About Self-Healing from a Surgeon's Experience with Exceptional Patients*. New York, Harper Perennial.

Seto, A., C. Kusaka, et al. (1992). "Detection of extraordinary large bio-magnetic field strength from human hand during external Qi emission." *Acupunct Electrother Res* **17**(2): 75–94.

Shang, C. (1993). "Bioelectrochemical oscillations in signal transduction and acupuncture – an emerging paradigm." *Am J Chin Med* **21**(1): 91–101.

Shang, C. (2001). "Emerging paradigms in mind-body medicine." *J Altern Complement Med* **7**(1): 83–91.

Sharma, H.M., C. Dwivedi, et al. (1990). "Antineoplastic properties of Maharishi-4 against DMBA-induced mammary tumors in rats." *Pharmacol Biochem Behav* **35**(4): 767–773.

Sharrard, W.J. (1990). "A double-blind trial of pulsed electromagnetic fields for delayed union of tibial fractures." *J Bone Joint Surg Br* **72**(3): 347–355.

Shen, J., N. Wenger, et al. (2000). "Electroacupuncture for control of myeloablative chemotherapy-induced emesis: A randomized controlled trial." *JAMA* **284**(21): 2755–2761.

Shen, Q. and P.H. Brown (2003). "Novel agents for the prevention of breast cancer: targeting transcription factors and signal transduction pathways." *Journal of Mammary Gland Biology & Neoplasia* **8**(1): 45–73.

Shin, H.R., J.Y. Kim, et al. (2000). "The cancer-preventive potential of Panax ginseng: a review of human and experimental evidence." *Cancer Causes Control* **11**(6): 565–576.

Simonton, O.C., S. Simonton, et al. (1978). *Getting Well Again: A Step-By-Step, Self-Help Guide to Overcoming Cancer for Patients and their Families*. Los Angeles, New York, J.P. Tarcher; distributed by St. Martin's Press.

Singh, R.H. (2002). "An assessment of the ayurvedic concept of cancer and a new paradigm of anticancer treatment in Ayurveda." *J Altern Complement Med* **8**(5): 609–614.

Sisken, B.F. and J. Walker (1995). Therapeutic aspects of electromagnetic fields for soft-tissue healing. *Electromagnetic fields: biological interactions and mechanisms*. M. Blank. Washington, DC, American Chemical Society. xiv, 497.

Sklar, L.S. and H. Anisman (1981). "Stress and cancer." *Psychol Bull* **89**(3): 369–406.

Sparreboom, A., M.C. Cox, et al. (2004). "Herbal remedies in the United States: potential adverse interactions with anticancer agents." *J Clin Oncol* **22**(12): 2489–2503.

Spiegel, D., J.R. Bloom, et al. (1989). "Effect of psychosocial treatment on survival of patients with metastatic breast cancer." *Lancet* **2**(8668): 888–891.

Struve, J.K. (2002). "Faith's impact on health. Implications for the practice of medicine." *Minn Med* **85**(12): 41–44.

Tatsumura, Y., G. Maskarinec, et al. (2003). "Religious and spiritual resources, CAM, and conventional treatment in the lives of cancer patients." *Altern Ther Health Med* **9**(3): 64–71.

Temoshok, L. (1987). "Personality, coping style, emotion and cancer: towards an integrative model." *Cancer Surv* **6**(3): 545–567.

Temoshok, L., B.W. Heller, et al. (1985). "The relationship of psychosocial factors to prognostic indicators in cutaneous malignant melanoma." *J Psychosom Res* **29**(2): 139–153.

Thompson, L.U., M.M. Seidl, et al. (1996). "Antitumorigenic effect of a mammalian lignan precursor from flaxseed." *Nutrition & Cancer* **26**(2): 159–165.

Tiller, W.A. (1997). *Science and Human Transformation: Subtle Energies, Intentionality and Consciousness*. Walnut Creek, CA, Pavior Publishing.

Tiller, W.A., W. Dibble, et al. (2001). *Conscious Acts of Creation*. Walnut Creek, CA, Pavior Publishing.

Trock, D.H., A.J. Bollet, et al. (1993). "A double-blind trial of the clinical effects of pulsed electromagnetic fields in osteoarthritis." *J Rheumatol* **20**(3): 456–460.

Tyler, V.E. (1993). *The Honest Herbal: A Sensible Guide to the Use of Herbs and Related Remedies*. New York, Pharmaceutical Products Press.

Vainio, H. and F. Bianchini (2003). *IARC Handbook of Cancer Prevention, Vol. 8, Fruits and Vegetables*. Lyon, France, IARC Press.

Visintainer, M.A., M.E.P. Seligman, et al. (1983). "Helplessness, chronic stress and tumor development." *Psychosomatic Medicine* **45**: 75–76.

Wang, C., J.P. Collet, et al. (2004). "The effect of tai chi on health outcomes in patients with chronic conditions." Arch Int Med 164:493–501.

Wardell, D.W. and J. Engebretson (2001). "Biological correlates of Reiki Touch(sm) healing." *J Adv Nurs* **33**(4): 439–445.

Waxler-Morrison, N., T.G. Hislop, et al. (1991). "Effects of social relationships on survival for women with breast cancer: a prospective study." *Soc Sci Med* **33**(2): 177–183.

Weil, A. (1995). *Spontaneous Healing: How to Discover and Enhance Your Body's Natural Ability to Maintain and Heal Itself*. New York, Knopf: Distributed by Random House.

Wilkinson, D.S., P.L. Knox, et al. (2002). "The clinical effectiveness of healing touch." *J Altern Complement Med* **8**(1): 33–47.

Williams, K.A., M.M. Kolar, et al. (2001). "Evaluation of a Wellness-Based Mindfulness Stress Reduction intervention: a controlled trial." *Am J Health Promot* **15**(6): 422–432.

Wirth, D.P., J.R. Cram, et al. (1997). "Multisite electromyographic analysis of therapeutic touch and qigong therapy." *J Altern Complement Med* **3**(2): 109–118.

Wong, B. and J. McKeen (2001). *The New Manual for Life*. Gabriola Island, BC, Canada, PD Publishing.

Worden, J.W. and A.D. Weisman (1975). "Psychosocial components of lagtime in cancer diagnosis." *J Psychosom Res* **19**(1): 69–79.

Wu, X., Beecher, G.R., Holden, J.M., Haytowitz, D.B., Gebhardt, S.E., Prior, R.L. (2004). "Lipophilic and Hydrophilic Antioxidant Capacities of Common Foods in the United States." *J Agric Food Chem* **52**(12): 4026–4037.

Xiaoguang, C., L. Hongyan, et al. (1998). "Cancer chemopreventive and therapeutic activities of red ginseng." *J Ethnopharmacol* **60**(1): 71–78.

Xu, H., W. Guomin, et al. (1988). Observation of T-lymphocytes by anae staining in the clinical application of qigong. *Proceedings of the First World Conference for Academic Exchange of Medical Qigong*, Beijing, China, Qigong Institute.

Xu, X.C. (2002). "COX-2 inhibitors in cancer treatment and prevention, a recent development." *Anticancer Drugs* **13**(2): 127–137.

Ye, F., S. Chen, et al. (2002). "Effects of electro-acupuncture on immune function after chemotherapy in 28 cases." *J Tradit Chin Med* **22**(1): 21–23.

Youssef, K.M., M.A. El-Sherbeny (2004). "Synthesis of curcumin analogues as potential antioxidant, cancer chemopreventive agents." *Archiv der Pharmazie* **337**(1): 42–54.

Yuan, J.M., R.K. Ross, et al. (1996). "Morbidity and mortality in relation to cigarette smoking in Shanghai, China. A prospective male cohort study." *Jama* **275**(21): 1646–1650.

Yun, T.K. (2001). "Panax ginseng – a non-organ-specific cancer preventive?" *Lancet Oncol* **2**(1): 49–55.

Yun, T.K. (2003). "Experimental and epidemiological evidence on non-organ specific cancer preventive effect of Korean ginseng and identification of active compounds." *Mutat Res* **523–524**: 63–74.

Yun, T.K., S.Y. Choi, et al. (2001). "Epidemiological study on cancer prevention by ginseng: are all kinds of cancers preventable by ginseng?" *J Korean Med Sci* **16 Suppl**: S19–27.

Yun, T.K., Y.S. Lee, et al. (2001). "Anticarcinogenic effect of Panax ginseng C.A. Meyer and identification of active compounds." *J Korean Med Sci* **16 Suppl**: S6–18.

Zarkovic, N., T. Vukovic, et al. (2001). "An overview on anticancer activities of the Viscum album extract Isorel." *Cancer Biother Radiopharm* **16**(1): 55–62.

Zimmerman, J. (1990). "Laying on hands healing and therapeutic touch: a testable theory." *BEMI Currents, Journal of the Bio-Electro-Magnetics Institute* **2**: 8–17.

Zorrilla, E.P., L. Luborsky, et al. (2001). "The relationship of depression and stressors to immunological assays: a meta-analytic review." *Brain Behav Immun* **15**(3): 199–226.

The Drug Development Process

Naja E. McKenzie

College of Medicine, University of Arizona, Tucson AZ 85724

The chemopreventive agent development process is a science in its infancy. Developers of chemopreventive agents face the same regulatory hurdles as do therapeutic drug developers. As in all drug development, chemoprevention scientists must demonstrate both safety and efficacy for an agent to be approved for marketing to the public. Historically, this has meant that developers must demonstrate reduced cancer incidence or mortality in order to show effectiveness. Needless to say, this would be a lengthy process given the 20 to 30-year trajectory of carcinogenesis. This requirement has been modified in recent years. The notion of targeted prevention of cancer is now based on the discovery of surrogate endpoint biomarkers, signal transduction pathways, and the ability to promote or inhibit specific molecules in those pathways with new molecular entities (NME) or drugs (O'Shaughnessy, Kelloff et al. 2002).

In the United States and internationally, the development and manufacture of drug products is regulated by government entities in order to protect general populations as well as research participants. In the United States (U.S.), the Food and Drug Administration (FDA) has this regulatory responsibility, while in Europe and Japan, the responsibility falls to individual governments using standards established and maintained by the International Conference of Harmonization (ICH). The regulatory agencies and the developers of drugs must balance the benefit of new drugs to the population as a whole against the risk to individuals participating in clinical trials and eventually to the general public. In the development of chemopreventive agents, the risk must be very low and the benefit very high, as, in order to be effective, large at-risk populations would need to use the drug, possibly for life, in order for a drug to be effective in preventing cancer (Anonymous 1999).

The process of developing chemopreventive agents consists of several systematic steps. First, NMEs are chosen based on basic science findings. Promising agents then undergo preclinical testing in animal models. Before human testing can begin, the science must be reviewed by the FDA or other regulatory agency. After the completion of clinical trials and prior to marketing, findings must be evaluated and communicated to the scientific community. This chapter outlines the process of developing chemopreventive agents and the standards that guide such development.

Selecting New Molecular Entities for Development as Chemopreventive Agents

New molecular entities are the focus of scientific study in cancer therapeutics as well as cancer prevention programs across the world. However, the selection of new molecular entities (NMEs) for development is not a random or serendipitous process. Rather, specific important criteria apply to the selection of NMEs for clinical development as potential chemopreventive agents. The major criteria include evidence of activity in preventing cancer at the target site, low toxicity to allow for potential use in large populations, the identification of the biomarkers associated with the effectiveness of the NME, and the availability of a pertinent population for clinical testing. The focus of these criteria is the real feasibility of giving a drug prophylactically to large populations at risk for a particular type of cancer (Kelloff, Hawk et al. 1996).

There are significant precedents for the notion of developing drugs that lessen the risk for a disease or the recurrence of disease and that can be given on a large scale. An example of such a precedent is the development and FDA approved marketing of lipid lowering drugs that aim to reduce the risk of cardiovascular disease. The process included research on cholesterol lowering and modulation of other markers. Lowering of cholesterol emerged as a definitive risk reduction marker and development of cholesterol lowering drugs followed. In the case of cancer chemopreventive agents, early associated biomarkers discovered by basic scientist must also form the basis for development. Examples of such markers are proliferation antigens [e.g., proliferating cell nuclear antigen (PCNA)], inhibition of growth factors [e.g., epidermal growth factor receptor (EGFR)] and apoptosis.

Discovery of related biomarkers is followed by research to demonstrate activity against proliferation of pre-cancer or intraepithelial neoplasias (IEN). Demonstration of activity is performed in vitro in cell lines and later in vivo in animal models. Satisfactory activity in both models can then be evaluated as justification for proceeding to clinical trials. In addition to peer review by other scientists, the FDA performs the function of approving clinical trials in humans using NMEs. The criteria used by the FDA to evaluate proposed drugs for development and marketing are safety and effectiveness viewed in a risk-benefit balancing framework.

An important requirement for chemoprevention agents is that while they must be highly effective, they must also be safe enough to be given to large populations at risk for a particular cancer. This is a marked departure from the usual thinking about therapeutic cancer drugs where the toxicity, unless major, is an expected fact that is mitigated by the effectiveness of the drug in treating the cancer. Therapeutic clinical trials, therefore, tend to seek the highest effective dose for which the toxicity can be justified by its effectiveness, while chemoprevention studies seek to find the highest safe dose that is also effective.

An important consideration for selecting a NME for development as a chemopreventive agent is the availability of the agent in quantities needed for all phases of testing. A supply can be assured by either synthesizing the drug, provided no patent rights are contravened, or acquired in bulk from the manufacturer or wholesaler of known compounds. Synthesis can be a computer assisted process in which a compound is simulated using enzymes that attach to the disease related target site on the cell membrane. Synthesis of a drug for research also requires attention to documentation of good laboratory practice (GLP). While formal GLP is not required for synthesis of drugs intended for laboratory use only, it becomes a consideration when applying for FDA approval for testing in humans.

Acquisition can be a more efficient way of getting a supply of a new drug substance for testing. Many known compounds are available from chemical suppliers and even proprietary drugs may be available in sample quantities or by agreement from the manufacturers. Academic institutions can be highly effective and less costly than commercial laboratories in basic and preclinical science portions of drug development. Such arrangements are usually managed by Materials Transfer Agreements (MTA). The FDA may require that a compound that is to be used in clinical trials be manufactured under current Good Manufacturing Practice (GMP). It may therefore be necessary for clinical researchers to limit drug development to the pre-clinical stage unless a GMP supply of the study compound can be found.

Some promising chemopreventive compounds may have been tested in countries where laws are less restrictive. Drugs thus studied may be of interest to drug development researchers in FDA or ICH regulated countries and may enter their list of potential drugs as a result of preclinical activity or safety and effectiveness in humans. However, any human testing must be repeated under US regulatory requirements. Under new guidance for botanicals, clinical data obtained in non-US safety trials can be used to support later and larger trials provided the botanical used is the same. However, the developer must be able to show bioequivalence. Likewise, agents may have been tested for other purposes and based on other activity and have subsequently yielded serendipitous findings. Repeating studies designed to explore those findings can lead to discovery of safety and effectiveness for those new indications. In all cases, scientifically sound animal testing must precede testing in humans in order to get a preliminary idea of what may be expected in regard to safety and effectiveness in humans and to get information to guide dose setting in clinical trials. In summary, agents selected for clinical trials are those which have shown the most activity in preclinical testing and at the same time have shown the least toxicity at doses that can be tolerated by large elements of the population.

Regulatory Requirements and the US Food and Drug Administration

Details of the legislative basis of the drug development regulatory authority of the US Food and Drug Administration (FDA) and the requirements of the regulatory process are the basis for an understanding of the Investigational New Drug application (IND) and the accepted phases of clinical trials research. Good Clinical Practice considerations are essential for drug trials in human and the requirements for the protection of human subjects in clinical trials. Specifics of the regulatory requirements outlined here can be found in the current Code of Federal Regulations, Title 21, Parts 50, 54, 56, and 312.

The FDA, an agency within the Department of Health and Human Services (DHHS), is authorized to regulate drug development by a series of federal laws. These laws, enacted over the past 150 years, are authorized under the Interstate Commerce Clause of the US Constitution. The first law enacted, the Drug Importation Act of 1848, was written in response to the perception that excessive mortality during the Mexican War was caused by harmful drugs entering the country and that such substances had to be regulated or prohibited. Virtually every subsequent law was passed in response to an actual or perceived problem. The Biologics Control Act was passed in reaction to a diphtheria vaccine developed from horses with tetanus that caused the death of many children, especially in St. Louis. This Act was designed to ensure purity and safety of serums and vaccines and included annual licensing requirements and inspections of manufacturing facilities (FDA 1999).

In 1906, the Pure Food and Drugs Act was passed as the foundation of modern food and drug law. It was, in large part, the creation of Harvey Washington Wiley, the chief chemist of the Bureau of Chemistry. The Act prohibited interstate commerce of mislabeled and adulterated drugs and food. The basic authorizing act of the FDA came in 1938 in the Federal Food, Drug and Cosmetic Act. Again, it was a reaction to an elixir of sulfonamide marketed by S.C. Massengill which used a solvent similar to antifreeze and caused the death of 107 people. It required new drugs, devices and cosmetics to be shown to be safe before they were brought to market. This Act required the filing of a New Drug Application (NDA) and adequate directions for safe use. Various refinements followed.

The next reactive legislation came about due to the thalidomide tragedy. Senator Estes Kefauver was holding hearings pertaining to the manufacturing of antibiotics and other development practices. An NDA was submitted for Kevadon, the brand of thalidomide that the William Merrell Company hoped to market in the U.S. Despite ongoing pressure from the firm, the FDA's medical officer, Dr. Frances Kelsey, refused to allow the NDA to become effective because of insufficient safety data. By 1962, thalidomide's horrifying effects on newborns became known. Even though Kevadon was never approved for marketing, Merrell had distributed over two million tablets for investigational use, use which the contemporary law and regulations left mostly unchecked. Once thalidomide's deleterious effects became known, namely major birth defects, the agency moved quickly to recover the supply from physicians, pharmacists, and patients. Henceforth, drug developers are required to provide sufficient preclinical data that a drug is safe to give to humans before commencing clinical trials. For her efforts, Dr. Kelsey received the President's Distinguished Federal Civilian Service Award in 1962, the highest civilian honor available to government employees.

Current regulations are contained in a series of laws including the FDA Modernization Act of 1997, renewed in 2002. Today, the FDA is responsible for the review of new products, keeping watch over the safety of the drug supply, developing standards and regulations, and correcting or preventing problems through regulatory compliance programs. Drug regulatory efforts are handled by the Center for Drug Evaluation and Research (CDER). The main areas of focus are safety, effectiveness and availability (FDA 1999).

The Investigational New Drug Application

An Investigational New Drug Application is required by anyone planning to test a new molecular entity in humans. An IND actually allows a developer to proceed by permitting the shipment of drug for the purpose of conducting clinical trials. The provisions of the Code of Federal Regulations (CFR) that pertain to INDs are found in Title 21 Section 312 [21 CFR Part 312 (1999)]. An IND is not needed to study a legally marketed drug, unless the studies will deal with new indications, new delivery methods or new labeling claims. This section is a global review of this process and is not intended to provide comprehensive information for drug developers to file an IND. For more specific details, please consult the CFR.

The FDA's primary IND review objective is to protect human subjects involved in initial clinical trials. In later phases of investigation, the FDA also reviews IND submissions for scientific rigor to permit assurance of effectiveness. In addition to information about the applicant's identity and qualifications, the IND must contain the following information:

- A general investigational plan
- An investigator's brochure
- Protocol for planned studies (Nestle, Alijagic et al.)
- Chemistry, manufacturing and control information
- Pharmacology and toxicology information
- Summary of previous human experience.

In a general investigational plan a developer provides background information on the drug to be tested and the rationale for testing it in the manner and for the duration proposed. The developer also indicates the number of research participants to be enrolled over the course of the development of the drug. Most importantly, the developer summarizes the likelihood and severity of risks anticipated in humans based on the results of testing in animals.

The investigators brochure (IB) is a set of documentation that provides detailed information to investigators who will be performing the clinical trials. The IB includes information on the drug substance and how it is formulated. It summarizes pharmacological and toxicological effects and pharmacokinetics of the drug as tested in animals and discloses any such findings available in humans and concludes with a discussion of anticipated risks, special precautions and monitoring needed in the clinical trial.

Protocols must contain the objectives of each proposed study with specific attention to the indications studied and desired endpoints. Protocols must be specific in detailing the number and characteristics of study participants to be recruited and those to be excluded for safety reasons. The design of the study must be described in detail and must be appropriate to the type of trial envisioned. In particular, details pertaining to randomization, blinding and control are specified in the protocol. Finally, the protocol must describe what the actual data will look like and how they will be analyzed and reported. The data collected must include specific measurements pertaining to the safety of study participants, so that adverse events related to the administration of the drug can be reported and evaluated.

Chemistry, manufacturing and control (CMC) information includes relatively complex information about the composition, manufacture and quality control of the drug substance (raw drug) and drug product (drug as formulated for use in humans). Identity, quality, purity and strength of the drug must be supplied to the FDA as well as the methods for validating each parameter. The FDA must be assured by the manufacturer that these parameters will remain stable over time and can be maintained from one batch to the next. As the scope of investigations increases, the FDA requires that new information pertaining to CMC be submitted in detail.

Pharmacology and toxicology information is very important in the IND as this is the basis for concluding that the drug can be reasonably assumed to be safe to study in humans. Pharmacology information includes the effects and mechanism (Nestle,

Alijagic et al.) of action of the drug in animals. To the extent known, the absorption, distribution, metabolism and excretion of the drug are included in this section. Toxicology information consists of an integrated summary of toxicological testing in animals. Specifically, results of acute, sub-acute and chronic toxicity testing in animals are reported as are reproductive or developmental effects of the drug. Full tabulations of data, not summaries, must be provided to the FDA.

If previous human studies have been performed with the drug, for example, by another route or for different indications, such data are to be summarized in the IND as should any human trials experience from other countries. Any published papers can be included in the submission. Certainly, if the drug to be studied is marketed or has previously been marketed in another country, experience from that population should also be included in the application. Finally, for drugs that are believed to have abuse potential, are radioactive or are to be studied in a pediatric population, submission of additional information illuminating those characteristics, as applicable, is required.

Phases of Clinical Research

The Phases of Investigation are a set of conventions the FDA requires developers to use when planning and reporting clinical trials. There are four phases of investigation, of which the first three are most commonly used. Phase I represents the first use of a given drug in humans. This kind of study is usually performed in a small sample, in the range of 20 to 80, and with normal volunteers, but it can also be done with patients. In this phase of study, the drug is tested in humans to establish a measure of safety and to provide enough information about metabolism and the pharmacokinetics of the drug to design a well-controlled, scientifically valid Phase II study. Phase I studies are typically closely monitored, especially if no previous experience in humans exists.

Phase II studies include studies to evaluate effectiveness for a particular indication in patients with the disease as well as continuing the evaluation of safety. Phase II a studies are usually small and fairly short in duration, typically three months, and are designed to evaluate dose-response on both pharmacological and intermediate endpoints. Phase II b studies are randomized, placebo-controlled, double-blinded trials in a larger group of patients, perhaps 75 to 100. In this phase, participants usually receive the same dose, possibly with dose-reduction provided for in the event of adverse study related effects. The investigational treatment may also be compared to standard treatment in this phase. Endpoints of Phase II trials in chemoprevention studies would include the biomarkers and pathways found to be affected in pre-clinical and animal studies.

Phase II studies are larger trials of more than 100 participants. This phase of study is specifically aimed at determining whether the new drug is more effective and/or safer than the standard treatment. Frequently, Phase III trials are conducted in multiple settings and locations across the country in order to supply evidence for effectiveness in a more heterogeneous population. Generally, participants are randomized to an investigational group, which receives the test agent, or a control group, which receives the standard treatment. Phase III trials data are the centerpiece of the New Drug Application (NDA) submitted to the FDA to obtain permission to market the new drug.

Phase IV studies are undertaken after approval of the NDA and marketing of the drug. These studies, which are not as common as Phase I through III trials, can be requested by the FDA as non-essential to the approval of the drug, but useful in providing additional information that could, for example, change the prescribing information or labeling of a drug. If requested, manufacturers commit to do such studies at the time of the approval of the NDA. The design of Phase IV studies depends on the research question. They generally resemble Phase III studies but participants come from a more defined population in order to support specific use of the drug. Phase IV studies can also be undertaken voluntarily by manufacturers to extend the marketing potential of the drug.

Good Clinical Practice

The term Good Clinical Practice (GCP) refers to a standard for the design, conduct, performance, monitoring, auditing, recording, analyses, and reporting of clinical trials that provides assurance that the data and reported results are credible and accurate, and that the rights, integrity and confidentiality of trial subjects are protected (ICH 1994). Developed by the International Conference on Harmonisation (ICH), GCP guidelines follow a set of fundamental principles for the ethical conduct clinical trials involving human subjects. These principles were formulated in the World Medical Association's Declaration of Helsinki in 1964 and revised in 1989 (WMA 1989). The principles cover the manner of conducting clinical trials as follows:

- Clinical trials should be conducted according to ethical principles based on the Declaration of Helsinki.
- Risks should be weighed against potential benefits prior to starting a trial.
- The rights, safety and well-being of study participants are primary considerations.
- All available clinical and non-clinical information should be presented for evaluation of a proposed trial.
- Trials should be scientifically sound and clearly described in a detailed protocol.
- Protocol should be approved by an ethics board and should be followed exactly as approved.
- Any medical care given to study participants should be performed by or under the direct authority of a qualified physician.
- Individuals involved in conduction clinical trials should be qualified by education, training and experience to perform their study tasks.
- Freely given informed consent should be obtained from every study participant.
- All trial information should be documented and stored in a way that assures accurate reporting, interpretation and verification.
- Investigational products should be manufactured, handled and stored according to approved standards.
- Quality assurance systems must be in place to assure quality of data.

Adherence to the principles of GCP is the responsibility of the sponsor, the principal investigator, and all study staff. Compliance is monitored by the FDA's Bioresearch monitoring department (BIMO). In the U.S., penalties for non-compliance can range from voluntary correction of deficiencies to fines and imprisonment in cases of deliberate fraud.

The New Drug Application

The New Drug Application (NDA) is submitted when all phases of investigation have been concluded. The NDA requires all the documentation necessary to present a complete picture of how the drug is made, formulated and checked for quality, how the drug performed in clinical testing, how the drug was tested in animals, and what happens to the drug in the body. The NDA also must include the proposed labeling so the FDA can ascertain that the claims made on the label do not exceed what can be reasonably supported by the clinical trials. Actual data and reports are part of the NDA so conclusions can be validated. The primary purpose of review is to evaluate safety and effectiveness in the context of the data presented and the claims made in the proposed marketing materials. The experiences gained in clinical trials provide the basis for telling health care providers how they should prescribe the drug. All this information is summarized on what becomes the package insert. If the documentation submitted to the FDA for review as an NDA is deemed insufficient, the application will be declined (FDA 1999). The company can then resubmit when the deficiencies have been addressed. Pharmaceutical companies pay a fee for the review of their NDA. Instituting this fee has shortened review times considerably and consequently has lessened the time it takes for new drugs to reach the consumer.

Clinical trials serve to promote safe and effective drugs and to eliminate those that turn out to be ineffective or too risky for the benefit they provide. Of the drugs tested for safety in Phase I, about 70% are successful. Of those, only about 33% successfully clear the effectiveness requirements of Phase 2. Of the drugs that successfully make it through Phase II, only about 25% make it through Phase III. In all, only about 20% of all INDs submitted are approved for marketing.

Conclusion

In this chapter we have reviewed the steps that are taken to develop a chemopreventive agent, from bench to market. While chemopreventive agents differ from therapeutic agents in their scope and intent, their development requires the same stringent adherence to laws, regulations and principles.

References

Anonymous (1999). "Prevention of cancer in the next millennium: Report of the Chemoprevention Working Group to the American Association for Cancer Research." *Cancer Research* **59**(19): 4743–4758.

FDA (1999). From test tube to patient: Improving health through human drugs. Rockville, MD, Food and Drug Administration, Center for Drug Evaluation and Research.

ICH (1994). International Conference on Harmonisation of Technical Requirements for Registration of Pharmaceuticals for Human Use. Geneva, ICH Secretariat.

Kelloff, G. J., E. T. Hawk, et al. (1996). "Strategies for identification and clinical evaluation of promising chemopreventive agents." *Oncology (Huntington)* **10**(10): 1471–1484; discussion 1484–1488.

Nestle, F. O., S. Alijagic, et al. (1998). "Vaccination of melanoma patients with peptide- or tumor lysate-pulsed dendritic cells." *Nature Medicine* **4**: 328–332.

O'Shaughnessy, J. A., G. J. Kelloff, et al. (2002). "Treatment and prevention of intraepithelial neoplasia: an important target for accelerated new agent development [comment]." *Clinical Cancer Research* **8**(2): 314–346.

WMA (1989) World Medical Association Declaration of Helsinki, World Medical Association.

Developing Topical Prodrugs for Skin Cancer Prevention

Elaine L. Jacobson, Hyuntae Kim, Moonsun Kim, Georg T. Wondrak, and Myron K. Jacobson

College of Pharmacy and Arizona Cancer Center, University of Arizona, Tucson, AZ 85724

The skin plays multiple roles in protection from environmental insults yet skin damage, particularly that derived from sunlight, constitutes a major public health problem. End stage skin damage in the form of non-melanoma skin cancers (NMSC) are the most frequent malignancies in the United States with more than 1,000,000 cases diagnosed annually (Karagas, Greenberg et al. 1999). Melanoma skin cancer is the most rapidly increasing cancer. Actinic keratosis (AK), skin lesions that can progress to NMSC are far more prevalent than skin cancers. The occurrence of DNA damage and cellular responses to DNA damage are major determinants of skin damage including skin cancer (Ames 2001; Ullrich 2002). A compelling body of evidence now indicates that there are multiple targets for reducing skin damage and that several key micronutrients are candidates for skin damage prevention. However, a major challenge for the development of prevention strategies for skin damage is the difficulty of delivering micronutrients to skin. Delivery to skin via the blood circulation of nutrients taken orally is inherently inefficient since this delivery is distal to other organs, particularly the liver, which removes many agents by first pass metabolism. In addition the major cell targets for prevention of skin cancer are located in the epidermis which is non-vascular.

Described here are strategies to limit skin damage and thus skin cancer by targeting multiple mechanisms that include preventing DNA damage, enhancing DNA repair, preventing immune suppression, and preventing migration of transformed cells from epidermis to dermis. Further, an approach for delivery of key protective agents to skin cells using prodrugs specifically tailored for topical delivery is described. Finally, this approach is illustrated using niacin as a model micronutrient demonstrating that topical delivery of this polar compound to skin cells via prodrugs is feasible and that targeted delivering provides prevention benefit for skin.

Strategies for Intervention

Genotoxic stress is known to be a major factor in skin damage. While the mechanisms that cause skin damage are complex and incompletely understood, genotoxic stress in the form of DNA damage is a major factor. Figure 1 shows the primary sources of genotoxic stress in both the dermis and epidermis of skin and the consequences of this stress. Three interrelated sources of genotoxic stress in skin are reactive oxygen species (ROS), reactive carbonyl species (RCS) and sunlight. Sunlight is the major source of skin damage as it leads to DNA damage directly via formation of pyrimidine

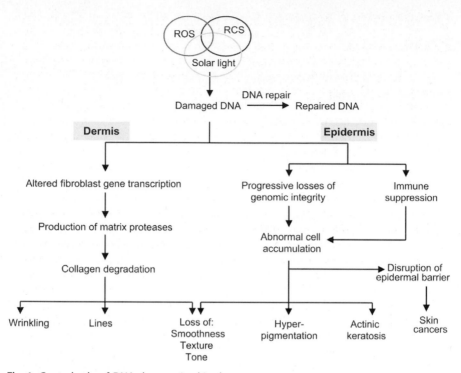

Fig. 1. Central role of DNA damage in skin damage

dimers and other photoproducts (Ullrich 2002) and indirectly via generation of ROS and RCS by photooxidation and photosensitization reactions (Wondrak, Cervantes-Laurean et al. 2002; Wondrak, Roberts et al. 2002; Roberts, Wondrak et al. 2003). Indeed, sunlight has been documented as a complete carcinogen. While the UVB region of sunlight, the region responsible for most of the direct DNA damage by sunlight, is the most effective at initiation of squamous cell carcinoma (SCC), recent studies have shown that solar simulated light containing more predominantly UVA rays that induce ROS also cause SCC formation (Pentland, Schoggins et al. 1999; Agar, Halliday et al. 2004). The involvement of ROS in the promotion and progression phases of skin cancer is well established (Perchellet and Perchellet 1989). ROS include superoxide, hydroxyl radical, hydrogen peroxide, singlet oxygen, nitric oxide, peroxynitrite, and hypochlorite. All cells are exposed to ROS during the normal course of energy metabolism and/or immune surveillance in addition to sunlight exposure. While ROS are involved in normal cell signaling pathways, increased ROS formation during oxidative stress disrupts signaling pathways causing negative consequences for normal cell function. In addition to DNA, proteins also are targets for damage by ROS in skin. Carbonyl stress, mediated by RCS from metabolic sources, lipid peroxidation, and glycoxidation targets skin cell DNA and extracellular matrix proteins with accumulation of protein advanced glycation end products (AGEs) during chronological and actinic aging of skin (Wondrak, Cervantes-Laurean et al. 2002; Wondrak, Jacobson et al. 2002; Wondrak, Roberts et al. 2002; Roberts, Wondrak et al. 2003). Recently AGEs have been identified as potent UVA sensitizers of photooxidative stress in human skin, establishing a vicious cycle of RCS and ROS formation in sunlight induced genotoxic stress.

Figure 1 also overviews two major consequences of genotoxic stress in skin. First, chronic DNA damage results in progressive losses of genomic integrity that result in and are required for end stage skin damage in the form of skin cancer. These progressive losses of genomic integrity lead to altered growth properties of damaged keratinocytes such as unresponsiveness to terminal differentiation signals leading to epidermal hyperplasia and progressively to detectable skin lesions diagnosed as actinic keratosis (Jeffes and Tang 2000; Lober, Lober et al. 2000). Cell populations present in actinic keratosis lesions can progress to transformed cell populations that represent epidermal carcinoma in situ (Horowitz and Monger 1995; Guenthner, Hurwitz et al. 1999). Subsequent cellular changes occur including induction of matrix proteases that facilitate disruption of the integrity of the epidermal barrier leading to invasion of the dermis, the point at which the damage process is diagnosed as SCC. A second major consequence of DNA damage in skin is the suppression of immune responses that would normally detect and remove damaged cells. While mechanisms of immune suppression extend well beyond DNA damage, the latter represents a major factor in immune sup-

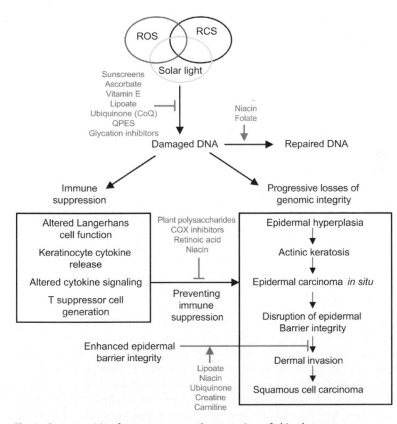

Fig. 2. Opportunities for treatment and prevention of skin damage

pression. The consequences of genotoxic stress include altered migration and antigen presentation by Langerhans cells, stimulation of cytokine release by keratinocytes that likely alters cytokine signaling required for normal immune surveillance including generation of T suppressor cells. Given the complexity of damage pathways and the down stream consequences, it seems likely that a combination strategy to prevent skin damage will be essential.

Figure 2 identifies opportunities for epidermal intervention by various agents where substantial evidence suggests the possibility of modulating the consequences of genotoxic stress. These opportunities include preventing DNA damage, enhancing DNA repair, preventing immune suppression both by preventing DNA damage and by mechanisms downstream from DNA damage, and strengthening the integrity of the epidermal barrier to prevent migration of transformed cells from the epidermis.

Strategy 1: Preventing DNA damage

Sunscreens. The value of sunscreens in preventing DNA damage has clearly been demonstrated in animal models in which sunscreens applied prior to solar simulated light (SSL) exposure prevented p53 mutations and dramatically reduced skin cancer incidence (Ananthaswamy, Ullrich et al. 1999). Further, sunscreens prevent photoimmune suppression in mice (Reeve, Bosnic et al. 1998) and man (Fourtanier, Gueniche et al. 2000). Despite growing use of sunscreens, their inability to protect across a broad spectrum of solar radiation combined with poor public knowledge of appropriate selection and use have not led to decreases in skin cancer incidence. While the use of sunscreens needs to be an integral part of an overall strategy to reduce skin damage, their inability as a single agent to reduce skin damage illustrates the need for a combination of prevention agents.

Ascorbate (Vitamin C). Vitamin C has been used widely in recent years as a skin protective agent. It is known to function as an antioxidant and likely serves multiple roles in collagen synthesis (Geesin, Darr et al. 1988). Further, this vitamin is important in recycling of reducing power in cells by exchange of electrons with vitamin E (Beyer 1994). A study in mice has shown inhibition of phorbol ester induced skin tumor promotion using a lipophilic ester of vitamin C which, in its free form, is unstable and has poor penetration through the stratum corneum (Smart and Crawford 1991). Further studies of stable, deliverable forms of vitamin C designed for optimal uptake by cells may prove beneficial in limiting DNA damage and improve skin cancer prevention. It is important to consider, however, that this compound can serve both as an antioxidant and a pro-oxidant.

Tocopherol (Vitamin E). Topical application of tocopherol has been shown to decrease the incidence of ultraviolet-induced skin cancer in mice (Berton, Conti et al. 1998; Burke, Clive et al. 2000). Vitamin E provides protection against UV-induced skin photodamage through a combination of antioxidant and UV absorptive properties (McVean and Liebler 1997). Topical application of alpha-tocopherol on mouse skin inhibits the formation of cyclobutane pyrimidine photoproducts (Chen, Barthelman et al. 1997). However, topically applied alpha-tocopherol is rapidly depleted by UVB radiation in a dose-dependent manner (Liebler and Burr 2000) as vitamin E in skin can absorb UV light and generate the tocopheryl radical (Kagan, Witt et al. 1992). Hence, vitamin E in skin may act in two conflicting manners, as a radical scavenger and possibly as a photosensitizer. Indeed, tocopherol has been shown to exacerbate UVA induced DNA damage in vitro (Nocentini, Guggiari et al. 2001). However, reductive antioxidants (ascorbate, thiols, ubiquinols, etc.) can reduce tocopherol radicals back to tocopherol (Kagan, Serbinova et al. 1990). Unlike the soluble vitamins that are too hydrophilic for optimal delivery through the stratum corneum, vitamin E is more lipophilic than is optimal for delivery into skin. Thus, when applied topically as the parent compound, residence time on the surface of skin is prolonged making the agent susceptible to UVB light absorption and possible conversion to a tocopheryl radical, which is a potential photosensitizer. On the other hand, when Vitamin E is stabilized by derivatization to a prodrug and effectively delivered into skin possessing an environment of reductive antioxidants (ascorbate, thiols, ubiquinols, etc.) or formulated with antioxidants, tocopherol radical formation can be eliminated by three mechanisms: (1) decreased exposure to UVB on the surface of skin due to rate of delivery, (2) stability of vitamin E due to derivatization to prodrug, and (3) rapid conversion back to tocopherol of any tocopheryl radicals formed due to the presence of reductive antioxidants in skin cells and/or in the delivery vehicle. While preclinical data demonstrate that tocopherol has photoprotective properties, clinical data do not yet convincingly show that dietary supplementation is of significant therapeutic value in protection from acute or chronic photodamage. Further, use of ester derivatives of vitamin E to date have stabilized the molecule, but have increased the lipophilicity of the compound thereby decreasing its delivery to skin. This illustrates the general lack of understanding of delivery mechanisms for micronutrient benefits in skin. Thus, it seems likely that cutaneous bioavailability of dietary and existing preparations of topical tocopherol may be insufficient to combat photodamage in skin.

Lipoate. While a clear role for direct ROS scavenging by lipoate has not been firmly established, lipoate has a redox potential of −0.32 V, allowing it to reduce oxidized glutathione and ascorbate nonenzymatically in the skin antioxidative network (Guo and Packer 2000). In keratinocytes, lipoate is reduced to its active form, dihydrolipoate, which results in significant inhibition of the consumption of tocopherol and ubiquinone following UVA irradiation (Guo and Packer 2000). This protection presumably occurs via the role of lipoate along with ascorbate and tocopherol in the maintenance of redox balance. Lipoate topically applied to hairless mouse skin shows penetration and conversion to dihydrolipoate demonstrating cellular delivery although the efficacy of delivery was not examined in detail (Podda, Rallis et al. 1996). Lipoate *per se* is much too hydrophilic for effective topical delivery.

Ubiquinone (Coenzyme Q10). Ubiquinone offers the potential to reduce DNA damage directly as an ROS scavenger and by supporting redox cycles that resist oxidative stress (Tomasetti, Littarru et al. 1999). Ubiquinone and tocopherol are the major lipophilic antioxidants in skin (Shindo, Witt et al. 1994). The content of ubiquinone is 9 times higher in the epidermis than in the dermis and a strong role in protection against skin damage is suggested by the observation that skin ubiquinone content decreases rapidly following solar irradiation (Shindo, Witt et al. 1994). A recent study has demonstrated that in vivo supplementation with ubiquinone enhances the recovery of human lymphocytes from oxidative DNA damage, supporting the hypothesis that this micronutrient can limit DNA damage in vivo (Tomasetti, Littarru et al. 1999). In addition to its role as a direct ROS scavenger, ubiquinone has been postulated to function as an integral part of antioxidant defense pathways that also include tocopherol, ascorbate, glutathione and NADPH (Podda and Grundmann-Kollmann 2001). Beneficial effects of topical ubiquinone on prevention and reversal of skin photoaging also have been reported although the same study reported that the extremely lipophilic nature of the molecule strongly limited bioavailability following topical application (Hoppe, Bergemann et al. 1999), again illustrating the desirability of an effective strategy for topical delivery of this micronutrient. As with the case of tocopherol, ubiquinone *per se* also is much too lipophilic for effective topical delivery.

Quenchers of Photoexcited States (QPES). We have coined the term QPES to refer to agents that physically quench or dissipate the energy transferred from sunlight to skin molecules, thereby inactivating photoexcited states that would ultimately interact with oxygen or other molecules to produce RCS and ROS, hydrogen peroxide and singlet oxygen in particular. UV and near visible chromophores in skin extracellular proteins (keratin, collagen, and elastin) are endogenous photosensitizers that mediate photodamage in human skin (Wondrak, Roberts et al. 2002; Wondrak, Roberts et al. 2003). Small molecule quenchers of this novel class of sun damage targets are predicted to serve a chemopreventive role in suppressing photooxidative pathways of photocarcinogenesis and photoaging by direct physical quenching of photoexcited states that occurs without chemical depletion or need for metabolic regeneration of the active compound. This represents intervention at a very early step in the production of these UV induced deleterious species upstream of ROS formation. We have identified small polar compounds that accomplish these goals and envision that derivatives suitable for topical delivery will be required for optimal protective benefit to limit skin damage.

Glycation Inhibitors. Among the chromophores in skin that serve as photosensitizers of UV light are the nonenzymatically formed AGE chromophores generated from chemical reactions between reducing sugars and other RCS with protein amino groups followed by rearrangements and oxidation reactions. These structures form during intrinsic aging and accumulate at accelerated rates in photoaged skin. Interaction of AGEs with UV light readily generates ROS and more RCS forming a vicious cycle of skin damage (Wondrak, Cervantes-Laurean et al. 2002; Wondrak, Jacobson et al. 2002; Wondrak, Roberts et al. 2002; Roberts, Wondrak et al. 2003). Identifying agents to inhibit the formation of AGEs and optimize delivery of such agents could be very beneficial in limiting DNA damage that contributes to skin cancer.

Strategy 2: Enhancing DNA repair

Niacin. A major target for niacin (nicotinic acid) with regard to enhancing DNA repair is poly(ADP-ribose) polymerase-1 (PARP-1) and downstream signaling pathways, whose activity is enhanced by niacin due to increased availability of NAD, the bioactive form of niacin and a substrate for PARP-1. The involvement of PARP-1 as a target for cancer prevention by niacin is based on studies that have demonstrated the involvement of PARP-1 in the maintenance of genomic integrity following genotoxic stress (Jacobson and Jacobson 1999; Rolli, Armin et al. 2000). PARP-1 functions in the synthesis of chromatin-associated polymers of ADP-ribose that function in cellular recovery from DNA damage and maintenance of genomic stability. The activation of PARP-1 by DNA strand breaks leads to complex signaling pathways that can enhance cell survival or result in cell death by apoptosis as shown in Figure 3. In cases where the amount of damage is relatively small, PARP-1 activation enhances cellular recovery by interaction with other proteins such as p53 and the nuclear proteosome to stimulate both DNA repair and histone degradation such that the cell can fully recover from the genotoxic stress. When the damage is relatively higher, PARP-1 plays a key role in effecting cell death by apoptosis through its transcriptional activation role involving the NF-κB pathway and by preventing ATP depletion and DNA repair through PARP-1 cleavage (Jacobson and Jacobson 1999). Of direct relevance to skin, PARP-1 has been shown to be required for Fas, FasL mediated apoptosis critical to removal of badly damaged and potentially carcinogenic 'sunburn' cells that arise following sunlight exposures that lead to erythema (Hill, Ouhtit et al. 1999). Validation of niacin as a chemoprevention agent has been obtained in a mouse model where high dose oral niacin intake resulted in dose-dependent (1) increased skin NAD content, (2) decreased skin tumor incidence 70%, and (3) reduced immune suppression 86% (Gensler, Williams et al. 1999).

Folate. A major prevention target for folate relates to its role in providing precursors for DNA repair synthesis. It may also promote genomic integrity through its role in the generation of methyl groups needed for control of gene expression. Its cancer protection potential has been demonstrated by large-scale epidemiological and nutritional studies indicating that decreased folate status increases the risk of developing stomach (Fang, Xiao et al. 1997), colorectal and breast cancer (Prinz-Langenohl, Fohr et al. 2001). Consistent with a role in DNA repair, chromosome breaks and centrosome abnormalities have been observed in patients deficient in folate (Heath 1966; Chen, Reidy et al. 1989). In vitro, DNA strand breakage and uracil misincorporation increased in a time and concentration dependent manner after human lymphocytes were cultured with decreasing amounts of folate (Duthie and Hawdon 1998). DNA breaks are associated with an increased risk of cancer in humans. Moreover, folate deficiency impairs DNA excision repair in rat colonic

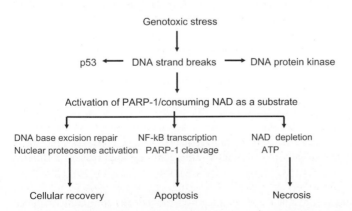

Fig. 3. Interrelationship of niacin metabolism and DNA damage and repair pathways

mucosa (Choi, Kim et al. 1998). These data indicate that folic acid deficiency affects the stability of cellular DNA at the chromosomal and molecular levels (Choi and Mason 2000). While folate deficiency has been extensively documented by analysis of human plasma, folate status within skin has not been widely investigated. Nevertheless, the inefficiency of delivery of nutrients to skin argues that documented folate deficiencies will extend to skin. Additionally, photolysis of folate appears likely to deplete this nutrient in sun-exposed skin (Jablonski and Chaplin 2000). It has been reported that fair-skinned patients undergoing photochemotherapy for dermatological conditions have low serum folate concentrations, suggesting that folate depletion may occur in vivo (Branda and Eaton 1978). With regard to delivery, folate *per se* is too hydrophilic for effective topical skin delivery.

Strategy 3: Preventing photoimmune suppression

While the mechanisms leading to photoimmune suppression are still poorly understood, DNA damage is a major factor leading to reduced immune surveillance (Ullrich 2002). Two major cell targets are Langerhans cells where DNA damage leads to suppression of cell migration and antigen presentation functions and keratinocytes where DNA damage results in altered cytokine signaling and reduced immune function potentially involved in generation of T suppressor cells (Elmets, Bergstresser et al. 1983; Cruz, Tigelaar et al. 1990). In addition to DNA, two other targets have been identified for immune suppression. The photoconversion of urocanic acid to cis-urocanic acid has been implicated in immune suppression, although the molecular mechanisms are still poorly defined (Moodycliffe, Norval et al. 1993). Also, ROS generation including membrane lipid peroxidation has been implicated in immune suppression (Ullrich 2002), possibly by altering signaling pathways at the membrane level, although DNA as the ultimate target is still a possibility. In view of the strong link between DNA damage and immune suppression, it is not surprising that agents that prevent DNA damage or enhance DNA repair reduce suppression (Gensler, Williams et al. 1999; Ullrich 2002). Additionally, several other agents offer promise for prevention of immune suppression at stages following DNA damage.

Plant Polysaccharides. A number of plant polysaccharides, such as those found in *Aloe barbadenis*, appear to prevent immune suppression by mechanisms distinct from those that do so by preventing DNA damage (Strickland 2001).

COX Inhibitors. Drugs that block production of PGE2 by cyclooxygenase activity have been shown to reduce photoimmune suppression, suggesting a role of overproduction of prostaglandins in immune suppression (Shreedhar, Giese et al. 1998).

Retinoic Acid. Defective dendritic cell function caused by abnormal differentiation of these cells is an important mechanism of tumor escape from immune system control. All-trans-retinoic acid has been shown to induce maturation of these cells in cancer patients and this may suggest a role in modulating immune suppression (Almand, Clark et al. 2001).

Niacin. As described above, niacin has been shown to prevent photoimmune suppression (Gensler, Williams et al. 1999). While the ability of niacin to prevent immune suppression may be due to its ability to limit DNA damage by enhancing DNA repair, it should be noted that niacin has recently been discovered to stimulate the release of leptin (Kim 2002). Leptin is emerging as a hormone that modulates numerous protective effects in skin including immune modulation. Thus, it is possible that niacin prevents immune suppression via effects on leptin secretion.

Strategy 4: Enhancing the Epidermal Barrier

The epidermis of skin is a constantly renewing tissue. This renewal involves a complex series of events that involves proliferation of keratinocytes in the basal layer followed by terminal differentiation that ultimately leads to an epidermal barrier whose integrity is crucial to the protection of the organism from environmental insults. Several points need to be considered with regard to micronutrients in epidermal turnover. First, there is a growing body of evidence indicating that a significant percentage of the American population is deficient in a number of micronutrients and the constant turnover of the epidermis makes this tissue particularly vulnerable to micronutrient depletion. While there is limited data on micronutrient content of skin, studies have demonstrated that micronutrient deficiencies observed in plasma also are observed in skin (Peng, Peng et al. 1993), a wide range of tissue NAD content has been observed in human skin (Jacobson, Shieh et al. 1999), and solar exposure has been demonstrated to deplete micronutrients (Jablonski and Chaplin 2000; Liebler and Burr 2000). Thus, skin is a likely site of micronutrient deficiencies with potentially adverse consequences leading to skin damage. Second, the constant renewal of the epidermal compartment places an important energy requirement on the organism. Thus, the nutritional status of micronutrients whose bioactive forms play important roles in cellular energy generation is important to the integrity of the epidermal barrier (Jacobson, Giacomoni et al. 2001). Micronutrients in this category include lipoate, niacin, ubiquinone, creatine, and carnitine. Third, the non-vascular nature of the epidermal compartment makes micronutrient delivery to this compartment inherently inefficient. The above considerations have led to the proposal that optimal energy metabolism will strengthen integrity of the epidermal barrier which in turn can lead to a decrease in skin cancer. Studies have shown that cell populations with altered growth properties within actinic keratosis lesions can be recognized by immune surveillance and removed. Alternatively, cell populations within such lesions can progress to cell populations (carcinoma in situ) that secrete proteases and other factors that allow escape from the epidermis. Thus, the status of the epidermal barrier integrity can be a deciding factor between the ultimate fates of removal or escape of abnormal cell populations from the epidermal compartment.

Innovative Agents for Skin Cancer Prevention are Needed

Several approaches have been taken to reduce the rate of skin damage and photodamage. Reducing the amount of damage that reaches critical biomolecules in the skin is the objective of sunscreens, antioxidants, and quenchers of photoexcited states (Figure 2). Sunscreens aim to directly absorb sunlight photons and thus lessen the amount of damage that reaches the skin, and quenchers are designed to deactivate excited state molecules in skin prior to interaction with oxygen to limit the amount of ROS formed.

Glycation inhibitors also are designed to limit ROS generation from solar irradiation of AGE-pigments in skin. Alternatively, antioxidants, which include vitamins C and E as active ingredients, are designed to intercept damage to the skin by capture of ROS generated by sunlight exposure. While the approaches designed to reduce damage to the skin are beneficial, they have inherent limitations, as neither sunscreens nor antioxidants can effectively eliminate oxidative stress. Sunscreens absorb only a portion of the rays of sunlight that cause damage, many are not photostable for more than a few minutes in sunlight, and the feasible levels of antioxidants in skin creams can only partially reduce oxidative stress. Another approach to treating skin deterioration involves accelerating the removal of the upper layers of damaged skin to allow replacement with undamaged skin. The application of retinoic acid (tretinoin, Renova and Retin A) results in an increased rate of cell turnover allowing new cells to mature and replace damaged cells, but a side effect is a weakened skin barrier and increased photosensitivity. Chemical peels using agents such as alpha-hydroxy acids or beta-hydroxy acids cause a chemical exfoliation of the top layers of skin, again allowing new cells to replace the damaged cells that have been removed. Topical formulations of 5-fluorouracil represent an aggressive therapy for removal of skin lesions and a topical formulation of the cyclooxygenase (COX) inhibitor diclofenac has been approved for treatment of actinic keratosis. Surgical or laser procedures also can remove damaged skin. While these approaches play important roles in the treatment of skin damage, the high irritation potential, increased sunlight sensitivity, and long downtime for patient recovery from facial disfiguration of most current treatments combined with the enormity of the problem indicates that new approaches to treat and prevent skin damage still are needed.

Lipophilic ester prodrugs have been used to increase the permeability of polar compounds for transdermal systemic drug delivery. With regard to micronutrients, some derivatives of vitamins C and E have been prepared and used in skin care products, but a systematic, scientific base for rational development of compounds and their evaluation demonstrating optimal delivery of protective agents to the cellular components of skin has not been reported. For example, the realization that vitamin E is more stable as an ester derivative resulted in the design of a compound that was less efficacious than the parent compound, but to our knowledge the flux rates into skin of vitamin E esters have not been studied (Alberts, Goldman et al. 1996). We predict that a more polar derivative of vitamin E also would stabilize the compound and improve delivery. This approach to optimize skin micronutrients and/or chemoprevent genotoxic stress in skin with multiple agents is complementary to and integrative with existing approaches and new developments such as designing more effective sunscreens to limit skin damage.

Topical Delivery: the Cornerstone of a Skin Damage Prevention Strategy

We have reviewed above evidence indicating that several agents are therapeutic candidates for skin damage prevention. However, a major challenge for the development of prevention strategies for skin damage relates to the difficulty of delivering small molecules to skin. Delivery to skin via the blood circulation of nutrients taken orally is inherently inefficient as delivery is distal to other organs and numerous cell targets for skin cancer prevention are located in the epidermis which is non vascular. The challenging in delivering many micronutrients topically is that they are small molecules that do not have optimal properties to insure prolonged skin residence time required for efficacy. For example, niacin, ascorbate, lipoate, creatine, carnitine, and folate are too polar for effective delivery while vitamin E, vitamin E acetate, and ubiquinone are too lipophilic. To resolve this problem, we have studied niacin (nicotinic acid) as a model nutrient to determine the feasibility of optimizing topical delivery to skin cells. Briefly, the strategy is as follows. Prodrugs designed for optimal delivery are synthesized as esters or thioesters of the parent micronutrient or drug. Once delivered to the epidermis, the abundant and nonspecific esterases present there rapidly cleave the prodrugs back to the parent compound. The delivery properties are designed to provide a slow, continuous supply of micronutrient to skin cells to allow increased uptake by the cells. This strategy takes into consideration two distinct barriers that influence the delivery of small molecules to skin, lipophilicity of the stratum corneum and skin metabolic activity. Our formulation strategy controls the rate of partitioning of the prodrug in and out of the stratum corneum by designing derivatives with an optimal lipophilicity for such partitioning. Figure 4 shows a multiple compartment model that serves as the framework for the development of this delivery strategy. Briefly described below are features of the topical delivery strategy that have emerged from our research.

A Pronutrient Must Effectively Partition from the Topical Formulation Into the Stratum Corneum. The highly lipophilic nature of the stratum corneum dictates that a pronutrient be sufficiently lipophilic to effectively partition into the stratum corneum from the donor compartment, which can be a skin cream or lotion (arrow #1 in Figure 4). As described in more detail below, the required lipophilicity needed for diffusion from the stratum corneum into the epidermis predicts that an efficacious pronutrient should be sufficiently lipophilic to rapidly partition from the cream or lotion into the stratum corneum. We have synthesized esters of nicotinic acid that are lipophilic derivatives that allow rapid diffusion from the topical formulation into the stratum corneum.

The Pronutrient Must be Stable in the Topical Formulation. The lipophilicity of a prodrug should allow it to be formulated in a skin cream or lotion and the linkage of the nutrient derivative must be very stable in these formulations. We have shown that the prodrug lipophilicity optimal for delivery is such that the prodrug is easy to formulate in a cream or lotion. Also, in the case of niacin prodrugs, our developmental research examined and identified compounds that were stable to chemical hydrolysis when formulated in a cream or lotion.

The Pronutrient must Partition from the Stratum Corneum into the Epidermis at an Optimal Rate to Achieve Effective Delivery to the Cellular Components of Skin (#2 in Figure 4). Studies of drug structure-penetration relationships have provided useful information concerning partitioning from the stratum corneum to the epidermis (Tsai, Tayar et al. 1992; Potts and Guy 1993; Webber, Meyer-Trumpener et al. 1994). This rate of flux is controlled by a diffusion constant and for small uncharged molecules lipophilicity is the major factor that determines the diffusion constant. A correlation between skin permeability (P_B) and the physicochemical properties of the drug, such as octanol/water partition coefficient ($P_{oct/w}$) have proven to be of great value in predicting drug transport across skin. Figure 5 illustrates the relationship be-

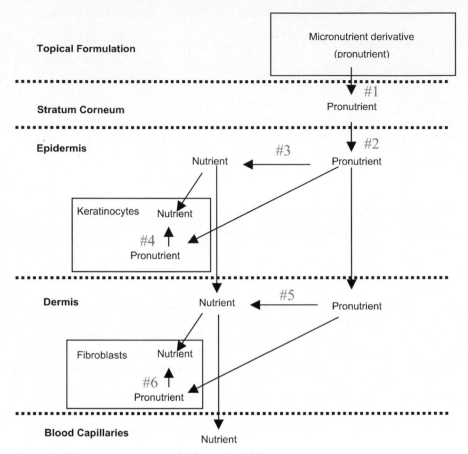

Fig. 4. Multiple compartment model for topical delivery

tween compound lipophilicity, rate of flux from stratum corneum, and skin residence time (Roberts, Anderson et al. 1978; Anderson, Higuchi et al. 1988).

A series of niacin esters were synthesized and their log $P_{oct/w}$ values were determined. The values demonstrated a linear relationship between alkyl chain length of the niacin ester and the logarithm of the octanol/water partition coefficient. These data allowed us to relate prodrug lipophilicity to niacin delivery and thus allowed identification of the lipophilicity range that provides an optimal rate of prodrug and thus drug delivery.

The Pronutrient must be Efficiently Bioconverted to Active Nutrient in Skin. The delivery approach that we designed for niacin involved the bioconversion of the pronutrient to niacin by the action of skin esterases. Studies on the esterase distribution of skin have shown that the stratum corneum has little or no esterase activity, the epidermis has the highest activity and the dermis has reduced activity relative to the epidermis (Sugibayashi, Hayashi et al. 1999). Delivery should be possible whether the

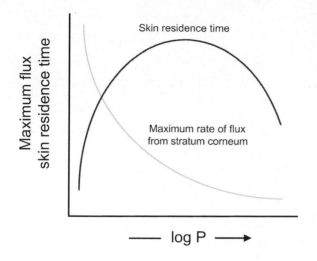

Fig. 5. Relationship between compound lipophilicity, rate of flux from stratum corneum, and skin residence time

Skin residence time

Maximum rate of flux from stratum corneum

Maximum flux skin residence time

— log P —→

bioconversion is extracellular (#3 and 5, Figure 4) or following uptake by the target cells (#4 and 6, Figure 4) since cells contain specific transport systems for niacin and the lipophilicity of the prodrug should make it readily bioavailable through passive diffusion also. Skin cells also contain esterases. Bioconversion was confirmed by experiments that determined the effect of niacin prodrugs on the content of the bioactive form of niacin, NAD, in skin cells. Thus, we have measured bioconversion of the prodrug to nutrient and then bioconversion of the nutrient to the active form of the vitamin in this case. In this manner, we were able to relate the major factor determining the rate of partitioning from stratum corneum to epidermis (prodrug lipophilicity) to the effectiveness of cellular delivery (skin cell NAD content).

Developing a Niacin Prodrug as a Potential Skin Cancer Prevention Agent Rationale. Nicotinic acid was selected for development as the first topical agent in a series of micronutrients based on its known effects in preclinical studies. The diagram in Figure 6 outlines the three predominant mechanisms of action of this compound. First, it has long been appreciated that nicotinic acid, as well as nicotinamide, can serve as the vitamin precursor of NAD and recent studies have demonstrated that NAD deficiency can occur in Western populations (Jacobson, Dame et al. 1995) and while the degree of deficiency may not reach that which elicits symptoms of pellagra, it may be relevant in the development of chronic disease states such as cancer. NAD is essential in energy metabolism and may be a very important factor in the continual epidermal renewal of skin, which is known to turnover approximately every 28–30 days. In addition, numerous dermal functions are energy demanding. Since skin is the largest organ of the body, maintenance of optimal NAD for energy in skin by dietary means could be challenging, particularly during aging and following photodamage. Secondly, NAD serves as a substrate for the enzyme PARP-1, which plays an essential role in maintenance of genomic integrity and NAD is rapidly consumed during genomic stresses such as UV radiation and environmental insults to skin (Jacobson, Antol et al. 1983). This pathway may also be important in immune function, which is criti-

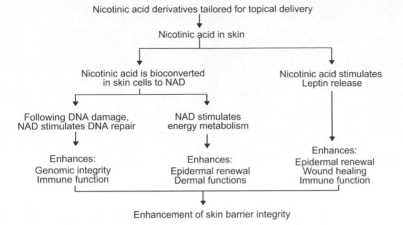

Fig. 6. Known effects of nicotinic acid in skin

cal following UV exposure. Thirdly, we have shown that nicotinic acid stimulates the release of the cytokine, leptin (Kim, Jacobson et al. 2002), which has been shown to function in epidermal renewal, wound healing, immune function, and inhibition of tumor promotion. Based on these findings, a development program for a topical prodrug of nicotinic acid was initiated.

Synthesis and Characterization of Niacin Prodrugs. The feasibility of developing a topical delivery system for skin protective agents was established by demonstrating that delivery of a niacin prodrug is controlled primarily by the rate of diffusion (lipophilicity). We synthesized, purified, and characterized niacin derivatives using alcohols varying in alkyl chain lengths from 8 to 18 carbon atoms to construct niacin derivatives.

To assess targeted delivery to skin, niacin derivatives were formulated in a compatible lotion and administered to the backs of hairless mice, once daily for three days. Skin samples from the site of application were evaluated for intracellular NAD content. This measurement assesses the net effect of diffusion of the prodrug through the stratum corneum to the cellular layers of skin, bioconversion to niacin, uptake by cells, and subsequent conversion to NAD. From Figure 7, it can be seen that derivatives having log P values ranging from around 6 to 10 were effective at targeting delivery to skin cells with tetradecyl nicotinate (TN or Nia-114) (Log $P_{oct/w}$ of 7.5) most effectively elevating NAD in mouse skin at the site of application. Also, it can be seen in Figure 7 that the free forms of the vitamin, nicotinamide and nicotinic acid did not effectively deliver to skin cells to increase skin cell NAD content.

The proposed topical delivery system was designed to target small molecules to skin with minimal systemic exposure. To evaluate this effect, skin samples taken from the abdominal area (distal to the application site) were compared to that taken from the back (site of application). Minimal changes in NAD occurred in abdominal samples while significant increases were observed in the samples from the back as shown in Figure 7. These data provide evidence for preferential delivery to the targeted tis-

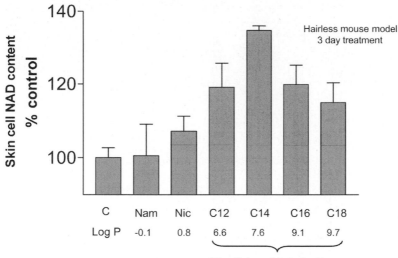

Fig. 7. Effect of niacin derivatives applied topically on skin cell NAD

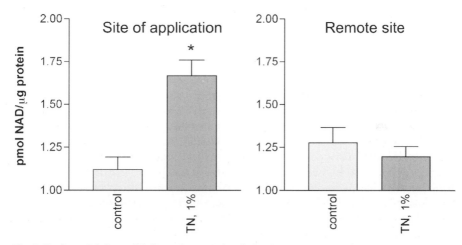

Fig. 8. Preferential dermal delivery by tetradecyl nicotinate in mouse skin

sue. These data show that tetradecyl nicotinate delivers niacin at a slow sustained rate at the site of delivery on the stratum corneum, allowing hydrolysis of the prodrug at a rate suitable for efficient uptake and bioconversion by skin cells. In contrast, lauryl nicotinate increased skin NAD content at both the site of application and at a distal site (data not shown), indicating tissue saturation at remote sites due to transdermal delivery. Using this lead candidate, tetradecyl nicotinate, dose- and time-response studies were carried out to determine the dosing concentration and schedule for optimal delivery to skin cells (Figure 9). Using 7 days as an end point, concentrations of tetrade-

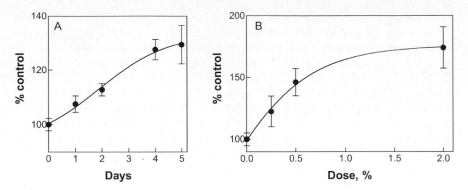

Fig. 9. Dose (A) and time (B) effects of topical tetradecyl nicotinate treatment on NAD content of hairless mouse skin

cyl nicotinate up to 1.0% increased NAD in skin. The time course of skin NAD content is shown for 1% tetradecyl nicotinate. A plateau was observed at about 5 days.

Tetradecyl nicotinate was found to be stable at room temperature and at elevated temperatures for extended periods of time appropriate to further development. In addition, bioconversion studies showed that it was readily converted to nicotinate and the free alcohol, demonstrating that tetradecyl nicotinate functions effectively as a prodrug of niacin for topical delivery.

Clinical Development of Tetradecyl Nicotinate (Nia-114)

Clinical Evaluation of Nia-114. This compound has undergone extensive safety evaluation in vitro and in vivo to determine the repetitive epidermal contact potential of a test material to induce primary or cumulative irritation and/or contact sensitization. The test material at 5% showed no potential for dermal irritation or allergic contact sensitization. Skin creams containing this compound are extremely well tolerated with daily use. No irritation was reported by study subjects or detected by study physicians. Measurements designed to detect even minimal irritation as skin redness showed a trend away from redness for Nia-114 treated skin. These data demonstrate that the controlled delivery of niacin using the prodrug strategy eliminates the vasodilation effects that occur when niacin is applied topically or taken orally. The prodrug strategy was designed to provide slow continuous delivery where the concentration of niacin reaching the circulation would be below the threshold to induce vasodilation. With these safety and tolerability evaluations completed, the clinical effects on skin of Nia-114 were then evaluated in multiple studies that have used a double blinded, placebo-controlled study design. Results of these studies are summarized below.

Nia-114 Simultaneously Increases Skin Cell Turnover and Skin Barrier Integrity. The effects of Nia-114 on stratum corneum turnover was measured by disappearance of Dansyl staining as a surrogate measure of the rate of skin cell turnover. Treatment with Nia-114 resulted in a highly statistically significant stimulation of skin cell turnover in the range of 7 to 11% compared to placebo. Thus, it is similar to other treatments for photodamage in its property to increase skin cell turnover; however, the magnitude of the effect is less than that observed for other treatments. The advantage of this approach to stimulate skin cell turnover is that the turnover occurs in a manner that strengthens skin barrier integrity as described below while other treatments that stimulate turnover do so to such a degree that skin barrier integrity is seriously compromised.

The effect of Nia-114 on the integrity of the skin barrier has been determined in a number of different ways that include determination of the rates of transepidermal water loss (TEWL), TEWL following a standard regimen of stratum corneum removal by tape stripping to assess effects on the upper epidermis, and by stratum corneum conductance determinations. Each of these methods has shown that Nia-114 strengthens the integrity of the skin barrier. The relationship between rates of TEWL and skin barrier integrity has been validated showing that decreased rates clearly reflect a more intact skin barrier (Reeve, Bosnic et al. 1998). Nia-114 treatment resulted in a highly statistically significant ($p = 0.006$ versus placebo) decrease in the rate of TEWL of nearly 20% above the effect of the placebo alone. The effect of Nia-114 on skin barrier integrity has been assessed following removal of the stratum corneum layer of skin using a standardized protocol of tape stripping. Nia-114 treated arms showed a 20% decrease in the rate of TEWL at 18 weeks of treatment ($p = 0.07$ versus placebo). Stratum corneum conductance measurements showed a highly statistically significant progressive increase in skin barrier integrity for Nia-114 treated skin compared to placebo of 10% at weeks 12 ($p = 0.05$) and 18 ($p = 0.01$). The unique ability of Nia-114 to simultaneously stimulate skin cell turnover and strengthen skin barrier integrity is consistent with the known roles of nicotinic acid (see Figure 6). It will be interesting to determine whether strengthening the integrity of the epidermal barrier will limit progression of in situ cancers to metastatic cancers. Further studies will be needed to verify this hypothesis.

Nia-114 Dramatically Increases Skin Barrier Integrity in Compromised Skin. Figure 10 shows the results of skin barrier assessment with placebo and Nia-114 treatment at 4 and 8 weeks in a group of atopic study subjects measuring rates of transepidermal

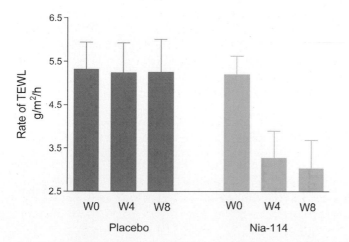

Fig. 10. Decrease in rate of treansepidermal water loss during treatment with Nia-114 in individuals with atopic skin

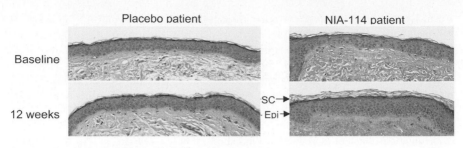

Fig. 11. Histological analyses of Nia-114 effects on skin

water loss (TEWL) to assess barrier integrity. Research has shown that rates of TEWL are strongly correlated with severity of clinical symptoms in atopic subjects (Chamlin, Kao et al. 2002). The results show that the placebo had no significant effect on barrier function while the Nia-114 treatment resulted in an approximately 35% and 45% increase in barrier function at 4 and 8 weeks. This effect of Nia-114 on skin barrier integrity in atopic subjects has exciting implications for clinical evaluation of benefits of this compound (Chamlin, Kao et al. 2002). Furthermore, it has been reported recently that low levels of leptin are strongly correlated with the risk of atopic skin, which is of interest with regard to the leptin releasing property of nicotinic acid (Jacobson, Kim et al. 2002) and the role of leptin release in preventing skin tumor promotion (Thuillier, Anchiraico et al. 2000). The data of Figure 11 show examples of histological analyses of skin punch biopsies from a clinical trial evaluating the effects of Nia-114 on skin. The increase in layers of corneocytes of the stratum corneum, responsible for barrier function, observed over 12 weeks of treatment as compared to the placebo is remarkable and correlates with effects measured by physical methods.

Nia-114 Confers Photoprotection. The effect of Nia-114 treatment on the minimum time of UV exposure to cause erythema also was determined in two separate sets of experiments. Nia-114 treatment results in a photoprotective effect of approximately 9% relative to control (data not shown). Erythema following UV exposure results from DNA damage, and the increased skin resilience following treatment is consistent with the known effects of nicotinic acid on enhancement of DNA repair and strengthening skin barrier integrity. The photoprotective effect of Nia-114 treatment contrasts sharply with other treatments for photodamage where photosensitivity is often observed.

Development of Nia-114 as a Skin Cancer Prevention Agent. Preclinical data has generated a body of evidence that has led to a RAPID Award from National Cancer Institute of the National Institutes of Health for development of Nia-114 as a skin cancer prevention agent. The RAPID program supports preclinical toxicology and pharmacology studies, filing an Investigational New Drug Application (IND) with the US Food and Drug Administration, and the planning and execution of Phase I clinical evaluation.

Conclusion

The complexity of processes that lead to skin damage are such that successful skin prevention strategies almost certainly will require a combination of agents that can provide prevention benefit by impacting different aspects of skin damage. Effective topical delivery of protective agents provides a solution to the difficulty of delivering to skin compounds taken orally. Topical delivery allows prevention to be targeted to the sites of damage, namely sun exposed skin, while minimizing systemic exposure. An increasing body of evidence indicates that key micronutrients can combat skin damage by multiple mechanisms including the reduction of genotoxic stress that is clearly a major factor in accumulated skin damage. A critical factor in any prevention strategy must be the safety of the prevention agent since long-term human exposure will be required. The tolerance and safety of micronutrients makes them excellent prevention candidates. The known protective effects of nicotinic acid summarized in Figure 6 have led us to develop a topical prodrug of this micronutrient and to begin development of this agent for skin cancer prevention. The data presented in this chapter indicate that the approach we have initiated allows effective delivery and provides benefit to skin with the potential to serve as a component of skin cancer prevention strategies. The approach is applicable to numerous other micronutrients and small molecule agents that have potential for skin cancer prevention.

References

Agar, N.S., G.M. Halliday, et al. (2004). "The basal layer in human squamous tumors harbors more UVA than UVB fingerprint mutations: A role for UVA in human skin carcinogenesis." *PNAS* **101**: 4954–4959.

Alberts, D.S., R. Goldman, et al. (1996). "Disposition and metabolism of topically administered alpha-tocopherol acetate: a common ingredient of commercially available sunscreens and cosmetics." *Nutr Cancer* **26**(2): 193–201.

Almand, B., J.I. Clark, et al. (2001). "Increased production of immature myeloid cells in cancer patients: a mechanism of immunosuppression in cancer." *J Immunol* **166**(1): 678–689.

Ames, B.N. (2001). "DNA damage from micronutrient deficiencies is likely to be a major cause of cancer." *Mutat Res* **475**(1–2): 7–20.

Ananthaswamy, H.N., S.E. Ullrich, et al. (1999). "Inhibition of solar simulator-induced p53 mutations and protection against skin cancer development in mice by sunscreens." *J Invest Dermatol* **112**(5): 763–768.

Anderson, B.D., W.I. Higuchi, et al. (1988). "Heterogeneity effects on permeability-partition coefficient relationships in human stratum corneum." *Pharm Res* **5**(9): 566–573.

Berton, T.R., C.J. Conti, et al. (1998). "The effect of vitamin E acetate on ultraviolet-induced mouse skin carcinogenesis." *Mol Carcinog* **23**(3): 175–184.

Beyer, R.E. (1994). "The role of ascorbate in antioxidant protection of biomembranes: interaction with vitamin E and coenzyme Q." *J Bioenerg Biomembr* **26**(4): 349–358.

Branda, R.F. and J.W. Eaton (1978). "Skin color and nutrient photolysis: an evolutionary hypothesis." *Science* **201**(4356): 625–626.

Burke, K.E., J. Clive, et al. (2000). "Effects of topical and oral vitamin E on pigmentation and skin cancer induced by ultraviolet irradiation in Skh:2 hairless mice." *Nutr Cancer* **38**(1): 87–97.

Chamlin, S.L., J. Kao, et al. (2002). "Ceramide-dominant barrier repair lipids alleviate childhood atopic dermatitis: changes in barrier function provide a sensitive indicator of disease activity." *J Am Acad Dermatol* **47**(2): 198–208.

Chen, A.T., J.A. Reidy, et al. (1989). "Increased chromosome fragility as a consequence of blood folate levels, smoking status, and coffee consumption." *Environ Mol Mutagen* **13**(4): 319–324.

Chen, W., M. Barthelman, et al. (1997). "Inhibition of cyclobutane pyrimidine dimer formation in epidermal p53 gene of UV-irradiated mice by alpha-tocopherol." *Nutr Cancer*
29(3): 205–211.

Choi, S.W., Y.I. Kim, et al. (1998). "Folate depletion impairs DNA excision repair in the colon
of the rat." *Gut* **43**(1): 93–99.

Choi, S.W. and J.B. Mason (2000). "Folate and carcinogenesis: an integrated scheme." *J Nutr*
130(2): 129–132.

Cruz, P. D., Jr., R. E. Tigelaar, et al. (1990). "Langerhans cells that migrate to skin after intravenous infusion regulate the induction of contact hypersensitivity." *J Immunol* **144**(7):
2486–2492.

Duthie, S.J. and A. Hawdon (1998). "DNA instability (strand breakage, uracil misincorporation, and defective repair) is increased by folic acid depletion in human lymphocytes in
vitro." *Faseb J* **12**(14): 1491–1497.

Elmets, C.A., P.R. Bergstresser, et al. (1983). "Analysis of the mechanism of unresponsiveness
produced by haptens painted on skin exposed to low dose ultraviolet radiation." *J Exp
Med* **158**(3): 781–794.

Fang, J.Y., S.D. Xiao, et al. (1997). "Relationship of plasma folic acid and status of DNA
methylation in human gastric cancer." *J Gastroenterol* **32**(2): 171–175.

Fourtanier, A., A. Gueniche, et al. (2000). "Improved protection against solar-simulated radiation-induced immunosuppression by a sunscreen with enhanced ultraviolet A protection." *J Invest Dermatol* **114**(4): 620–627.

Geesin, J.C., D. Darr, et al. (1988). "Ascorbic acid specifically increases type I and type III
procollagen messenger RNA levels in human skin fibroblast." *J Invest Dermatol* **90**(4):
420–424.

Gensler, H.L., T. Williams, et al. (1999). "Oral niacin prevents photocarcinogenesis and
photoimmunosuppression in mice." *Nutr Cancer* **34**(1): 36–41.

Guenthner, S.T., R.M. Hurwitz, et al. (1999). "Cutaneous squamous cell carcinomas consistently show histologic evidence of in situ changes: a clinicopathologic correlation." *J Am
Acad Dermatol* **41**(3 Pt 1): 443–448.

Guo, Q. and L. Packer (2000). "Ascorbate-dependent recycling of the vitamin E homologue
Trolox by dihydrolipoate and glutathione in murine skin homogenates." *Free Radic Biol
Med* **29**(3–4): 368–374.

Heath, C.W., Jr. (1966). "Cytogenetic observations in vitamin B12 and folate deficiency."
Blood **27**(6): 800–815.

Hill, L.L., A. Ouhtit, et al. (1999). "Fas ligand: a sensor for DNA damage critical in skin cancer
etiology." *Science* **285**(5429): 898–900.

Hoppe, U., J. Bergemann, et al. (1999). "Coenzyme Q10, a cutaneous antioxidant and ener-
gizer." *Biofactors* **9**(2-4): 371–378.

Horowitz, R.M. and L.E. Monger (1995). "Solar keratosis: an evolving squamous cell carcinoma: benign or malignant?" *Dermatol Surg* **21**: 183.

Jablonski, N.G. and G. Chaplin (2000). "The evolution of human skin coloration." *J Hum Evol*
39(1): 57–106.

Jacobson, E.L., K.M. Antol, et al. (1983). "Poly(ADP-ribose) metabolism in ultraviolet irradiated human fibroblasts." *J Biol Chem* **258**(1): 103–107.

Jacobson, E.L., A.J. Dame, et al. (1995). "Evaluating the role of niacin in human carcinogenesis." *Biochimie* **77**(5): 394–398.

Jacobson, E.L., P.U. Giacomoni, et al. (2001). "Optimizing the energy status of skin cells during solar radiation." *J Photochem Photobiol B* **63**(1–3): 141–147.

Jacobson, E.L., W.M. Shieh, et al. (1999). "Mapping the role of NAD metabolism in prevention and treatment of carcinogenesis." *Mol Cell Biochem* **193**(1–2): 69–74.

Jacobson, M.K. and E.L. Jacobson (1999). "Discovering new ADP-ribose polymer cycles: protecting the genome and more." *Trends Biochem Sci* **24**(11): 415–417.

Jacobson, M.K., H. Kim, et al. (2002). "A topical niacin prodrug enhances wound healing by
stimulation of leptin secretion." *J Invest Dermatol* **118**: 840.

Jeffes, E.W., 3rd and E.H. Tang (2000). "Actinic keratosis. Current treatment options." *Am J
Clin Dermatol* **1**(3): 167–179.

Kagan, V., E. Serbinova, et al. (1990). "Antioxidant effects of ubiquinones in microsomes and mitochondria are mediated by tocopherol recycling." *Biochem Biophys Res Commun* **169**(3): 851–857.

Kagan, V., E. Witt, et al. (1992). "Ultraviolet light-induced generation of vitamin E radicals and their recycling. A possible photosensitizing effect of vitamin E in skin." *Free Radic Res Commun* **16**(1): 51–64.

Kagan, V.E., E.A. Serbinova, et al. (1990). "Generation and recycling of radicals from phenolic antioxidants." *Arch Biochem Biophys* **280**(1): 33–39.

Karagas, M.R., E.R. Greenberg, et al. (1999). "Increase in incidence rates of basal cell and squamous cell skin cancer in New Hampshire, USA. New Hampshire Skin Cancer Study Group." *Int J Cancer* **81**(4): 555–559.

Kim, H., M.K. Jacobson, et al. (2002). "A Topical Niacin Prodrug Enhances Wound Healing by Stimulation of Leptin Secretion." *Journal of Investigative Dermatology* **119**: 8405.

Kim, H., Kim, M., Qasem, J.G., Coyle, D.L., Jacobson, M.K. and Jacobson, E.L. (2002). "A Topical Niacin Prodrug for Skin Cancer Prevention." *Proc Am Asso Cancer Res* **43**: 1144.

Liebler, D.C. and J.A. Burr (2000). "Effects of UV light and tumor promoters on endogenous vitamin E status in mouse skin." *Carcinogenesis* **21**(2): 221–225.

Lober, B.A., C.W. Lober, et al. (2000). "Actinic keratosis in squamous cell carcinoma." *J Am Acad Dermatol* **43**(5): 881.

McVean, M. and D.C. Liebler (1997). "Inhibition of UVB induced DNA photodamage in mouse epidermis by topically applied alpha-tocopherol." *Carcinogenesis* **18**(8): 1617–1622.

Moodycliffe, A.M., M. Norval, et al. (1993). "Characterization of a monoclonal antibody to cis-urocanic acid: detection of cis-urocanic acid in the serum of irradiated mice by immunoassay." *Immunology* **79**(4): 667–672.

Nocentini, S., M. Guggiari, et al. (2001). "Exacerbating effect of vitamin E supplementation on DNA damage induced in cultured human normal fibroblasts by UVA radiation." *Photochem Photobiol* **73**(4): 370–377.

Peng, Y.M., Y.S. Peng, et al. (1993). "Micronutrient concentrations in paired skin and plasma of patients with actinic keratoses: effect of prolonged retinol supplementation." *Cancer Epidemiol Biomarkers Prev* **2**(2): 145–150.

Pentland, A.P., J.W. Schoggins, et al. (1999). "Reduction of UV-induced skin tumors in hairless mice by selective COX-2 inhibition." *Carcinogenesis* **20**(10): 1939–1944.

Perchellet, J.P. and E.M. Perchellet (1989). "Antioxidants and multistage carcinogenesis in mouse skin." *Free Radic Biol Med* **7**(4): 377–408.

Podda, M. and M. Grundmann-Kollmann (2001). "Low molecular weight antioxidants and their role in skin ageing." *Clin Exp Dermatol* **26**(7): 578–582.

Podda, M., M. Rallis, et al. (1996). "Kinetic study of cutaneous and subcutaneous distribution following topical application of [7,8-14C]rac-alpha-lipoic acid onto hairless mice." *Biochem Pharmacol* **52**(4): 627–633.

Potts, R.O. and R. Guy (1993). The prediction of precutaneous penetration, a mechanistic model. *Dermal and Transdermal Drug Delivery*. R. Gurny and A. Teubner, Wiss Verlagsges. 153–160.

Prinz-Langenohl, R., I. Fohr, et al. (2001). "Beneficial role for folate in the prevention of colorectal and breast cancer." *Eur J Nutr* **40**(3): 98–105.

Reeve, V.E., M. Bosnic, et al. (1998). "Ultraviolet A radiation (320–400 nm) protects hairless mice from immunosuppression induced by ultraviolet B radiation (280-320 nm) or cis-urocanic acid." *Int Arch Allergy Immunol* **115**(4): 316–322.

Roberts, M.J., G.T. Wondrak, et al. (2003). "DNA damage by carbonyl stress in human skin cells." *Mutat Res* **522**(1-2): 45–56.

Roberts, M.S., R.A. Anderson, et al. (1978). "The percutaneous absorption of phenolic compounds: the mechanism of diffusion across the stratum corneum." *J Pharm Pharmacol* **30**(8): 486–490.

Rolli, V., R. Armin, et al. (2000). Poly(ADP-ribose) polymerase: structure and function. *Poly ADP-ribosylation reactions: From DNA damage and stress signalling to cell death*. G.d.M.a.S. Shall. Oxford, Oxford University Press. 35–67.

Shindo, Y., E. Witt, et al. (1994). "Enzymic and non-enzymic antioxidants in epidermis and dermis of human skin." *J Invest Dermatol* **102**(1): 122–124.

Shreedhar, V., T. Giese, et al. (1998). "A cytokine cascade including prostaglandin E2, IL-4, and IL-10 is responsible for UV-induced systemic immune suppression." *J Immunol* **160**(8): 3783–3789.

Smart, R. C. and C. L. Crawford (1991). "Effect of ascorbic acid and its synthetic lipophilic derivative ascorbyl palmitate on phorbol ester-induced skin-tumor promotion in mice." *Am J Clin Nutr* **54**(6 Suppl): 1266S–1273S.

Strickland, F. M. (2001). "Immune regulation by polysaccharides: implications for skin cancer." *J Photochem Photobiol B* **63**(1–3): 132–410.

Sugibayashi, K., T. Hayashi, et al. (1999). "Simultaneous transport and metabolism of ethyl nicotinate in hairless rat skin after its topical application: the effect of enzyme distribution in skin." *J Control Release* **62**(1–2): 201–218.

Thuillier, P., G. J. Anchiraico, et al. (2000). "Activators of peroxisome proliferator-activated receptor-alpha partially inhibit mouse skin tumor promotion." *Mol Carcinog* **29**(3): 134–142.

Tomasetti, M., G. P. Littarru, et al. (1999). "Coenzyme Q10 enrichment decreases oxidative DNA damage in human lymphocytes." *Free Radic Biol Med* **27**(9–10): 1027–1032.

Tsai, R. S., N. E. Tayar, et al. (1992). "Physicochemical properties and transport behavior of piridil: considerations on its membrane-crossing potential." *Int J Pharm* **80**: 39–49.

Ullrich, S. E. (2002). "Photoimmune suppression and photocarcinogenesis." *Front Biosci* **7**: D684–703.

Webber, H., K. Meyer-Trumpener, et al. (1994). "Ester des Naproxens als potentielle prodrugs zur Hautpenetration." *Arch Pharm* **327**: 337–345.

Wondrak, G. T., D. Cervantes-Laurean, et al. (2002). "Identification of alpha-dicarbonyl scavengers for cellular protection against carbonyl stress." *Biochem Pharmacol* **63**(3): 361–373.

Wondrak, G. T., E. L. Jacobson, et al. (2002). "Photosensitization of DNA damage by glycated proteins." *Photochem Photobiol Sci* **1**(5): 355–363.

Wondrak, G. T., M. J. Roberts, et al. (2003). "Proteins of the extracellular matrix are sensitizers of photo-oxidative stress in human skin cells." *J Invest Dermatol* **121**(3): 578–586.

Wondrak, G. T., M. J. Roberts, et al. (2002). "Photosensitized growth inhibition of cultured human skin cells: mechanism and suppression of oxidative stress from solar irradiation of glycated proteins." *J Invest Dermatol* **119**(2): 489–498.

Skin Cancer Prevention

Maria Lluria-Prevatt and David S. Alberts

College of Medicine, University of Arizona, Tucson AZ 85724

Epidemiology of Skin Cancer

Skin cancer is the most common malignancy in the world. One out of three new cancers is a skin cancer (Diepgen and Mahler 2002). More than 1 million cases of non-melanoma skin cancer (NMSC) (basal cell carcinoma [BCC] and squamous cell cancers [SCC]) occur annually (Jermal, Tiwan et al. 2004). Approximately 800,000 of these cancers are BCC and about 200,000 are SCC (Diepgen and Mahler 2002). In Australia, NMSC accounts for 75% of all cancers and is 30 times more prevalent than lung cancer among men and 10 times more prevalent than breast cancer among women (Burton 2000). Incidence rates for NMSC are increasing. An average increase of 3 to 8% per year since the 1960s has occurred in the white populations of Europe, the U.S., Canada and Australia (Glass and Hoover 1989; Green 1992). Incidence data for NMSC are sparse because traditional cancer registries do not track NMSC, however it has been estimated that the incidence of NMSC is 18 to 20 times greater than that of melanoma. Incidence rates of NMSC increase proportionally with the proximity to the equator, with high cumulative Ultraviolet radiation (UVR) light exposure and with age (Diepgen and Mahler 2002). The incidence of NMSC has until most recently affected the older population – especially men who have worked outdoors, however the age of onset has steadily decreased. While the incidence rates for non-melanoma skin cancers continues to rise the mortality rate has decreased in recent years however there continues to be a substantial impact on morbidity, health and health care costs. In 2001, approximately 2000 deaths were reported due to NMSC mostly due to metastasis of SCC to the lymph nodes and other sites. Early diagnosis and appropriate therapy result in a 95% cure rate. Prevention is the key management tool for NMSC.

The most serious form of skin cancer is melanoma. Worldwide the number of melanoma cases is increasing faster than any other cancer. In 2004, an estimated 55,100 persons are expected to be diagnosed with melanoma and 10,250 deaths will occur due to melanoma (Jermal, Tiwan et al. 2004). Data from the US Surveillance, Epidemiology and End Results (SEER) registry demonstrated that melanoma was the most rapidly increasing malignancy in both sexes in the U.S. during 1973–1997 (Lens and Dawes 2004). In the last few decades, the incidence rate of melanoma has substantially increased especially among the Caucasian population. During the 1970s, the incidence rate of melanoma was approximately 6% a year. However, the rate of increase has slowed to less than 3% per year. The rate of melanoma incidence is 10 times higher in whites than in African Americans (Jermal, Tiwan et al. 2004). In Australia, melanoma is the fourth most common cancer among males and the third most common among females. Statistical data suggests that the lifetime risk for melanoma in Australia is now one in 25 for men and 1 in 34 for women (Burton 2000). In the United States the lifetime risk of developing melanoma was 1 in 1500 individuals in the year 1935 while in 2002 the risk was 1 in 68 individuals (Rigel 2002) and in 2004 the estimated risk is 1 in 55 for males and 1 in 82 for females (Jermal, Tiwan et al. 2004). It has been estimated that melanoma will be the fifth most common cancer among males and the seventh most common cancer among females in the U.S. in the year 2004 (Jermal, Tiwan et al. 2004).

Non-melanoma skin cancer arises from keratinocytes and originates in the epidermis. BCC originates from the basal cells of the epidermis and occasionally those of the infundibular and outer root sheath of the hair follicles (Lang 1991). BCCs are rarely fatal and seldom metastasize however they can be locally invasive and destructive (Randle 1996). SCC originates from keratinizing cells of the epidermis. These tumors are more aggressive than BCC and more likely to metastasize. While death rates remain low for NMSC, the incidence is very high and therefore treatment is very costly. The Medicare cost of treating NMSC between 1992 and 1995 was nearly $500 million consuming 4.5% of all Medicare cancer costs (Housman, Feldman et al. 2003). Of additional concern, individuals who develop NMSC are at increased risk for the development of new skin cancers within the next few years following diagnosis (Diepgen and Mahler 2002). A follow-up study found that 52% of individuals diagnosed with SCC developed subsequent NMSC within five years of initial therapy (Frankel, Hanusa et al. 1992). Prevention of NMSC is a sensible strategy to lowering these costs.

Melanoma arises from melanocytes, the pigment producing cells, which reside in the dermal and epidermal junction of the skin. Survival is strongly associated with the thickness of the lesion. If caught early, melanoma can be cured by surgical excision of thinner lesions (0.75 mm or less) and has a five-year survival rate of 99% (Koh 1991). Patients with thicker melanoma (more than 3.5 mm) have a steep decrease in survival rates (Lens and Dawes 2004). Tumors greater than 4 mm in depth are associated with a five-year survival rate of less than 50%. If the disease spreads the survival of five years after diagnosis is only about 30 to 40%. Estimated annual cost for the treatment of melanoma in 1997 was estimated to be $563 million (Tsao 1998). Stage I and II disease comprised 5% of the total while stage II and stage IV disease consumed 34% and 55% of the total cost, respectively. Aggressive primary prevention could substantially reduce this economic burden.

Risk Factors

Ultraviolet Radiation Exposure. Aside from genetics, the major risk factors for all skin cancers are exposure to ultraviolet radiation and skin color or the inability to tan. All skin cancers have been associated with exposure to sunlight however the pattern of sun exposure may vary between skin cancers types.

UVR is comprised of wavelengths from 200 to 400 nm. The ozone of the earth's atmosphere absorbs most light wavelengths below 290 nm. Therefore, UVB (290–320 nm) and UVA (320–400 nm) are the only portions reaching the earth's surface. UVR light reaching the earth's surface is comprised of 90–99% UVA and one to 10% UVB. UVR causes many biological reactions in the skin, including inflammatory response in a sunburn, hindrance of immune activity, premature aging and damage to DNA resulting in potential development of skin cancer (Dissanayake, Greenoak et al. 1993).

UVR can result in mutations in genes that regulate cell proliferation and repair. UVR-induced linkage between two adjacent pyrimidines (cytosine or thymine) on the same DNA strand is usually repaired by nucleotide excision repair enzymes before replication. However, if the repair fails or is delayed fixed DNA mutations can occur when DNA polymerase inserts adenine dinucleotide (AA) opposite the unrepaired dimer. The erroneous pairing of AA with CC or CT linked photoproducts mutations are observed as CC→TT and C→T, respectively. These are characteristically induced by only UVR and as such are designated UVR signature mutations (Wikonkal and Brash 1999).

In the past, UVB was thought to be more important than UVA in the generation of sun damage and skin cancer. However, UVA has become increasingly suspect in the development of skin cancer (Runger 1999). The photocarcinogenesis of UVA differs from UVB in that UVA is not readily absorbed by DNA, but is absorbed by other molecules within the cell, giving rise to reactive oxygen species, which in turn damage DNA, membranes and other cellular constituents (de Gruijl 2000). UVA has been shown to induce mutations in DNA including p53, which is discussed later in this chapter as an important genetic marker for NMSC (Burren, Scaletta et al. 1998). UVA has been found to be an important factor in the development of melanoma. Several investigators have argued that UVA is more relevant in melanoma causation than the UVB range (Setlow, Grist et al. 1993). Much of the evidence of UVA exposure as a risk factor for melanoma has come from epidemiological studies of users of sunbeds or tanning equipment with spectral output that is in the UVA range (Swerdlow and Weinstock 1998; Wang, Setlow et al. 2001). A recent study of women from Norway and Sweden found that the women who visited a tanning parlor at least once a month were 55% more likely to later develop melanoma than women who did not artificially suntan. Those who used sunlamps during their 20s had the greatest risk, approximately 150% higher than similarly aged women who did not use tanning beds (Veierod, Weiderpass et al. 2003). Further contributing to the controversy, a preclinical study showed that UVB, and not UVA, exposure promoted melanoma growth in a mouse model (De Fabo, Noonan et al. 2004).

Chronic exposure to UVR is the predominant cause of NMSC. Over 80% of these cancers develop on parts of the body exposed to the sun including the face, neck and arms (Diepgen and Mahler 2002). Incidence rates for NMSC correspond well with increased UVR exposure as demonstrated by the increased incidence among individuals with occupational or recreational outdoor exposure or who reside at latitudes closer to the equator (Diepgen and Mahler 2002). Many studies have shown an inverse relationship between latitude and NMSC incidence (Almahroos and Kurban 2004). A report from Southeastern Arizona suggests the incidence rates of NMSC in Arizona are three to six times higher than those in subjects with similar skin type and living in regions of higher latitude (Harris 2001). A compilation of these and several other studies demonstrates a more than 50-fold difference in rates of NMSC incidence between Australia and Arizona (low latitude) and Finland (high latitude), with the higher incidence occurring in the lower latitudes (Almahroos and Kurban 2004). Several Australian studies have demonstrated that people in countries with high ambient solar radiation have a higher incidence of NMSC than migrants with the same genetic background from countries with lower ambient solar radiation (Almahroos and Kurban 2004). People who move during childhood to the countries of high ambient solar radiation from countries with

Table 1. Predictors of incident squamous cell carcinoma (Foote, Harris et al. 2001)

Predictors	Relative risk (95% confidence interval)
Age	1.04 (1.02–1.07)
Gender	
Female	1.00
Male	1.63 (1.04–2.55)
Hair color	
Dark brown/black	1.00
Light brown/blonde	0.97 (0.63–1.50)
Red	1.82 (1.01–3.31)
Residence in Arizona (number of years after age 30)	
<10 years	1.00
≥10 years	1.96 (1.27–3.04)

low ambient solar radiation have equal incidence of NMSC as natives (English, Armstrong et al. 1998). However, individuals who make this same move later in life have a lower incidence. This data supports the idea that NMSC develops from a chronic exposure of UVR. The risk factor of skin color for the development of NMSC is demonstrated by the lower risk of ethnically darker skinned migrants.

Melanoma incidence is also associated with exposure to UVR. Childhood sunburns and intense intermittent sun exposure are major risk factors for melanoma (Gilchrest, Eller et al. 1999). Anatomic locations of melanoma development support the basis for intermittent UVR exposure as a risk factor. Melanoma is most commonly found on the trunk of men and the trunk and lower extremities of women. These sites are not normally acclimated to the sun by chronic exposure, but rather tend to be exposed during outdoor recreational activities. The effects of the sun on the development of melanoma are modulated by skin type. Light pigmentation increases the risk of the development of melanoma.

In a study conducted at the University of Arizona, risk factors for SCC were evaluated among 918 Arizona residents with sun-damaged skin (at least 10 clinically assessable AK lesions) who had been randomized to the placebo arm of a skin cancer chemoprevention trial (Foote, Harris et al. 2001). As shown in Table 1, risk factors for BCC included older age, male gender, red hair color and at least 10 years' residence in the state of Arizona, which is located in a lower-latitude region of the U.S. with documented rates of SCC and BCC that are among the highest in the world (Harris 2001).

Other Risk Factors. The presence of precancerous lesions increases the risk of developing skin cancer. For SCC the precancerous lesion is actinic keratosis (AK) and for melanoma the precancerous lesions is thought to be dysplastic nevi (DN). BCC does not appear to have a precancerous lesion however the presence of AK can often be an indicator of risk. Additional risk for skin cancer includes genetics, immune suppressive disease, past history of skin cancer and occupational exposure to coal tar, pitch, creosote, arsenic compounds or radium. Age, male gender, and DNA repair disorders such as xeroderma pigmentosum are also risk factors for skin cancer. For melanoma, additional risk factors include one or more family members who had melanoma and a large number of moles (risk increases with number of moles) or the presence of DN. Approximately five to 12% of patients with melanoma have a family history of melanoma in one or more first-degree relatives (Goldstein and Tucker 2001). Mutations in two melanoma susceptibility genes, CDKN2A (p16) located on chromosome 9 (9p21) and CDK4 located on chromosome 12 (12q13) have been identified. Mutations in p16 have been identified in 20% of tested melanoma families (Bishop, Demenais et al. 2002).

Genetic Alterations in NMSC. Genetic studies of AK and SCC have found alterations on possible tumor suppressor genes of chromosomes 9p, 13q, 17p, 17q and 3p (Quinn, Sikkink et al. 1994; Hunter 1997). The targets for most of these mutations have not been identified except for p53, which lies on chromosome 17p. Recognized genetic targets in NMSC include p53 mutations demonstrated in a progression of normal skin to sun damaged skin to AK to SCC (Einspahr, Alberts et al. 1999). p53 mutations have also been identified in BCC (Matsumura, Nishigori et al. 1996). Many of these mutations are $CC \rightarrow TT$ or $C \rightarrow T$ changes at dipyrimidine sites suggestive of UVR damage (Tsao 2001).

Results from an analysis of genetic changes in 36 AKs and 23 invasive SCCs (Rehman, Takata et al. 1996) suggest that the relationship between the accumulation of genetic change and behavior for NMSC is complex. However, the overall pattern of autosome loss in AKs was similar to that seen for SCCs. Loss of chromosome 17p was the most frequent target of loss of heterozygosity (LOH), which is consistent with data showing a high rate of UVR-induced mutations in p53 (Brash, Rudolph et al. 1991), detection of p53 mutations in irradiated skin and cultured keratinocytes (Nakazawa, English et al. 1994), and evidence showing p53 mutations in pre-invasive lesions (Einspahr, Alberts et al. 1999). However, the number of SCCs with chromosome 17p loss far exceeded the number in which mutations were detected in p53 exons 5–8, consistent with the presence of other targets of inactivation on chromosome 17 (Wales, Biel et al. 1995). Increased p21$^{WAF1/CIP1}$ immunostaining and p53 immunostaining were observed in 97% and 83% of AKs, respectively, and were observed in lesions without any detectable LOH or p53 mutation, suggesting that changes in proliferation, p21$^{WAF1/CIP1}$ expression, and p53 expression may precede allelic loss or p53 mutation. A large number of AKs showing multiple areas of LOH and p53 mutation may not have acquired the relevant genetic change to allow invasion of the underlying dermis (Wales, Biel et al. 1995).

Genetic alterations in NMSC also include mutations in the ras gene. The frequency of ras mutations in SCC ranges up to almost 50% and up to 30% in BCC (Pierceall, Goldberg et al. 1991). Mutations in ras have also been identified in AKs (Spencer, Kahn et al. 1995). Different rates reported for SCC and BCC ras mutations may reflect different techniques, different study populations and/or the differing molecular epidemiology of low and high sun exposure.

Although more commonly reported in melanoma, recent studies suggest alterations in p16 can be found in up to 24% of SCCs and 3.5% of BCC (Soufir, Moles et al. 1999). Several of the detected mutations were UVR signature mutations. These mutations may account for alterations observed on chromosome 9p21 in SCC (Tsao 2001).

Genetic alterations in BCC are found in both hereditary and sporadic cases. The PTCH gene is found in patients with nevoid BCC syndrome, characterized by the rapid development of numerous BCCs early in life (Tsao 2001). Recent studies have demonstrated that 15–39% of these patients harbor mutations in the PTCH gene (Aszterbaum, Rothman et al. 1998).

Genetic Alterations in Melanoma. Linkage studies of families with multiple cases of melanoma have been important in pursuing genetic analysis however the genetic relationship between melanoma and the dysplastic nevus syndrome are complex. Karyotype studies of both familial and sporadic melanomas frequently showed large deletions of band region 1p36, del(1)(p36.1-p36.3) (Dracopoli, Bruns et al. 1994), suggesting that multiple tumor suppressor genes in this region were deleted. The PITSLRE protein kinase gene locus maps to band region 1p36. Several of its products may affect apoptotic signaling (Lahti, Xiang et al. 1995). Studies have demonstrated alterations in the PITSLRE protein kinase gene complex in melanomas (Wymer 1997).

Another frequently altered chromosome region, 9p21, contains a group of genes involved in cell cycle regulation. Among several potential tumor suppressor genes located on 9p21, p16 (CDKN2A/p16^{ink4a}) is the most important melanoma susceptibility gene identified to date with germline mutations present in 9p-linked melanoma families (Hussussian, Struewing et al. 1994; Kamb, Shattuck-Eidens et al. 1994) and in 30–50% of members of melanoma kindreds (Halachmi and Gilchrest 2001). p16 inhibits the ability of cyclin dependent kinases, CDK-4 and CDK-6, to activate substrates needed for progression past G1 of the cell cycle and therefore acts as a cell cycle check point protein (Liggett and Sidransky 1998). Germline mutations in the gene encoding CDK4 have also been described in a small number of melanoma-prone cases (Zou 1996; Soufir, Avril et al. 1998). In sporadic tumors, loss of p16 protein expression has been shown to occur only in invasive and metastatic stages of melanoma and to be infrequent in primary thick nodular melanoma (Reed, Loganzo et al. 1995; Straume and Akslen 1997). The loss of p16 also seems to be associated with recurrent disease and has been the most useful marker for progressive disease. Alterations in p16 include CpG island methylation and translation repression mutations in the five prime untranslated regions (Haluska and Hodi 1998).

The phosphatases PTEN/MMAC1, located at 10q23,3, have been found deleted in more than 40% of melanoma cell lines (Ortonne 2002). Bcl-2 has been demonstrated to be over expressed in melanoma cells (Jansen, Wacheck et al. 2000). The transcription factor AP-2, and three of its downstream targets, c-kit, E-cadherin and p21, were found to be involved in later phases of melanoma progression (Baldi, Santini et al. 2001).

Dr. Arbiser of Emory University School of Medicine identified the activation of Mitogen-Activated Protein Kinase (MAPK) as an early event in melanoma progression (Cohen, Zavala-Pompa et al. 2002). One hundred and thirty one melanocytic lesions, ranging from atypical nevi to metastatic melanoma, were studied for the expression of phosphorylated (active) MAPK and two target genes known to be induced by MAPK signaling, tissue factor and vascular endothelial growth factor. While MAPK activation was positive in only 21.5% of benign nevi (with mild atypia), MAPK activation was seen in both radial and vertical growth phase melanomas. These findings suggest MAPK signaling as a potential target of chemoprevention in early melanoma.

In one study, five to 35% of various graded melanomas or nevi had some type of ras mutation (Yasuda, Kobayashi et al. 1989). Within the Ras family, N-Ras has the most significant association with melanoma progression. Herlyn et al. found a role for Ras in approximately 15-20% of melanomas with a positive association with sun exposure (Herlyn and Satyamoorthy 1996). Developments from the Cancer Genome Project have revealed that 66% of melanomas tested had a mutation in BRAF with the same single substitution occurring in 80% of the melanomas (Davies, Bignell et al. 2002). BRAF is known to play a role in cell growth and division. Most recently, investigators observed this same BRAF mutation (resulting in the V599E amino-acid substitution) in 63 of 77 (82%) histologically diverse nevi including 4 of 5 (80%) dysplastic nevi (Pollock, Harper et al. 2003). This mutation was observed in 68% of melanoma metastases and 80% of primary melanoma. These findings demonstrate that the mutation of BRAF and activation of the RAS-RAF-MEK-ERK-MAP kinase pathway, which mediates cellular responses to growth signals, is a crucial and early step in the progression of melanoma.

Screening and Early Detection

Early screening of SCC is often done by the diagnosis of AK. Self exams are strongly recommended. Warning signs include a skin growth that increases in size or changes color or thickness or a sore that continues to crust, bleed or itch. Identification of these changes warrants a more extensive check up from a dermatologist. A precursor lesion to SCC, AK often requires treatment. AKs can be difficult to treat and require frequent visits to a dermatologist, since patients usually have multiple AKs that present at different times. The treatment for AK is usually cryosurgery with liquid nitrogen, excision or topical 5-FU cream (International Medical News Group 2002). Cryosurgery is the most common treatment but is associated with blistering, scabbing, hypopigmentation, inflammation and occasionally pain. Treatment with 5-FU often results in severe blistering. Other options for AK treatment include dermabrasion or chemical peeling (Dinehart 2000). Topical diclofenac (Del Rosso 2003) and imiquimod (Berman, Ricotti et al. 2004) have also been approved by the US Food and Drug Administration for the treatment of AK. Appropriate chemoprevention strategies of AK or pre-AK treatment would not only reduce incidence of SCC but also eradicate the need for these disagreeable treatments mentioned above.

Screening for early melanoma includes a dermatological assessment however self-examinations are strongly recommended as well. This assessment includes a review of ones moles carefully looking for what the Skin Cancer Foundation calls the ABCD of melanoma: Asymmetry, Borders, Color and Diameter. Most early melanomas are asymmetrical where the common mole is round and symmetrical. Early melanomas often have irregular borders with scalloped or notched edges. Normal moles have smooth borders. The color of early melanoma tends to have several shades of brown, tan or black and as the melanoma progresses the colors red, white or blue may appear. Normal moles tend to be a single shade of color. Early melanomas tend to grow larger than normal moles with diameters of at least 6 mm. The discovery of any of these characteristics should be promptly reported to a physician preferably one that specializes in skin cancer and is trained to identify early signs of melanoma.

It is apparent with the increase of skin cancer incidence, incomplete resolution by early detection and the current treatments, there is an urgent need to develop well-tolerated and effective prevention strategies for NMSC and melanoma.

Prevention of Skin Cancer

Primary Prevention. Since exposure to UVR is a major risk factor in the development of skin cancer, the focus of primary prevention has been to limit exposure to UVR. The recommendation from the American Academy of Dermatology, the American College of Preventive Medicine and the American Cancer Society are: (1) to reduce sun exposure during peak hours of intense ultraviolet exposure (usually 10 am to 4 pm); (2) to wear protective clothing to cover as much of the skin as possible, including long sleeved shirts and hats with wide brims; and (3) to seek shade (Manson, Rexrode et al. 2000). Public health campaigns have been underway since the 1980's for the prevention of skin cancers. These campaigns recommend limited exposure to sun, the use of sunscreen, and early detection through screening. In Australia, where skin cancer is of epidemic proportions (2 out of 3 people born in Australia will likely require treatment for at least one skin cancer in their lifetime) (Giles, Marks et al. 1988), major campaigns have taken place such as the "Slip! Slop! Slap!" ("slip" on a shirt, "slop" on sunscreen, "slap" on a hat), "Sunsmart," and "Me No Fry." While 90% of Australians now recognize the dangers of skin cancer and the associated risks (Borland, Marks et al. 1992; Hill, White et al. 1993), the relationship between education and incidence reduction is still unclear. In an article by a leading Australian academic dermatologist, several cohort studies are reviewed and indicate some leveling or reduction in skin cancer incidence in younger populations of Australia, potentially associated with the success of the skin cancer awareness public campaigns (Marks 1999).

The 2003 Cancer Progress Report from the US Department of Health and Human Services and related departments reports limited success in the US population's attitudes toward sun exposure (2001). This report contains data gathered by the Centers for Disease Control and Prevention/National Center for Health Statistics. In the year 2000, 60 percent of adults said they were likely to seek some sort of sun protection, 31% were likely to use sunscreen, 26% were likely to use sunscreen with a sun protection factor (SPF) of 15 or higher, 32% very likely to wear protective clothing and 28% were very likely to seek shade. This data shows an increase from 1998 where there was an actual decline in the sun protection from previous years. In the June 3rd 2002 issue of the Philadelphia Inquirer (Uhlman 2002) the author remarks "Most adolescents avoid sunscreen like a summer reading list." The desire for a golden tan and the messy inconvenience of sunscreen outweighs the distant threat of skin cancer in the minds of these adolescents. In a study of sun protection practices in adolescents, only one third of the respondents reported routine sunscreen use during the past summer (Geller, Colditz et al. 2002). Eighty three percent reported sun burning at least once and 36% reported three or more burns during the previous summer. Nearly 10% of all respondents used tanning beds during the previous year, with 24.6% of girls age 15–18 reporting tanning bed use. Many girls who used tanning beds reported a belief that it was worth getting burned. These findings are very alarming considering that tanning in the teen years is a key factor for lifetime cumulative sun exposure and increased risk for skin cancer, particularly melanoma, which is clearly related to early age sunburns.

While advocated as an important protection against sun exposure, sunscreen use has created some controversy. Most sunscreen products may not offer adequate protection against the harmful effects of the sun's ultraviolet radiation. Protection provided by sunscreen is based on the SPF (sun protection factor); however, this is only indicative of a reduction in erythema. Therefore, individuals who apply sunscreen often expose themselves for longer periods of times in the sun because of the lack of uncomfortable effects due to erythema. As discussed earlier, UVA exposure is an important risk factor in development of skin cancer. Most sunscreens are inadequate in absorbing the longer wavelengths of the UVA portion of the sun's spectral output and, therefore, may only provide a portion of the protection needed for skin cancer prevention.

Observational studies of melanoma suggest that sunscreen use may be associated with increased risk, potentially due to fair-skinned individuals spending more time in the sun without the visible effects of a sunburn (Autier, Dore et al. 1995). Other studies also have found that frequent use of sunscreens was associated with a relative risk of 1.8 to 2.8 for cutaneous melanoma (Klepp and Magnus 1979; Graham, Marshall et al. 1985; Beitner, Norell et al. 1990). Consistent with these epidemiologic studies, one study in mice treated with sunscreen demonstrated a lack of protection toward UVR-induced melanoma growth (Wolfe 1994). In this study, C3H mice were transplanted with K1735 melanoma cells and exposed to UVR subsequent to sunscreen application. The sunscreen preparations contained o-PABA (octyl-N-dimethyl-p-aminobenzoate), 2-EHMC (2-ethylhexyl-p-methoxycinnamate) and BP-3 (benzophenone-3). This formulation was effective in reducing histopathologic alterations in the mouse ear skin but failed to prevent UVR-induced inflammation and melanoma growth.

Secondary Prevention. The current primary methods for skin cancer prevention, including behavioral modification and the use of sunscreens, have not proven sufficient to protect against rise in skin cancer incidence. Therefore, other strategies of prevention need to be coupled with primary prevention. The most promising of these strategies are the development of chemopreventive agents, which target early stage or precancerous lesions. Sporn (Sporn and Suh 2000) describes chemoprevention as a "pharmacological approach to intervention in order to arrest or reverse the process of carcinogenesis." He emphasizes the importance of an increased cancer research effort to control carcinogenesis "rather than attempting to cure end-stage disease." Control of carcinogenesis should be targeted at early stages because "it is easier to fix anything when the smallest numbers of its components are broken." The control of carcinogenesis through chemoprevention has gained credibility due to the FDA approval of tamoxifen for reducing breast cancer (Fisher, Costantino et al. 1998; Lippman and Brown 1999) and from FDA approvals of agents for treating intraepithelial neoplasias (IENs) such as diclofenac for AK (O'Shaughnessy, Kelloff et al. 2002) and celecoxib for FAP (Steinbach, Lynch et al. 2000). Agents for chemoprevention are ultimately applied to the general healthy population at high risk for particular cancers. Safety and efficacy must be established in large-scale prospective randomized clinical trials. Furthermore, agents need to be non-toxic, inexpensive and available in oral or topical form (for skin). Clinical trials in patients with premalignant lesions are initially performed to investigate the modulation of biomarkers as surrogate endpoints. Lippman and Hong equate the current cancer chemoprevention studies to a delay in cancer development where the measures include a reduction in the rate of tumor development and overall decrease in the incidence of number of tumors (Lippman and Hong 2002). Meyskens described chemoprevention as an interaction between sciences of carcinogenesis, cellular biology and cancer screening/early detection and cancer prevention/

treatment (Meyskens 1988). Clearly, all of these scientific disciplines are required to develop highly efficacious chemopreventive strategies for skin cancer.

For skin cancer, the eradication of AK and DN would most likely reduce the incidence of NMSC and melanoma, respectively. The approach employed in the development of chemopreventive agents include: (1) availability of precancerous lesions (AK or DN) to evaluate the potential reduction in risk of progression; (2) identifying target molecules that are often modified and subsequently contribute to skin carcinogenesis; (3) developing animal model systems to test potential chemopreventive agents in skin; (4) delivery of highly potent agents directly into the epidermis even more specifically through the development of prodrug formulations (discussed in Chapter 8), and (5) availability of intermediate molecular or histologic markers of the carcinogenic process to be used as endpoints.

Targeting Precursor Lesions for Chemoprevention. Current chemoprevention trials evaluate the efficacy of chemoprevention agents by the eradication or reduction of intraepithelial neoplasias (IENs). In skin the IEN used include AK for SCC and DN for melanoma because individuals with AK are at increased risk for developing NMSC, and the presence of DN is the single most important risk factor for developing melanoma.

In general, IENs are near-obligate cancer precursor lesions that have genetic abnormalities, loss of cellular control function, similar phenotypic characteristics of invasive cancer and are risk markers for cancer. The presence of IENs in an individual is indicative of an increased likelihood of developing invasive cancer as compared to unaffected individuals (O'Shaughnessy, Kelloff et al. 2002). The American Association for Cancer Research (AACR) Task Force on the Treatment and Prevention of Intraepithelial Neoplasia recommends targeting individuals with or at risk for IENs for new agent development because of the potential preventive consequence on developing invasive cancer (O'Shaughnessy, Kelloff et al. 2002). IENs have been described for many types of cancers including: colorectal adenomas for colorectal cancer; dysplastic oral leukoplakia for head and neck cancers; Barrett's esophagus for esophageal cancer; cervical intraepithelial neoplasia for cervical cancer; prostatic intraepithelial neoplasia for prostate cancer; transitional cell carcinoma in situ for bladder cancer; and actinic keratosis for NMSC.

Targeting precancerous lesions for chemoprevention is a rational strategy for the reduction of SCC incidence. Evidence for this rational includes: (1) the recent FDA approval of Diclofenac for treating AK as a preventive measure against SCC (O'Shaughnessy, Kelloff et al. 2002) and (2) the recent report from the Southeastern Arizona Skin Cancer Registry that suggests the leveling of SCC incidence in southeastern Arizona could be due to the removal of the precursor lesion, AK, while BCC incidence appears to continue to rise because there is no known precursor lesion for BCC to be removed or treated (Harris 2001).

AK, also known as solar or senile keratoses, are cutaneous lesions with chromosomal abnormalities that occur primarily on sun-exposed skin surfaces (Callen 2000). AK is a proliferating mass of transformed neoplastic keratinocytes confined to the epidermis. AKs develop on the surface of the skin as thickened cornified, scaly lesions (O'Shaughnessy, Kelloff et al. 2002). Papules and plaques are often found on a background of sun-damaged skin with telangiectasias, hyper or blotchy pigmentation, and a yellowish hue. The lesions range in size from 1–2 mm papules to large plaques (Callen 2000). AKs are most often diagnosed by histopathologic examination, since diagnosis by appearance can often be unclear as to whether the lesion is an AK or SCC. Typical histologic characteristics of AKs include irregular arrangement of cells with atypical, pleomorphic keratinocytes at the basal cell layer demonstrating nuclear pleomorphism, loss of polarity, crowding of nuclei and disordered maturation (Callen 2000).

The lack of significant cytological differences between AK and SCC gives rise to the premise that AKs represent early SCCs (Dinehart, Nelson-Adesokan et al. 1997). Several investigators consider AKs to be precursors or early forms of SCC (Glogau 2000; Salasche 2000). Inasmuch as AK is well accepted as a precursor to SCC, the Centers for Medicare and Medicaid Services have added a national coverage policy to include the treatment of AK (2002). The percent at which AK progresses to SCC have been demonstrated up to 16% (Glogau 2000). Approximately 60% of SCCs have been demonstrated to arise from preexisting AKs and/or the contiguous skin surface (Sober and Burstein 1995). Therefore, AK can be defined as a potential risk factor for the development of SCC.

Based on histological features, melanoma development has been described by Li and Herlyn as follows: (1) common acquired and congenital nevi with normal melanocytes that have a finite lifespan and no cytogenetic abnormalities; (2) DN that display both cellular and architectural atypia; (3) radial growth of a melanoma; (4) vertical growth phase of the primary melanoma; and (5) metastatic melanoma (Li and Herlyn 2000).

In 10 of 11 case-control studies, DN has emerged as one of the most important risk factors for melanoma (Greene 1997). On average, 34% of patients with melanoma had DN, in comparison with 11% of control subjects. Relative risk ranged from 1.0 to 16.7 for melanoma in the presence of DN. Several studies also reported an increased risk for melanoma with an increase in the number of DN. Cohort studies of patients with familial DN have also provided evidence for presence of DN as a risk factor for the development of new melanomas (Greene 1997). In a retrospective study drawn from 820 patients diagnosed with a first primary cutaneous melanoma, 82% of 50 examined patients with multiple melanomas were clinically diagnosed with dysplastic nevi (Stam-Posthuma, van Duinen et al. 2001). Histological confirmation was demonstrated in 78.0% of these patients and 16 of 37 patients had more than 30 clinically diagnosed DN, eight patients had 11 to 20 DN, four patients had 21 to 30 DN and nine patients had one DN. Finally, prospective studies have concluded that patients with DN and no family history also have an increased risk of melanoma (Greene 1997).

Other studies have investigated the idea that melanoma actually arises from DN (Marras, Faa et al. 1999). One such report performed cytogenetic analyses of DN in a young patient with a family history of melanoma (Marras, Faa et al. 1999). A t(6;15)(q13;q21) translocation found in one of the DN was similar to a translocation, with a breakpoint at 6q13 reported in a benign, nondysplastic nevi (Richmond, Fine et al. 1986) and in a cutaneous metastatic melanoma (Thompson, Emerson et al. 1995). The repeated occurrence of this rearrangement provides initial support for the hypothesis that melanoma progresses from normal melanocytes to benign nevus, to DN, to early melanoma, to late melanoma, and then to metastatic melanoma.

In a study by investigators at the National Cancer Institute and the University of Pennsylvania, almost all members of a family cohort with melanoma also had DN. New melanomas were only diagnosed in family members with DN (Greene, Clark et al. 1985; Greene, Clark et al. 1985). These data suggest that not only are DNs risk factors for melanoma, but they may also be the precursor lesions from which new melanoma evolve.

The use of dysplastic nevi, as a precancerous lesion and an indication of chemoprevention efficacy, has been used in previous research and is proposed in upcoming trials. To date, four chemoprevention trials with topical tretinoin have been performed on individuals with dysplastic nevi (Stam-Posthuma 1998). In these trials, DNs were targeted as surrogate markers for chemoprevention of melanoma.

Molecular Targets for Chemoprevention Identified in UVR Signaling Pathways. Skin carcinogenesis caused by UVR is a multi-step process of initiation, promotion and progression (Figure 1). The best phases to intervene are the tumor promotion and progression phases, which are slow, rate-limiting stages. The initiation phase occurs rapidly. The targeting of AK and DN are at the promotion phase where several specific genetic alterations can occur. In order to produce specific chemopreventive agents it is necessary to first identify important molecular targets, which are modified in the carcinogenesis process. For both NMSC and melanoma many of these targets can be identified by understanding the UVR signaling pathways and identifying the points where alterations occur due to UVR signaling. An extensive review of prevention of SCC by targeting UVR signaling can be found elsewhere (Bowden 2004). Bachelor and Bowden have recently reviewed UVA mediated signaling which may be involved in skin tumor promotion and progression and eventually provide additional targets for chemoprevention (Bachelor and Bowden 2004). The identification of these targets has been revealed by in vitro and in vivo model systems in the laboratory. The initiating events in skin cancer appear to involve gene mutations in proto-oncogenes or tumor suppressor genes. In the case of UVR induced skin carcinogenesis, these initiating mutations have been identified in the TP53 tumor suppressor gene as UVR signature mutations (Ziegler, Leffell et al. 1993). These mutations have been identified in AK and SCC (Nelson, Einspahr et al. 1994). The initiated cell undergoes a clonal expansion during the promotion phase at which point it is most likely that AK and DN in human skin arise. UVR tumor promotion is carried out by signaling molecules that give rise to altered gene expression. For SCC development, the UVR-induced clonal expansion signaling has been demonstrated to lead to the activation of activator protein-1 (AP-1) transcription factor or to cyclooxygenase-2 (COX2) expression (Bowden 2004). Three signaling molecules identified in the UVR signaling cascade (Figure 2) during the promotion stage of SCC include mitogen-activated protein kinases (MAPKs) (Chen, Tang et al. 2001), phosphatidylinositol 3-kinase (PI3K) (Kabayama, Hamaya et al. 1998), and epidermal growth factor (EGF) receptors (Wan, Wang et al. 2001). These three molecules serve as excellent targets for the development of chemoprevention.

AP-1 is upregulated in response to UVR-induced MAPK signaling in human keratinocytes in vitro (Chen and Bowden 2000). The transcription factor, AP-1, mediates the transcription of genes containing a 12-O-tetradecanoylphorbol-13-acetate (TPA) response element (TRE) (Lee, Haslinger et al. 1987). AP-1 is made up of homo- and heterodimers of proteins from the Jun and Fos families (Curran and Franza 1988).

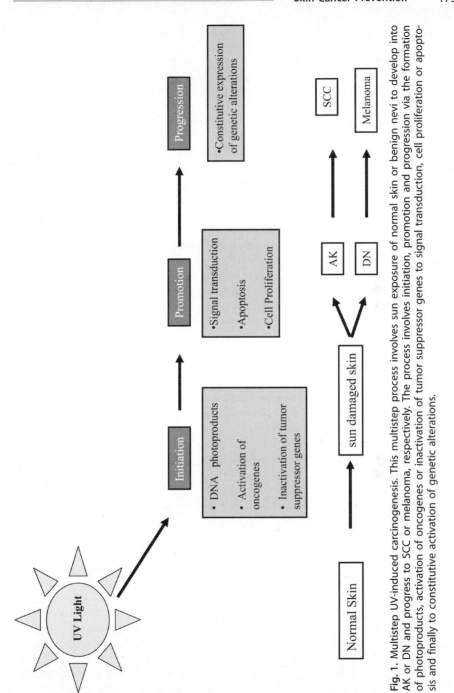

Fig. 1. Multistep UV-induced carcinogenesis. This multistep process involves sun exposure of normal skin or benign nevi to develop into AK or DN and progress to SCC or melanoma, respectively. The process involves initiation, promotion and progression via the formation of photoproducts, activation of oncogenes or inactivation of tumor suppressor genes to signal transduction, cell proliferation or apoptosis and finally to constitutive activation of genetic alterations.

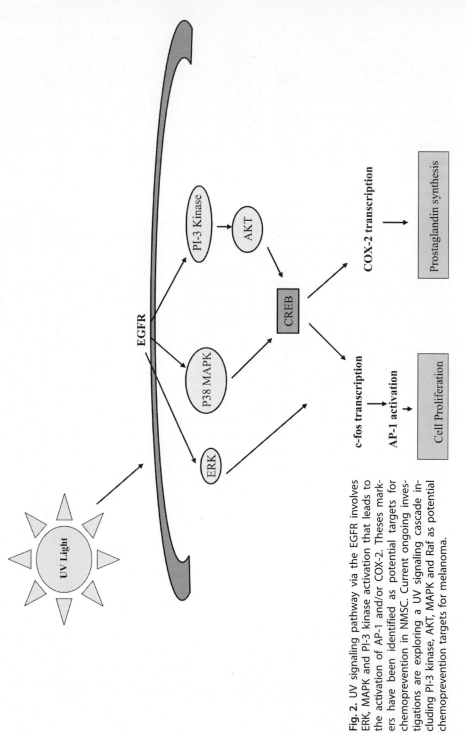

Fig. 2. UV signaling pathway via the EGFR involves ERK, MAPK and PI-3 kinase activation that leads to the activation of AP-1 and/or COX-2. Theses markers have been identified as potential targets for chemoprevention in NMSC. Current ongoing investigations are exploring a UV signaling cascade including PI-3 kinase, AKT, MAPK and Raf as potential chemoprevention targets for melanoma.

These genes are considered early response genes because of their rapid response to environmental changes, such as growth factors, stress, or DNA damage (Angel, Hattori et al. 1988; Ryseck, Hirai et al. 1988). Induction of Jun and Fos results from post-translational modification (Stein, Angel et al. 1992). In contrast, UVR activation of AP-1-dependent genes, such as the metalloproteinase genes and c-Fos appears to require new protein synthesis of Jun and Fos (Konig, Ponta et al. 1992).

c-Fos is constitutively expressed in both rodent and human epidermis (Basset-Seguin, Escot et al. 1990; Fisher, Byers et al. 1991) as demonstrated by immunohisto-chemical localization, suggesting that c-Fos has a role in growth and cell proliferation (Basset-Seguin, Escot et al. 1990). Additionally, UVB (Chen, Borchers et al. 1998) and UVA irradiation (Silvers and Bowden 2002) has been shown to induce c-Fos expression in human keratinocytes. Similarly, in rat epidermis, single doses of UVB produced a rapid and sustained increase in c-Fos and c-Jun mRNA and protein throughout the epidermis at early time points, but were restricted to the basal layer at later time points. This suggests their possible role in the induction of both apoptosis and cell proliferation (Gillardon, Eschenfelder et al. 1994).

Investigators have demonstrated the important role of AP-1 in UVR carcinogenesis in human and mouse keratinocytes as well as transgenic mice. UVB (Chen, Borchers et al. 1998) and UVA (Silvers and Bowden 2002) were shown to activate AP-1 in Ha-CaT cells (human keratinocyte cell line) with a correlative increase in c-Fos expression. The blocking of AP-1 transactivation in malignant mouse SCC cell lines inhibits the formation of tumors in athymic nude mice (Domann, Levy et al. 1994). c-Fos and junD were identified as the main components of the AP-1 complex induced by UVB. The upregulation of AP-1 by UVB has been demonstrated in mouse skin (Barthelman, Chen et al. 1998) and human skin (Fisher and Voorhees 1998). In studies with mouse epidermal JB6 cells, it has been demonstrated that blocking tumor promoter-induced AP-1 activity inhibited neoplastic transformation by an AP-1-inhibiting dominant negative Jun (Dong, Birrer et al. 1994). UVB irradiation studies have demonstrated an induction of AP-1 through the MAPK signaling cascade in human keratinocytes (Chen and Bowden 1999). A critical role for MAPK signaling (p38 and JNK) in AP-1 transactivation has also been demonstrated by UVA irradiation (Silvers, Bachelor et al. 2003). A mouse model that was used for testing the hypothesis that AP-1 activation has a functional role in the promotion of UVB-induced skin tumors is a TAM67 mouse crossed with a mouse expressing an AP-1 luciferase reporter gene. The TAM67 transgenic mouse contains a dominant-negative c-JUN mutant transgene (TAM67) under the control of the human keratin 14 promoter expressed in the epidermis of SKH-1 hairless mice. These mice show a decrease in UVB light-induced AP-1 activation with a signal UVB exposure. The expression of the TAM67 delayed the appearance of tumors, reduced the number of tumors per mouse and reduced the size of the tumors subsequent to chronic UVB exposure. The data demonstrated that the expression of the TAM67 inhibited UVB-induced AP-1 activation in the epidermis and inhibited UVB-induced skin tumor development. Information gathered from these studies have enabled the formulation of a UVB signaling pathway that leads to AP-1 activation and provides a good molecular target for the development of new chemoprevention strategies to prevent UVR-induced skin cancers (Bowden 2004).

The MAPKs are part of signaling cascades that involve the regulation of cell proliferation and differentiation in human epidermis (Geilen, Wieprecht et al. 1996). Mitogen-activated protein (MAP) kinases are a family of serine/threonine protein kinases. These kinases have been found to be important in cellular response to growth stimuli (Peyssonnaux and Eychene 2001). MAP kinases are activated by translocation to the nucleus, where kinases phosphorylate their targets substrates such as transcription factors (Coso, Chiariello et al. 1995). The MAP kinase family includes c-Jun-NH$_2$ terminal kinases (JNKs/SAPKs), extracellular signal-regulated protein kinases (ERKs) and p38 MAP kinases. JNKs/SAPKs and p38 kinases are activated by stress, including UVR irradiation (Kallunki, Su et al. 1994). Investigators have demonstrated that UVA and UVB irradiation causes activation of ERKs, JNKs and p38 kinases in cell culture (Huang 1997; Huang, Ma et al. 1997; Dong, Huang et al. 1998).

p38 MAP kinase plays an important role in UVB-induced c-Fos expression in human keratinocytes (Chen and Bowden 1999). Both p38 and ERK were significantly activated by UVB irradiation in human keratinocytes. Treatment of these cells with a p38 inhibitor, SB202190, inhibited UVB-induced p38 activation but did not induce ERK activation. In addition the treatment of the cells with MEK1 inhibitor, PD98059, inhibited UVB-induced ERK activation but not UVB-induced p38 activation (Chen and Bowden 1999). The blocking of p38 almost completely abrogates UVB-induced c-Fos gene transcription and c-FOS protein synthesis. Inhibition of ERK partially abrogates UVB-induced c-fos transcriptional and protein levels. Inhibiting both p38 and ERK completely blocked UVB-induced c-fos expression but also decreased c-Fos basal gene expression. The p38 inhibitor, SB202190, strongly inhibited UVB-induced AP-1 transactivation as well as AP-1 DNA binding (Chen and Bowden 2000). These data together suggests that the upstream molecules of C-Fos and AP-I signaling, p38 and ERK are potential targets for chemoprevention in NMSC.

Another target gene in UVB signaling is COX-2. COX-2 is a key enzyme involved in the synthesis of prostaglandins. Prostaglandins have been linked to several important events of the carcinogenesis process. An increase in COX-2 expression occurs after UVB exposure in both human skin (Buckman, Gresham et al. 1998) and cultured human keratinocytes (An et al. 2002). There is also an increase expression of COX-2 protein in human squamous cell carcinoma biopsies and when compared to normal non-sun exposed control skin. Selective inhibition of COX-2 in hairless mice has resulted in a significant reduction of UVR-induced skin tumors in hairless mice (Pentland, Schoggins et al. 1999). Of particular interest is another study which demonstrated that p38 is required for UVB-induced COX-2 gene expression in human keratinocytes (Chen, Tang et al. 2001). Inhibition of p38 with SB202190 markedly inhibited UVB-induced COX-2 mRNA. There was no effect when the Mek inhibitor PD98059 was used. UVA has also been shown to induce COX-2 in keratinocytes (Bachelor, Silvers et al. 2002). Since p38 MAPK appears to be an important step in two UV-induced signaling pathways (ending in the transcription factors AP-1 and COX-2), it is an excellent candidate as a target for chemoprevention.

JNK phosphorylates c-Jun (Derijard, Hibi et al. 1994; Kallunki, Su et al. 1994), a component of the AP-1 transcription factor. There are three JNK genes (JNK-1, -2 and -3) that have been identified in humans. It has been demonstrated that JNK2 knockout (JNK2$^{-/-}$) mice, in a two-stage tumor promotion skin carcinogenesis model with DMBA and TPA, exhibited significant reduction in papilloma burden compared with wild-type controls (Chen, Nomura et al. 2001). Further studies to look at the UVR signaling pathway for skin carcinogenesis may point toward JNK as another potential target for chemoprevention of skin cancer.

The Phosphatidylinositol-3 kinase (PI-3 kinase) pathway regulates cellular proliferation, growth, apoptosis and cytoskeletal rearrangement. PI-3 kinases are heterodimeric lipid kinases composed of regulatory and catalytic domains (Vivanco and Sawyers 2002). PI-3 kinase is an important enzyme associated with a variety of receptors or protein-tyrosine kinases and acts as a direct biochemical link between a novel phosphatidylinositol pathway and a number of receptor proteins, including the receptors for insulin or platelet-derived growth factor (Downes and Carter 1991). This enzyme is a heterodimer of a 110-kDa unit (Auger, Serunian et al. 1989). It can phosphorylate phosphatidylinositol (Ptdins), Ptdins (4) phosphate [Ptdins (4) P], or Ptdins(4,5) bisphosphate [Ptdins(4,5)P2] to produce Ptdins(3)P, Ptdins(3,4)P2, or Ptdins(3,4,5) trisphosphate [Ptdins(3,4,5)P3], respectively (Whitman, Downes et al. 1988; Cohen, Liu et al. 1990; Nomura, Kaji et al. 2001). Insulin or growth factor stimulation of the associated tyrosine kinase results in phosphorylation of the p85 subunit of PI-3 kinase. This phosphorylation is important for activation of PI-3 kinase (Huang, Ma et al. 1997). Akt works downstream in the PI-3 kinase pathway to regulate proliferation, apoptosis and growth (Vivanco and Sawyers 2002). Akt, a serine/threonine kinase, is activated by recruitment to the plasma membrane. Clinical evidence of PI-3 kinase activation has been reported in various cancers and the identification of downstream kinases provides a potential target for mediating tumorigenesis (Vivanco and Sawyers 2002). Investigators have shown that UVB irradiation activates Akt in JB6, mouse epidermal cells. This activation was attenuated by inhibitors for MAP kinase/ERK kinase-1 and p38 (Nomura, Kaji et al. 2001). It has been reported that PI-3 kinase plays an important role in UVB-induced AP-1 and Akt activation (Huang, Ma et al. 1997; Nomura, Kaji et al. 2001). Inhibition of PI-3 kinase was found to block UVB-induced activation of p90 ribosomal protein S6 kinase (P70S6K), known to be associated with AP-1 in tumor promoter-induced cell transformation (Zhang, Zhong et al. 2001).

Wan et al. demonstrated that solar UVR irradiation of human skin activated EGFR as well as other downstream signals including MAP kinases, ERK, JNK and p38 (Wan, Wang et al. 2001; Wan, Wang et al. 2001). Their investigations revealed activation of the PI3-kinase/AKT survival pathway via EGFR. They also found that EGF crosstalks with cytokine receptors such as IL-1 receptor leading to the activation of c-Jun kinase in response to UVR irradiation of human keratinocytes. Additional investigators have shown that UVA-induced EGFR signaling is required for activation of p90RSK/p70S6K, PI-3 kinase and ERK (Zhang, Dong et al. 2001).

Signaling cascades due to UVR stimulation that leads to skin carcinogenesis of melanoma are not defined as extensively as for NMSC. Investigators have outline UVR signaling pathways for melanogenesis (Tada, Pereira et al. 2002). However, there is a thus far only a few identified molecules that could potentially serve as molecular targets (Raf and MAPK) for chemoprevention of melanoma. The Raf kinases were the first Ras effectors identified and have been the most extensively studied (Hunter 1997). Ras associates with and activates Raf-1, which in turn phosphorylates and activates MEK kinase, which in turn phosphorylates the MAP kinases, ERK1 and ERK2 (Liaw 1993; Samuels, Weber et al. 1993; Warne, Viciana et al. 1993; Ghosh, Xie et al. 1994). Activated MAP kinases translocate to the nucleus where they can modulate gene expression (Hill and Treisman 1995; Marshall 1995). Raf-1 has also been shown to interact with PKC, a key regulatory protein associated with a second signal transduction pathway (Kolch, Heidecker et al. 1993). Two well-established biological events that are associated with activation of the Raf/MEK/ERK pathway are cell proliferation and cell cycle progression. Halaban and colleagues have observed that several of the mitogenic factors for melanocytes, bFGF, MCGF, and HGF/SF, stimulate ERK1/ERK2 phosphorylation (Funasaka, Boulton et al. 1992; Halaban 1992; Halaban, Rubin et al. 1992). Investigators have demonstrated that Raf plays an important role in progression of melanoma (Pollock, Harper et al. 2003). The data from these studies identified a particular mutation that was found in 68% of metastatic melanoma, 80% of primary melanoma and 82% of a diverse set of nevi. These findings implicate Raf as a potential target for chemoprevention of melanoma, since Raf mutations are evident at the early stage of primary melanoma and nevi. The identification of MAPK as an early event in melanoma progression (Cohen, Zavala-Pompa et al. 2002) provides another potential target for the chemoprevention of melanoma.

Animal Models for Studying Chemoprevention Agents. In order to understand the mechanism of carcinogenesis and investigate efficacy of chemoprevention agents prior to clinical application, animal models that closely resemble human disease must be developed. The SKH-1 hairless mouse is a model for the studies of skin cancer pathogenesis and the evaluation of chemoprevention of UVB-induced skin cancer (Bowden 2004). The most obvious advantage of these mice is that they are hairless and therefore do not require any removal of hair that may actually protect the skin from UVR light. With increasing dose level, three times a week for 25 weeks nearly 100% of the mice develop at least one skin tumor with an average of 7–9 tumors per mouse. Most of these tumors are SCC, which arise from benign papillomas. UVB irradiation is used as a complete carcinogen in these mice. Another protocol used with these mice is UVB exposure twice a week for 20 weeks. This results in epidermal hyperplasia; no immediate tumors occur but a high risk of developing skin tumors during the next several months in the absence of any further UVR. This latter model system resembles humans who are heavily exposed to UVR early in life with reduced exposure later in life. Chemoprevention agents can be tested in these models.

A mouse strain with abnormalities in the hedgehog signaling pathway develops neoplasms which closely resembles human BCC. These mice contain a heterozygous allele in the PTCH gene (ptc+/–). Chemoprevention studies with green and black tea have been studied in this mouse model (Herbert, Khugyani et al. 2001).

Multiple animal models of melanoma have been reported however difficulties with these models for studies of chemoprevention are that tumors develop at a low incidence rate and the latency period is often very long. There are two models for melanoma, which are useful for the studies of chemoprevention agents. Powell et al. report the development of a transgenic mouse for which when chemically induced develops melanoma. The mouse line expresses a mutated human Ha-ras (TPras) gene driven by a mouse tyrosinase promoter. This transgene is therefore expressed in pigment producing cells of the mice. The protocol for inducing melanoma in these mice is topical application of 50 µg 7,12-dimethylbenz-[a]anthracene (DMBA) once a week for five weeks. Development of melanoma occurs around 15 weeks. Tumors only occur in the mice expressing the transgene and no tumors develop in the negative littermates. Tumors develop in >80% of the treated mice. No spontaneous cutaneous melanoma or other skin cancers develop in these mice. Metastatic lesions have been observed in the skin, lungs and lymph nodes of the DMBA-treated transgenic mice (Powell 1999). Melanomas isolated from TPras transgenic mice display alterations and/or losses of p16 (Gause, Lluria-Prevatt et al. 1997) much like human melanoma. Another model is a transgenic model, which utilizes a metallothionein-gen promoter driving a hepatocyte growth factor/scatter factor (c-Met receptor tyrosine kinase ligand) gene based on the albino FVB background. Development of melanoma occurs in this model system after a single acute exposure of an erythemal dose of UVR irradiation. Development of invasive melanoma occurs in 80% of the animals. These melanoma closely resemble human melanoma in terms of the development between the dermis and epidermis.

Endpoints for Evaluating Efficacy of Chemoprevention Agents. Because the process of carcinogenesis can take many years, assessment of clinical chemoprevention trials using cancer incidence as an endpoint requires a long follow-up period and large sample sizes. The rationale for the use of intermediate biomarkers is to circumvent these issues in chemoprevention trials (Einspahr, Alberts et al. 1997), since biomarkers occur at steps preceding the occurrence of malignancy. As discussed by Lippman et al. (Lippman, Lee et al. 1990), biomarkers of intermediate endpoints can be defined as measurable markers of cellular or molecular events associated with specific stages of the multi-step progression of carcinogenesis. Thus, the risk of carcinogenic transformation, whether in the skin or other sites, can be correlated with the quantitative degree and pattern of biomarker expression. Criteria for identifying and evaluating the potential efficacy of biomarkers are as follows:

- Variability of expression between phases of the carcinogenesis process (i.e., normal, premalignant, malignant)
- Ability for early detection in the carcinogenesis pathway
- Association with risk of developing cancer or recurrence of the precancer
- Potential for modification by a chemopreventive agent
- Presence in tissues that are easily accessible for multiple biopsies
- Capability to develop adequate assay quality control procedures.

Markers of cellular proliferation can be used as intermediate biomarker to evaluate the efficacy of chemoprevention agents in clinical trials and animal model systems. Enhanced cellular proliferation has been closely associated with the process of tumorigenesis in numerous tissues including skin (Einspahr, Alberts et al. 1996). Proliferating cellular nuclear antigen (PCNA) functions as an auxiliary protein to DNA polymerase d and e in DNA replication and repair (Hall, Levison et al. 1990). Expression of PCNA increases late in G1, is maximally expressed in S, and decreases in the G2/M phases of the cell cycle. Therefore, PCNA can be used to evaluate cell proliferation and chemoprevention efficacy.

Apoptosis also serves as biomarker for the efficacy of chemoprevention agents in clinical trials and animal model systems. Apoptosis is a unique mode of cell death, characterized by ultrastructural changes distinct from necrosis (Kerr, Wyllie et al. 1972). In the developing animal, programmed cell death removes cells during remodeling of a number of organs (Haake and Polakowska 1993). Apoptosis is also involved in tissue regression following hormone stimulation or deprivation in hormone-sensitive tissues, such as the prostate, and functions in development of the immune system (Haake and Polakowska 1993). In continually renewing tissues such as the epidermis, homeostasis is maintained through a balance between cellular proliferation and cell death. Apoptosis may also play an important role in regression of neoplasms (Haake and Polakowska 1993). Alterations in either cell proliferation or cell death can lead to loss of growth control, thereby playing major roles in the process of tumorigenesis. Apoptosis is characterized by cell shrinkage, plasma membrane blebbing, nuclear fragmentation and chromatin condensation. Apoptotic cells are rapidly phagocytosed by neighboring cells in order to prevent the release of cell contents. In contrast to necrosis, apoptosis is an organized and controlled process of cell death (Kerr, Wyllie et al. 1972).

Investigators have shown that p53 mutations increase through the progression of normal skin, sun damaged skin, AK and SCC. While the frequency of p53 mutations was 14% in normal skin, this percentage rose to 38.5% in sun-damaged skin, 63% in AK and 54% in SCC. Proliferation was also increased through this same progression. SCC samples demonstrated an increased presence of BAX compared to AK (Einspahr, Alberts et al. 1999). This data supports the use of p53 as a biomarker for disease progression when evaluating the efficacy of chemoprevention agents.

Karyometric evaluation of the epidermis has been used as a developmental secondary endpoint in clinical studies (Bozzo, Alberts et al. 2001). Nuclear chromatin patterns can be used diagnostically to assess changes in the development of cells, particularly the development into a cancerous cell, which could then be correlated with the prognosis of individual patients. Image analysis of nuclear chromatin patterns provides a quantitative approach (Weyn, Jacob et al. 2000). With image analysis, karyometric features are described by the arrangement of a combination of pixels. These features are then combined by means of multivariate analysis of criteria used for prognosis. Digital microscopic studies of epithelia from ectocervix (Wied, Bartels et al. 1980), lung mucosa (MacAulay, Lam et al. 1995), colonic mucosa (Bibbo, Michelassi et al. 1990), glandular epithelium of the thyroid (Bibbo, Bartels et al. 1986), breast (Susnik, Worth et al. 1995), bladder (Sherman and Koss 1983), and the prostate (Irinopoulou, Rigaut et al. 1993) have detected very subtle, possibly pre-neoplastic changes in the organization of nuclear chromatin in biopsies from individuals with premalignant and malignant lesions of these organ sites. When these same tissue sections were examined with standard histopathological techniques, no abnormalities were detected. Thus, digital microscopy can provide highly sensitive detection of early change and may provide novel diagnostic clues. Digital imagery can reliably detect very early subtle changes in the organization of nuclear chromatin in epithelial cells that appear to be entirely normal during histopathologic examination. This technology, which uses high resolution imagery of cell nuclei to assign values to karyometric features, may enable the quantitative assessment of progressive change from normal appearing to severely sun damaged skin to AK to SCC as well as from DN to melanoma. Nuclear karyometric measurements have been performed on both benign and malignant melanocytic lesions (Bjornhagen, Bonfoco et al. 1994; Stolz, Vogt et al. 1994). Using imprint specimens, Stolz et al. (Stolz, Vogt et al. 1994) found five features (mean value and standard deviation of nuclear area and the 80th, 90th and 95th percentile of the DNA distribution) to be significantly different between benign melanocytic lesions and melanoma. A second report (Stolz, Vogt et al. 1994) found significant differences between benign melanocytic tumors and malignant melanoma for the following features: mean nuclear area; coefficient of variation (cv) of nuclear area; cv of nuclear shape; nuclear contour index; mean and cv of nucleolar area; and DNA distribution rates. Investigators have conducted feasibility studies for the karyometric assessment of skin shave biopsies of AKs and for the assessment of the effects of chemopreventive intervention, using quantitative characterization by digital microscopy (Bozzo, Vaught et al. 1998). Sections of shave skin biopsies were digitized and a minimum of 100 nuclei from each was recorded per case. After image segmentation, feature extraction software produced 93 karyometric features per nucleus that were stored for analysis. Discriminant functions were derived according to differences between normal nuclei and those with sun damage. Profiles commonly found in malignant cells were seen in the AK lesions. Using these features, a grading score was developed based on a plot of degree of solar damage versus the mean discriminant function. While upper inner arm (minimally sun exposed) skin biopsies demonstrated as few as 3% of nuclei affected by sun damage, the AK lesions included approximately 50% affected nuclei. Discriminant functions derived from values obtained from samples ranging from normal to sun damaged to premalignant (AK or DN) to malignant (SCC or melanoma) phenotypes establish a progression curve that can be used to determine the efficacy of applied chemopreventive agents (Bozzo, Alberts et al. 2001) (Figure 3). They have also applied this novel technology to demonstrate the efficacy of two chemoprevention agents, a-DFMO and Vitamin A, in patients with moderately severe sun damaged skin (Bozzo, Alberts et al. 2001; Alberts, Ranger-Moore et al. 2004).

Optical Coherence Tomography (OCT) is a potentially new technique for identifying and characterizing AKs and monitoring their response to chemoprevention agents (Barton, Gossage et al. 2003). Based on Michelson interferometry, this technique was first in-

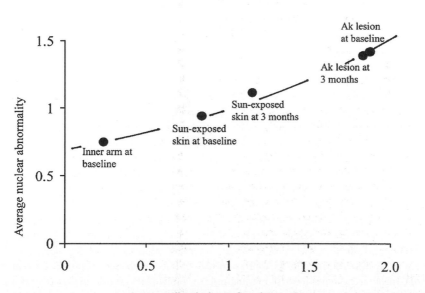

Fig. 3. Average nuclear abnormality versus average discriminant function scores for the 10% worst nuclei from the upper inner arm at baseline, sun-exposed skin at baseline and three months, and AK lesions at baseline and three months (Ranger-Moore 2002).

troduced for investigations of the human eye (Fercher, Mengedoht et al. 1988). This non-invasive technique uses coherent light operating in the near infrared region of 1300 nm to produce two-dimensional images of the skin (Welzel 2001). The resulting photons have a typical penetrating depth of 1.0 to 1.5 mm allowing for multiple layers and structures to be distinguished. The resolution afforded by this technique makes it possible to distinguish features such as stratum cornea, epidermal layer, hair follicles, sebaceous glands and blood vessels. In addition, it is possible to evaluate the efficacy of topical application of ointments and similar treatments, as these compounds tend to increase the detection/penetrating depth of the coherent light (Welzel 2001). In OCT, images of epithelial skin tumors and cell aggregation from the epidermis are visible. In some cases, lateral borders of the tumor adjacent to healthy skin are detectable and BCC can be distinguished from fibrous stroma. It is also possible to diagnose various inflammatory skin diseases such as psoriasis and eczema. The OCT measurement is an unobtrusive and safe technique with no side effects for the patient.

In a pilot study on 20 subjects to investigate the OCT appearance of upper inner arm, sun-damaged skin and mild AKs (Barton, Gossage et al. 2003) and to determine if features or quantitative measures in OCT images could be used to reliably differentiate between these categories, OCT images of upper inner arm showed skin layers and features (stratum corneum, epidermis, dermis, blood vessels) seen in previous studies; additionally in this subject base the subcutaneous fat layer was usually seen. Sundamaged skin was characterized by increased signal in the epidermis and rapid attenuation of light. AKs were diverse in appearance but frequently characterized by high surface reflection, the presence of a low-signal band in the stratum corneum, and heterogeneous appearance in the epidermis/dermis. Significant differences were found between skin categories using measures of stratum corneum and epidermal/dermal depths and intensities. The presence of a dark band in the stratum corneum was 79% sensitive and 100% specific for AK. This study suggests that OCT may be a useful non-invasive technique for monitoring AK during the clinical studies to evaluate the efficacy of chemoprevention agents.

Potential Chemoprevention Agents for Skin Cancer. The investigators at the Arizona Cancer Center use a decision tree which results in leads for chemoprevention agents that will potentially result in a clinical trial (Einspahr, Bowden et al. 2003). The agents are selected based on epidemiological literature and activity in in vitro and in vivo models of UV skin carcinogenesis. Agents with novel mechanisms of action that are active against identified molecular targets are tested for their ability to modify the target and inhibit tumorigenesis in the animal models. Subsequent to toxicological evaluation and proper formulation, promising agents then progress to human phase I and then to phase II trials in subjects with AKs, DNs or sun-damaged skin. Intermediate endpoints are evaluated to identify efficacy of the select agent. The following discussion provides an overview of chemoprevention agents for skin cancer which have been or are currently in clinical trials as well as future agents which may result in clinical trials due to their activity toward modulation of molecular targets previously discussed for NMSC and melanoma in in vitro or in vivo models systems.

A few potential chemopreventive agents have been taken through Phase III clinical trials in people at high risk for NMSC (Stratton 2001; Bowden 2004). The agents are beta-carotene (Greenberg, Baron et al. 1990), selenium (Clark, Combs et al. 1996), retinol (Moon, Levine et al. 1997) and 13-cis-retinoic acid (Tangrea, Edwards et al. 1992). Of these trials, the only one with positive results involved oral administration of 25,000 U/day of retinol in 2297 subjects with moderate to severe AK (Moon, Levine et al. 1997). This trial resulted in a reduction in SCC but not in BCC. The hazard ratio for first new SCC was 0.74 when comparing subjects from the retinol supplemented group to placebo. Vitamin A (retinol) has been demonstrated to be necessary for cell growth and differentiation of human epithelial tissues, reproduction and visual function (Gudas 1994). Retinoids have been shown to be involved in cell growth, cell differentiation and carcinogenesis, all mediated in part by nuclear retinoic acid receptors and retinoid X receptors (Mangelsdorf, Unesonso et al. 1994; Xu, Clifford et al. 1994).

There have been several smaller phase II trials in subjects at risk for NMSC that have resulted in positive outcomes. Recently, a phase IIa/IIb safety, dose-finding and efficacy study of orally administered Vitamin A in participants with sun damaged skin resulted in a positive outcome (Alberts, Ranger-Moore et al. 2004). The results were evaluated using karyometric analysis (described previously). One hundred twenty randomized participants were given daily oral placebo, 25K, 50K or 75K units of Vitamin A (retinyl palmitate) for 12 months. The primary endpoints included quantitative, karyometric image analysis and assessment of retinoid receptors in sun-damaged skin. This analysis suggests that orally administered Vitamin A is effective as a skin cancer chemopreventive agent by reducing levels of actinic nuclear damage as measured by average nuclear abnormality levels and discriminant function scores derived from ap-

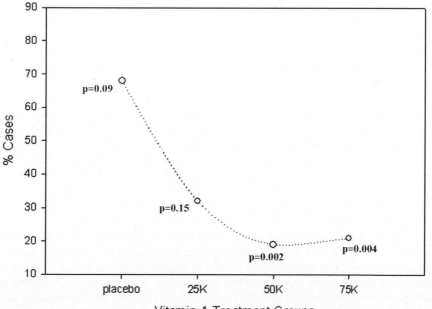

Fig. 4. Dose response to vitamin A treatment as demonstrated by percent of cases with increased actinic damage decreases based on karyometric analysis, adapted from Bartels et al. (Bartels, Ranger-Moore et al. 2002).

propriate karyometric features (Figure 4). The dose effects of Vitamin A correlated with increases in retinoid receptors, RAR-α, RAR-β and RXR-α, at the 50,000 IU per day vitamin A dose.

Another clinical trial performed by Alberts and colleagues demonstrated that topical 2-(Difluoromethyl)dl-ornithine (α-DFMO) can reduce spermidine concentrations and the number of AK lesions in patients at high risk of skin cancer (Alberts, Dorr et al. 2000). Forty-eight participants with moderately severe AKs on their forearms were assigned randomly to topical α-DFMO treatment. A reduction of 23.5% in the number of AK lesions was seen from baseline to the six-month follow up. Spermidine concentration was reduced by 26% in skin biopsies from α-DFMO-treated arms. No systemic toxicities were detected; however, seven of the forty-eight (14.6%) participants experienced severe (4.2%) or moderate (10.4%) inflammatory reaction on their α-DFMO-treated arms. In skin biopsies from this study, investigators were able to demonstrate a significant reduction of 22% in p53-positive cells (Einspahr, Nelson et al. 2002). However, there were no significant changes in proliferation cell nuclear antigen (PCNA) index, apoptotic indices or p53 mutation frequencies. With karyometric analysis, α-DFMO treatment markedly decreased the discriminant function score indicating effectiveness in reducing nuclear abnormalities. α-DFMO is an irreversible inhibitor of ornithine decarboxylase (ODC), the rate-limiting enzyme in polyamine synthesis, and may exert its chemoprevention effects by inhibiting growth and/or inducing apoptosis. α-DFMO inhibits polyamine biosynthesis by covalently binding to ODC, thus inhibiting proliferation and inducing apoptosis. Leads for the use of α-DFMO came from previous studies where α-DFMO had been demonstrated as an antitumor agent in several animal models for carcinogenesis including a report that oral α-DFMO inhibited cutaneous carcinogenesis and immunosuppression in a mouse model (Gensler 1991). In Xpa knockout mice, α-DFMO, given in drinking water, reduced UVR-induced skin tumors in mice (Takigawa, Enomoto et al. 1990). Tumor-suppressive activity was demonstrated for α-DFMO in melanoma (in vitro and in metastatic melanoma in a clinical trial) (Bregman and Meyskens 1986; Meyskens 1986).

Diclofenac is a nonsteroidal anti-inflammatory drug (NSAID) often used alone for degenerative arthritis management or with opioids in the treatment of pain associated with cancer. Investigations have shown that diclofenac has activity in the treatment of actinic keratosis, thereby potentially preventing progression to SCC. An early study of 29 subjects assessed the efficacy and safety of topical diclofenac (Solaraze). Three percent diclofenac in 2.5% hyaluronic acid gel was generally well tolerated with the exception of 7 (24%) patients who experienced irritant-type contact dermatitis (Rivers and McLean 1997). Additional clinical trials have further explored the potential therapeutic effect of this gel formulation. One randomized double-blind controlled trial of 130 patients, which did not include a follow up period, did not find a significant difference between the use of diclofenac/hyaluronan and placebo in the eradication of AKs (McEwan and Smith 1997). However, two other randomized, double-blind, placebo-controlled studies found treatment with 3.0% diclofenac to be effective in the treatment of AK. A study of 195 patients with at least five AKs investigated the duration of treatment for 30 or 60 days with two daily applications of the gel (Rivers, Arlette et al. 2002). While no significant difference was seen after 30 days, the 60-day treatment group showed a statistically significant difference in the number of patients (33% to 10%) with complete resolution of all target lesions in treated areas when compared to placebo group. The 60-day treatment group was also significantly different than place-bo in the number of patients with resolution of target and new lesions in treated area, visible but no longer palpable lesions and investigator and patient global improvement indices. Another study of 96 subjects also demonstrated a statistically significant dif-ference in a 60-day treatment regimen when comparing the above criteria (Wolf, Tay-lor et al. 2001). In both these studies, the gel was well tolerated with only a few sub-jects reporting skin reactions. The mechanism of action of the 3.0% diclofenac, with regard to tumor resolution, is unknown. As an NSAID, diclofenac inhibits cyclooxy-genase enzymes (COX-1 and COX-2). A case control study in women found an inverse association of NSAIDS intake and malignant melanoma (Harris, Beebe-Donk et al. 2001). One group demonstrated that 26 to 28 primary melanoma cell lines expressed COX-2 (Denkert, Kobel et al. 2001). Finally, a UVR-induced tumor mouse model dem-onstrated a lengthening in tumor latency period and reduced tumor multiplicity when mice were treated with a COX-2 inhibitor, Celecoxib (Orengo, Gerguis et al. 2002). An increase in arachidonic acid metabolism in keratinocytes due to exposure to UVB (Buckman, Gresham et al. 1998) may be a target for this type of chemoprevention.

An agent developed at the University of Arizona, Melanotan-1 (MT-1) could poten-tially be used as a chemopreventive agent against melanoma and NMSC. This agent is a superpotent melanotropic peptide that results in darkening of the skin. In clinical studies with MT-1 there was no improvement of tanning in doses greater than 0.16 mg/kg/day for ten days by subcutaneous (SC) injection. No moderate toxicities occurred at this dose as in the higher doses (Levine 1999); a single exposure of three MED of UVB did not enhance eumelanin content of the skin either before or after MT-1 administration (Dorr, Dvorakova et al. 2000). While treatment showed darken-ing of the skin on days 14 and 21, there was no significant difference from baseline to four weeks after dosing. Investigators found that the most effective delivery was by SC administration, which resulted in an increase in eumelanin and measured tanning by reflectance in the forearm and forehead. For the purpose of prolonging skin darkening by the use of MT-1, investigators formulated a controlled release MT-1 implant formu-lation based on a PLGA polymer. In studies with an in vitro frog skin bioassay, they found that the implants (1 mg of peptide) showed that the melanophores migrated to the dendritic processes of the pigment cells, which resulted in skin darkening. In vivo studies using pigmented haired and hairless guinea pigs with the MT-1 implants (4 mg peptide), increase of skin darkening was observed for up to three months and eumelanin content demonstrated a 2.5 fold increase one month and persisted for three months. This prolonged increase in pigment, specifically eumelanin, can be favorable to the prevention against photodamage induced by UVR radiation.

Currently, MT-1 is under development in Australia. Two objectives are underway: (1) clinical testing of multiple daily subcutaneous injections to reduce sun damage in high risk individuals with precancerous lesions; and (2) the development of a slow re-lease depot formulation designed to release drug from a single subcutaneous injection over several months. Phase I/II trials in Adelaide, Australia found that the 0.16 mg/kg/day injection dose caused increased eumelanin deposition in the skin, similar to re-sults reported in the Arizona studies. No dose limiting side effects were noted. The next phase II trial will be performed in three cities (Melbourne, Sydney and Brisbane) evaluating the effect of MT-1 on patients with multiple AK in an attempt to reduce the total number of lesions and improve overall skin condition. Of additional interest, patients will be phenotyped for melanocortin-1 receptor (MCR) variants (these are most often individuals who do not respond to UVR light with melanin production, including red-haired, freckled, and easily-burned people) to evaluate the response to the drug with receptor type. This will assess if the drug will benefit this type of individual known to be at high risk for sun-induced skin cancers. The second objective with MT-1 with a slow release depot formulation will begin phase I clinical studies after the conclusion of animal toxicology studies that are now underway.

Dellavalle and colleagues (Dellavalle, Nicholas et al. 2003) review the role of statins or fibrates in melanoma chemoprevention. Results from two large clinical trials demonstrated a decrease in melanoma incidence in subjects given lipid-lowering medications for coronary artery disease. In another study 27 melanomas were newly diagnosed in 3301 placebo-treated patients, whereas only 14 melanomas were diagnosed in 3304 lovastatin-treated patients (Buchwald 1992). The incidence of all other cancers was not statistically different. Another study with gemfibrozil, a hypolipidemic medication, nine melanomas were diagnosed in 1267 patients treated with placebo and only one melanoma was diagnosed in a five-year period in 1264 gemfibrozil-treated patients (Rubins, Robins et al. 1999). Again, all other cancers were not significantly different. Statins are known to inhibit the isoprenoid protein modification and therefore may be inhibiting ras farnesylation and cause a downregulation of ras oncogenic potential in melanoma.

Other phase II trials have focused on the potential chemoprevention activity of topical green tea extracts (e.g., polyphenon E) in patients with AK on their arm (Stratton 2001). Animal studies have demonstrated a chemopreventive effect of Epigallocatechin gallate (EGCG). Investigators have reported a reduction in tumor incidence with topical application of EGCG in UVB-irradiated mice. Mice were irradiated at a total dose of 2.1×10^6 J/m^2. Skin cancer developed in 96% of control mice and 62% of mice given 10 mg of EGCG and 39% of mice given 50 mg of EGCG. EGCG did not affect immunosuppression and oral administration did not decrease UVR-induced skin tumor incidence. In the investigation of a mechanism of action for EGCG, it was demonstrated that EGCG can inhibit UVB-induced AP-1 activity in a dose range of 5.45 nM to 54.5 µM in human keratinocytes when applied before, after or both before and after UVB irradiation (Barthelman 1998). Inhibition of AP-1 by topical EGCG application was also evident in a transgenic mouse model. EGCG inhibited UVB-induced steady state message and transcriptional activation of the c-fos gene as well as the accumulation of the c-Fos protein. Upstream of c-Fos, EGCG significantly inhibited activation of p38 MAPK yet did not affect JNK or ERK activation. AP-1 inhibition potentially, through the reduction of c-Fos by EGCG, may be the mechanism by which EGCG inhibits UVB-induced tumor formation in mice (Chen, Dong et al. 1999). Theaflavins demonstrated a stronger inhibition of AP-1 than EGCG and inhibition of the activation of ERK and JNK was also significant with theaflavin treatment (Nomura, Ma et al. 2000).

Investigators have developed a 10% (w/w) EGCG formulation in Hydrophilic ointment USP for topical application. An intradermal uptake of 19% and 0.9% of the applied dose was evident in the mouse and human skin, respectively, while transdermal penetration was observed only in the mouse skin (Dvorakova, Dorr et al. 1999). The 10% EGCG formulation was used in a phase I clinical trial to assess safety and the sun protection factor (SPF). An SPF of 3.6 was recorded for this ointment, applied to buttock skin. No systemic toxicities with topical application to the arms were seen in 19 participants that completed the study. However, 42% of the participants reported moderately severe skin reaction and histological evaluation corroborated the clinical findings.

The chemopreventive activity of aspirin and sodium salicylate were investigated in a UVB-induced NMSC hairless SKH-1 mouse model (Bair, Hart et al. 2002). While sodium salicylate significantly inhibited UVB-induced tumor formation, aspirin had only a moderate effect. The protection supplied by sodium salicylate appears to be in part due to its sunscreen effect, which was demonstrated by the reduction of thymine dimers in the epidermis of mice treated with sodium salicylate. Aspirin was unable to prevent dimer formation (Bair, Hart et al. 2002).

In vitro studies revealed that a derivative of NDGA, tetra-O-methylnordihydroguaiaretic acid, inhibited growth of several tumor cell lines, including a melanoma line where there was morphologic evidence of apoptosis. This compound also inhibited the synthesis of DNA and caused cell cycle arrest in G_0/G_1 and G_2/M phases of the cell cycle. Growth inhibitory effects of this compound were also exhibited in vivo (Lambert, Meyers et al. 2001). Bowden and colleagues have also identified NDGA as an inhibitor of UVB-induced c-Fos and AP-1 transactivation by inhibiting the PI-3 kinase signal transduction pathway (Gonzales and Bowden 2002).

A potential chemopreventive agent for melanoma, Apomine, has been studied in a clinical and preclinical setting. Apomine is a bisphosphonate ester that has been reported to activate the farnesoid X receptor, increase the rate of degradation of HMG-CoA reductase and induce apoptosis (Niesor, Flach et al. 1999). Apomine has been shown to inhibit the growth of many tumor cell lines, including those derived from leukemia, colon, liver, ovary and breast (Falch, Antoni et al. 2000). Growth inhibition and apoptotic activity were compared to those of simvastatin, farnesol and 25-hydroxycholesterol, which all affect HMG-CoA reductase. Apomine was most like farnesol, a non-steriol regulator of cholesterol synthesis. In a phase I trial at the Arizona Cancer Center, it was demonstrated by plasma pharmacokinetics that a daily dose of 125 mg/m^2 of apomine was sufficiently bioavailable to levels used in in vitro studies that demonstrated activity against fresh human solid cancers. In preliminary studies in a TPras transgenic melanoma mouse model (Powell, Alberts et al. 2002), apomine caused a 55% reduction in melanoma development induced by DMBA. In vitro studies with melanoma cell lines derived from the transgenic TPras mouse model and treated with apomine demonstrated a significant reduction in Ras detected in the membrane fraction (activated Ras). Apomine was also able to reduce UVR-induced Akt phosphorylation but had no effect on phosphorylation of ERK1/2 (Powell, Alberts et al. 2002). In a phase I clinical trial at the Arizona Cancer Center, apomine expressed prolonged cancer stabilization in patients with metastatic melanoma and recurrent ovarian cancer with minimal or no toxicity (Powell, Alberts et al. 2002).

Another agent with potential chemopreventive activity in both melanoma and NMSC is Perillyl Alcohol (POH). POH is a cyclic monoterpene that reduces the amount of Ras and Ras-related proteins and has been reported to induce apoptosis. POH is found in the essential oils of numerous plants including citrus fruit, cherries and mint. Limonene (a precursor of POH) has been demonstrated to reduce the incidence of spontaneous lymphomas in p53 –/– mice and to inhibit the development of chemically-induced rodent mammary, liver, lung and forestomach tumors (Crowell

1999). Ras oncogene-induced mammary carcinoma development has also been inhibited by limonene (Gould, Moore et al. 1994). POH has demonstrated chemopreventive properties in several types of cancers, including liver cancer in rats (Mills, Chari et al. 1995), pancreatic cancer in hamsters (Stratton, Dorr et al. 2000) and mammary tumors in rats (Haag and Gould 1994). Perillyl alcohol and limonene as oral agents have also been used in clinical trials (Gould, Moore et al. 1994; Crowell 1999). Chemopreventive properties of topical POH have been demonstrated in a nonmelanoma and a melanoma mouse model (Barthelman, Chen et al. 1998; Lluria-Prevatt, Morreale et al. 2002). In both models, topically applied POH significantly reduced the incidence of tumors. Investigators also reported that POH reduced detectable levels of Ras, inhibited the activation of Akt and MAPK and reduced UVR-induced reactive oxygen species in melanoma cells (Lluria-Prevatt, Morreale et al. 2002). The mechanisms of action for POH identified thus far include inhibition of cell proliferation, induced tumor cell differentiation (Morse and Stoner 1993) and increased apoptosis (Mills, Chari et al. 1995). POH has been shown to inhibit protein isoprenylation in Ras (Hohl and Lewis 1995; Stayrook, McKinzie et al. 1998). Evidence of chemopreventive activity in mouse models and the suspected molecular targets for POH makes it an ideal compound for potential chemoprevention studies in melanoma and NMSC.

Future agents will most likely be identified by their mechanism of action. The selected agents will have specific targets such as those described earlier as important in the UV signaling pathways and carcinogenesis process of skin cancer development (Figure 2). For p38 MAPK, there are inhibitors which are a group of polycyclic pyridinylimidazole compounds. SFK86002, a bicyclic pyridinylimidazole, first reported to inhibit LPS-stimulated cytokine production (Lee, Kumar et al. 2000). Early reports indicated a role of cytokine inhibition as a potential mechanism for the potent anti-inflammatory activity of these compounds (Lee, Griswold et al. 1988). Subsequently, SB203580 and other 2,4,5-triaryl imidazoles were prepared as a tool for finding the molecular target involved in cytokine regulation (Lee, Badger et al. 1993). Later discoveries indicated p38/CSBP as the molecular target of these compounds (Gallagher, Seibel et al. 1997). One such compound, SB202190, inhibits p38 phosphorylation of myelin basic protein (MBP) while not effecting ERK or JNK MAP kinases. The compound also inhibits p38 phosphorylation of activating transcription factor 2 and blocks LPS-induced TNF and interleukin biosynthesis as well as inducing LDL receptors in vitro (2002). Investigators have used SB202190 to understand the mechanisms of UVB- and UVA-mediated p38 MAPK.

SP600125, an anthrapyrazole, is an inhibitor of JNK catalytic activity (Bennett, Sasaki et al. 2001). This inhibitor was identified in a high-throughput biochemical screen by using purified recombinant JNK2 and c-Jun. SP600125 demonstrated inhibitory activity consistent with the role of JNK in CD4+ cell activation and differentiation, CD14+ cell gene expression and in thymocyte death. SP600125 inhibits c-Jun phosphorylation in cells and also COX-2, IL-2, IFN-γ, TNF-α, IL-10 and also MMP gene expression (Han 2001). In vivo studies demonstrated that SP600125 inhibited LPS-induced TNF-α expression in mice (Bennett, Sasaki et al. 2001). SP600125 also prevented anti-CD3-mediated thymocyte apoptosis in a C57BL/6 mouse model (Bennett, Sasaki et al. 2001). In addition, this inhibitor of JNK blocked cell proliferation but did not kill CD4+ cells, resulting in a cytostatic effect on T cell proliferation. Although several anthrapyrazoles have been identified as chelators of DNA (i.e., doxorubicin), SP600125 did not exhibit characteristics of a strong interchelator of DNA in competitive binding assays. SP600125 also did not induce apoptosis (Bennett, Sasaki et al. 2001). Both compounds, MAPK inhibitor, SB202190, and the JNK inhibitor, SP600125, were able to inhibit UVA-induced AP-1 and c-fos transactivation as well as c-fos expression in the HaCat cell line transfected with a luciferase reporter (Silvers, Bachelor et al. 2003).

Inositol hexaphosphate (InsP$_6$) is a direct inhibitor of PI-3 kinase in vitro (Huang, Ma et al. 1997). This agent has also demonstrated inhibition of EGF-induced AP-1 activation and cell transformation of JB6 epidermal cells (Huang 1997). InsP$_6$ also inhibits UVB-induced AP-1 and NF-κB transcriptional activity. This compound is similar in structure to a potent PI-3 kinase inhibitor, D-3-deoxy-3-fluoro-PtdIns (Powis, Berggren et al. 1995).

LY294002 is a morpholino derivative of the broad-spectrum kinase inhibitor, quercetin. This compound is also an inhibitor of PI-3 kinase. This agent has been shown to cause inhibition of UVB-induced COX-2 promoter activity and protein expression of COX-2 in human keratinocytes (Tang, Gonzales et al. 2001).

Three specific inhibitors of EGFR tyrosine kinase, PD153035, AG1478 and ZD1839, may be potentially useful as chemopreventive agents. PD153035 is a 4-anilinoquinazoline compound that acts via competitive binding at the ATP site with the RGF receptor (Fry 1994). AG1478 is a member of a family of tyrosine phosphor kinase inhibitors called tyrophostins (Gazit 1996), which were designed to mimic the tyrosine substrates. Investigators have shown that these inhibitors (Zhang, Dong et al. 2001) can block UVA-induced EGFR signaling. ZD1839 (Iressa; AstraZeneca Pharmaceuticals) is another inhibitor of EGFR, which could be considered for topical formulation development as a chemoprevention agent. ZD1839 has been shown to inhibit activation in a variety of human skin cell types in vivo subsequent to oral therapy (Albanell, Rojo et al. 2002). In association with the EGFR inhibition, MAP kinase activation and keratinocyte proliferative rates decreased and an increase in the apoptotic index also occurred during therapy. ZD1839 is a substituted anilinoquinazoline that selectively inhibits EGF-stimulated tumor cell growth and blocks EGF-stimulated autophosphorylation in tumor cells (Wakeling, Simon et al. 2002). Clinical trials with oral ZD1839 have shown this compound to provide well-tolerated antiumor activity in patients (Wakeling 2002; Lorusso 2003).

As discussed earlier BRAF is a potential molecular target for the chemoprevention of melanoma. BAY 43-9006 is a potent inhibitor of Raf kinase (Lyons, Wilhelm et al. 2001). Oral administration of this compound has shown significant activity in four different human tumor types including colon (Gianpaolo-Ostravage 2001), pancreatic, lung and ovarian tumors carried out in xenograft models. Clinical testing of this compound in cancer patients began in July 2000 (Strumberg 2001). Preliminary clinical data reported the compound to be well tolerated. At least 37% of patients in the initial study had stable disease lasting longer than 12 weeks. This compound could be a promising agent for chemoprevention specifically for melanoma.

Meyskens et al. (Meyskens, Farmer et al. 2004) present a review of studies that suggest that ROS may be central to the pathogenesis of melanocyte transformation and melanoma progression. They suggest a critical early pathogenic event is the change of anti-oxidant to pro-oxidant melanin, the pigment produced by melanocytes. Once the melanin is oxidized by ROS generated by UV, an accumulation of metals occurs and the antioxidant response is depleted, the build up of ROS occurs. This, in turn, leads to melanosomal damage, DNA mutations, transcription activation and enhancement and activation of an anti-apoptotic (drug resistant) phenotype of melanocytes. Chemoprevention of melanoma within the context of this etiological hypothesis may involve the early use of antioxidants.

Conclusion

Skin cancer is a major health problem in the U.S. as well as in countries such as Australia. With high health care costs, increasing incidence, limited treatments, and a significant loss of life specifically for melanoma, prevention of this disease is imminent. Primary prevention strategies focus on an avoidance of sun exposure and the use of sunscreen compounds. Significant advances in molecular biology in combination with pharmaceutical developments have opened the door for research in the field of chemoprevention. For skin cancer, the formulation of a UV-induced signal transduction pathway (Figure 2) that identifies important molecules involved in the carcinogenesis process has provided molecular targets for the development of target-specific agents. This pathway has been developed by the use of animal and cellular model systems of skin carcinogenesis. These targets include AP-1 and COX-2, as well as upstream targets such as EGFR, PI-3 kinase, MAPK, JNK and Raf. Ongoing and future clinical trials will evaluate agents that act specifically to block molecules that are altered early in the development of skin cancer. These agents will most likely be delivered in a topical formulation using technology (e.g. prodrug development) that allows for maximum epidermal delivery with minimal systemic toxicity. The combination of several chemoprevention agents working in a synergistic fashion in these topical formulations will provide a promising strategy for the prevention of skin cancer.

References

Cancer Progress Report 2001 (2001). U.S. Department of Health and Human Services, Public Health Service, National Institutes of Health, National Cancer Institute. **2001**.

(2002). "Discussed in Calbiochem online catalog (Catalog No. 559388)."

(2002). "Treatment of actinic keratosis now covered under Medicare." *Oncology*: 141.

Albanell, J., F. Rojo, et al. (2002). "Pharmacodynamic studies of the epidermal growth factor receptor inhibitor ZD1839 in skin from cancer patients: histopathologic and molecular consequences of receptor inhibition." *J Clin Oncol* **20**(1): 110–124.

Alberts, D., J. Ranger-Moore, et al. (2004). "Safety and efficacy study of dose intensive oral vitamin A in participants with sun damaged skin." *Clin Cancer Res* **10**: 1875–1880.

Alberts, D.S., R.T. Dorr, et al. (2000). "Chemoprevention of human actinic keratoses by topical 2-(difluoromethyl)-dl-ornithine." *Cancer Epidemiol Biomarkers Prev* **9**(12): 1281–1286.

Almahroos, M. and A.K. Kurban (2004). "Ultraviolet Carcinogenesis in Nonmelanoma Skin Cancer. Part 1: Incidence Rates in Relation to Geographic Locations and in Malignant Populations." *SKINmed* **3**(1): 29–35.

An, K.P. et al. (2002). "Cyclooxygenase-2 expression in murine and human nonmelanoma skin cancers: implications for therapeutic approaches." *Photochem Photobiol* **76**: 73–80.

Angel, P., K. Hattori, et al. (1988). "The jun proto-oncogene is positively autoregulated by its product, Jun/AP-1." *Cell* **55**(5): 875–885.

Aszterbaum, M., A. Rothman, et al. (1998). "Identification of mutations in the human PATCHED gene in sporadic basal cell carcinomas and in patients with the basal cell nevus syndrome." *J Invest Dermatol* **110**(6): 885–888.

Auger, K.R., L.A. Serunian, et al. (1989). "PDGF-dependent tyrosine phosphorylation stimulates production of novel polyphosphoinositides in intact cells." *Cell* **57**(1): 167–175.

Autier, P., J.F. Dore, et al. (1995). "Melanoma and use of sunscreens: an EORTC case-control study in Germany, Belgium and France. The EORTC Melanoma Cooperative Group." *Int J Cancer* **61**(6): 749–755.

Bachelor, M.A. and G.T. Bowden (2004). "UVA-mediated activation of signaling pathways involved in skin tumor promotion and progression." *Semin Cancer Biol* **14**(2): 131–138.

Bachelor, M.A., A.L. Silvers, et al. (2002). "The role of p38 in UVA-induced cyclooxygenase-2 expression in the human keratinocyte cell line, HaCaT." *Oncogene* **21**(46): 7092–7099.

Bair, W.B., 3rd, N. Hart, et al. (2002). "Inhibitory effects of sodium salicylate and acetylsalicylic acid on UVB-induced mouse skin carcinogenesis." *Cancer Epidemiol Biomarkers Prev* **11**(12): 1645–1652.

Baldi, A., D. Santini, et al. (2001). "Expression of AP-2 transcription factor and of its downstream target genes c-kit, E-cadherin and p21 in human cutaneous melanoma." *J Cell Biochem* **83**(3): 364–372.

Bartels, P.H., J. Ranger-Moore, et al. (2002). "Statistical analysis of chemopreventive efficacy of vitamin A in sun-exposed, normal skin." *Anal Quant Cytol Histol* **24**(4): 185–197.

Barthelman, M., W. Bair, K. Kramer-Strickland, W. Chen, B. Timmerman, S. Valic, Z. Dong, G.T. Bowden (1998). "(–)-epigallocatechin-3-gallate inhibition of ultraviolet B-induced AP-1 activity." *Carcinogenesis* **19**(12): 2001–2204.

Barthelman, M., W. Chen, et al. (1998). "Inhibitory effects of perillyl alcohol on UVB-induced murine skin cancer and AP-1 transactivation." *Cancer Res* **58**(4): 711–716.

Barton, J.K., K. Gossage, et al. (2003). "Investigating sundamaged skin and actinic keratosis with optical coherence tomography: a pilot study." *Technol Cancer Res Treat* **2**(6): 1–11.

Basset-Seguin, N., C. Escot, et al. (1990). "High levels of c-fos proto-oncogene expression in normal human adult skin." *J Invest Dermatol* **94**(4): 418–422.

Beitner, H., S.E. Norell, et al. (1990). "Malignant melanoma: aetiological importance of individual pigmentation and sun exposure." *Br J Dermatol* **122**(1): 43–51.

Bennett, B.L., D.T. Sasaki, et al. (2001). "SP600125, an anthrapyrazolone inhibitor of Jun N-terminal kinase." *Proc Natl Acad Sci* **98**(24): 13681–13686.

Berman, B., C.A. Ricotti, Jr., et al. (2004). "Determination of the area of skin capable of being covered by the application of 250 mg of 5% imiquimod cream." *Dermatol Surg* **30**(5): 784–786.

Bibbo, M., P.H. Bartels, et al. (1986). "Markers for malignancy in the nuclear texture of histologically normal tissue from patients with thyroid tumors." *Anal Quant Cytol Histol* **8**(2): 168–176.

Bibbo, M., F. Michelassi, et al. (1990). "Karyometric marker features in normal-appearing glands adjacent to human colonic adenocarcinoma." *Cancer Res* **50**(1): 147–151.

Bishop, D.T., F. Demenais, et al. (2002). "Geographical variation in the penetrance of CDKN2A mutations for melanoma." *J Natl Cancer Inst* **94**: 894–903.

Bjornhagen, V., E. Bonfoco, et al. (1994). "Morphometric, DNA, and proliferating cell nuclear antigen measurements in benign melanocytic lesions and cutaneous malignant melanoma." *Am J Dermatopathol* **16**(6): 615–623.

Borland, R., R. Marks, et al. (1992). "Public knowledge about characteristics of moles and melanomas." *Aust J Public Health* **16**(4): 370–375.

Bowden, G.T. (2004). "Prevention of non-melanoma skin cancer by targeting ultraviolet-B-light signalling." *Nat Rev Cancer* **4**(1): 23–35.

Bozzo, P., D.S. Alberts, et al. (2001). "Measurement of chemopreventive efficacy in skin biopsies." *Anal Quant Cytol Histol* **23**(4): 300–312.

Bozzo, P.D., L.C. Vaught, et al. (1998). "Nuclear morphometry in solar keratosis." *Anal Quant Cytol Histol* **20**(1): 21–28.

Brash, D.E., J.A. Rudolph, et al. (1991). "A role for sunlight in skin cancer: UV-induced p53 mutations in squamous cell carcinoma." *Proc Natl Acad Sci USA* **88**(22): 10124–10128.

Bregman, M.D. and F.L. Meyskens, Jr. (1986). "Difluoromethylornithine enhances inhibition of melanoma cell growth in soft agar by dexamethasone, clone A interferon and retinoic acid." *Int J Cancer* **37**(1): 101–107.

Buchwald, H. (1992). "Cholesterol inhibition, cancer and chemotherapy." *Lancet* **339**: 1154–1156.

Buckman, S.Y., A. Gresham, et al. (1998). "COX-2 expression is induced by UVB exposure in human skin: implications for the development of skin cancer." *Carcinogenesis* **19**(5): 723–729.

Burren, R., C. Scaletta, et al. (1998). "Sunlight and carcinogenesis: expression of p53 and pyrimidine dimers in human skin following UVA I, UVA I + II and solar simulating radiations." *Int J Cancer* **76**(2): 201–206.

Burton, R.C. (2000). "Malignant Melanoma in the year 2000." *CA Cancer J Clin* **50**: 209–213.

Callen, J.P. (2000). "Statement on Actinic Keratosis." *J Am Acad Dermatol* **42**(1 Part 2): 1.

Chen, N., M. Nomura, et al. (2001). "Suppression of skin tumorigenesis in c-Jun NH(2)-terminal kinase-2-deficient mice." *Cancer Res* **61**(10): 3908–3912.

Chen, W., A.H. Borchers, et al. (1998). "UVB irradiation-induced activator protein-1 activation correlates with increased c-fos gene expression in a human keratinocyte cell line." *J Biol Chem* **273**(48): 32176–32181.

Chen, W. and G.T. Bowden (1999). "Activation of p38 MAP kinase and ERK are required for ultraviolet-B induced c-fos gene expression in human keratinocytes." *Oncogene* **18**(52): 7469–7476.

Chen, W. and G.T. Bowden (2000). "Role of p38 mitogen-activated protein kinases in ultraviolet-B irradiation-induced activator protein 1 activation in human keratinocytes." *Mol Carcinog* **28**: 196–202.

Chen, W., Z. Dong, et al. (1999). "Inhibition of ultraviolet B-induced c-fos gene expression and p38 mitogen-activated protein kinase activation by (–)-epigallocatechin gallate in a human keratinocyte cell line." *Mol Carcinog* **24**(2): 79–84.

Chen, W., Q. Tang, et al. (2001). "Role of p38 MAP kinases and ERK in mediating ultraviolet-B induced cyclooxygenase-2 gene expression in human keratinocytes." *Oncogene* **20**(29): 3921–3926.

Clark, L.C., G.F. Combs, et al. (1996). "Effects of selenium supplementation for cancer prevention in patients with carcinoma of the skin. A randomized controlled trial. National Prevention of Cancer Study Group." *JAMA* 276(1957–1963).

Cohen, B., Y.X. Liu, et al. (1990). "Characterization of p85, a target of oncogenes and growth factor receptors." *Mol Cell Biol* **10**(6): 2909–2915.

Cohen, C., A. Zavala-Pompa, et al. (2002). "Mitogen-activated protein kinase activation is an early event in melanoma progression." *Clin Cancer Res* **8**(12): 3728–3733.

Coso, O.A., M. Chiariello, et al. (1995). "Transforming G protein-coupled receptors potently activate JNK (SAPK). Evidence for a divergence from the tyrosine kinase signaling pathway." *J Biol Chem* **270**(10): 5620–5624.

Crowell, P.L. (1999). "Prevention and therapy of cancer by dietary monoterpenes." *J Nutr* **129**(3): 775S–778S.

Curran, T. and B.R. Franza, Jr. (1988). "Fos and Jun: the AP-1 connection." *Cell* **55**(3): 395–397.

Davies, H., G.R. Bignell, et al. (2002). "Mutations of the BRAF gene in human cancer." *Nature* **417**(6892): 949–954.

De Fabo, E.C., F.P. Noonan, et al. (2004). "Ultraviolet B but not ultraviolet A radiation initiates melanoma." *Cancer Res* **64**(18): 6372–6376.

de Gruijl, F.R. (2000). "Photocarcinogenesis: UVA vs UVB." *Methods Enzymol* **319**: 359–366.

Del Rosso, J.Q. (2003). "New and emerging topical approaches for actinic keratoses." *Cutis* **72**(4): 273–276, 279.

Dellavalle, R.P., M.K. Nicholas, et al. (2003). "Melanoma Chemoprevention: A role for statins of fibrates." *Am J Ther* **10**: 203–210.

Denkert, C., M. Kobel, et al. (2001). "Expression of cyclooxygenase 2 in human malignant melanoma." *Cancer Res* **61**(1): 303–308.

Derijard, B., M. Hibi, et al. (1994). "JNK1: a protein kinase stimulated by UV light and Ha-Ras that binds and phosphorylates the c-Jun activation domain." *Cell* **76**(6): 1025–1037.

Diepgen, T.L. and V. Mahler (2002). "The epidemiology of skin cancer." *Br J Dermatol* **146**(Suppl 61): 1–6.

Dinehart, S.M. (2000). "The treatment of actinic keratoses." *J Am Acad Dermatol* **42**(1 Pt 2): 25–28.

Dinehart, S.M., P. Nelson-Adesokan, et al. (1997). "Metastatic cutaneous squamous cell carcinoma derived from actinic keratosis." *Cancer* **79**(5): 920–923.

Dissanayake, N.S., G.E. Greenoak, et al. (1993). "Effects of ultraviolet irradiation on human skin-derived epidermal cells in vitro." *J Cell Physiol* **157**(1): 119–127.

Domann, F.E., J.P. Levy, et al. (1994). "Stable expression of a c-JUN deletion mutant in two malignant mouse epidermal cell lines blocks tumor formation in nude mice." *Cell Growth Differ* **5**: 9–16.

Dong, Z., M.J. Birrer, et al. (1994). "Blocking of tumor promoter-induced AP-1 activity inhibits induced transformation in JB6 mouse epidermal cells." *Proc Natl Acad Sci USA* **91**(2): 609–613.

Dong, Z., C. Huang, et al. (1998). "Increased synthesis of phosphocholine is required for UV-induced AP-1 activation." *Oncogene* **17**(14): 1845–1853.

Dorr, R.T., K. Dvorakova, et al. (2000). "Increased eumelanin expression and tanning is induced by a superpotent melanotropin [Nle4-D-Phe7]-alpha-MSH in humans." *Photochem Photobiol* **72**(4): 526–532.

Downes, C.P. and A.N. Carter (1991). "Phosphoinositide 3-kinase: a new effector in signal transduction?" *Cell Signal* **3**(6): 501–513.

Dracopoli, N.C., G.A. Bruns, et al. (1994). "Report and abstracts of the First International Workshop on Human Chromosome 1 Mapping 1994. Bethesda, Maryland, March 25–27, 1994." *Cytogenet Cell Genet* **67**(3): 144–165.

Dvorakova, K., R.T. Dorr, et al. (1999). "Pharmacokinetics of the green tea derivative, EGCG, by the topical route of administration in mouse and human skin." *Cancer Chemother Pharmacol* **43**(4): 331–335.

Einspahr, J., D.S. Alberts, et al. (1996). "Evaluation of proliferating cell nuclear antigen as a surrogate end point biomarker in actinic keratosis and adjacent, normal-appearing, and non-sun-exposed human skin samples." *Cancer Epidemiol Biomarkers Prev* **5**(5): 343–348.

Einspahr, J.G., D.S. Alberts, et al. (1997). "Surrogate end-point biomarkers as measures of colon cancer risk and their use in cancer chemoprevention trials." *Cancer Epidemiol Biomarkers Prev* **6**(1): 37–48.

Einspahr, J.G., D.S. Alberts, et al. (1999). "Relationship of p53 mutations to epidermal cell proliferation and apoptosis in human UV-induced skin carcinogenesis." *Neoplasia* **1**(5): 468–475.

Einspahr, J.G., G.T. Bowden, et al. (2003). "Skin cancer chemoprevention: strategies to save our skin." *Recent Results Cancer Res* **163**: 151–164.

Einspahr, J.G., M.A. Nelson, et al. (2002). "Modulation of biologic endpoints by topical difluoromethylornithine (DFMO), in subjects at high-risk for nonmelanoma skin cancer." *Clin Cancer Res* **8**(1): 149–155.

English, D.R., B.K. Armstrong, et al. (1998). "Demographic characteristics, pigmentary and cutanous risk factors of squamous cell carcinoma of the skin. A case-control study." *Int J Cancer* **76**: 628–634.

Falch, J., I. Antoni, et al. (2000). "The mevalonate/isoprenoid pathway inhibitor apomine (SR-45023A) is antiproliferative and induces apoptosis similar to farnesol." *Biochem Biophys Res Commun* **270**: 240–246.

Fercher, A., K. Mengedoht, et al. (1988). "Eye length measurement by interferometry with partially coherent Light." *Opt Lett* **13**: 186–188.

Fisher, B., J.P. Costantino, et al. (1998). "Tamoxifen for prevention of breast cancer: report of the National Surgical Adjuvant Breast and Bowel Project P-1 Study." *J Natl Cancer Inst* **90**(18): 1371–1388.

Fisher, C., M.R. Byers, et al. (1991). "Patterns of epithelial expression of Fos protein suggest important role in the transition from viable to cornified cell during keratinization." *Development* **111**(2): 253–258.

Fisher, G.J. and J.J. Voorhees (1998). "Molecular mechanisms of photoaging and its prevention by retinoic acid: ultraviolet irradiation induces MAP kinase signal transduction cascades that induce Ap-1-regulated matrix metalloproteinases that degrade human skin in vivo." *J Investig Dermatol Symp Proc* **3**(1): 61–68.

Foote, J.A., R.B. Harris, et al. (2001). "Predictors for cutaneous basal- and squamous-cell carcinoma among actinically damaged adults." *Int J Cancer* **95**(1): 7–11.

Frankel, D.H., B.H. Hanusa, et al. (1992). "New primary nonmelanoma skin cancer in patients with a history of squamous cell carcinoma of the skin. Implications and recommendations for follow-up." *J Am Acad Dermatol* **26**(5 Pt 1): 720–726.

Fry, D.W., A.J. Kraker, et al. (1994). "A specific inhibitor of the epidermal growth factor receptor tyrosine kinase." *Science* **265**: 1093–1095.

Funasaka, Y., T. Boulton, et al. (1992). "c-Kit-kinase induces a cascade of protein tyrosine phosphorylation in normal human melanocytes in response to mast cell growth factor and stimulates mitogen-activated protein kinase but is down-regulated in melanomas." *Mol Biol Cell* **3**(2): 197–209.

Gallagher, T.F., G.L. Seibel, et al. (1997). "Regulation of stress-induced cytokine production by pyridinylimidazoles; inhibition of CSBP kinase." *Bioorg Med Chem* **5**(1): 49–64.

Gause, P.R., M. Lluria-Prevatt, et al. (1997). "Chromosomal and genetic alterations of 7,12-dimethylbenz[a]anthracene-induced melanoma from TP-ras transgenic mice." *Mol Carcinog* **20**(1): 78–87.

Gazit, A. et al. (1996). "Tyrphostins IV – highly potent inhibitors of EGF receptor kinase. Structure-activity relationship study of 4-anilidoquinazolines." *Bioorg Med Chem* **4**: 1203–1207.

Geilen, C.C., M. Wieprecht, et al. (1996). "The mitogen-activated protein kinases system (MAP kinase cascade): its role in skin signal transduction. A review." *J Dermatol Sci* **12**(3): 255–262.

Geller, A.C., G. Colditz, et al. (2002). "Use of sunscreen, sunburning rates, and tanning bed use among more than 10,000 US children and adolescents." *Pediatrics* **109**(6): 1009–1014.

Gensler, H.L. (1991). "Prevention by alpha-difluoromethylornithine of skin carcinogenesis and immunosuppression induced by ultraviolet irradiation." *J Cancer Res Clin Oncol* **117**(4): 345–350.

Ghosh, S., W.Q. Xie, et al. (1994). "The cysteine-rich region of raf-1 kinase contains zinc, translocates to liposomes, and is adjacent to a segment that binds GTP-ras." *J Biol Chem* **269**(13): 10000–10007.

Gianpaolo-Ostravage, C., D. Bankston, et al. (2001). "Anti-tumor efficacy of the orally active Raf kinase inhibitor BAY 43-9006 in human tumor xenograft models." *AACR* **92**(4954).

Gilchrest, B.A., M.S. Eller, et al. (1999). "The pathogenesis of melanoma induced by ultraviolet radiation [comment]." *N Engl J Med* **340**(17): 1341–1348.

Giles, G.G., R. Marks, et al. (1988). "Incidence of non-melanocytic skin cancer treated in Australia." *Br Med J (Clin Res Ed)* **296**(6614): 13–17.

Gillardon, F., C. Eschenfelder, et al. (1994). "Differential regulation of c-fos, fosB, c-jun, junB, bcl-2 and bax expression in rat skin following single or chronic ultraviolet irradiation and in vivo modulation by antisense oligodeoxynucleotide superfusion." *Oncogene* **9**(11): 3219–3225.

Glass, A.G. and R.N. Hoover (1989). "The emerging epidemic of melanoma and squamous cell skin cancer." *JAMA* **262**: 2097–2100.

Glogau, R.G. (2000). "The risk of progression to invasive disease." *J Am Acad Dermatol* **42**(1 Pt 2): 23–24.

Goldstein, A.M. and M.A. Tucker (2001). "Genetic epidemiology of cutaneous melanoma. A global perspective." *Arch Dermatol* **137**: 1493–1496.

Gonzales, M. and G.T. Bowden (2002). "Nordihydroguaiaretic acid-mediated inhibition of ultraviolet B-induced activator protein-1 activation in human keratinocytes." *Mol Carcinog* **34**(2): 102–111.

Gould, M.N., C.J. Moore, et al. (1994). "Limonene chemoprevention of mammary carcinoma induction following direct in situ transfer of v-Ha-ras." *Cancer Res* **54**(13): 3540–3543.

Graham, S., J. Marshall, et al. (1985). "An inquiry into the epidemiology of melanoma." *Am J Epidemiol* **122**(4): 606–619.

Green, A. (1992). "Changing patterns in incidence of non-melanoma skin cancer." *Epithelial Cell Biol* **1**(1): 47–51.

Greenberg, E.R., J.A. Baron, et al. (1990). "A clinical trial of beta carotene to prevent basal-cell and squamous cell cancers of the skin." *N Engl J Med* **323**: 789–795.

Greene, M.H. (1997). "Genetics of cutaneous melanoma and nevi." *Mayo Clin Proc* **72**(5): 467–474.

Greene, M.H., W.H. Clark, Jr., et al. (1985). "Acquired precursors of cutaneous malignant melanoma. The familial dysplastic nevus syndrome." *N Engl J Med* **312**(2): 91–97.

Greene, M.H., W.H. Clark, Jr., et al. (1985). "High risk of malignant melanoma in melanoma-prone families with dysplastic nevi." *Ann Intern Med* **102**(4): 458–465.

Gudas, L.J. (1994). "Retinoids and vertebrate development." *J Biol Chem* **269**(22): 15399–15402.

Haag, J.D. and M.N. Gould (1994). "Mammary carcinoma regression induced by perillyl alcohol, a hydroxylated analog of limonene." *Cancer Chemother Pharmacol* **34**(6): 477–483.

Haake, A.R. and R.R. Polakowska (1993). "Cell death by apoptosis in epidermal biology." *J Invest Dermatol* **101**(2): 107–112.

Halaban, R., Fan, B., Ahn, J., Funasaka, Y., Gitay-Goren, H., Neufeld, G. (1992). "Growth factors, receptor kinases, and protein tyrosine phosphatases in normal and malignant melanocytes." *J Immunother* **12**: 154–161.

Halaban, R., J.S. Rubin, et al. (1992). "Met and hepatocyte growth factor/scatter factor signal transduction in normal melanocytes and melanoma cells." *Oncogene* **7**(11): 2195–2206.

Halachmi, S. and B.A. Gilchrest (2001). "Update on genetic events in the pathogenesis of melanoma." *Curr Opin Oncol* **13**(2): 129–136.

Hall, P.A., D.A. Levison, et al. (1990). "Proliferating cell nuclear antigen (PCNA) immunolocalization in paraffin sections: an index of cell proliferation with evidence of deregulated expression in some neoplasms." *J Pathol* **162**(4): 285–294.

Haluska, F.G. and F.S. Hodi (1998). "Molecular genetics of familial cutaneous melanoma." *J Clin Oncol* **16**(2): 670–682.

Han, H., Boyle, D., Chang, L., Bennett, B., Karin, M., Manning, A., Firestein, G. (2001). "c-Jun N-terminal kinase is required for metalloproteinase expression and joint destruction in inflammatory arthritis." *J Clin Invest* **108**: 73–81.

Harris, R.B., Griffith, K., Moon, T.E. (2001). "Trends in the incidence of nonmelanoma skin cancers in southeastern Arizona, 1985–1996." *J Am Acad Dermatol* **45**(4): 528–536.

Harris, R.E., J. Beebe-Donk, et al. (2001). "Inverse association of non-steroidal anti-inflammatory drugs and malignant melanoma among women." *Oncol Rep* **8**(3): 655–657.

Herbert, J.L., F. Khugyani, et al. (2001). "Chemoprevention of basal cell carcinomas in the ptc1 +/– mouse – green and black tea." *Skin Pharmacol Appl Skin Physiol* **14**(6): 358–362.

Herlyn, M. and K. Satyamoorthy (1996). "Activated ras. Yet another player in melanoma?" *Am J Pathol* **149**(3): 739–744.

Hill, C.S. and R. Treisman (1995). "Transcriptional regulation by extracellular signals: mechanisms and specificity." *Cell* **80**(2): 199–211.

Hill, D., V. White, et al. (1993). "Changes in sun-related attitudes and behaviours, and reduced sunburn prevalence in a population at high risk of melanoma." *Eur J Cancer Prev* **2**(6): 447–456.

Hohl, R.J. and K. Lewis (1995). "Differential effects of monoterpenes and lovastatin on RAS processing." *J Biol Chem* **270**(29): 17508–17512.

Housman, T.S., S.R. Feldman, et al. (2003). "Skin Cancer is among the most costly of all cancers to treat for the Medicare population." *J Acad Dermatol* **48**: 425–429.

Huang, C., W. Ma, et al. (1997). "Direct evidence for an important role of sphingomyelinase in ultraviolet-induced activation of c-Jun N-terminal kinase." *J Biol Chem* **272**(44): 27753–27757.

Huang, C., W.Y. Ma, et al. (1997). "Inositol hexaphosphate inhibits cell transformation and activator protein 1 activation by targeting phosphatidylinositol-3' kinase." *Cancer Res* **57**(14): 2873–2878.

Huang, C., W.Y. Ma, C.A. Ryan, Z. Dong (1997). "Proteinase inhibitors I and II from potatoes specifically block UV-induced activator protein-1 activation through a pathway that is independent of extracellular signal-regulated kinases, c-Jun N-terminal kinases, and p38 kinases." *Proc Natl Acad Sci USA* **94**: 11957–11962.

Hunter, T. (1997). "Oncoprotein networks." *Cell* **88**(3): 333–346.

Hussussian, C.J., J.P. Struewing, et al. (1994). "Germline p16 mutations in familial melanoma." *Nat Genet* **8**(1): 15–21.

International Medical News Group (2002). "Nonmelanoma skin cancer new solutions to treatment." *Supplement to Skin and Allergy News.*

Irinopoulou, T., J.P. Rigaut, et al. (1993). "Toward objective prognostic grading of prostatic carcinoma using image analysis." *Anal Quant Cytol Histol* **15**(5): 341–344.

Jansen, B., V. Wacheck, et al. (2000). "Chemosensitisation of malignant melanoma by BCL2 antisense therapy." *Lancet* **356**(9243): 1728–1733.

Jermal, A., R.C. Tiwan, et al. (2004). "Cancer Statistics 2004." *CA Cancer J Clin* **54**: 8–29.

Kabayama, Y., M. Hamaya, et al. (1998). "Wavelength specific activation of PI3-kinase by UVB irradiation." *FEBS Letters* **441**: 297–301.

Kallunki, T., B. Su, et al. (1994). "JNK2 contains a specificity-determining region responsible for efficient c-Jun binding and phosphorylation." *Genes Dev* **8**(24): 2996–3007.

Kamb, A., D. Shattuck-Eidens, et al. (1994). "Analysis of the p16 gene (CDKN2) as a candidate for the chromosome 9p melanoma susceptibility locus." *Nat Genet* **8**(1): 23–26.

Kerr, J.F., A.H. Wyllie, et al. (1972). "Apoptosis: a basic biological phenomenon with wide-ranging implications in tissue kinetics." *Br J Cancer* **26**(4): 239–257.

Klepp, O. and K. Magnus (1979). "Some environmental and bodily characteristics of melanoma patients. A case-control study." *Int J Cancer* **23**(4): 482–486.

Koh, H.K. (1991). "Cutaneous melanoma [comment]." *N Engl J Med* **325**(3): 171–182.

Kolch, W., G. Heidecker, et al. (1993). "Protein kinase C alpha activates RAF-1 by direct phosphorylation." *Nature* **364**(6434): 249–252.

Konig, H., H. Ponta, et al. (1992). "Interference between pathway-specific transcription factors: glucocorticoids antagonize phorbol ester-induced AP-1 activity without altering AP-1 site occupation in vivo." *Embo J* **11**(6): 2241–2246.

Lahti, J.M., J. Xiang, et al. (1995). "PITSLRE protein kinase activity is associated with apoptosis." *Mol Cell Biol* **15**(1): 1–11.

Lambert, J.D., R.O. Meyers, et al. (2001). "Tetra-O-methylnordihydroguaiaretic acid inhibits melanoma in vivo." *Cancer Lett* **171**(1): 47–56.

Lang, P.G., Maize, J.C. (1991). Basal Cell Carcinoma. *Cancer of the Skin.* R. Friedman, D.S. Rigel, A.W. Kopf, M.N. Harris and D. Baker. Philadelphia, W.B. Saunders. 14–24.

Lee, J.C., A.M. Badger, et al. (1993). "Bicyclic imidazoles as a novel class of cytokine biosynthesis inhibitors." *Ann NY Acad Sci* **696**: 149–170.

Lee, J.C., D.E. Griswold, et al. (1988). "Inhibition of monocyte IL-1 production by the anti-inflammatory compound, SK&F 86002." *Int J Immunopharmacol* **10**(7): 835–843.

Lee, J.C., S. Kumar, et al. (2000). "Inhibition of p38 MAP kinase as a therapeutic strategy." *Immunopharmacology* **47**(2–3): 185–201.

Lee, W., A. Haslinger, et al. (1987). "Activation of transcription by two factors that bind promoter and enhancer sequences of the human metallothionein gene and SV40." *Nature* **325**(6102): 368–372.

Lens, M.B. and M. Dawes (2004). "Global perspectives of contemporary epidemiological trends of cutaneous malignant melanoma." *Br J Cancer* **150**(2): 179–185.

Levine, N., R.T. Dorr, G.A. Ertl, C. Brooks, D.S. Alberts (1999). "Effects of a potent synthetic melanotropin, NI[4]-D-Phe[7]-MSH (Melanotant-1) on tanning: a dose range study." *J Dermatol Treatment* **10**: 127–132.

Li, G. and M. Herlyn (2000). "Dynamics of intercellular communication during melanoma development." *Mol Med Today* **6**(4): 163–169.

Liaw, G.J., E. Steingrimsson, F. Pignoni, A.J. Courey, J.A. Lengyel (1993). "Characterization of downstream elements in Raf-1 pathway." *Proc Natl Acad Sci USA* **90**: 858–862.

Liggett, W.H., Jr. and D. Sidransky (1998). "Role of the p16 tumor suppressor gene in cancer." *J Clin Oncol* **16**(3): 1197–1206.

Lippman, S.M. and P.H. Brown (1999). "Tamoxifen prevention of breast cancer: an instance of the fingerpost." *J Natl Cancer Inst* **91**(21): 1809–1819.

Lippman, S.M. and W.K. Hong (2002). "Cancer prevention by delay. Commentary: J.A. O'Shaughnessy et al., Treatment and Prevention of Intraepithelial Neoplasia: An Important Target for Accelerated New Agent Development. *Clin Cancer Res* **8**: 314–346, 2002." *Clin Cancer Res* **8**(2): 305–313.

Lippman, S.M., J.S. Lee, et al. (1990). "Biomarkers as intermediate end points in chemoprevention trials." *J Natl Cancer Inst* **82**(7): 555–560.

Lluria-Prevatt, M., J. Morreale, et al. (2002). "Effects of perillyl alcohol on melanoma in the TPras mouse model." *Cancer Epidemiol Biomarkers Prev* **11**(6): 573–579.

Lorusso, P.M. (2003). "Phase I studies of ZD1839 in patients with common solid tumors." *Semin Oncol* **30**(Suppl 1): 21–29.

Lyons, J.F., S. Wilhelm, et al. (2001). "Discovery of a novel Raf kinase inhibitor." *Endocr Relat Cancer* **8**(3): 219–225.

MacAulay, C., S. Lam, et al. (1995). "Malignancy-associated changes in bronchial epithelial cells in biopsy specimens." *Anal Quant Cytol Histol* **17**(1): 55–61.

Mangelsdorf, D., K. Unesonso, et al. (1994). The Retinoid Receptors. *The Retinoids*. M.B. Sporn, A.B. Roberts and D.S. Goodman. New York, Raven Press. 319–349.

Manson, J.E., K.M. Rexrode, et al. (2000). "The case for a comprehensive national campaign to prevent melanoma and associated mortality." *Epidemiology* **11**(6): 728–734.

Marks, R. (1999). "Two decades of the public health approach to skin cancer control in Australia: why, how and where are we now?" *Australas J Dermatol* **40**(1): 1–5.

Marras, S., G. Faa, et al. (1999). "Chromosomal changes in dysplastic nevi." *Cancer Genet Cytogenet* **113**(2): 177–179.

Marshall, C.J. (1995). "Specificity of receptor tyrosine kinase signaling: transient versus sustained extracellular signal-regulated kinase activation." *Cell* **80**(2): 179–185.

Matsumura, Y., C. Nishigori, et al. (1996). "Characterization of p53 gene mutations in basal-cell carcinomas: comparison between sun-exposed and less-exposed skin areas." *Int J Cancer* **65**(6): 778–780.

McEwan, L.E. and J.G. Smith (1997). "Topical diclofenac/hyaluronic acid gel in the treatment of solar keratoses." *Australas J Dermatol* **38**(4): 187–189.

Meyskens, F.L., Jr. (1988). "Thinking about cancer causality and chemoprevention." *J Natl Cancer Inst* **80**(16): 1278–1281.

Meyskens, F.L., Jr., P.J. Farmer, et al. (2004). "Etiologic pathogenesis of melanoma: a unifying hypothesis for the missing attributable risk." *Clin Cancer Res* **10**(8): 2581–2583.

Meyskens, F.L., E.M. Kingsley, T. Glattke, et al. (1986). "A phase II study of alpha-difluoromethylornithine (DFMO) for the treatment of metastatic melanoma." *Inv New Drugs* **4**: 257–262.

Mills, J.J., R.S. Chari, et al. (1995). "Induction of apoptosis in liver tumors by the monoterpene perillyl alcohol." *Cancer Res* **55**(5): 979–983.

Moon, T.E., N. Levine, et al. (1997). "Effect of retinol in preventing squamous cell skin cancer in moderate-risk subjects: a randomized, double-blind, controlled trial. Southwest Skin Cancer Prevention Study Group." *Cancer Epidemiol Biomarkers Prev* **6**(11): 949–956.

Morse, M.A. and G.D. Stoner (1993). "Cancer chemoprevention: principles and prospects." *Carcinogenesis* **14**(9): 1737–1746.

Nakazawa, H., D. English, et al. (1994). "UV and skin cancer: specific p53 gene mutation in normal skin as a biologically relevant exposure measurement." *Proc Natl Acad Sci USA* **91**(1): 360–364.

Nelson, M.A., J.G. Einspahr, et al. (1994). "Analysis of the p53 gene in human precancerous actinic keratosis lesions and squamous cell cancers." *Cancer Letters* **85**(1): 23–29.

Niesor, E., J. Flach, et al. (1999). "Synthetic Farnesoid X Receptor (FXR) agonists: a new class of cholesterol synthesis inhibitors and antiproliferative drugs." *Drugs Future* **24**: 431–438.

Nomura, M., A. Kaji, et al. (2001). "Mitogen- and stress-activated protein kinase 1 mediates activation of Akt by ultraviolet B irradiation." *J Biol Chem* **276**(27): 25558–25567.

Nomura, M., W.Y. Ma, et al. (2000). "Inhibition of ultraviolet B-induced AP-1 activation by theaflavins from black tea." *Mol Carcinog* **28**(3): 148–155.

Orengo, I.F., J. Gerguis, et al. (2002). "Celecoxib, a cyclooxygenase 2 inhibitor as a potential chemopreventive to UV-induced skin cancer: a study in the hairless mouse model." *Arch Dermatol* **138**(6): 751–755.

Ortonne, J.P. (2002). "Photobiology and genetics of malignant melanoma." *Br J Dermatol* **146** (Suppl) 61: 11–16.

O'Shaughnessy, J.A., G.J. Kelloff, et al. (2002). "Treatment and prevention of intraepithelial neoplasia: an important target for accelerated new agent development [comment]." *Clin Cancer Res* **8**(2): 314–346.

Pentland, A.P., J.W. Schoggins, et al. (1999). "Reduction of UV-induced skin tumors in hairless mice by selective COX-2 inhibition." *Carcinogenesis* **20**: 1939–1944.

Peyssonnaux, C. and A. Eychene (2001). "The Raf/MEK/ERK pathway: new concepts of activation." *Biol Cell* **93**(1–2): 53–62.

Pierceall, W.E., L.H. Goldberg, et al. (1991). "Ras gene mutation and amplification in human nonmelanoma skin cancers." *Mol Carcinog* **4**(3): 196–202.

Pollock, P.M., U.L. Harper, et al. (2003). "High frequency of BRAF mutations in nevi." *Nat Genet* **33**(1): 19–20.

Powell, M.B., D.S. Alberts, et al. (2002). "Preclinical and clinical activity of Apomine, a novel biophosphonate ester in the prevention and treatment of melanoma". *Proc AACR*.

Powell M.B., P. Hyman, J. Gregus, M. Lluria-Prevatt, R. Nagle, G.T. Bowden (1999). "Induction of melanoma in TPras transgenic mice." *Carcinogenesis* **20**(9): 1747–1753.

Powis, G., M. Berggren, et al. (1995). "Advances with phospholipid signalling as a target for anticancer drug development." *Acta Biochim Pol* **42**(4): 395–403.

Quinn, A.G., S. Sikkink, et al. (1994). "Basal cell carcinomas and squamous cell carcinomas of human skin show distinct patterns of chromosome loss." *Cancer Res* **54**(17): 4756–4759.

Randle, H. (1996). "Basal Cell Carcinoma. Identification and treatment of the high-risk patient." *Dermatolog Surg* **22**: 255–261.

Reed, J.A., F. Loganzo, Jr., et al. (1995). "Loss of expression of the p16/cyclin-dependent kinase inhibitor 2 tumor suppressor gene in melanocytic lesions correlates with invasive stage of tumor progression." *Cancer Res* **55**(13): 2713–2718.

Rehman, I., M. Takata, et al. (1996). "Genetic change in actinic keratoses." *Oncogene* **12**(12): 2483–2490.

Richmond, A., R. Fine, et al. (1986). "Growth factor and cytogenetic abnormalities in cultured nevi and malignant melanomas." *J Invest Dermatol* **86**(3): 295–302.

Rigel, D.S. (2002). "The effect of sunscreen on melanoma risk." *Dermatol Clin* **20**: 601–606.

Rivers, J.K., J. Arlette, et al. (2002). "Topical treatment of actinic keratoses with 3.0% diclofenac in 2.5% hyaluronan gel." *Br J Dermatol* **146**(1): 94–100.

Rivers, J.K. and D.I. McLean (1997). "An open study to assess the efficacy and safety of topical 3% diclofenac in a 2.5% hyaluronic acid gel for the treatment of actinic keratoses." *Arch Dermatol* **133**(10): 1239–1242.

Rubins, H.B., S.J. Robins, et al. (1999). "Gemifibrozil for the secondary prevention of coronary heart disease in men with low levels of high density lipoprotein cholesterol." *N Engl J Med* **341**: 410–418.

Runger, T.M. (1999). "Role of UVA in the pathogenesis of melanoma and non-melanoma skin cancer. A short review." *Photodermatol Photoimmunol Photomed* **15**(6): 212–216.

Ryseck, R.P., S.I. Hirai, et al. (1988). "Transcriptional activation of c-jun during the G0/G1 transition in mouse fibroblasts." *Nature* **334**(6182): 535–537.

Salasche, S.J. (2000). "Epidemiology of actinic keratoses and squamous cell carcinoma." *J Am Acad Dermatol* **42**(1 Pt 2): 4–7.

Samuels, M.L., M.J. Weber, et al. (1993). "Conditional transformation of cells and rapid activation of the mitogen-activated protein kinase cascade by an estradiol-dependent human raf-1 protein kinase." *Mol Cell Biol* **13**(10): 6241–6252.

Setlow, R.B., E. Grist, et al. (1993). "Wavelengths effective in induction of malignant melanoma." *Proc Natl Acad Sci USA* **90**(14): 6666–6670.

Sherman, A. and L. Koss (1983). "Morphometry of benign urothelial cells in the presence of cancer." *Analyt Quant Cytol Histol* **5**: 221.

Silvers, A.L., M.A. Bachelor, et al. (2003). "The role of JNK and p38 MAPK activities in UVA-induced signaling pathways leading to AP-1 activation and c-Fos expression." *Neoplasia* **5**(4): 319–329.

Silvers, A.L. and G.T. Bowden (2002). "UVA irradiation-induced activation of activator protein-1 is correlated with induced expression of AP-1 family members in the human keratinocyte cell line HaCaT." *Photochem Photobiol* **75**(3): 302–310.

Sober, A.J. and J.M. Burstein (1995). "Precursors to skin cancer." *Cancer* **75**(2 Suppl): 645–650.

Soufir, N., M.F. Avril, et al. (1998). "Prevalence of p16 and CDK4 germline mutations in 48 melanoma-prone families in France. The French Familial Melanoma Study Group." *Hum Mol Genet* **7**(2): 209–216.

Soufir, N., J.P. Moles, et al. (1999). "P16 UV mutations in human skin epithelial tumors." *Oncogene* **18**(39): 5477–5481.

Spencer, J.M., S.M. Kahn, et al. (1995). "Activated ras genes occur in human actinic keratoses, premalignant precursors to squamous cell carcinomas." *Arch Dermatol* **131**(7): 796–800.

Sporn, M.B. and N. Suh (2000). "Chemoprevention of cancer." *Carcinogenesis* **21**(3): 525–530.

Stam-Posthuma, J.J. (1998). "Effect of topical tretinoin under occlusion on atypical nevi." *Melanoma Research* **8**: 539–548.

Stam-Posthuma, J.J., C. van Duinen, et al. (2001). "Multiple primary melanomas." *J Am Acad Dermatol* **44**(1): 22–27.

Stayrook, K.R., J.H. McKinzie, et al. (1998). "Effects of the antitumor agent perillyl alcohol on H-Ras vs. K-Ras farnesylation and signal transduction in pancreatic cells." *Anticancer Res* **18**(2A): 823–828.

Stein, B., P. Angel, et al. (1992). "Ultraviolet-radiation induced c-jun gene transcription: two AP-1 like binding sites mediate the response." *Photochem Photobiol* **55**(3): 409–415.

Steinbach, G., P.M. Lynch, et al. (2000). "The effect of celecoxib, a cyclooxygenase-2 inhibitor, in familial adenomatous polyposis." *N Engl J Med* **342**(26): 1946–1952.

Stolz, W., T. Vogt, et al. (1994). "Differentiation between malignant melanomas and benign melanocytic nevi by computerized DNA cytometry of imprint specimens." *J Cutan Pathol* **21**(1): 7–15.

Stratton, S.P. (2001). "Prevention of non-melanoma skin cancer." *Curr Oncol Rep* **3**: 295–300.

Stratton, S.P., R.T. Dorr, et al. (2000). "The state-of-the-art in chemoprevention of skin cancer." *Eur J Cancer* **36**(10): 1292–1297.

Straume, O. and L.A. Akslen (1997). "Alterations and prognostic significance of p16 and p53 protein expression in subgroups of cutaneous melanoma." *Int J Cancer* **74**(5): 535–539.

Strumberg, D., W. Schuehly, J.F. Moeller, D. Hedler, R. Hilger, W. Stellberg, H. Richly, R. Heinig, G. Ahr, G. Wensing, J. Kuhlmann, M.E. Scheulen, S. Seeber (2001). "Phase I clinical, pharmacokinetic and pharmacodynamic study of the Raf kinase inhibitor BAY 49-9006 in patients with locally advanced or metastatic cancer." *Proc AACR* **330**.

Susnik, B., A. Worth, et al. (1995). "Malignancy-associated changes in the breast. Changes in chromatin distribution in epithelial cells in normal-appearing tissue adjacent to carcinoma." *Anal Quant Cytol Histol* **17**(1): 62–68.

Swerdlow, A.J. and M.A. Weinstock (1998). "Do tanning lamps cause melanoma? An epidemiologic assessment." *J Am Acad Dermatol* **38**(1): 89–98.

Tada, A., E. Pereira, et al. (2002). "Mitogen- and Ultraviolet-B-Induced Signaling Pathways in Normal Human Melanocytes." *J Invest Dermatol* **118**(2): 316–322.

Takigawa, M., M. Enomoto, et al. (1990). "Tumor angiogenesis and polyamines: alpha-difluoromethylornithine, an irreversible inhibitor of ornithine decarboxylase, inhibits B16 melanoma-induced angiogenesis in vivo and the proliferation of vascular endothelial cells in vitro." *Cancer Res* **50**(13): 4131–4138.

Tang, Q., M. Gonzales, et al. (2001). "Roles of Akt and glycogen synthase kinase 3beta in the ultraviolet B induction of cyclooxygenase-2 transcription in human keratinocytes." *Cancer Res* **61**(11): 4329–4332.

Tangrea, J.A., B.K. Edwards, et al. (1992). "Long-term therapy with low-dose isotretinoin for prevention of basal cell carcinoma: a multicenter clinical trial." *J Natl Cancer Inst* **84**: 328–332.

Thompson, F.H., J. Emerson, et al. (1995). "Cytogenetics of 158 patients with regional or disseminated melanoma. Subset analysis of near-diploid and simple karyotypes." *Cancer Genet Cytogenet* **83**(2): 93–104.

Tsao, H. (2001). "Genetics of nonmelanoma skin cancer." *Arch Dermatol* **137**(11): 1486–1492.

Tsao, H., G.S. Roers, A.J. Sober (1998). "An estimate of the annual direct cost of treating cutaneous melanoma." *J Am Acad Dermatol* **38**: 669–680.

Uhlman, M. (2002). Teens take risks for tans: Sunscreen often goes by the wayside, a study shows. FDA is evaluating labeling. *Philadelphia Inquirer.* Philadelphia, PA. A08.

Veierod, M.B., E. Weiderpass, et al. (2003). "A prospective study of pigmentation, sun exposure, and risk of cutaneous malignant melanoma in women." *J Natl Cancer Inst* **95**(20): 1530–1538.

Vivanco, I. and C.L. Sawyers (2002). "The phosphatidylinositol 3-Kinase AKT pathway in human cancer." *Nat Rev Cancer* **2**(7): 489–501.

Wakeling, A.E. (2002). "Epidermal growth factor receptor tyrosine kinase inhibitors." *Curr Opin Pharmacol* **24**(4): 382–387.

Wakeling, A.E., G.P. Simon, et al. (2002). "An orally active inhibitor of epidermal growth factor signaling with potential for cancer therapy." *Cancer Res* **62**: 5749–5754.

Wales, M.M., M.A. Biel, et al. (1995). "p53 activates expression of HIC-1, a new candidate tumour suppressor gene on 17p13.3." *Nat Med* **1**(6): 570–577.

Wan, Y.S., Z.Q. Wang, et al. (2001). "Ultraviolet irradiation activates PI 3-kinase/AKT survival pathway via EGF receptors in human skin in vivo." *Int J Oncol* **18**: 461–466.

Wan, Y.S., Z.Q. Wang, et al. (2001). "EGF receptor crosstalks with cytokine receptors leading to the activation of c-Jun kinase in response to UV irradiation in human keratinocytes." *Cell Signal* **13**: 139–144.

Wang, S.Q., R. Setlow, et al. (2001). "Ultraviolet A and melanoma: a review [comment]." *J Am Acad Dermatol* **44**(5): 837–846.

Warne, P.H., P.R. Viciana, et al. (1993). "Direct interaction of Ras and the amino-terminal region of Raf-1 in vitro." *Nature* **364**(6435): 352–355.

Welzel, J. (2001). "Optical coherence tomography in dermatology: a review." *Skin Res Technol* **7**(1): 1–9.

Weyn, B., W. Jacob, et al. (2000). "Data representation and reduction for chromatin texture in nuclei from premalignant prostatic, esophageal, and colonic lesions." *Cytometry* **41**(2): 133–138.

Whitman, M., C.P. Downes, et al. (1988). "Type I phosphatidylinositol kinase makes a novel inositol phospholipid, phosphatidylinositol-3-phosphate." *Nature* **332**(6165): 644–646.

Wied, G.L., P.H. Bartels, et al. (1980). "Cytomorphometric markers for uterine cancer in intermediate cells." *Analytical & Quantitative Cytology* **2**(4): 257–263.

Wikonkal, N.M. and D.E. Brash (1999). "Ultraviolet radiation induced signature mutations in photocarcinogenesis." *J Investig Dermatol Symp Proc* **4**: 6–10.

Wolf, J.E., Jr., J.R. Taylor, et al. (2001). "Topical 3.0% diclofenac in 2.5% hyaluronan gel in the treatment of actinic keratoses." *Int J Dermatol* **40**(11): 709–713.

Wolfe, P., C.K. Donawho, M.L. Kripke (1994). "Effects of sunscreen on UV radiation-induced enhancement of melanoma growth in mice." *J Natl Cancer Inst* **86**(2): 99–105.

Wymer, J.A., R. Taetle, J.M. Yang, J.M. Lahti, V.J. Kidd, M.A. Nelson (1997). "Alterations in the PITSLRE protein kinase gene complex on chromosome band 1p36 in melanoma." *Proc AACR.*

Xu, X.C., J.L. Clifford, et al. (1994). "Detection of nuclear retinoic acid receptor mRNA in histological tissue sections using nonradioactive in situ hybridization histochemistry." *Diagn Mol Pathol* **3**(2): 122–131.

Yasuda, H., H. Kobayashi, et al. (1989). "Differential expression of ras oncogene products among the types of human melanomas and melanocytic nevi." *J Invest Dermatol* **93**(1): 54–59.

Zhang, Y., Z. Dong, et al. (2001). "Induction of EGFR-dependent and EGFR-independent signaling pathways by ultraviolet A irradiation." *DNA Cell Biology* **20**: 769–779.

Zhang, Y., S. Zhong, et al. (2001). "UVA induces Ser381 phosphorylation of p90RSK/MAP-KAP-K1 via ERK and JNK pathways." *J Biol Chem* **276**(18): 14572–14580.

Ziegler, A., D.J. Leffell, et al. (1993). "Mutation hotspots due to sunlight in the p53 gene of nonmelanoma skin cancers." *Proc Natl Acad Sci USA* **90**(9): 4216–4220.

Zou, L., Weger, J., Yang, Q., et al. (1996). "Germline mutations in the p16INK4a binding domain of CDK4 familial melanoma." *Nat Genet* **7**: 209–216.

Colorectal Cancer Prevention

Ayaaz Ismail, Eugene Gerner, and Peter Lance

College of Medicine, University of Arizona, Tucson, AZ 85724

Adenocarcinomas of the colon and rectum (colorectal cancer, CRC) are malignant epithelial neoplasms. A polyp is a localized lesion that projects above the surrounding mucosa. Adenomatous polyps (adenomas) are benign neoplasms that arise from colorectal glandular epithelium. In the United States (U.S.), colorectal adenoma (CRA) prevalence is approximately 25% by age 50 and rises to around 50% by age 70. The histological hallmarks of a CRA are altered glandular architecture and dysplasia of the epithelium. The great majority of CRCs develop from CRAs in a process called the adenoma-carcinoma sequence. This process may take from years to decades for the earliest CRA to progress to CRC (Leslie, Carey et al. 2002). A CRA progresses to become a CRC when the dysplastic cells invade through the muscularis mucosa. While most CRCs develop from CRAs, fewer than 10% of CRAs ever progress to CRC. Hyperplastic colorectal polyps are histologically distinct from CRAs, occur most frequently in the rectum and sigmoid colon, are not neoplastic and do not progress to CRC. Besides CRAs, the inflammatory bowel diseases, ulcerative colitis (UC) and Crohn's disease of the colon (Crohn's colitis), predispose to CRC.

In 5% or fewer of cases, predisposition to CRC is inherited as an autosomal dominant or other Mendelian disorder, often with associated predispositions to benign or malignant tumors of other organs (Kinzler and Vogelstein 1996; Lindor 2004). Familial adenomatous polyposis (FAP) and hereditary nonpolyposis colorectal cancer (HNPCC) account for most of the autosomal dominantly inherited CRC cases. With the exception of the chromosomes that determine sex, a diploid nucleus contains two very similar versions of each chromosome, one from each parent. It follows that each diploid nucleus carries two versions (alleles) of each autosomal gene. In FAP, the inherited, germline abnormality (mutation) is in the *Adenomatosis Polyposis Coli (APC)* gene, a tumor suppressor gene. In HNPCC, the germline abnormality is in one of the mismatch repair (MMR) genes, whose products coordinate to repair defective DNA. Colorectal tumorigenesis does not occur in individuals with germline FAP or MMR gene mutations while the other, wild-type allele of the mutated gene functions normally. Tumorigenesis occurs when an inactivating mutation occurs in the wild-type FAP or MMR gene in the somatic, colorectal epithelial cell from which the neoplasm arises.

Most CRC cases arise outside the context of one of the inherited CRC syndromes and are termed sporadic. It is now clear that the molecular pathogenesis of most sporadic CRCs involves either the *APC* or MMR gene pathway. The difference between familial and sporadic cases is that in the latter, both "hits" to the *APC* or MMR alleles are somatic and occur in the colorectal epithelial cell where tumorigenesis originates.

But *APC* or MMR malfunction alone does not cause malignant transformation. A developing neoplasm must acquire sequential malfunction of multiple genes, usually four to six or more, before progression to invasive malignancy occurs (Hanahan and Weinberg 2000; Hahn and Weinberg 2002).

CRCs evolve through distinct genetic pathways involving genetic instability, which is the driving force for tumor development (Lengauer, Kinzler et al. 1998). Three genetic instability pathways have been identified in CRC. They are called chromosomal instability (Rajagopalan, Nowak et al. 2003), microsatellite instability (MSI), and the CpG island methylator phenotype (CIMP). Chromosomal instability is the tumorigenic mechanism in FAP and in approximately 85% of sporadic CRCs that develop as a result of losses of both *APC* alleles and other tumor suppressor genes (Vogelstein, Fearon et al. 1988). HNPCC and the remaining 15% of sporadic CRCs develop because of MSI that results from inactivation of the DNA MMR system (Ionov, Peinado et al. 1993). Clusters of cytosine-guanosine pairs, termed CpG islands, in the promoter regions of many genes are prone to age-related methylation. Such "hypermethylation" can lead to gene silencing. In a proportion of CRCs, functional loss of certain tumor suppressor genes is caused by CpG island methylation and silencing rather than mutations (Toyota, Ho et al. 1999).

Epidemiology

CRC is the second most frequent fatal malignant neoplasm in the U.S. It is estimated that in 2004 there will be 146,940 new cases and 56,730 deaths from the disease (Jemal, Tiwari et al. 2004). Sporadic CRC is uncommon below the age of 50 years (Cooper, Yuan et al. 1995). The incidence rises to 159 per 100,000 by age 65 to 69 and 387 per 100,000 for those over the age of 85. CRC affects men and women at approximately equal rates (Jemal, Tiwari et al. 2004). Rates are highest among African Americans, with intermediate rates observed among whites, Asians, Pacific Islanders and Hispanics (Ward, Jemal et al. 2004). Low incidence rates have been observed among American Indians and Alaska Natives.

Worldwide, the incidence of CRC varies 20-fold, with the highest rates reported in the U.S. and other western countries and the lowest in India (Bingham and Riboli 2004). The incidence is increasing rapidly in some countries where previously rates were low. For example, 40 years ago, CRC was rare in Japan whereas incidence in Japanese men at ages 55 to 60 years is now twice that of men in the United Kingdom (UK) (Bingham and Riboli 2004).

The risk for developing CRC increases with migration from a low-risk area to a high-risk area (Potter 1999). This was seen in Japanese migrants to the U.S. and Hawaii in the 1950s and 1960s, whose risk became greater than native Japanese living in Japan. Furthermore, offspring of the Japanese migrants developed risks similar to U.S. white populations. Similar increases in risk were seen in Europeans that migrated to Australia and in Jews that migrated to Israel from North Africa.

Approximately 50% of CRCs occur in the rectum and sigmoid, 25% in the cecum and ascending colon, 15% in the transverse colon and 10% in the descending colon. This distribution pattern changes with age. There is an increased propensity for proximal neoplasms with increased age. At age 65 to 69 years, 36% of CRCs occur proximal to the splenic flexure but by age 85 and older, 50% are proximal to the splenic flexure.

This has implications for the optimal screening modality in CRC prevention programs (Cooper, Yuan et al. 1995).

Risk Factors

The wide range of CRC incidence rates around the world is attributed largely to dietary differences (Potter 1999; Mason 2002; Bingham and Riboli 2004). Diets rich in foods from plant sources, low in saturated fat and red meat, and low in calories and alcohol (Giovannucci, Rimm et al. 1995) are generally considered protective against CRC. Conversely, consumption of a Western diet high in calories, animal fat and refined carbohydrates, and a high body mass index (BMI) combine to increase CRC risk. These lifestyle factors, also risk factors for type 2 diabetes, are associated with hyperinsulinemia, insulin resistance and elevated levels of insulin-like growth factors (IGFs), which are mitogenic in normal and neoplastic cells (LeRoith, Baserga et al. 1995). Circulating IGF-1 (formerly called somatomedin-C) level is associated positively with CRC risk (Ma, Pollak et al. 1999; Palmqvist, Hallmans et al. 2002) and elevated insulin production may predict CRC risk independently of body mass index and IGF-1 level (Ma, Giovannucci et al. 2004). Most of the clinical and biochemical effects of acromegaly result from stimulation of IGF-1 production by unregulated growth hormone secretion. CRC risk is increased over two-fold in acromegalics, presumably as a result of sustained elevations of IGF-1 level (Baris, Gridley et al. 2002).

Physical Activity. The evidence that a high level of physical activity protects against colon cancer is convincing (Colditz, Cannuscio et al. 1997; Friedenreich 2001). At low levels of activity, obesity may be an additional independent risk factor. Physical activity may protect against rectal (Slattery, Edwards et al. 2003) as well as colon cancer but the evidence is less emphatic.

Family History of Colorectal Adenoma or Colorectal Carcinoma. As discussed, the predisposition to CRC is autosomal dominantly inherited in kindreds with FAP or HNPCC. CRAs numbering in the hundreds or thousands usually develop during the second decade in individuals with FAP. Without prophylactic panproctocolectomy the likelihood of malignant transformation approaches 100%. An attenuated form of FAP (AFAP) has been described (Spirio, Samowitz et al. 1998). AFAP is characterized by lifetime accumulation of 10 to 20 rather than hundreds or thousands of CRAs and a later age of onset than unmodified FAP. Gene penetrance in HNPCC is 75 to 80%. Diagnosis of CRC in these patients is rare before the age of 25 years, occurs on average at age 45 years and has occurred in 70 to 80% of those affected by age 70 years. The majority of CRCs are in the proximal colon in HNPCC patients, who usually develop no more than tens of CRAs and very rarely more than 100.

FAP and HNPCC account for less than 5% of CRC cases, but familial clustering outside the context of well-characterized CRC family syndromes is considerably more common so that a familial component contributes to 20 to 30% of cases (Grady 2003). Risk for CRC can be increased up to eight-fold in individuals with one or more first-degree relatives (parents, siblings or children) who have had CRC (Grady 2003). The magnitude of risk depends on the age at diagnosis of the index case and the number of affected relatives.

Inflammatory Bowel Disease. Ulcerative colitis (UC) and Crohn's disease comprise the chronic idiopathic inflammatory conditions termed inflammatory bowel disease. Patients with inflammatory bowel disease are thought to be at increased risk for CRC. The evidence of this connection is more robust for UC than Crohn's disease (Jess, Winther et al. 2004). The major determinants of CRC risk in patients with UC are the duration and extent of disease. Risk is not elevated for the first 8 to 10 years after diagnosis but thereafter increases by 0.5 to 1.0% yearly (Munkholm 2003). Patients with pancolitis (total colitis as judged by appearances at colonoscopy) are at greatest risk and this is corroborated by evidence that the severity of inflammation due to UC is an important determinant of risk for CRC (Rutter, Saunders et al. 2004). Primary sclerosing cholangitis complicating UC compounds the risk for CRC, leading to cumulative rates as high as 50% after 25 years (Jayaram, Satsangi et al. 2001).

CRC-related mortality rates in patients with UC reported in recent years have been lower than in older reports. This apparent improvement reflects several factors. Most large recent reports are population-based studies as opposed to many of the earlier studies, which reported selected series of patients with mostly severe disease from specialist referral centers. Some of the lowest reported rates are from countries, such as Denmark, or regions where prophylactic colectomy rates are high. It is also possible that the now widely applied use of prolonged aggressive therapy with 5-aminosalicylic acid has chemopreventive benefit against progression to CRC. Recent population-based studies suggest an overall normal life expectancy in patients with UC (Winther, Jess et al. 2003) and a modest reduction of life expectancy in younger patients with Crohn's disease that is not attributable to CRC (Card, Hubbard et al. 2003).

Other Risk Factors. Risk of CRC is increased by 100 to 7,000 times in patients with a ureterosigmoidostomy (urinary diversion procedure by surgical placement of the ureter into the colon) (Woodhouse 2002). The most reliable estimate of excess risk is probably near the lower end of this range. The latency period is long with an average of 20 years but shorter periods have been reported. Nitrosamines generated from the diverted urine are thought to be important etiologic factors.

Asymptomatic CRAs and CRCs have been reported in patients diagnosed with *Streptococcus bovis* infective endocarditis. Although the frequency of this association is controversial (Gonzalez-Juanatey, Gonzalez-Gay et al. 2003), screening colonoscopy is usually recommended for these patients. A similar association has also been reported with *Streptococcus agalactiae* infection.

Single nucleotide polymorphisms (SNPs) in genes other than *APC* or those of the MMR family are increasingly recognized as determinants of risk for developing CRAs and CRC. For example, a SNP affecting the expression of *ornithine decarboxylase* (*ODC*), a downstream gene in the *APC*-dependent pathway to CRC, is associated with risk of CRA recurrence (Martinez, O'Brien et al. 2003).

Screening and Early Detection

Currently, the U.S. Preventive Services Task Force recommends approximately 50 different preventive services, with CRC screening being one of the most important. In an analysis of these 50 services, it was estimated that CRC screening by fecal occult blood testing (FOBT), flexible sigmoidoscopy or the combination (at appropriate intervals) when delivered to 100% of the target population would result in 225,000 to 450,000 quality-adjusted life-years (QALY) saved at a cost of $ 12,000 to $ 18,000 per QALY saved (Coffield, Maciosek et al. 2001). Of the 50 preventive services, only nine others, including childhood and influenza vaccinations, tobacco cessation counseling, and cervical cancer screening, achieved an equal or greater QALY savings and cost-effectiveness rating. (Please refer to Chapter 2 for a thorough discussion of QALYs.)

The rationale for CRC screening is based on two premises. First, the proportion of early-stage CRCs with favorable prognosis is greater for CRCs detected by screening than for those diagnosed after symptoms have developed (Niv, Lev-El et al. 2002; Whynes, Frew et al. 2003). Second, most CRCs develop from CRAs and most screen-detected CRAs can be removed endoscopically by polypectomy. The observed subsequent incidence of CRC is reduced by as much as 90%, compared to the predicted incidence, following CRA polypectomy (Winawer, Zauber et al. 1993; Citarda, Tomaselli et al. 2001). Thus, the evidence to support population-wide CRC screening is compelling.

An individual's risk for developing CRC is considered as either average or increased. Groups at increased risk include: (1) patients with a past history of CRA or CRC; (2) patients with inflammatory bowel disease; (3) members of FAP or HNPCC kindreds; and (4) individuals with one or more first-degree relatives who have had CRAs or CRCs. The American Cancer Society and other authorities agree that average-risk men and women age 50 years and over should adopt one of the following screening strategies (Winawer, Fletcher et al. 2003; Smith, Cokkinides et al. 2004):
1. Annual FOBT; or
2. Flexible sigmoidoscopy every 5 years; or
3. Annual FOBT and flexible sigmoidoscopy every 5 years; or
4. Double contrast barium enema every 5 years; or
5. Colonoscopy every 10 years.

A problem affecting decisions on CRC screening policy is that FOBT is the only tool for which supportive evidence in the form of statistically significant outcomes of randomized controlled trials (RCTs) exists. Evidence for the other strategies comes only from case-control studies or mere conjecture and is, therefore, less secure. Another major problem is delivery. Screening rates among Americans are unacceptably low. The highest CRC screening rates are among whites (41% for sigmoidoscopy and 34% for FOBT), the lowest are among Hispanics (28% for sigmoidoscopy and 21% for FOBT) and rates for African Americans and American Indians/Alaskan Natives are intermediate (BRFSS 2002). The lowest rates of screening occur among uninsured individuals, with 10 to 15% for FOBT and 15 to 20% for flexible sigmoidoscopy. Furthermore, individuals with lower levels of education have lower rates of screening: 29% for sigmoidoscopy among people with 11 or fewer years of education as opposed to 46% among those with 13 or more years of education.

Fecal Occult Blood Test (FOBT). Much of the published experience with FOBT has come from Hemoccult guaiac-based stool tests, which detect the peroxidase activity of heme and other stool peroxidases. The American Cancer Society and other authorities in the U.S. recommend annual FOBT without rehydration (Winawer, Fletcher et al. 2003; Smith, Cokkinides et al. 2004). To reduce test inaccuracy, patients are asked to follow certain guidelines for several days before and during stool collection. They should avoid aspirin or other nonsteroidal anti-inflammatory drugs, vitamin C and iron supplements, and red meat. The evidence-based protocol for FOBT CRC screening involves the patient sampling two separate regions of three consecutive spontaneously evacuated stool specimens. Each Hemoccult card has two windows, one for each of the regions sampled from a single stool, giving a total of six windows for a complete FOBT. For optimum quality control, cards should be sent for development to an appropriately monitored laboratory. When this is done, cards are usually not read until several days after defecation and sampling of the stool. FOBT positivity is recorded if a positive reaction is seen in one or more of the six windows to which stool was applied in a complete test. Structural evaluation of the rectum and colon, usually by total colonoscopy, is indicated in all patients with a positive FOBT.

The delay between the time of applying stool to FOBT cards and application of developing reagents in the laboratory further compromises an already insensitive test. Some sensitivity can be retrieved by card rehydration before applying the developing reagent but this drastically reduces test specificity, thereby leading to an unacceptable increase in the number of negative colonoscopies. The current unequivocal recommendation is that guaiac-based cards should not be rehydrated before development.

Besides rehydration, various FOBT modifications have been made to improve test performance. Hemoccult SENSA is a more sensitive guaiac-based test than the original Hemoccult and the more recent Hemoccult II version of this test. More expensive immunochemical tests that are specific for human haemoglobin have been introduced to improve specificity. These include HemeSelect, and the more recent InSure and Flex-Sure occult blood tests.

Longitudinal RCTs of FOBT have not included a criterion standard examination, such as a "gold-standard" colonoscopy. A few studies have compared performance of a single three-card application of FOBT among asymptomatic subjects to findings at a contemporaneous colonoscopy or air-contrast barium enema. Under these circumstances, the sensitivity of an unrehydrated FOBT for invasive CRC is approximately 30% (Ahlquist, Wieand et al. 1993). In other words, FOBT is negative in two-thirds or more of patients who undergo a structural evaluation of the rectum and colon shortly after a positive FOBT.

Nonetheless, multiple-card hemoccult FOBT at one- or two-year intervals, respectively, has been shown to reduce CRC incidence and mortality, by 17 to 20% (Mandel, Church et al. 2000) and 21 to 33% (Mandel, Bond et al. 1993; Mandel, Church et al. 1999). FOBT-related reductions in CRC incidence and mortality occur as a result of the diagnostic and therapeutic interventions implemented because of a positive FOBT. It is noteworthy that in the study reporting the largest (33%) reduction in CRC mortality, FOBT was performed annually and greater than 80% of hemoccult cards were rehydrated before development (Mandel, Bond et al. 1993). Contributions to FOBT sensitivity and specificity from restrictions of medications and diet before and during stool collection have not been evaluated in a RCT. Likewise, performance characteristics of Hemoccult SENSA® and the immunochemical FOBTs have not been assessed in randomized trials (Young, St John et al. 2003).

Physicians often perform a digital rectal exam (DRE), which is appropriate, but then smear stool from the gloved finger used for the DRE on a FOBT card, which is developed and read immediately in the office without quality control. Performance of

FOBT in this manner is inappropriate and has never been evaluated rigorously. However, from indirect evidence the sensitivity and specificity of FOBT performed this way are so inferior that the practice cannot be supported. Fewer than 10% of CRCs arise within reach of the examining finger at DRE (Winawer, Fletcher et al. 1997).

Flexible Sigmoidoscopy. A 60-cm flexible endoscope is used for screening sigmoidoscopy. Flexible sigmoidoscopy is an office-based procedure, usually performed by primary care physicians or their non-physician assistants (Schoenfeld, Lipscomb et al. 1999) without intravenous conscious sedation. An enema is administered immediately before the procedure. Complete examination of the rectum and sigmoid colon is routinely accomplished by appropriately trained practitioners but insertion of the flexible sigmoidoscope proximal to the junction of the sigmoid and descending colon is often not achieved. Authorities in the U.S. recommend colonoscopy for all patients with any adenoma at screening sigmoidoscopy and repeat flexible sigmoidoscopy five years after a negative examination. Once-per-lifetime screening flexible sigmoidoscopy for colorectal cancer is being assessed in a nationwide program in the UK (Atkin, Cuzick et al. 1993). Prevalence of distal adenomas and CRCs in an interim report of the UK trial was 12.1 and 0.3%, respectively (Atkin, Cuzick et al. 2002). In this trial, small polyps were removed during screening and colonoscopy was undertaken if high-risk polyps (three or more adenomas, 10 mm or greater in diameter, villous, severely dysplastic, or malignant) were found.

Case-control studies indicate that mortality from CRCs within reach of the instrument may be reduced by 60 to 80% as a result of therapy implemented for findings at flexible sigmoidoscopy (Newcomb, Norfleet et al. 1992; Selby, Friedman et al. 1992). The disadvantage of screening flexible sigmoidoscopy is failure to identify proximal CRAs and CRCs, which are accessible only with the colonoscope. A proportion of these proximal lesions are identified at colonoscopies performed because of distal CRAs or CRCs found at flexible sigmoidoscopy. Adenomas of at least 10 mm in diameter and all those with villous histology or high-grade dysplasia are termed "advanced." Advanced adenomas are those at greatest risk for progression to CRC. New (metachronous) adenomas can develop in the years after adenoma polypectomy or CRC resection. Patients from whom advanced adenomas or CRCs were removed are those most likely to develop metachronous CRAs or CRCs. Thus, advanced adenomas as well as early-stage CRCs are crucial target lesions for CRC screening programs. From 46 to 52% of patients with proximal advanced adenomas or CRCs do not have synchronous distal CRAs or CRCs (Imperiale, Wagner et al. 2000; Lieberman, Weiss et al. 2000). The overall sensitivity of flexible sigmoidoscopy for diagnosing advanced adenomas and CRCs, using colonoscopy as the criterion standard, is estimated at 70 to 80% (Pignone, Rich et al. 2002).

The recommendation that a repeat screening flexible sigmoidoscopy need not be performed until five years after a negative examination is based on evidence of a low yield of advanced lesions at the second procedure. In one study, adenomas were reported in 6% of screenees at a second examination five years after the first but none had CRCs or advanced adenomas (Rex, Lehman et al. 1994). In another study, the interval between examinations was three years. CRAs or CRCs were found in 3.1% of patients at the second examination, including 0.8% with advanced adenomas or CRCs (Schoen, Pinsky et al. 2003).

Combining annual FOBT and flexible sigmoidoscopy every five years is an accepted screening strategy (Winawer, Fletcher et al. 2003; Smith, Cokkinides et al. 2004). In years that flexible sigmoidoscopy is due, the annual FOBT should be done first; if positive, the patient is referred for colonoscopy and should not undergo an unnecessary sigmoidoscopy as well. The combination of FOBT and sigmoidoscopy been evaluated in neither randomized controlled trials nor case-control studies. Combined once-only FOBT and a surrogate for flexible sigmoidoscopy were evaluated in a study of screening colonoscopy (Lieberman and Weiss 2001). FOBT was performed before colonoscopy in all patients and those distal lesions identified within 60 centimeters of the anal verge at colonoscopy, the surrogate lesions, were designated as accessible by flexible sigmoidoscopy. FOBT was negative and distal, sigmoidoscopy-accessible CRAs or CRCs were absent in 24% of patients with proximal advanced CRAs or CRCs. Without colonoscopy, advanced proximal lesions would have been missed in these patients.

Barium Enema. The double contrast barium enema (DCBE) is a radiologic test in which barium and air are introduced into the rectum and colon. Radiographs are taken with the patient in various positions and mass lesions (CRAs or CRCs) are identified as projections outlined by a thin layer of barium against a dark background of air contrast. Patients with DCBE appearances of a polyp or cancer should undergo colonoscopy. Repeat DCBE in five years is recommended after a negative test.

DCBE is inferior to optical colonoscopy for detection of CRAs. In a study comparing the two procedures, approximately 50% of CRAs over 6 mm that were seen at colonoscopy were diagnosed by DCBE (Winawer, Stewart et al. 2000). No randomized trials have been conducted to determine if DCBE reduces CRC incidence or mortality. DCBE is retained for the time being as a screening option because it offers the opportunity to visualize the entire colon. Its major application is for patients who are medically unsuitable candidates for invasive procedures. Virtual colonoscopy is likely to replace DCBE before long as the non-invasive method of choice for structural evaluation of the colon.

Colonoscopy. The American Cancer Society and other authorities recommend optical colonoscopy, to be repeated in ten years following a negative study (Winawer, Fletcher et al. 2003; Smith, Cokkinides et al. 2004) as a primary screening tool. Careful bowel preparation with nonabsorbable lavage fluid is essential before colonoscopy, which is performed under conscious intravenous sedation. Because of the sedation, patients must be accompanied after the procedure and are not allowed to drive or return to work until the following day.

Assessment of the accuracy of optical colonoscopy is problematic because it is considered the criterion standard for other CRC screening modalities. To tackle this problem, the miss rate of colonoscopy was determined from findings at same-day, back-to-back colonoscopy performed by different endoscopists (Rex, Cutler et al. 1997). Sensitivity for large adenomas was 90% and for small adenomas (less than 10 mm) was 75%. It is reasonable to assume that sensitivity for CRC is at least 90%. Studies reporting 90% or similar rates of sensitivity for detecting advanced colorectal lesions have almost invariably been conducted in specialist centers (Rex, Cutler et al. 1997). It is unclear whether similar accuracy prevails in the community settings where most colonoscopies are performed.

There are no studies evaluating whether screening colonoscopy alone reduces the incidence or mortality from CRC but indirect evidence suggests substantial benefit. Estimates from the National Polyp Study were that up to 90% of CRCs could be prevented by regular colonoscopic surveillance examinations (Winawer, Zauber et al. 1993). In a study of cost-effectiveness using models based on multiple assumptions, it was estimated that colonoscopic screening every 10 years would reduce CRC incidence and mortality by 58 and 61%, respectively (Frazier, Colditz et al. 2000). These estimates of the benefits of screening optical colonoscopy await more rigorous confirmation.

Optical colonoscopy has several disadvantages as a primary screening tool. The obligatory bowel preparation is unpleasant and patients may experience discomfort during the procedure. Costs and logistical challenges of providing colonoscopy for the whole population over the age of 50 years are daunting. Complications can occur, the most serious being bowel perforation, which necessitates emergency abdominal surgery and can very rarely be fatal. Perforation rates due to colonoscopy vary quite widely. In the Veterans Administration Cooperative Study of 3,196 patients undergoing screening colonoscopy there were no perforations (Nelson, McQuaid et al. 2002). In a 5% sample of Medicare beneficiaries from regions of the United States covered by the Surveillance, Epidemiology, and End Results (SEER) Program there were 77 perforations after 39,286 colonoscopies for a rate of 1.96 of every 1000 procedures (Gatto, Frucht et al. 2003). In a recent prospective study of 9,223 colonoscopies performed over a four month period in three regions of the UK National Health Service, the perforation rate was 1.30 in 1000 (Bowles, Leicester et al. 2004).

History of CRAs or CRC. Management of patients who have had one or more CRAs removed at colonoscopy is based on findings from that procedure (Winawer, Fletcher et al. 2003). Those with three or more CRAs or an advanced CRA should have a surveillance colonoscopy at three years. Patients with one or two non-advanced CRAs should have the first follow-up colonoscopy at 5 years. If total colonoscopy was not performed preoperatively, patients should have the procedure six months after surgical resection of a CRC. For those who had a preoperative colonoscopy, a surveillance colonoscopy should be performed three years after surgery.

Inflammatory Bowel Disease. Patients with a history of UC or Crohn's colitis for more than 8 to 10 years should undergo colonoscopic surveillance (Winawer, Fletcher et al. 2003). Objectives are to remove polyps, sample elevated lesions (the dysplasia-associated lesion or mass, DALM) and obtain multiple biopsies over the full length of the colon. Biopsies should be read by pathologists with specialist expertise in gastroenterology for the presence and degree of dysplasia, which is used as an index of risk for future invasive cancer. The purpose of surveillance is to offer and perform prophylactic surgery before frank malignancy, which is often multi-focal, develops. Optimal care for these patients can best be provided by a multidisciplinary team of experts. High-grade dysplasia is usually an indication for panproctocolectomy, which may also be indicated for low-grade dysplasia and for patients with UC or Crohn's colitis under other circumstances.

Surveillance programs have been shown to improve the survival of UC patients in a case-control study (Choi, Nugent et al. 1993). All patients with UC or Crohn's colitis should undergo a first surveillance colonoscopy to re-assess the extent of colonic involvement after 8 to 10 years of disease. The extent of disease and presence or absence of dysplasia will dictate the frequency of subsequent surveillance colonoscopy.

FAP and HNPCC Kindreds. Annual sigmoidoscopy starting at age 10 to 12 years to look for development of CRAs is recommended for children of a parent with FAP (Grady 2003). Clinical testing for *APC* germline mutations is widely available but should only be offered in conjunction with genetic counselling by qualified individuals. When a family's *APC* mutation has been identified, children born to the family can be tested for that mutation. If negative, they will not develop FAP and need not undergo surveillance sigmoidoscopy. Colonoscopy is recommended every one to two years starting at age 25, or 10 years earlier than the youngest age of colon cancer diagnosis in the family for children born to HNPCC kindreds (Winawer, Fletcher et al. 2003). Genetic testing can be offered to children at risk in HNPCC families for which the MMR gene mutation has been identified. If positive, the importance of surveillance for the gastrointestinal and other HNPCC-related cancers is emphasized to the patient and family. (Please refer to Chapter 4 for a complete discussion of genetic testing and the hereditary risk of cancer.)

First-Degree Relatives of People with CRAs or CRCs. People with a first-degree relative with CRC or CRAs diagnosed before the age of 60 years or two first-degree relatives diagnosed with CRC at any age should have screening colonoscopy starting at age 40 years or 10 years younger than the earliest diagnosis in their family, whichever comes first (Winawer, Fletcher et al. 2003). Colonoscopy should be repeated every five years. People with a first-degree relative with CRC or CRAs diagnosed at the age of 60 years or older or two second-degree relatives with CRC should be screened as average-risk individuals, but from the age of 40 rather than 50 years.

Emerging Screening Tests

Fecal DNA. With appropriate processing and the polymerase chain reaction (PCR), it is now possible to isolate and detect DNA from colorectal epithelial cells shed into the bowel lumen in stool specimens (Ahlquist, Skoletsky et al. 2000). Proof of concept studies have shown that mutated DNA from *APC*, K-*ras* and other genes from neoplastic colorectal cells can be detected in this way (Ahlquist, Skoletsky et al. 2000; Traverso, Shuber et al. 2001). High throughput technology pioneered by EXACT Sciences (Maynard, MA) has made it possible to process sufficient samples to begin trials of fecal DNA testing for CRC screening. In a recent study the PreGen-Plus[TM] fecal DNA test was performed on patients who underwent colonoscopy (Tagore, Lawson et al. 2003). The sensitivity of PreGen-Plus[TM] for invasive CRC and advanced adenomas, respectively, in these patients was 64 and 57%. Preliminary results of a screening study comparing PreGen-Plus[TM] and FOBT to colonoscopy in 2,507 asymptomatic subjects at average risk for CRC were reported at a meeting but have not yet been published (Rex 2004). Sensitivity of PreGen-Plus[TM] and FOBT, respectively, for invasive CRC was 52 and 13% and for advanced adenomas was 15 and 11%. PreGen-Plus[TM] is commercially available. At this stage of development, the sensitivity of fecal DNA testing is intermediate between FOBT and colonoscopy but the cost is prohibitive. As the technology matures, this situation may change in favor of fecal DNA testing.

Virtual Colonoscopy. Thin-section, helical computed tomography (CT) followed by off-line processing, a technique termed CT colonography or virtual colonoscopy, can yield high-resolution, three-dimensional images of the colon. For good resolution, at present the same bowel preparation as for optical colonoscopy must be administered, and the colon must be insufflated with air or carbon dioxide via a rectal tube. Expectations have been raised that the sensitivity and specificity of virtual colonoscopy may approach those of optical colonoscopy. Results from early studies comparing the two techniques lead to conflicting conclusions. For example, Pickhardt et al. reported almost identical sensitivities of around 90% for detection of adenomas at least 6 millimeters in diameter by virtual and optical colonoscopy (Pickhardt, Choi et al. 2003). In contrast, Cotton et al. reported a sensitivity of only 39% for detection of adenomas at least 6 mm in diameter by virtual colonoscopy compared to 99% sensitivity for the same lesions by optical colonoscopy (Cotton, Durkalski et al. 2004).

Various explanations have been proposed for these discrepant results. Patients in the Pickhardt study received double the usual volume of sodium phosphate for bowel preparation. This group used superior computer software for a virtual "fly-through" of the colon that has not been used by other groups. The sensitivity of optical colonoscopy achieved by the Cotton group is superior to most published reports and almost certainly not matched in routine daily practice.

Clearly, the role of virtual colonoscopy as a primary screening tool has not been finalized. Where available it is now the procedure of choice for structural evaluation of the colon in patients who are unsuitable for optical colonoscopy or in whom optical colonoscopy could not be completed. Disadvantages of virtual colonoscopy are the bowel preparation that is required, insufflation of the colon, which is uncomfortable, and the need for a second procedure, optical colonoscopy, to biopsy or remove lesions identified at a positive virtual procedure. It is agreed that patients with lesions at least 6 mm in diameter should be referred for optical colonoscopy. Consensus has not been reached on the management of patients diagnosed with small polyps at virtual colonoscopy. Most CRAs of diameter less than 6 millimeters in older average-risk individuals are of trivial significance. Some advocate that patients in this category with one or two small adenomas diagnosed at virtual colonoscopy need not be referred for optical colonoscopy and polypectomy. The question of appropriate follow up if this "watchful waiting" approach is taken is unresolved. Options include optical colonoscopy or repeat virtual colonoscopy at intervals to be determined.

The field of CRC screening is evolving rapidly. Optical colonoscopy is the current criterion standard but whether it is feasible to aim for delivery of this procedure to the entire population over age 50 years is unclear. A major effort is under way to develop less invasive triaging tools, such as fecal DNA testing and virtual colonoscopy, with sufficient sensitivity and specificity that optical colonoscopy in the average-risk population could be restricted to people with a positive triaging test. Fecal tagging techniques using orally administered contrast agents are under development for the purpose of doing away with the need for bowel preparation before virtual colonoscopy. Successful development of fecal tagging would probably lead to more widespread use of virtual colonoscopy for CRC screening in the average-risk population.

Chemoprevention

The wealth of epidemiologic data implicating diet in colorectal carcinogenesis has provided the rationale for numerous efforts at reducing CRC risk by dietary and related interventions. The term chemoprevention is used to cover this topic, meaning the long-term use of oral agents to prevent colorectal neoplasms (Lamprecht and Lipkin 2003). The adenoma-carcinoma sequence and the fact that new (metachronous) CRAs develop in people from whom CRCs have been resected or CRAs removed have been exploited in the design of chemoprevention studies. Thus, randomized trials have been conducted in patients who have undergone removal of baseline CRAs by colonoscopic polypectomy. The subsequent rates of adenoma recurrence in the intervention and control groups are compared to determine the efficacy of the intervention.

Fiber. RCTs of wheat bran fiber supplements (13.5 g versus 2 g per day) (Alberts, Martínez et al. 2000) and consumption of a diet low in animal fat and high in fiber, fruit and vegetables (Schatzkin, Lanza et al. 2000) for 3 to 5 years failed to reduce adenoma recurrence rate. However, the validity of adenoma recurrence trials as surrogates for evaluating chemopreventive efficacy against CRC has been challenged on several grounds. Patients with baseline advanced adenomas have been in the minority in many CRA recurrence trials yet these are the patients in whom chemoprevention would be most applicable. It is possible that alternative factors influence recurrence in patients with advanced and non-advanced baseline CRAs. Many CRA recurrence trials have insufficient power to exclude significant benefit from the intervention(s) in the subgroup with baseline advanced adenomas. In addition, only the early, initiation stage of the adenoma-carcinoma sequence is examined in CRA recurrence trials. Agents that do not inhibit CRA initiation and do not reduce CRA recurrence rate could, nonetheless, inhibit the more important events of adenoma progression and malignant transformation to CRC. Furthermore, the relatively short duration of CRA recurrence trials may be insufficient for anti-carcinogenic actions to take effect. Lastly, most participants in CRA recurrence trials are in their sixth decade or older. To be active, it is possible that chemopreventive agents must be introduced much earlier in life.

High intake of dietary fiber has been associated with decreased risk for CRAs (Peters, Sinha et al. 2003) and CRCs (Bingham and Riboli 2004) in observational studies. It is possible that exercise and other healthy-lifestyle factors were important confounding variables in these studies.

The American Gastroenterological Association recommends a total fiber intake of at least 30 to 35 grams of fiber per day (Kim 2000). Fiber should be from all sources, including fruits, vegetables, cereals, grains and legumes, because of possible interactions between fiber and anti-carcinogens present in fiber-rich foods.

Folate. In its chemically reduced form of tetrahydrofolate, folate is essential for cellular integrity (Lamprecht and Lipkin 2003). Folate plays important antineoplastic roles in the control of DNA methylation and DNA synthesis and maintenance. Folate consumption by participants in the Nurses' Health Study cohort was assessed by questionnaire. Relative risk for developing CRC was 0.25 for those with consumption in the highest quintile (more than 400 μg/day) compared to those in the lowest quintile (200/day or less) after 15 years of use (Giovannucci, Stampfer et al. 1998). Further analysis of these data showed that the greatest protection conferred by high folate consumption against developing CRC was in people with a family history of the disease (Fuchs, Willett et al. 2002). This suggests that inherited characteristics related to folate metabolism, the genotype, influence risk for CRC, the phenotype.

Polymorphisms are alternative alleles of a gene. There may be subtle functional differences among the respective protein products of different polymorphic alleles. An individual can be homozygous or heterozygous for polymorphic genes. If homozygous, both copies of the gene are the same allele. If heterozygous, each copy is a different allele. Multiple enzymes (gene products), such as 5, 10-methylenetetrahydrofolate reductase (*MTHFR*), are involved in the pathways of folate metabolism. A role for folate in preventing colorectal carcinogenesis has been shown in individuals homozygous for a common polymorphism of *MTHFR* (Lamprecht and Lipkin 2003).

Calcium. Calcium is an important micronutrient that controls a large number of intracellular processes with antineoplastic potential (Lamprecht and Lipkin 2003). Dietary calcium also binds to bile and fatty acids with the effect of curbing intestinal cell proliferation. Calcium supplements (1200 mg daily) reduced CRA recurrence by 19% compared to placebo (Baron, Beach et al. 1999) in subjects with adequate vitamin D levels (Grau, Baron et al. 2003).

Selenium. Selenium as selenomethionine is an essential micronutrient, which is incorporated into at least 30 selenoproteins after absorption. On the basis of epidemiologic data suggesting that high selenium levels might protect against non-melanoma skin cancer, a randomized trial of selenium supplementation in the form of brewer's yeast was conducted in patients at high risk for this cancer (Clark, Combs et al. 1996). The incidence of non-melanoma skin cancer, the primary endpoint of the trial, was not reduced but significant results were reported for several secondary endpoints (Duffield-Lillico, Reid et al. 2002). These included reductions in total cancer mortality of 41% and colon cancer incidence of 54%. A phase III trial of selenium supplementation with CRA recurrence as the primary endpoint is now in progress.

Aspirin and Nonsteroidal Antiinflammatory Drugs. There is extensive epidemiological, clinical and experimental evidence that aspirin and other nonsteroidal antiinflammatory drugs (NSAIDs) reduce CRC risk and may reduce mortality from the disease by as much as 40 to 50% (Thun, Henley et al. 2002). NSAIDs inhibit the cyclooxygenase (COX) enzymes, COX-1 and COX-2. The colorectal and other antineoplastic actions of NSAIDs have been attributed largely to inhibition of COX-2 but other actions of these agents that are not related to COX inhibition contribute to their antineoplastic activity (Chan, Morin et al. 1998; He, Chan et al. 1999).

Management of patients with familial adenomatous polyposis (FAP) can consist of colectomy with construction of an ileorectal anastomosis in order to preserve the anal sphincter, thus obviating the need for a permanent ileostomy. In a cohort study, long-term use of sulindac, a non-selective COX inhibitor, reduced CRA burden in the retained rectal segment of most FAP patients following colectomy and ileorectal anastomosis (Cruz-Correa, Hylind et al. 2002). However, in a prospective RCT, sulindac did not prevent the development of CRAs in subjects with FAP prior to colectomy (Giardiello, Yang et al. 2002).

Aspirin has been shown to significantly reduce the risk of developing new CRAs over a period of one to three years in RCTs of patients from whom CRCs were recently resected (Sandler, Halabi et al. 2003) or CRAs were removed colonoscopically (Baron, Cole et al. 2003; Benamouzig, Deyra et al. 2003). A single daily dose level (325 mg) was used in the study of patients who had undergone CRC resection. Two daily dose levels of aspirin (81 mg, low-dose and 325 mg, standard-dose) were tested in one of the CRA recurrence trials (Baron, Cole et al. 2003). Low-dose aspirin, as used for cardiovascular prophylaxis, reduced CRA recurrence by 19% but, rather surprisingly, the recurrence rate was not decreased in the group that received the 325 mg dose.

The effect of aspirin dose and duration of use on CRA risk was clarified in another report from the Nurses' Health Study (Chan, Giovannucci et al. 2004). The greatest effect was evident at a weekly total dosage of at least 14 standard-dose tablets, which is much higher than is recommended for cardiovascular prophylaxis. Similar dose-response relationships were found among regular short-term users (5 years or less) and long-term users (more than 5 years). Genetic factors may further modify dose-related effects of aspirin on CRA and CRC risk. As mentioned, a polymorphism of the *ornithine decarboxylase* gene was found to enhance substantially the protective effect of aspirin against CRA recurrence (Martinez, O'Brien et al. 2003).

Potentially life-threatening gastrointestinal (hemorrhage), cerebrovascular (hemorrhagic stroke) and renal complications occur with sufficient frequency to preclude the unrestricted long-term use of standard-dose aspirin therapy for chemoprevention of CRC. Even low-dose aspirin is associated with some risk for hemorrhagic stroke (He, Whelton et al. 1998) and gastrointestinal hemorrhage (Cryer 2002). The complications of aspirin are attributed largely to inhibition of COX-1 and the chemopreventive activity to inhibition of COX-2. Selective COX-2 inhibitors, the coxibs, were developed in the hope that complications would be minimized. The first two clinically available coxibs were celecoxib and rofecoxib. Although sulindac did not prevent the development of CRAs in subjects with FAP (Giardiello, Yang et al. 2002), celecoxib at the higher of two dose levels (400 mg twice daily) significantly reduced polyp burden after six months in patients with FAP (Steinbach, Lynch et al. 2000). Celecoxib and rofecoxib were shown in a nested case-control study using data from a government insurance database to protect against the development of colorectal neoplasia (Rahme, Barkun et al. 2003). On the basis of the promising results from observational studies, several RCTs of coxibs using the CRA recurrence model were initiated but have yet to be reported. The process of evaluating coxib antineoplastic efficacy was recently jolted by an interim report of an excess of 16 myocardial infarctions or strokes per 1000 patients in a rofecoxib (VIOXX®) CRA recurrence trial (Fitzgerald 2004; Topol 2004). As a result, Merck, the manufacturer, abruptly withdrew VIOXX® from the worldwide market. Although celcecoxib-related cardiovascular toxicity has so far not been reported from CRA recurrence trials of this agent, a definitive statement on the antineoplastic efficacy and safety of the coxibs as a class would be premature.

Ursodeoxycholic Acid. Deoxycholic acid (DCA) is the predominant fecal secondary bile acid. Combined epidemiological, experimental and clinical data support the hypothesis that fecal DCA concentration is positively associated with CRC risk. Ursodeoxycholic acid (UDCA) is physiologically present in very low concentrations in human bile and at pharmacological oral doses given long-term can dissolve small, translucent gall stones. UDCA also reduces fecal DCA concentration, providing the rationale for its potential use as a chemopreventive agent for colorectal neoplasia, and is devoid of significant toxicity. The current main clinical indication for chronic UDCA use is treatment of the potentially fatal primary disorders of bile ducts, primary biliary cirrhosis and primary sclerosing cholangitis. UDCA reduced the rate of CRA recurrence in an observational study of primary biliary cirrhosis patients taking UDCA (Serfaty, De Leusse et al. 2003). UC is associated with primary biliary cirrhosis and also, as described, with increased CRC risk. UDCA was strongly associated with decreased prevalence of colonic dysplasia in patients with UC and primary sclerosing cholangitis in an observational study (Tung, Emond et al. 2001) and a RCT (Pardi, Loftus et al. 2003). UDCA (13 to 15 mg/kg daily) significantly decreased CRC risk in patients with UC and primary sclerosing cholangitis (Pardi, Loftus et al. 2003). The magnitude of this effect, first apparent approximately three years after starting UDCA therapy, continued to increase with lengthening duration of therapy.

In a recently completed RCT, although UDCA (8 to 10 mg/kg daily for three years) did not reduce the rate of CRA recurrence, there was a statistically significant 39% reduction in the recurrence of CRAs with high-grade dysplasia (Alberts, Martinez et al. 2004). It is possible that the relatively low UDCA dose and short three-year duration of the trial contributed to the lack of a significant effect on total CRA recurrence.

Current Status of CRC Chemoprevention. RCT evidence for macronutrient interventions to reduce risk for colorectal neoplasia is lacking. However, diets that are high in fiber, fruit and vegetable content and low in unsaturated fats confer multiple other well validated preventive health benefits. It remains possible that they reduce CRC risk and there are no significant adverse effects. Micronutrient folate and calcium supplements can safely be taken by people in the general population and have been shown to protect against colorectal neoplasia, besides their other benefits. There are no grounds for recommending pharmacological chemoprevention to the population at average CRC risk and the same applies for those average-risk people who have had one or two non-advanced adenomas removed. The latter group should follow current recommendations for surveillance colonoscopy. People taking low-dose aspirin for cardiovascular prophylaxis may also be protected against colorectal neoplasia.

Standard-dose aspirin chemoprevention should be restricted to people at increased CRC risk, for whom the decision to recommend aspirin chemoprevention should usually be individualized by a specialist. The risks of peptic ulceration, complicated by perforation or hemorrhage, and hemorrhagic stroke must be considered. Screening and surveillance protocols should not be relaxed in subjects at increased risk for CRC who are taking chemopreventive therapy. UDCA continues to show promise for CRC chemoprevention and is remarkably safe. Approaches to chemoprevention are likely to change substantially as the results of RCTs become available.

References

Ahlquist, D. A., J. E. Skoletsky, et al. (2000). "Colorectal cancer screening by detection of altered human DNA in stool: Feasability of a multitarget assay panel." *Gastroenterology* **119**: 1219–1227.

Ahlquist, D. A., H. S. Wieand, et al. (1993). "Accuracy of fecal occult blood screening for colorectal neoplasia." *JAMA* **269**: 1262–1267.

Alberts, D.S., M.E. Martínez, et al. (2004). "Phase III trial of ursodeoxycholic acid to prevent colorectal adenoma recurrence." *Submitted for publication*.

Alberts, D.S., M.E. Martínez, et al. (2000). "Lack of effect of a high-fiber cereal supplement on the recurrence of colorectal adenomas." *N Engl J Med* **342**: 1156–1162.

Atkin, W.S., J. Cuzick, et al. (2002). "Single flexible sigmoidoscopy screening to prevent colorectal cancer: baseline findings of a UK multicentre randomised trial." *Lancet* **359**: 1291–1300.

Atkin, W.S., J. Cuzick, et al. (1993). "Prevention of colorectal cancer by once-only sigmoidoscopy." *Lancet* **341**: 736–740.

Baris, D., G. Gridley, et al. (2002). "Acromegaly and cancer risk: a cohort study in Sweden and Denmark." *Cancer Causes Control* **13**(5): 395–400.

Baron, J.A., M. Beach, et al. (1999). "Calcium supplements for the prevention of colorectal adenomas. Calcium Polyp Prevention Study Group." *N Engl J Med* **340**(2): 101–107.

Baron, J.A., B.F. Cole, et al. (2003). "A randomized trial of aspirin to prevent colorectal adenomas." *N Engl J Med* **348**: 891–899.

Benamouzig, R., J. Deyra, et al. (2003). "Daily soluble aspirin and prevention of colorectal adenoma recurrence: One-year results of the APACC trial1." *Gastroenterology* **125**(2): 328–336.

Bingham, S. and E. Riboli (2004). "Diet and cancer – the European Prospective Investigation into Cancer and Nutrition." *Nat Rev Cancer* **4**(3): 206–215.

Bowles, C.J., R. Leicester, et al. (2004). "A prospective study of colonoscopy practice in the UK today: are we adequately prepared for national colorectal cancer screening tomorrow?" *Gut* **53**(2): 277–283.

BRFSS (2002). Colorectal Cancer Screening – 2002. Division of Adult and Community Health, National Center for Chronic Disease Prevention and Health Promotion, Centers for Disease Control and Prevention, Behavioral Risk Factor Surveillance System Online Prevalence Data, 1995–2002.

Card, T., R. Hubbard, et al. (2003). "Mortality in inflammatory bowel disease: a population-based cohort study." *Gastroenterology* **125**(6): 1583–1590.

Chan, A.T., E.L. Giovannucci, et al. (2004). "A prospective study of aspirin use and the risk for colorectal adenoma." *Ann Intern Med* **140**(3): 157–166.

Chan, T.A., P.J. Morin, et al. (1998). "Mechanisms underlying nonsteroidal antiinflammatory drug-mediated apoptosis." *Proc Natl Acad Sci USA* **95**: 681–686.

Choi, P.M., F.W. Nugent, et al. (1993). "Colonoscopic surveillance reduces mortality from colorectal cancer in ulcerative colitis." *Gastroenterology* **105**(2): 418–424.

Citarda, F., G. Tomaselli, et al. (2001). "Efficacy in standard clinical practice of colonoscopic polypectomy in reducing colorectal cancer incidence." *Gut* **48**(6): 812–815.

Clark, L., J. Combs, J.F., et al. (1996). "Effects of selenium supplementation for cancer prevention in patient with carcinomas of the skin." *JAMA* **276**: 1957–1963.

Coffield, A.B., M.V. Maciosek, et al. (2001). "Priorities among recommended clinical preventive services." *Am J Prev Med* **21**(1): 1–9.

Colditz, G.A., C.C. Cannuscio, et al. (1997). "Physical activity and reduced risk of colon cancer: implications for prevention." *Cancer Causes Control* **8**(4): 649–667.

Cooper, G.S., Z. Yuan, et al. (1995). "A national population-based study of incidence of colorectal cancer and age. Implications for screening in older Americans." *Cancer* **75**(3): 775–781.

Cotton, P.B., V.L. Durkalski, et al. (2004). "Computed tomographic colonography (virtual colonoscopy): a multicenter comparison with standard colonoscopy for detection of colorectal neoplasia." *JAMA* **291**(14): 1713–1719.

Cruz-Correa, M., L.M. Hylind, et al. (2002). "Long-term treatment with sulindac in familial adenomatous polyposis: a prospective cohort study." *Gastroenterology* **122**(3): 641–645.

Cryer, B. (2002). "Gastrointestinal safety of low-dose aspirin." *Am J Manag Care* **8**(22 Suppl): S701–708.

Duffield-Lillico, A.J., M.E. Reid, et al. (2002). "Baseline characteristics and the effect of selenium supplementation on cancer incidence in a randomized clinical trial: a summary report of the Nutritional Prevention of Cancer Trial." *Cancer Epidemiol Biomarkers Prev* **11**(7): 630–639.

Fitzgerald, G.A. (2004). "Coxibs and cardiovascular disease." *N Engl J Med* **351**(17): 1709–1711.

Frazier, A.L., G.A. Colditz, et al. (2000). "Cost-effectiveness of screening for colorectal cancer in the general population." *JAMA* **284**: 1954–1961.

Friedenreich, C.M. (2001). "Physical activity and cancer prevention: from observational to intervention research." *Cancer Epidemiol Biomarkers Prev* **10**: 287–301.

Fuchs, C.S., W.C. Willett, et al. (2002). "The influence of folate and multivitamin use on the familial risk of colon cancer in women." *Cancer Epidemiol Biomarkers Prev* **11**: 227–234.

Gatto, N.M., H. Frucht, et al. (2003). "Risk of perforation after colonoscopy and sigmoidoscopy: a population-based study." *J Natl Cancer Inst* **95**(3): 230–236.

Giardiello, F.M., V.W. Yang, et al. (2002). "Primary chemoprevention of familial adenomatous polyposis with sulindac." *N Engl J Med* **346**: 1054–1059.

Giardiello, F.M., V.W. Yang, et al. (2002). "Primary chemoprevention of familial adenomatous polyposis with sulindac." *N Engl J Med* **346**(14): 1054–1059.

Giovannucci, E., E.B. Rimm, et al. (1995). "Alcohol, low-methionine–low-folate diets, and risk of colon cancer in men." *J Natl Cancer Inst* **87**(4): 265–273.

Giovannucci, E.L., M.J. Stampfer, et al. (1998). "Multivitamin use, folate, and colon cancer in women in nurses' health study." *Ann Intern Med* **129**: 517–524.

Gonzalez-Juanatey, C., M.A. Gonzalez-Gay, et al. (2003). "Infective endocarditis due to Streptococcus bovis in a series of nonaddict patients: clinical and morphological characteristics of 20 cases and review of the literature." *Can J Cardiol* **19**(10): 1139–1145.

Grady, W.M. (2003). "Genetic testing for high-risk colon cancer patients." *Gastroenterology* **124**(6): 1574–1594.

Grau, M.V., J.A. Baron, et al. (2003). "Vitamin D, calcium supplementation, and colorectal adenomas: results of a randomized trial." *J Natl Cancer Inst* **95**(23): 1765–1771.

Hahn, W.C. and R.A. Weinberg (2002). "Rules for making human tumor cells." *N Engl J Med* **347**: 1593–1603.

Hanahan, D. and R.A. Weinberg (2000). "The hallmarks of cancer." *Cell* **100**(1): 57–70.

He, J., P.K. Whelton, et al. (1998). "Aspirin and risk of hemorrhagic stroke." *JAMA* **280**: 1930–1935.

He, T.-C., T.A. Chan, et al. (1999). "PPARδ is an APC-regulated target of nonsteroidal anti-inflammatory drugs." *N Engl J Med* **99**: 335–345.

Imperiale, T.F., D.R. Wagner, et al. (2000). "Risk of advanced proximal neoplasms in asymptomatic adults according to the distal colorectal findings." *N Engl J Med* **343**: 169–174.

Ionov, Y., M.A. Peinado, et al. (1993). "Ubiquitous somatic mutations in simple repeated sequences reveal a new mechanism for colonic carcinogenesis." *Nature* **363**(6429): 558–561.

Jayaram, H., J. Satsangi, et al. (2001). "Increased colorectal neoplasia in chronic ulcerative colitis complicated by primary sclerosing cholangitis: fact or fiction?" *Gut* **48**(3): 430–434.

Jemal, A., R.C. Tiwari, et al. (2004). "Cancer statistics, 2004." *CA Cancer J Clin* **54**(1): 8–29.

Jess, T., K.V. Winther, et al. (2004). "Intestinal and extra-intestinal cancer in Crohn's disease: follow-up of a population-based cohort in Copenhagen County, Denmark." *Aliment Pharmacol Ther* **19**(3): 287–293.

Kim, Y.I. (2000). "AGA technical review: impact of dietary fiber on colon cancer occurrence." *Gastroenterology* **118**(6): 1235–1257.

Kinzler, K.W. and B. Vogelstein (1996). "Lessons from hereditary colorectal cancer." *Cell* **87**: 159–170.

Lamprecht, S.A. and M. Lipkin (2003). "Chemoprevention of colon cancer by calcium, vitamin D and folate: molecular mechanisms." *Nat Rev Cancer* **3**(8): 601–614.

Lengauer, C., K.W. Kinzler, et al. (1998). "Genetic instabilities in human cancers." *Nature* **396**: 643–649.

LeRoith, D., R. Baserga, et al. (1995). "Insulin-like growth factors and cancer." *Ann Intern Med* **122**(1): 54–59.

Leslie, A., F.A. Carey, et al. (2002). "The colorectal adenoma-carcinoma sequence." *Br J Surg* **89**: 845–860.

Lieberman, D.A. and D.G. Weiss (2001). "One-time screening for colorectal cancer with combined fecal occult-blood testing and examination of the distal colon." *N Engl J Med* **345**: 555–560.

Lieberman, D.A., D.G. Weiss, et al. (2000). "Use of colonoscopy to screen asymptomatic adults for colorectal cancer." *N Engl J Med* **343**: 162–168.

Lindor, N.M. (2004). "Recognition of genetic syndromes in families with suspected hereditary colon cancer syndromes." *Clin Gastroenterol Hepatol* **2**(5): 366–375.

Ma, J., E. Giovannucci, et al. (2004). "A prospective study of plasma C-peptide and colorectal cancer risk in men." *J Natl Cancer Inst* **96**(7): 546–553.

Ma, J., M.N. Pollak, et al. (1999). "Prospective study of colorectal cancer risk in men and plasma levels of insulin-like growth factor (IGF)-I and IGF-binding protein-3." *J Natl Cancer Inst* **91**(7): 620–625.

Mandel, J.S., J.H. Bond, et al. (1993). "Reducing mortality from colorectal cancer by screening for fecal occult blood." *N Engl J Med* **328**: 1365–1371.

Mandel, J.S., T.R. Church, et al. (2000). "The effect of fecal occult-blood screening on the incidence of colorectal cancer." *N Engl J Med* **343**(22): 1603–1607.

Mandel, J.S., T.R. Church, et al. (1999). "Colorectal cancer mortality: effectiveness of biennial screening for fecal occult blood." *J Natl Cancer Inst* **91**: 434–437.

Martinez, M.E., T.G. O'Brien, et al. (2003). "Pronounced reduction in adenoma recurrence associated with aspirin use and a polymorphism in the ornithine decarboxylase gene." *Proc Natl Acad Sci USA* **100**(13): 7859–7864.

Mason, J.B. (2002). "Nutritional chemoprevention of colon cancer." *Semin Gastrointest Dis* **13**(3): 143–153.

Munkholm, P. (2003). "Review article: the incidence and prevalence of colorectal cancer in inflammatory bowel disease." *Aliment Pharmacol Ther* **18 Suppl 2**: 1–5.

Nelson, E.B., K.R. McQuaid, et al. (2002). "Procedural success and complications of large-scale screening colonoscopy." *Gastrointest Endosc* **55**: 307–314.

Newcomb, P.A., R.G. Norfleet, et al. (1992). "Screening sigmoidoscopy and colorectal cancer mortality." *J Natl Cancer Inst* **84**(20): 1572–1575.

Niv, Y., M. Lev-El, et al. (2002). "Protective effect of faecal occult blood test screening for colorectal cancer: worse prognosis for screening refusers." *Gut* **50**(1): 33–37.

Palmqvist, R., G. Hallmans, et al. (2002). "Plasma insulin-like growth factor 1, insulin-like growth factor binding protein 3, and risk of colorectal cancer: a prospective study in northern Sweden." *Gut* **50**(5): 642–646.

Pardi, D.S., E.V. Loftus, Jr., et al. (2003). "Ursodeoxycholic acid as a chemopreventive agent in patients with ulcerative colitis and primary sclerosing cholangitis." *Gastroenterology* **124**: 889–893.

Peters, U., R. Sinha, et al. (2003). "Dietary fibre and colorectal adenoma in a colorectal cancer early detection programme." *Lancet* **361**(9368): 1491–1495.

Pickhardt, P.J., J.R. Choi, et al. (2003). "Computed tomographic virtual colonoscopy to screen for colorectal neoplasia in asymptomatic adults." *N Engl J Med* **349**(23): 2191–2200.

Pignone, M., M. Rich, et al. (2002). "Screening for colorectal cancer in adults at average risk: a summary of the evidence for the U.S. Preventive Services Task Force." *Ann Intern Med* **137**(2): 132–141.

Potter, J.D. (1999). "Colorectal cancer: molecules and populations." *J Natl Cancer Inst* **91**(11): 916–932.

Rahme, E., A.N. Barkun, et al. (2003). "The cyclooxygenase-2-selective inhibitors rofecoxib and celecoxib prevent colorectal neoplasia occurrence and recurrence." *Gastroenterology* **125**(2): 404–412.

Rajagopalan, H., M.A. Nowak, et al. (2003). "The significance of unstable chromosomes in colorectal cancer." *Nat Rev Cancer* **3**(9): 695–701.

Rex, D.K. (2004). "American college of gastroenterology action plan for colorectal cancer prevention." *Am J Gastroenterol* **99**(4): 574–577.

Rex, D.K., C.S. Cutler, et al. (1997). "Colonoscopic miss rates of adenomas determined by back-to-back colonoscopies." *Gastroenterology* **112**: 24–28.

Rex, D.K., G.A. Lehman, et al. (1994). "The yield of a second screening flexible sigmoidoscopy in average-risk persons after one negative examination." *Gastroenterology* **106**: 593–595.

Rutter, M., B. Saunders, et al. (2004). "Severity of inflammation is a risk factor for colorectal neoplasia in ulcerative colitis." *Gastroenterology* **126**(2): 451–459.

Sandler, R.S., S. Halabi, et al. (2003). "A randomized trial of aspirin to prevent colorectal adenomas in patients with previous colorectal cancer." *N Engl J Med* **348**: 883–890.

Schatzkin, A., E. Lanza, et al. (2000). "Lack of effect of a low-fat, high-fiber diet on the recurrence of colorectal adenomas." *N Engl J Med* **342**: 1149–1155.

Schoen, R.E., P.F. Pinsky, et al. (2003). "Results of repeat sigmoidoscopy 3 years after a negative examination." *JAMA* **290**(1): 41–48.

Schoenfeld, P., S. Lipscomb, et al. (1999). "Accuracy of polyp detection by gastroenterologists and nurse endoscopists during flexible sigmoidoscopy: A randomized trial." *Gastroenterology* **117**: 312–318.

Selby, J.V., G.D. Friedman, et al. (1992). "A case-control study of screening sigmoidoscopy and mortality from colorectal cancer." *N Engl J Med* **326**: 653–657.

Serfaty, L., A. De Leusse, et al. (2003). "Ursodeoxycholic acid therapy and the risk of colorectal adenoma in patients with primary biliary cirrhosis: an observational study." *Hepatology* **38**(1): 203–209.

Slattery, M.L., S. Edwards, et al. (2003). "Physical activity and colorectal cancer." *Am J Epidemiol* **158**(3): 214–224.

Smith, R.A., V. Cokkinides, et al. (2004). "American Cancer Society guidelines for the early detection of cancer, 2004." *CA Cancer J Clin* **54**(1): 41–52.

Spirio, L.N., W. Samowitz, et al. (1998). "Alleles of *APC* modulate the frequency and classes of mutations that lead to colon polyps." *Nat Genet* **20**: 385–388.

Steinbach, G., P.M. Lynch, et al. (2000). "The effect of celecoxib, a cyclooxygenase-2 inhibitor, in familial adenomatous polyposis." *N Engl J Med* **342**: 1946–1952.

Tagore, K.S., M.J. Lawson, et al. (2003). "Sensitivity and specificity of a stool DNA multitarget assay panel for the detection of advanced colorectal neoplasia." *Clin Colorectal Cancer* **3**(1): 47–53.

Thun, M.J., S.J. Henley, et al. (2002). "Nonsteroidal anti-inflammatory drugs as anticancer agents: Mechanistic, pharmacologic, and clinical issues." *J Natl Cancer Inst* **94**: 252–266.

Topol, E.J. (2004). "Failing the public health–rofecoxib, Merck, and the FDA." *N Engl J Med* **351**(17): 1707–1709.

Toyota, M., C. Ho, et al. (1999). "Identification of differentially methylated sequences in colorectal cancer by methylated CpG island amplification." *Cancer Res* **59**(10): 2307–2312.

Traverso, G., A.P. Shuber, et al. (2001). "Detection of *APC* mutations in fecal DNA from patients with colorectal tumors." *N Engl J Med* **346**: 311–320.

Tung, B.Y., M.J. Emond, et al. (2001). "Ursodiol use is associated with lower prevalence of colonic neoplasia in patients with ulcerative colitis and primary sclerosing cholangitis." *Ann Intern Med* **134**: 89–95.

Vogelstein, B., E.R. Fearon, et al. (1988). "Genetic alterations during colorectal-tumor development." *N Engl J Med* **319**(9): 525–532.

Ward, E., A. Jemal, et al. (2004). "Cancer disparities by race/ethnicity and socioeconomic status." *CA Cancer J Clin* **54**(2): 78–93.

Whynes, D.K., E.J. Frew, et al. (2003). "Colorectal cancer, screening and survival: the influence of socio-economic deprivation." *Public Health* **117**(6): 389–395.

Winawer, S.J., R.H. Fletcher, et al. (1997). "Colorectal cancer screening: Clinical guidelines and rationale." *Gastroenterology* **112**: 594–642.

Winawer, S.J., R.H. Fletcher, et al. (2003). "Colorectal cancer screening and surveillance: clinical guidelines and rationale-update based on new evidence." *Gastroenterology* **124**: 544–560.

Winawer, S.J., E.T. Stewart, et al. (2000). "A comparison of colonoscopy and double-contrast barium enema for surveillance after polypectomy." *N Engl J Med* **342**: 1766–1772.

Winawer, S.J., A.G. Zauber, et al. (1993). "Prevention of colorectal cancer by colonoscopic polypectomy." *N Engl J Med* **329**: 1977–1981.

Winther, K.V., T. Jess, et al. (2003). "Survival and cause-specific mortality in ulcerative colitis: follow-up of a population-based cohort in Copenhagen County." *Gastroenterology* **125**(6): 1576–1582.

Woodhouse, C.R. (2002). "Guidelines for monitoring of patients with ureterosigmoidostomy." *Gut* **51**(Suppl 5): V15–16.

Young, G.P., D.J. St John, et al. (2003). "Prescreening evaluation of a brush-based faecal immunochemical test for haemoglobin." *J Med Screen* **10**(3): 123–128.

Lung Cancer Prevention

Iman Hakim and Linda Garland

College of Medicine and College of Public Health, University of Arizona, Tucson AZ 85724

Lung cancer continues to exact a huge toll on the health status of Americans and people worldwide. In the United States (U.S.), the number of new lung cancer cases diagnosed per year has reached epidemic proportions. In 2004, an estimated 173,770 new cases of lung cancer were diagnosed, representing 12.7% of the 1,368,030 new cases of all cancers diagnosed in 2004 (Jemal, Tiwari et al. 2004). While prostate cancer and breast cancer lead new cancer cases in American men and women respectively in 2004, lung cancer remains the leading cause of cancer-related death for both men and women, with an estimated 160,440 of all 563,700 cancer deaths, or 28.5%, attributable to lung cancer. While once thought to be mainly a man's disease, lung cancer is now represented in a nearly equal fashion between the sexes, with women diagnosed with lung cancer in 2004 representing a full 46% of all new cases (Jemal, Tiwari et al. 2004).

The Epidemiology of Lung Cancer

Trends in Tobacco Use in the United States

The lung cancer epidemic that has now manifested in the U.S. had its roots in the tremendous increase in smoking prevalence through the 1900s. In the early 1900s, smoking, especially among women, was relatively rare (USDHHS 1980). Over the next 50 years, smoking prevalence increased dramatically, influenced by expanding tobacco marketing initiatives by the tobacco industry. Both male and female smokers were cultivated; in fact, as early as the 1920s the tobacco industry first began its targeting of women utilizing the concept of 'image advertising,' offering lipstick-colored cigarette tips for the woman smoker and developing advertising campaigns illustrated by the slogan, "Reach for a Lucky instead of a sweet" to create the association between cigarette use with staying slim, a theme particularly appealing to women (Wallace 1929). There was a significant increase in the numbers of men and women who took up the habit of smoking cigarettes during World War II, with cigarettes being included in government issue ration kits, and image advertising capitalizing on the war effort to promote smoking in women.

The Narrowing of the Gender Gap in Smoking Prevalence

While early in the century a large gender gap in smoking prevalence existed, the gap narrowed significantly over the middle and latter parts of the century as a consequence of several trends. First, women's use of cigarettes virtually soared over the mid-1900s in the face of aggressive niche marketing that linked women's smoking to their burgeoning social and political independence, a marketing effort best typified by the Virginia Slims advertising slogan, "You've Come a Long Way, Baby." Second, in the 1950s, the first epidemiologic studies were conducted that definitively linked tobacco exposure and lung cancer (Levin, Goldstein et al. 1950; Doll and Hill 1952). In 1964, the influential report of the Advisory Committee to the Surgeon General cited evidence of the adverse health effects of tobacco use (USDEW 1964). At that time, 51.9% of men and 33.9% of women were smoking (Giovino, Schooley et al. 1994).

In 1964, the Surgeon General's Report on Smoking and Health became the first national declaration of the association between cigarette smoking as a cause of cancer and other diseases. The publication of this report was followed in 1965 by a congressional act requiring a general health warning on all cigarette packaging regarding the dangers of cigarette smoking. The landmark 1964 Surgeon General's Report on Smoking and Health (USDHHS 1964) provided official evidence that cigarette smoking is a cause of cancer and other serious diseases. The following year, Congress passed the Federal Cigarette Labeling and Advertising Act, requiring health warnings on all cigarette packages: "Caution: Cigarette Smoking May be Hazardous to Your Health."

A wave of aggressive private, state and federal-based tobacco control initiatives followed, promoting smoking cessation and placing restrictions on some venues for tobacco advertisements such as broadcast advertising on televisions, bans on billboard advertising, and restrictions on sales and advertising to children and adolescents. For men, the latter part of the century saw a decline in smoking prevalence; for women, smoking prevalence continued to increase. Thus, at the very end of the 20th century, the gender gap had narrowed to only around 5%, with 22% of women aged 18 or old-

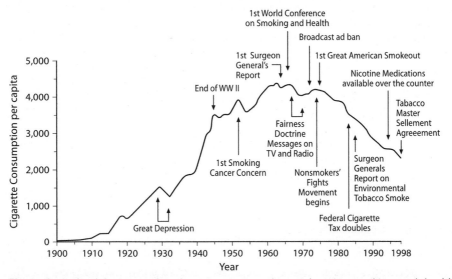

Fig. 1. Annual adult per capita cigarette consumption and major smoking and health events – Unites States, 1990–1998 – Source of data: US Department of Agriculture, 2000 Surgeon, General's Report.

er in the U.S. smoking cigarettes, compared to 26.4% of U.S. men. Figure 1 illustrates the trend in all adult cigarette smoking over the 20th century in relation to public health milestones.

While the decline in overall cigarette use in the U.S. over the latter part of the 20th century is considered to have been one of great public health achievements of that century, there continues to be about 48 million adult smokers, half of whom will die of smoking-related disease. Economically, the burden of tobacco use continues to exact a staggering $50 billion in medical expenditures and another $50 billion in indirect costs such as lost wages (1999). To continue to aggressively address the tremendous public health burden derived from tobacco use, the Department of Health and Human Services has recently issued a national health objective for the United States for the year 2010 to reduce the prevalence of cigarette smoking among adults to less than 12% (USDDHS 2000).

Demographic Variables and Tobacco Use

Tobacco use varies by a number of variables apart from gender; these include age, education, socioeconomic status and ethnicity/race. A Centers for Disease Control (CDC) analysis of self-reported data from the 2000 National Health Interview Survey (NHIS) sample showed smoking prevalence was highest among adults aged 18–44 years and lowest among adults aged greater than 65 years. Cigarette use varied inversely with level of education, with a prevalence of 47.2% in adults with a general education degree as compared to a prevalence of 8.4% among adults with a master's, professional or doctoral degree. Persons living below the poverty level had higher prevalence of smoking than persons at or above the poverty level (31.7% versus 22.9%, respectively) (2002).

Cigarette use varies widely by ethnic/racial groups. Factors that have been implicated in the complex interactions that influence tobacco use by ethnic group include socioeconomic status, cultural factors and norms, acculturation, biologic factors, impact of advertising targeted by ethnicity, price of tobacco products, and variation in the ability of communities to implement effective tobacco-control initiatives (2004). Smoking prevalence among five defined ethnic/racial groups varies widely (Table 1), with Asians (14.4%) and Hispanics (18.6%) having the lowest prevalence of cigarette use while American Indians/Alaska Natives having the highest prevalence (36.0%) (2002). The need to tailor tobacco control interventions by cultural demographics is underscored by a further analysis of the NHIS data showing that even within each of the four primary racial/ethnic minority populations (non-Hispanic blacks, American Indians/Alaska Natives, Asians/Pacific Islanders, and Hispanics), cigarette use by youth and adults varies widely (2004).

Etiology of Lung Carcinogenesis

Oxidative Damage

Oxidative damage is implicated in several chronic diseases including cancer and chronic inflammation. Oxidative reactions have been implicated as important modulators of human health and can play a role in both disease prevention and disease devel-

Table 1. Percentage of persons aged ≥18 years who were current smokers[a], by selected characteristics – National Health Interview Survey, United States, 2000, reprinted with permission from Morbidity and Mortality Weekly Report (2002)

Characteristic	Men (n = 13,986) %	(95% CI[b])	Women (n = 18,388) %	(95% CI)	Total (n = 32,374) %	(95% CI)
Race/Ethnicity[c]						
White, non-Hispanic	25.9	(±1.0)	22.4	(±0.8)	**24.1**	**(±0.7)**
Black, non-Hispanic	26.1	(±2.5)	20.9	(±1.7)	**23.2**	**(±1.5)**
Hispanic	24.0	(±2.1)	13.3	(±1.6)	**18.6**	**(±1.3)**
American Indian/ Alaska Native[d]	29.1	(±11.0)	42.5	(±11.0)	**36.0**	**(±8.0)**
Asian[e]	21.0	(±4.6)	7.6	(±2.8)	**14.4**	**(±2.8)**
Education[f]						
0–12 (no diploma)	33.2	(±2.2)	23.6	(±1.7)	**28.2**	**(±1.4)**
≤8	26.1	(±3.1)	14.2	(±2.2)	**20.0**	**(±1.9)**
9–11	37.6	(±3.5)	30.8	(±2.7)	**33.9**	**(±2.2)**
12	40.1	(±6.8)	25.3	(±5.1)	**32.7**	**(±4.4)**
GED[g] diploma	50.1	(±6.2)	44.3	(±5.7)	**47.2**	**(±4.3)**
12 (diploma)	31.7	(±1.9)	23.5	(±1.4)	**27.2**	**(±1.2)**
Associate Degree	21.9	(±2.8)	20.4	(±2.4)	**21.1**	**(±1.8)**
Some College	25.8	(±2.1)	21.6	(±1.7)	**23.5**	**(±1.3)**
Undergraduate Degree	14.2	(±1.7)	12.4	(±1.5)	**13.2**	**(±1.1)**
Graduate Degree	9.1	(±1.8)	7.5	(±1.6)	**8.4**	**(±1.2)**
Age Group (yrs)						
18–24	28.5	(±2.7)	25.1	(±2.4)	**26.8**	**(±1.8)**
25–44	29.7	(±1.4)	24.5	(±1.1)	**27.0**	**(±0.9)**
45–64	26.4	(±1.5)	21.6	(±1.3)	**24.0**	**(±1.0)**
≥65	10.2	(±1.3)	9.3	(±1.0)	**9.7**	**(±0.8)**
Poverty Status[h]						
At or above	25.4	(±1.0)	20.4	(±0.9)	**22.9**	**(±0.7)**
Below	35.3	(±3.2)	29.1	(±2.3)	**31.7**	**(±1.9)**
Unknown	23.6	(±1.8)	19.5	(±1.4)	**21.4**	**(±1.1)**
Total	**25.7**	**(±0.8)**	**21.0**	**(±0.7)**	**23.3**	**(±0.5)**

[a] Smoked ≥100 cigarettes during their lifetime and reported at the time of interview smoking everyday or some days. Excludes 301 respondents for whom smoking status was unknown.
[b] Confidence interval.
[c] Excludes 287 respondents of unknown, multiple, and other racial/ethnic categories.
[d] Wide variances among estimates reflect limited sample sizes.
[e] Does not include Native Hawaiians and Other Pacific Islanders.
[f] Persons aged ≥25 years. Excludes 305 persons with unknown years of education.
[g] General Education Development.
[h] The 1999 poverty thresholds from the Bureau of the Census were used in these calculations.

opment. Small-cell carcinoma of the lung (SCLC) is a highly malignant systemic disease characterized by rapid and widespread dissemination of tumor cells at the time of diagnosis (Erhola, Toyokuni et al. 1997). Decreased plasma peroxyl radical trapping capacity was reported in SCLC patients (Erhola, Toyokuni et al. 1997). The most enhanced lipid peroxidation in tumor tissue was noted in specimens of adenocarcinoma and SCLC tissue, in case of which 'early' dissemination and fast growth are common features (Zieba, Suwalski et al. 2000). Thus it appears that lung cancer of these histologic types is associated with an increased oxidative stress that is most likely due to the systemic nature of the disease (Erhola, Toyokuni et al. 1997). Oxidative damage to the DNA of key cellular genes is a fundamental event leading to malignancy (Ames, Gold et al. 1995), whereas cellular generation of oxidants is important in the control of infectious agents (Peterhans 1997; Akaike, Suga et al. 1998) and eliminating newly developed tumors (Farias-Eisner, Sherman et al. 1994; Filep, Baron et al. 1996; Yamashita, Uchida et al. 1997). Cellular-generated small molecules, such as nitrogen oxides and oxygen radicals, have the potential to cause significant genetic and cellular damage (Ames and Shigenaga 1992; Keefer and Wink 1996), yet they are also key cellular signaling molecules (Lane and Gross 1999), which may either protect against or enhance the development of malignancy.

The sources of increased oxidative stress derive from the increased burden of oxidants present in cigarette smoke, or from the increased amounts of reactive oxygen species released from leukocytes into the airspaces and blood (MacNee 2001). Oxidative processes have fundamental roles in inflammation through redox-sensitive transcription factors, such as NF-kappaB and AP-1, that regulate the genes for proinflammatory mediators and through protective mechanisms, such as antioxidant gene expression. In addition to the oxidative stress produced by cigarette smoking, dietary deficiency in antioxidants is shown to be related to the development of airflow limitation (MacNee 2001). Hence dietary supplementation may be a beneficial therapeutic intervention in this condition.

A common oxidative damage to DNA is the highly mutagenic 7,8-dihydro-8-oxoguanine adduct, which can be repaired by 8-oxoguanine glycosylase I (OGG1). The human homologue of the yeast OGG1 gene, hOGG1, has been cloned, and its genetic structure has been determined. Several polymorphisms in the hOGG1 gene were detected in humans. The distributions of this polymorphism varies for different populations, and among the different polymorphisms, the Ser-Cys polymorphism at codon 326 has been been suggested to reduce the activity of the enzyme. Because many environmental carcinogens produce 8-hydroxyguanine residue and mismatching to this modified base potentially causes oncogenic mutations, the capacity to repair these lesions can be involved in cancer susceptibility in human beings. Published data suggest that the presence of two hOGG1 326Cys alleles confers a 2-fold increased risk of lung cancer (Le Marchand, Donlon et al. 2002).

Although the specific mechanisms by which oxidative stress contributes to the development of carcinogenesis are largely unknown, oxidative DNA damage is thought to play a role in the development of carcinogenesis via at least two different mechanisms. In the first mechanism, genetic alterations induced by oxidants, such as mutations and chromosomal rearrangements, can play a role in the initiation and malignant conversion stages of carcinogenesis (Guyton and Kensler 1993). Most oxidative DNA damage results in a wide range of chromosomal abnormalities, causing a blockage of DNA replication and wide cytotoxicity (Bohr, Taffe et al. 1995). Mutations can occur through misrepair or due to incorrect replication past a damaged site, while chromosomal rearrangements can result from strand breakage misrepair (Halliwell and Aruoma 1991; Bohr, Taffe et al. 1995). These genetic alterations can result in permanent DNA damage and a population of initiated cells that must escape repair processes, overcoming cytotoxicity in order to be carried on to the progeny. The initiation potential of oxidants may be due to their ability to induce DNA base changes in certain oncogenes and tumor suppressor genes, contributing to carcinogenesis (Jackson 1994). Hydroxy radicals have been demonstrated to activate certain oncogenes, such as K-ras and C-Raf-1, respectively, through the induction of DNA point mutations in GC base pairs and N-terminal deletions in these genes (Jackson 1994). Base point mutations in CpG dinucleotides are also frequently found in certain tumor suppressor genes, such as p53 and retinoblastoma, leading to their inactivation (Nigro, Baker et al. 1989; Yandell, Campbell et al. 1989). Furthermore, hydroxy radical exposure of cells that contain mutant or absent p53 resulted in a failure to arrest in G1, reducing their capacity to repair damaged DNA (Jackson 1994). This increase in replication errors can compromise DNA fidelity, predisposing initiated cells to undergo additional oncogene activation and tumor suppressor gene inactivation, ultimately contributing to malignancy (Jackson 1994). Oxidant-induced cytotoxicity may also contribute to the initiation of carcinogenesis by depleting the normal cell population, promoting the clonal expansion of more resistant initiated cells, thus increasing the probability of mutation.

Among various markers of DNA damage, 8-hydroxydeoxyguanosine (8-OHdG), an oxidative adduct form of deoxyguanosine, is considered to be one of the most sensitive (Floyd, Watson et al. 1986). 8-OHdG is induced by several carcinogens and tumor promoters (Floyd 1990; Takeuchi, Nakajima et al. 1994; Shen, Ong et al. 1995) and causes mutation both *in vitro* and *in vivo* (Wood, Dizdaroglu et al. 1990; Cheng, Cahill et al. 1992). 8-OHdG occurs specifically in DNA and appears to be a reasonable marker for oxidative DNA damage (assuming a steady state) because the rate of output of 8-OHdG by repair should balance the rate of input of damage. Toyokuni and co-workers (Toyokuni, Okamoto et al. 1995) reported that human carcinoma cells (breast, lung, liver, kidney, brain, stomach, ovary) have a higher content of 8-OHdG than adjacent non-tumorous tissues. Moreover, investigators have reported a high concentration of 8-OHdG in lung cancer tissues (Inoue, Osaki et al. 1998). They hypothesized that the tumor cells themselves produce ROS spontaneously, which results in an increase of 8-OHdG in DNA. 8-OHdG levels in DNA of leukocytes and the central part of the lung were significantly associated with the number of cigarette smoked (Kasai 1998). An increased level of 8-OHdG was found in peripheral part of the lung from lung cancer patients when compared to non-cancer controls (Inoue, Osaki et al. 1998). Lung cancer patients showed higher levels of urinary 8-OHdG/creatinine than the controls. Furthermore, patients with complete or partial response to chemotherapy showed a significant decrease in urinary 8-OHdG/creatinine while patients with no change or progressive disease showed an increase. Nevertheless, 8-OHDG in blood DNA rather than urinary 8-OHdG might be a better marker of oxidative damage because the latter might reflect the repair process.

Recently, a new group of prostaglandin (PG)-like compounds, known as isoprostanes, has been discovered. 8-F2 isoprostanes (8-epi-PGF2) have been measured as indices of lipid peroxidation in body fluids such as urine, blood, bile (Leo, Aleynik et al. 1997; Pratico, Iuliano et al. 1998) pericardial (Mallat, Philip et al. 1998) and cerebrospinal fluid (Pratico et al. 1998; Montine, Beal et al. 1999), and lung condensate (Montuschi, Ciabattoni et al. 1998). Isoprostanes are formed from arachidonic acid *in vivo*, not by involvement of oxidizing enzymes, such as cyclooxygenase, but by free radical-catalyzed peroxidation. Free F2-isoprostanes are released from the esterified stores on the cell surface by the action of phospholipases (Ohashi and Yoshikawa 2000). Therefore, the amount of isoprostanes should reflect the levels of oxidant stress and free radicals *in vivo* (Morrow, Minton et al. 1994; Awad, Roberts et al. 1996).

Cell Proliferation and Lung Carcinogenesis

Lung cancer, like many other epithelial malignancies, is thought to be the outcome of genetic and epigenetic changes that result in a constellation of phenotypic abnormalities in bronchial epithelium. These include morphologic epithelial dysplasia, angiogenesis, increased proliferative rate, and changes in expression of cell surface proteins, particularly overexpression of epidermal growth factor receptor (EGFR) family proteins. EGFR overexpression is pronounced in virtually all squamous carcinomas and is also found in 65% of large cell and adenocarcinomas. Overexpression of EGFR is one of the earliest and most consistent abnormalities in bronchial epithelium of high-risk smokers. It is present at the stage of basal cell hyperplasia and persists through squamous metaplasia, dysplasia, and carcinoma in situ (Khuri, Lee et al. 2001).

The expression level of the proliferating cell nuclear antigen (PCNA) was associated with the histological grade of the bronchial biopsy site. Intervention with 13-cic-retinoic acid augmented the decreased proliferation status and decreased metaplasia index associated with discontinuation of smoking but had little impact on the proliferation status of the bronchial epithelium in those who continued to smoke (Khuri, Lee et al. 2001). The level of PCNA expression in the bronchial epithelium correlated with the degree of EGFR expression, which is also found to be increased in metaplastic lesions (Hommura, Dosaka-Akita et al. 2000). Another proliferation marker, Ki-67, has been shown to be increased in lung tumors and to provide some prognostic information (Nguyen, Jing et al. 2000; Hittleman 2002). In patients who had stopped smoking, the Ki-67 labeling index dropped significantly within a year and continued to drop thereafter. However, abnormal levels of Ki-67 labeling are detectable for more than 20 years after smoking cessation (Lee, Chaudhary et al. 1998). The Activator Protein-1 (AP-1) complex is a dimeric transcription factor composed of fos and jun proteins that regulates cellular growth and differentiation. Lee and co-workers (Lee, Chaudhary et al. 1998) demonstrated a reduction in basal AP-1 transcriptional activity was associated with the malignant transformation of human bronchial epithelial cells that was, in part, a consequence of decreased c-fos expression.

Apoptosis and Lung Carcinogenesis

Use of biomarkers to predict induction of apoptosis allows identification of biological signs that may indicate increased risk for disease. In cells undergoing apoptosis, the release of cytochrome c from the mitochondria to the cytoplasm and the activation of caspase-3, a key enzyme in the execution stage of apoptotic pathway, have been studied as biomarkers of apoptosis (Koomagi and Volm 2000). A significant correlation was observed between the expression of caspase-3, survival and metastasis in 135 non-small cell lung carcinomas. Caspase-3 expression correlated with a lower incidence of lymph node involvement ($p = 0.0007$). The median survival was longer for patients with caspase-3-positive carcinomas than for those with caspase-3-negative tumors (Chen, Sato et al. 1999).

Apoptosis is a highly programmed process regulated by many genes, including Bcl-2 family genes (Wang, Zhou et al. 2000). The Bcl-2 proto-oncogene, an indirect measure of apoptosis, is known to promote cell survival and to act as a negative regulator of the biological cascade that leads to apoptosis and to provide a growth advantage eventually leading to neoplastic transformation (Lee, Chaudhary et al. 1998). The mRNA expressions of the Bcl-2 gene were studied in a series of 137 pulmonary tissues collected at various sites and with different properties. According to the observations on benign lesions, non-cancer tissues distant from tumor, para-tumor tissues and cancer tissues, there was a trend toward increased Bcl-2 mRNA expression. Among them, Bcl-2 mRNA expression in lung cancer tissues was significantly increased as compared to benign lesions and tissues distant from tumor ($p < 0.01$) (Yang, Yang et al. 1998). Expression of the Bcl-2 protein has been reported for a variety of tumors, including the lung. The overexpression of Bcl-2 is thought to be early event in carcinogenesis, allowing cells with DNA damage to escape the normal mechanisms of apoptotic cell death. Conversely, the loss of Bcl-2 expression may be relatively late in the pathogenesis of lung cancer (Wang, Zhou et al. 2000).

Genetic Factors in Carcinogen Metabolism

Cigarette smoke contains numerous compounds that generate reactive oxygen species (ROS) that can damage DNA directly or indirectly via inflammatory processes (Frenkel, Donahue et al. 1988; Wei, Wei et al. 1993; Hecht 1999). Oxidants, either present in cigarette smoke and/or formed in the lungs of smokers, may trigger oxidative damage to DNA and cellular components, contributing to carcinogenesis. Free radical attack upon DNA generates a multiplicity of DNA damage, including modified bases. Some of these modifications have considerable potential to damage the integrity of the genome.

DNA damage was proposed as a useful parameter for assessing the genotoxic properties of environmental pollutants. The correlation between exposure to carcinogenic substance and the level of DNA damage is essential. ROS are highly biologically active chemicals. They may interact with DNA and damage its structure. Because the human population is biologically diverse and genetically heterogeneous, it is not surprising that differences in susceptibility to disease among individuals with or without exposure to environmental agents exist. Individuals vary greatly in their susceptibility to disease. This is true of adults and children. The etiologies of many diseases of childhood are due to a combination of factors, including genetic susceptibility and environmental exposures during vulnerable periods of development. Genes regulate cellular growth and development, DNA replication and repair, the metabolism of endogenous agents in the body, and the metabolism and excretion of exogenous agents that the body comes in contact with in the environment. This regulation varies over the life span, contributing to the cellular consequences of the environmental exposures.

DNA Hypermethylation and Lung Carcinogenesis

Methylation is the main epigenetic modification in humans; changes in methylation patterns play an important role in tumorigenesis. Aberrant promoter methylation has been described for several genes in various malignant diseases including lung cancer (Esteller, Corn et al. 1998; Esteller, Hamilton et al. 1999; Esteller, Tortola et al. 2000). In a large study of primary resected non-small cell lung cancer (NSCLC), a high frequency of methylation was observed, demonstrating that methylation may be the most common mechanism to inactivate cancer-related protection genes in NSCLC (Zoch-bauer-Muller, Fong et al. 2001).

The tumor suppressor gene (p16), DNA repair gene (MGMT), and genes related to metastasis and invasion (DAP-K and TIMP3) are well characterized. Each possess a CpG island in the 5′ region which is unmethylated in normal tissues, as expected for a typical CpG island (Esteller, Corn et al. 2001). Methylation of p16, MGMT, DAP-K and TIMP3 has been described in lung cancer cell lines and a small number of primary lung tumors (Esteller, Hamilton et al. 1999). Furthermore, when these CpG islands were hypermethylated in cancer cells, expression of the corresponding gene was silenced. The silencing was partially reversed by demethylation of the promoter region (Esteller, Hamilton et al. 1999). Thus, chemopreventive agents that have the ability to demethylate these genes may be able to restore their function and help slow or prevent carcinogenesis.

Belinsky and co-workers (Belinsky, Nikula et al. 1998) were the first to demonstrate that inactivation of the p16 tumor suppressor gene by aberrant methylation is an early and likely critical event in the development of NSCLC. Palmisano et al. (Palmisano, Divine et al. 2000) corroborated Belinsky's work, reporting that p16 hypermethylation was detected in 60–80% of squamous cell carcinoma (SCC), and 30–45% of adenocarcinomas. Several other studies have shown that inactivation of the p16 tumor gene is common in lung cancer (Belinsky, Nikula et al. 1998; Kersting, Friedl et al. 2000) and that methylation of the p16 gene is clearly associated with loss of gene transcription in lung tumors (Belinsky, Nikula et al. 1998). P16 methylation has also been observed in the precursor lesions of SCC, including basal cell hyperplasia, squamous metaplasia and carcinoma in situ of the lung. The frequency of p16 methylation increased from the lowest to highest-grade precursor lesions to SCC (Kersting, Friedl et al. 2000). The high frequency of p16 methylation in alveolar hyperplasias and adenomas – precursor lesions with an extremely high conversion rate to adenocarcinomas in NNK-treated rats – indicates that p16 hypermethylation is an early molecular event in lung carcinogenesis and thus a sound candidate biomarker for lung chemoprevention trials (Belinsky, Nikula et al. 1998).

The DNA repair protein, O^6-methylguanine DNA methyltransferase (MGMT), is a major determinant of susceptibility to methylating carcinogens and of tumor resistance to chloroethylating drugs (Danam, Qian et al. 1999). MGMT protein expression is decreased in some human tumors, including lung, with respect to their normal tissue counterparts. Loss of expression is rarely due to deletion, mutation or rearrangement of the MGMT gene. However, the methylation of discrete regions of the CpG island of MGMT is associated with the silencing of the gene in cell lines (Esteller, Hamilton et al. 1999). Aberrant methylation of MGMT was detected in 21–29% of NSCLCs (Esteller, Hamilton et al. 1999; Esteller, Corn et al. 2001). Palmisano et al. (Palmisano, Divine et al. 2000) detected MGMT methylation in epithelial cells shed from the airways in persons at risk for lung cancer, and reported a frequency of 16% in samples investigated. In contrast, methylation of MGMT has not been observed in normal lung tissue (Esteller, Hamilton et al. 1999).

Death-associated protein (DAP) kinase, also known as DAP-2, is a novel serine/ threonine kinase required for interferon gamma-induced apoptotic cell death (Tang, Khuri et al. 2000) that may function as a metastasis suppressor. Expression of DAP kinase was repressed in human cancers by hypermethylation in the promoter CpG region (Esteller, Sanchez-Cespedes et al. 1999; Tang, Khuri et al. 2000). Esteller (Esteller, Sanchez-Cespedes et al. 1999) studied primary NSCLC samples from 22 patients and found that DAP kinase was hypermethylated in five (23%) of the 22 tumors. In 135 lung tumors, 44% of the tumors were hypermethylated at the CpG sites of the DAP kinase gene; DAP kinase methylation was negatively associated with the expression of DAP kinase in lung cancer cell lines and demethylation restored DAP kinase gene expression (Tang, Khuri et al. 2000).

DNA repair plays a critical role in protecting the genome of the cell from insults of cancer-causing agents, such as those found in tobacco smoke. Reduced DNA repair capacity, therefore, can increase the susceptibility to smoking-related cancers. Recently, three coding polymorphisms in X-ray cross-complementing group 1 (XRCC1) DNA repair gene have been identified, and it is possible that these polymorphisms may affect DNA repair capacity and thus modulate cancer susceptibility. Polymorphisms of XRCC1 appear to influence risk of lung cancer and may modify risk attributable to environmental exposures. A recent published study suggests that XRCC1 codon 399 polymorphism may be an important genetic determinant of SCC of the lung in persons with lower amounts of cigarette use (Park, Lee et al. 2002).

Risk Factors for Lung Cancer

Tobacco Products

Cigarette smoking, the primary risk factor for lung cancer, accounts for approximately 90% of cases in men and 70% of cases in women (Shopland 1995; Jemal, Chu et al. 2001). A dose-response relationship between daily tobacco smoking and risk of death from lung cancer has been established in prospective analyses, with the relative risk of lung cancer mortality ranging from 4.6 to 7.8 in users of less than 10 cigarettes per day, compared to never smokers. This relative risk increases to more than 20 in individuals who smoke 25 to 40 or more cigarettes per day (Hammond 1966; Rogot and Murray 1980).

Cigarette smoking may result in chronic bronchitis, chronic obstructive pulmonary disease, and/or lung cancer. In the early 1960s, Passey (Passey 1962) hypothesized that it was the irritating properties of tobacco smoke, resulting in chronic bronchitis and inflammatory destruction of lung tissue, that was of pathogenic significance in the causal pathway of lung cancer, rather than any direct action by volatile and particulate carcinogens in tobacco smoke. The experiments of Kuschner (Kuschner 1968), however, suggested an alternative explanation; namely, that bronchial and bronchiolar inflammation, accompanied by reactive proliferation, squamous metaplasia, and dysplasia in basal epithelial cells, provided a cocarcinogenic mechanism for neoplastic cell transformation upon exposure to polycyclic aromatic hydrocarbons.

Currently, 40–50 million Americans are former smokers (Resnicow, Kabat et al. 1991). The risk of former smokers developing lung cancer actually increases during the first 3–5 years after smoking cessation; many smokers stop because they are symptomatic and may already have the disease (Hammond 1966). Eventually and gradually, over at least a decade or more, the risk of lung cancer for these individuals will come to approach that of never smokers (Halpern, Gillespie et al. 1993). In several studies, the risk of lung cancer in former smokers had not reached that of lifetime never smokers, even after 20 years since cessation (Khuri 1995; Burns 2000; Ebbert, Yang et al. 2003).

Current and former smokers older than 40 years with a smoking history of 20 pack-years or more and airflow obstruction, defined as a forced expiratory volume in one second/forced vital capacity (FEV1/FVC) of 70% or less and a FEV1 lower than 70%, are at high risk of developing lung cancer (Kennedy, Proudfoot et al. 1996). Patients with chronic obstructive pulmonary disease (COPD) have a four- to six-fold increased risk of lung cancer independent of their smoking history. The chronic inflammation associated with COPD appears to enhance lung cancer risk. At least ten cohort studies have reported that COPD is an independent predictor of lung cancer risk (Tenkanen, Hakulinen et al. 1987; Tockman, Anthonisen et al. 1987).

Reactive oxygen species (ROS) play an important role in toxicity of environmental chemicals. During passive smoking, the body is attacked by an excess of free radicals inducing oxidative stress. In non-smokers, even a short period of passive smoking breaks down serum antioxidant defense and accelerates lipid peroxidation (Zhang, Jiang et al. 2001). Tobacco smoke contains many carcinogens that exert their biological effects through interaction of reactive intermediates with DNA to form DNA adducts. The same electrophilic species also react with cellular proteins. The effects of smoking are evident by the detection of elevated levels of carcinogen-DNA adducts in many human tissues and of carcinogen-protein adducts in blood. Components of tobacco smoke also induce oxidative DNA damage (Phillips 2002). Exposure to environmental tobacco smoke resulted in a statistically significant increase of 63% of the oxidative DNA mutagen, 8-OHdG, in the blood of exposed subjects. This oxidative DNA damage has been linked to an increased risk of developing several degenerative chronic diseases, including coronary heart disease and cancer (Howard, Briggs et al. 1998). Significant effects on oxygen free radical production were found for gender and ethnicity, with men having greater values than women ($p < 0.001$) and white subjects having greater values than black subjects ($p = 0.025$).

Environmental tobacco smoke (ETS) constitutes both a residential and an occupational exposure. Animal data show that ROS introduced by passive smoking may contribute to K-ras activation as an initiator of a tumor model, possibly through the oxygen-induced DNA damage, and may also contribute to an initial activation and the subsequent down-regulation of protein kinase as a promoter (Maehira, Zaha et al. 2000). Rats exposed to sidestream cigarette smoke, the major component of ETS, showed significant increases in the accumulation of 8-OHdG in lung DNA (Maehira, Zaha et al. 2000; Izzotti, Balansky et al. 2001). Similarly, exposure to sidestream cigarette smoke significantly increased oxidative stress in mouse heart, liver, and lung tissues. In all three tissues, ETS increased the presence of 8-OHdG above the control levels (Howard, Briggs et al. 1998). The assessment of pathological effects produced by ETS in humans is controversial in epidemiological studies. However, based on a collection of studies, there is an association between exposure to ETS and lung cancer, with a relative risk around 1.2 (Boffetta and Nyberg 2003).

Environmental Exposures

Occupational exposures have been estimated to account for up to 20% of all lung cancer diagnoses. Many studies that comprise the body of literature on occupational exposure and lung cancer risk have been based on exposures in male smokers, thus introducing confounders in the analysis of pure exposure risk. Little data is available on the effect of occupational exposures in women and nonsmokers. Strong evidence exists for asbestos, ETS, radon prodigy and arsenic as occupational carcinogens in nonsmokers (Neuberger and Field 2003). Nonetheless, the International Agency for Research on Cancer (IARC) maintains a much longer list of workplace-related carcinogens, including both chemical and physical agents, implicated in the risk of lung cancer.

Because women have only recently been assimilated into many occupational environments formerly reserved for men, the role of occupational exposures has been estimated to be lower than that for men, around 5%. A more current analysis of occupational risk of lung cancer for women is needed so that a more accurate risk assessment for women in the workplace can be generated.

Worldwide, an increased risk of lung cancer independent of tobacco exposure has been documented for exposure to environmental carcinogens, a term that includes both outdoor and indoor air pollutants as well as contaminants of soil and drinking water. Persons are exposed to environmental carcinogens from both natural and man-made exposures, and exposures occur in both residential and occupational settings. While there appear overall to be relatively small relative risks of cancer following environmental exposure, the impact on worldwide health is great, given a high prevalence of exposures to these carcinogens.

The naturally-occurring radioactive gas radon and its radioactive progeny are sources of exposure to inhaled radioactive substances. Radon exposure occurs in occupational settings such as uranium and tin mines, and in homes built on radon-containing soil. Studies have consistently shown an excess of lung cancer risk in radon-exposed populations. Studies of radon-exposed underground miners have predicted that residential radon would be an important cause of non-tobacco related lung cancer; in fact, residential exposure to radioactive radon and its decay products are estimated to account for 10–12% of all lung cancer deaths in the U.S. (Lubin and Steindorf 1995). Radon mitigation programs for homes and improved workplace measures to mitigate exposure to radon and other radioactive elements will likely impact favorably on lung cancer risk.

A high incidence of lung cancer has been reported in some Asian women who have a traditionally low prevalence of cigarette smoking. This elevated risk of lung cancer has been related to indoor pollution from cooking and heating sources with chronic exposure to non-vented, potentially mutagenic cooking oil fumes and the carcinogenic metabolic products of heterocyclic amines aerosolized during the cooking of meat at high temperatures (He, Chen et al. 1991; Seow, Zhao et al. 2001).

Outdoor air pollution is composed of complex mixtures of chemical compounds, radionuclides, gas and particulate combustion products and fibers, a number of which are known carcinogens. Major sources of air pollution include industrial and automobile-related fossil fuel combustion, diesel exhaust, power plants and residential sources of emissions. Air pollution as a contributor to the risk of lung cancer has been supported by occupational studies of workers exposed to fossil fuel combustion products. After adjusting for smoking history, exposed workers had a two-fold risk of lung cancer relative to non-exposed workers (Doll 1972). Other studies have looked at lung cancer occurrence in populations with differential exposure to air pollutants (e.g., rural versus urban). Other studies have measured tissue biomarkers of exposure to respiratory carcinogens such as levels of benzo(a)pyrene, carcinogenic DNA adducts, chromosomal abnormalities and other measures of genetic damage in relation to exposure to air pollutants. Epidemiologic studies of lung cancer risk related to air pollution must account for a number of variables that are often difficult to quantify, such as concentration of pollutant carcinogens, length of exposure, geographic variables, genetic variables and individual tobacco smoke-related exposure within the study population. Nevertheless, there is a large body of data that supports a role for air pollution contributing independently to the risk of lung cancer, although estimates of lung cancer attributed to air pollutants range from less than 1% (Doll 1978) to 12% (Karch 1981). The causal relationship between air pollution and lung cancer risk remains of great public health import, given the migration of populations from rural into more urban settings, and the increasing expanding populations worldwide residing in highly polluted cities in many developing parts of the world (Cohen 2000).

Family History

There appears to be a small contribution to an individual's risk of developing lung cancer from family history, suggesting a role for genetic susceptibility that is independent of tobacco exposure. A number of studies have shown an increased risk of cancers in relatives of persons with lung cancer. A landmark study reported in 1963 showed suggestive evidence of familial aggregation of lung cancer specifically, with an excess of lung cancer mortality reported in relatives of 270 lung cancer probands (Tokuhata and Lilienfeld 1963). A number of more recent studies have also found an increase in both lung cancer and total cancers in the first-degree relatives of persons with lung cancer; these familial aggregations of cancer risk have been seen in both smoking *and nonsmoking* persons with lung cancer. In an investigation of family cancer history as a risk factor for lung cancer in nonsmoking men and women, a population-based case-control study showed an excess of certain cancers, especially lung, aerodigestive tract and female breast cancer in first-degree relatives of non-smoking cases (Mayne, Buenconsejo et al. 1999).

Lung cancer risk in families is influenced by familial aggregation of smoking habits; this variable is an important potential confounder of studies investigating pure genetic risk related to lung cancer. A recently reported large case-control study of persons with lung cancer and their first degree relatives investigated tobacco exposure-specific familial risk of lung and other smoking-related cancers. Eight hundred and six persons with lung cancer and 663 controls matched to the cases on age (within 5 years), sex, ethnicity, and smoking history addressed whether there was an excess of cancer in relatives of persons with lung cancer (Etzel, Amos et al. 2003). Cancer family history data were available for 6,430 first-degree relatives of the cases and 4,936 first-degree relatives of the controls. Adjustment was made for smoking history and age of lung cancer cases and their relatives. In first degree relatives of lung cancer cases, there was an significantly increased risk of smoking-related cancers (defined as cancers of the lung, bladder, head and neck, kidney, and pancreas) and lung cancer specifically. Relative risks were 1.28 for smoking-related cancer and 1.33 for lung cancer. Additionally, there was a 7-fold increased risk of breast cancer among daughters of lung cancer cases (Etzel, Amos et al. 2003). These data suggest that genetic factors modulate lung cancer risk independent of tobacco exposure, and that a better understanding of these factors may influence the way in which the health of families of lung cancer patients are monitored.

Genetic Susceptibility

Although smoking is the major risk factor for lung cancer, other factors, such as nutrition or genetic predisposition, may be involved. Genetic susceptibility to environmental carcinogens is thought to be attributable to genetic polymorphisms in metabolism enzymes, which have been found to substantially alter the activation and elimination of carcinogens (Smith, Smith et al. 1994).

Glutathione S-transferases (GSTs) constitute a complex multigene family that, in most instances, deactivates carcinogens, environmental pollutants, drugs, and a broad spectrum of other xenobiotics through conjugation with glutathione (Hayes and Pulford 1995). Therefore, GST induction may improve detoxification and excretion of potentially harmful compounds. Polymorphic variants in GSTs, μ (GSTM1), θ (GSTT1), and π (GSTP) have been studied extensively in relation to cancer etiology. Complete gene deletions in GSTM1 and GSTT1 and single nucleotide polymorphism in GSTP may result in a significant change in the function of the enzymes.

Both GSTM1 and GSTT1 are polymorphic, and the null alleles of these genes have deletions of the entire protein-coding region (Seidegard, Vorachek et al. 1988; Pemble, Schroeder et al. 1994). The GSTM1-null and GSTT1-null alleles are transmitted as autosomal recessive, with the phenotypic absence of the isozymes resulting from inheritance of a null allele from both parents. The prevalence of GSTM1-null and GSTT1-null genotypes differ markedly across ethnic and racial groups (GSTM1, 30–60%; GSTT1, 9–64%) (Bell, Taylor et al. 1993; Katoh, Nagata et al. 1996). GSTM1-null and GSTT1-null genotypes have been associated with increased risk of cancer in a number of studies, and it is hypothesized that individuals with putative high-risk genotypes suffer higher levels of carcinogen-induced genotoxic damage (Bell, Taylor et al. 1993; Rebbeck 1997).

Among the several classes of GSTs, GSTμ enzyme activity has been found to vary substantially between individuals because of an inherited deletion of the GSTM1 gene. GSTM1 is involved in the detoxification of tobacco smoke carcinogens including the polyaromatic hydrocarbons (PAHs) such as benzo(a)pyrene (Ketterer, Harris et al. 1992). Up to 50% of Caucasians have no GSTM1 enzyme because of the homozygous deletion of the gene (Seidegard, Vorachek et al. 1988), referred to as the GSTM1-null genotype. Individuals with the null genotype are unable to detoxify PAHs through this particular glutathione pathway. Although several epidemiological studies have found the null genotype to be associated with increased risk for the development of lung and other tobacco-related cancers (Hirvonen, Husgafvel-Pursiainen et al. 1993; Kihara and Noda 1994; Saarikoski, Voho et al. 1998), the findings in other studies are conflicting, and this association remains controversial (Zhong, Howie et al. 1991; Brockmoller, Kerb et al. 1993).

Screening for Early Detection

The ideal method for decreasing the burden of lung cancer in the near and distant future is through primary prevention (i.e., decreasing the initiation of cigarette use), especially in children and adolescents. Nevertheless, there are more than 40 million current smokers who are at risk for the development of lung cancer, only some of whom will successfully stop smoking. Additionally, there are 40–50 million former smokers in the United States who remain at an increased risk for the development of lung cancer even decades after quitting smoking (Hammond 1966; Doll and Peto 1976; Rogot and Murray 1980). Therefore, the development of effective lung cancer screening programs have been the focus of much interest in scientific research and public health domains. Early strategies for screening for lung cancer included the use of chest x-rays with or without cytologic analysis of sputum. More recent strategies have looked at the use of more sophisticated chest imaging and the incorporation of molecular biomarkers of lung carcinogenesis.

Preneoplasia and Intraepithelial Neoplasia

Risk of lung cancer among long-term heavy smokers continues even years after stopping smoking and is highest in smokers with chronic obstructive pulmonary disease. The prevalence of pre-invasive lesions did not change substantially for more than 10 years after cessation of smoking. Lung function was associated with the prevalence of pre-invasive lesions (Lam, leRiche et al. 1999). Numerous recent studies have indicated that lung cancer is not the result of a sudden transforming event in the bronchial epithelium but a multi-step process in which gradually accruing sequential genetic and cellular changes result in the formation of an invasive (i.e., malignant) tumor. Mucosal changes in the large airways that may precede or accompany invasive squamous carcinoma include hyperplasia, metaplasia, dysplasia, and carcinoma in situ (CIS) (Franklin 2000). Hyperplasia of the bronchial epithelium and squamous metaplasia are generally considered reversible and are believed to be reactive changes in the bronchial epithelium, as opposed to true preneoplastic changes (Wistuba, Behrens et al. 1999). In contrast, moderate-to-severe dysplasia and CIS lesions seldom regress after smoking cessation (Lam, leRiche et al. 1999) and frequently precede squamous cell carcinoma of the lung (Colby 1999). Advances in the understanding of lung cancer biology have led to observations that specific genetic changes occur in pre-malignant dysplasia (Kennedy, Proudfoot et al. 1996).

Standard Chest x-Rays and Sputum Cytology

Lung cancer screening programs were first initiated in the early 1950s, around the time that the link between tobacco exposure and lung cancer was reported in the scientific literature. Since then, 10 prospective trials have been designed and implemented that have utilized chest x-rays or sputum cytology in high-risk populations. Of note, nine of these trials did not include women. Three studies sponsored by the National Cancer Institute in the 1970s utilized a randomized trial design. Two of these studies, the Memorial-Sloan Kettering Study and the Johns Hopkins Lung Project, looked at the addition of cytology to chest x-ray screening (Melamed, Flehinger et al. 1984; Tockman 1986). While no benefit in terms of reduction of lung cancer mortality (considered the optimal endpoint due to absence of bias of screening efficacy) was gained with the addition of cytology, there were improvements in resectability and 5-year survival in the study population as compared to the Surveillance, Epidemiology and End Results database. The Mayo Lung Project (Fontana, Sanderson et al. 1984) evaluated chest x-ray plus cytology on an intensive schedule as compared to a control group, a portion of whom did receive chest x-rays on an annual or less frequent schedule outside of the study setting. There was no significant reduction in lung cancer mortality in the screened arm, and therefore the trial was originally deemed a negative screening trial. However, more recent analysis has shown that survival as an endpoint, which was improved in the screened arm, was not subject to biases (length, lead-time and overdiagnosis); as such, the reanalysis argues for a positive effect for this screening intervention (Strauss, Gleason et al. 1997).

Helical Computed Tomography

A step forward in the development of lung cancer screening technologies is the low-dose helical or spiral computed tomography (CT) scan. Developed in the 1990s, this scan allows for x-ray scanning of the entire chest in approximately 15–25 seconds. Images approximating a three-dimensional model of the lungs are generated via a computer program. Additionally, this technology employs a low dose of radiation and eliminates use of an intravenous contrast material, thus making it safer than the traditional high resolution contrasted CT scan. Limitations of this technology include a decreased sensitivity for detecting imaging abnormalities in the central regions of the lung, where more squamous cell lung cancers are located, and in the soft tissues of the middle of the thorax, where lymph nodes that may be involved by metastatic lung cancer are detected. Another potential limitation in the utilization of CT imaging in populations at risk for lung cancer is the detection of benign abnormalities, which may provoke unwarranted invasive and costly diagnostic procedures, such as biopsy.

A landmark study of the use of helical CT imaging in the screening of persons at risk for lung cancer has yielded important new data in lung cancer screening and early detection. The New York Early Lung Cancer Project (ELCAP) evaluated the usefulness of helical low-dose CT imaging in finding early stage lung cancers (Henschke, McCauley et al. 1999). The ELCAP Study evaluated a non-randomized cohort of 1,000 smokers over the age of 60 and with a history of significant cigarette use with both annual chest x-rays and low-dose helical CT scans. The main outcome measure was the frequency of detection of non-calcified lung nodules by imaging technique. The superiority of helical low-dose CT scanning over chest x-ray in the detection of non-calcified lung nodules (found in 233 persons by CT compared with 68 persons by chest x-ray). By an algorithm that included the use of an additional high resolution CT scan to better assess the nodules and by assigning either a close follow-up program with re-imaging of the nodules versus proceeding directly to biopsy, spiral CT imaging detected close to six times more malignant nodules than did chest x-ray (2.3

versus 0.4%). Of 28 nodules biopsied, 27 were malignant; thus only one biopsy was performed for a benign nodule. Eighty percent of those lung cancers found by helical CT imaging were Stage I cancers (less than 3 cm in greatest dimension, without lymph node involvement or distant metastases), which have the highest potential for cure via surgical resection or radiation therapy. In general, chest x-ray detected the larger tumors. Of the 27 nodules detected by CT imaging, 26 were resectable. Importantly, the cost effectiveness of this strategy thus far has been impressive. The cost of a screening program consisting of a single baseline low-dose CT scan in a fit person at least 60 years of age with at least 10 pack-years of smoking was only $2,500 per year of life saved (Wisnivesky, Mushlin et al. 2003). The cost of treating an early stage lung cancer is at least half the cost of treating an advanced stage lung cancer.

National Early Detection Initiatives

The provocative findings of the ELCAP study, in concert with re-analyses of earlier chest x-ray-based screening studies, have prompted a large screening initiative sponsored by the National Cancer Institute and the American Cancer Society. Initiated in 2002, the National Lung Screening Trial (NSLT), has reached its accrual goal of 50,000 current or former smokers who are randomized to receive annual screening with either spiral CT or traditional x-ray imaging for three years, followed by annual monitoring of participant health status through 2009. Collection of relevant biologic samples (blood, urine and sputum) for use with diagnostic markers of lung cancer currently in development, as well as biomarkers of the carcinogenic pathway, is being conducted in a subset of participants (NCI 2004).

While these early data are suggestive of a benefit, in terms of decreasing the morbidity and mortality from lung cancer through screening for early lung cancers with CT imaging, there remains no clear consensus position with regard to use of imaging technologies for lung cancer screening; therefore, at this time, screening with CT or other imaging in current and former smokers is not considered a standard health care practice.

Chemoprevention

Prevention of lung cancer altogether is preferable to screening for early detection. The most effective means of preventing lung cancer is avoidance or elimination of tobacco use. Although the prevalence of cigarette smoking in the U.S. has declined, the age-adjusted mortality of lung cancer has not shown a comparable decrease, partly due to the increased risk of lung cancer in former smokers. A central concept of chemoprevention is that intervention is likely to be most effective during identifiable premalignant steps of carcinogenesis. Lung cancer is an important public health concern in the U.S. and the need for an effective chemopreventive agent against this cancer is tremendous.

At present, approximately 25% of the U.S. adult population smokes. Primary prevention, through the reduction of cigarette smoking, is likely to be the most successful strategy in reducing lung cancer incidence. However, even if all current smokers in the U.S. quit today, more than a million cases of lung cancer would develop over the next decade because of cigarettes already smoked (Wagner and Ruckdeschel 1995). Therefore, a strategy to prevent cancers before they develop is a critical element in reducing the burden of lung cancer.

Chemopreventive Agents Under Investigation

There has been explosive growth in the understanding of the molecular and genetic mechanisms underlying the carcinogenic process. This has allowed for identification of critical genes that may be mutated, silenced epigenetically, or overexpressed in preneoplastic and neoplastic tissue; additionally, key proteins, growth receptors and cellular pathways have been identified that may be aberrantly expressed in the carcinogenic pathway and/or invasive cancer. Consequently, agents have been rationally selected or designed to target these critical elements. Given that molecular targets relevant to cancer are often not highly nor aberrantly expressed in normal tissue, targeted agents often have good safety profiles for normal tissues and many agents currently in development have good oral availability. Listed in Table 2 are a number of molecular targets that been identified in the molecular pathogenesis of lung cancer; additionally, some representative targeted chemopreventive agents currently in development are listed. While this table lists agents that have been developed synthetically, the target mole-

Table 2. Chemopreventive agents under investigation for the prevention of lung cancer

Molecular target/pathway	Proposed role(s) in lung carcinogenesis	Targeted chemopreventive agent: Class (Representative agents)
Cyclooxygenase-2 (COX-2)	Product of arachidonic acid metabolism involved in tumor promotion-related events including cellular hyperproliferation, inhibition of pro-grammed cell death (anti-apoptosis), new blood vessel formation (angiogenesis), inhibition of immune surveillance (Gridelli, Maion et al. 2000; Marks, Muller-Decker, et al. 2000)	Non-selective prostaglandin inhibitors (NSAIDs) Selective COX-2 inhibitors (Celebrex^{TM})
Lipoxygenases	Enzyme products of arachidonic acid metabolism involved in growth-related signal transduction (Cuendet and Pezzuto 2000)	5-, 8- and 12-lipoxygenase inhibitors
Ras protein farnesylation	The Ras protooncogene protein product requires farnesylation or related enzyme modification in order to relay signals for cell growth, differentiation, proliferation and survival. Mutated Ras is common in cancer and is associated with tumorigenesis. Other key proteins require farnesylation for function as well (Hahn, Bernhard, et al. 2001; Sebti 2003)	Farnesyl transferase inhibitors (Lonafarnib^{TM}, Zarnestra^{TM})
Cyclin D1	Regulatory molecule involved in cell cycle regulation; frequent aberrant expression of cyclin D1 resulting in unregulated cellular growth (Petty, Dragnev, et al. 2003)	Non-selective retinoids: all-trans-retinoic acid (ATRA); retinoid receptor selective agonists: (RAR) beta and retinoid X receptor (RXR) agonists
Epidermal Growth Factor Receptor (EGFR)	Cell transmembrane receptor; activation by growth factors causes signal transduction involved in tumor cell proliferation, anti-apoptosis, angiogenesis, and metastatic potential (Grandis and Sok 2004; Yano, Kondo, et al. 2003)	EGFR inhibitors: Monoclonal antibodies (Erbitux®), tyrosine kinase oral inhibitors (Iressa^{TM}, Tarceva^{TM})

cules or pathways have also been identified as targets of natural agents, such as botanicals and phytonutrients, that are being actively developed for lung cancer chemoprevention.

Various histological changes in the bronchial epithelium have been reported in association with chronic smoking and lung cancer. Furthermore, molecular changes have been found not only in the lungs of patients with lung cancer, but also in the lungs of current and former smokers without lung cancer. These observations are consistent with the multi-step model of carcinogenesis and "field cancerization" process, whereby the whole region is repeatedly exposed to carcinogenic damage (tobacco smoke) and is at risk for developing multiple, separate, clonally unrelated foci of neoplasia. The widespread aneuploidy that occurs throughout the respiratory tree of smokers supports this theory. However, the presence of the same somatic p53 point mutation at widely dispersed preneoplastic lesions in a smoker without invasive lung cancer indicates that expansion of a single progenitor clone may spread throughout the respiratory tree. These molecular alterations might thus be important targets for use in the early detection of lung cancer and for use as surrogate biomarkers in the follow up of chemoprevention studies.

However, at present, no biomarker of lung carcinogenesis has been fully validated in a clinical trial using cancer as an endpoint. Because the multi-step process of carcinogenesis can take many years, assessment of clinical chemoprevention trials using cancer incidence as an endpoint requires lengthy follow-up period and large sample sizes. The use of surrogate endpoint biomarkers (SEBs) potentially circumvents these issues by evaluating a biologic event that takes place between a carcinogen or external exposure and the subsequent development of cancer. Because of field cancerization and the fact that the multipath process of carcinogenesis is not regarded as a series of linear steps but rather as overlapping networks, multiple surrogate endpoint markers are preferable to identify potential epigenetic or genetic alterations leading to cancer. In order to be valid, the quantitative degree and pattern of the SEBs should correlate with carcinogenic transformation, respond to the intervention in a timely manner, and should reflect reversible events.

Dietary Supplements

In today's society, human activities and lifestyles generate numerous forms of environmental oxidative stress. Oxidative stress is defined as a process in which the balance between oxidants and antioxidants is shifted toward the oxidant side. This shift can lead to antioxidant depletion and potentially to biological damage if the body has an insufficient reserve to compensate for consumed antioxidants. The "antioxidant hypothesis" proposes that vitamin C, vitamin E, carotenoids, and other antioxidants in fruit and vegetables afford protection against heart disease and cancer by preventing oxidative damage to lipids and to DNA, respectively. Therefore, an increased oxidative stress accompanied by reduced endogenous antioxidant defenses may have a role in the pathogenesis of cancer.

The ability to evaluate any reduction in the primary endpoint of lung cancer requires large studies with large samples and lengthy follow up. The few phase III trials completed, including the Alpha-Tocopherol Beta Carotene Cancer Prevention Study (ATBC) (1994) and the beta-Carotene and Retinol Efficacy Trial (CARET) (Omenn,

Goodman et al. 1996), designed to prevent the occurrence of lung cancer in male current smokers, were negative. The CARET study evaluated beta-carotene and retinol in two populations at risk for lung cancer, including male asbestos workers and female and male cigarette smokers with 20 pack-years or greater history (either current or former smoker within 6 years of cessation). This was a randomized trial utilizing a 2 by 2 factorial design. An increase in lung cancer in the cohort receiving study vitamins was noted, although it did not reach statistical significance. With further analysis, it appeared that the beta-carotene supplemented cohort of current smokers had a 28% increase in rate of lung cancer (Omenn, Goodman et al. 1996).

The surprising detrimental effect of beta-carotene in the CARET trial was in accordance with findings of another large 2 by 2 factorial design study in Finnish male smokers utilizing beta-carotene and vitamin E (the Alpha Tocopherol Beta Carotene, or ATBC, Study). This study reported that the group taking beta-carotene supplements had an 18% increase in lung cancer as well as an 8% increase in total mortality (1994). There did not appear to be a benefit, in terms of lowering lung cancer risk, for α-tocopherol. It has been since hypothesized that oxidation products of beta-carotene formed in the presence of smoke may have procarcinogenic effects, with some *in vitro* and *in vivo* data supportive of this hypothesis (Wang and Russell 1999). These studies illustrate the importance of testing hypotheses derived from epidemiologic and laboratory data in the setting of large, randomized controlled trials, with careful consideration of potential and possibly unexpected interaction in the populations to be studied. Despite the less than encouraging results with retinoids in the earlier trials, there is continued interest in the development and testing of novel natural and synthetic retinoids as lung chemopreventive agents.

Results have been published from an intergroup phase III placebo-controlled, randomized trial in which 1,166 patients with pathological stage I NSCLC were treated with retinoid isotretinoin or placebo. Treatment did not improve the overall rates of second primary tumors, recurrences, or mortality (Lippman, Lee et al. 2001). Furthermore, secondary multivariate and subset analyses suggested that isotretinoin was in fact harmful to current smokers and beneficial only in never smokers. Despite the unexpected results from the CARET and similar supplementation trials showing that supplementation with micronutrients increased, rather than decreased, lung cancer incidence, considerable interest remains in investigating how other compounds in fruits and vegetables may affect lung cancer risk.

Chemopreventive treatments using other agents are currently being studied for the prevention of lung cancer. Vitamin E and aspirin are being evaluated in female nurses greater than 45 years of age in a randomized chemoprevention trial, using 9-cRA or 13-cRA and alpha-tocopherol or placebo (Kurie, Lotan et al. 2003). This study is evaluating individuals at high risk with no previous history of lung cancer and may help to determine if active chemoprevention efforts can reduce the risk for developing aero-digestive cancer.

Selenium

Selenium is an essential mineral, though only in trace amounts. Overt and pathology-inducing selenium deficiency among humans is extremely rare except for parts of China. In most areas of the world, normal food consumption is adequate to saturate the selenoenzyme systems identified to date. Results from epidemiological studies, human clinical intervention trials, and *in vitro* and *in vivo* animal models clearly support a protective role of selenium against cancer development (Combs 1999; Nelson, Reid et al. 2002). Although selenium compounds have been shown to suppress carcinogenesis in many animal models and cell line systems, the mechanisms by which selenium may exert its chemopreventive activity still remain unclear.

El-Bayoumy (El-Bayoumy 2001) recently reviewed potential mechanisms for the protective role of selenium against cancer. Different forms of selenium have been used in rodents, at multiple organ sites including the lung, to test hypotheses including inhibition of carcinogen-induced covalent DNA adduct formation (Prokopczyk, Cox et al. 1996) and retardation of oxidative damage to DNA, lipids and proteins (Narayanaswami and Sies 1990). The effects of these forms of selenium on cell growth and molecular targets of carcinogenesis have been extensively studied in cell culture and animal systems. Tumor cell growth, DNA, RNA and protein synthesis, apoptosis, cell death, cell cycle, p53, AP-1, and nuclear factor κB (NF-κB), aberrant crypt foci (ACF), COX-2, protein kinase C and A (PKC and PKA), thymidine kinase (TK), jun-N-kinase (JNK), DNA cytosine methyltransferase, cell proliferation and cell cycle biomarkers and 8-isoprostane have demonstrated the ability to be modified by selenium treatment (Ronai, Tillotson et al. 1995; Wu, Lanfear et al. 1995; Fiala, Staretz et al. 1998; Kawamori, El-Bayoumy et al. 1998; Ip, Thompson et al. 2000; Rao, Simi et al. 2000).

Ecologic studies suggest that dietary intakes of selenium are inversely associated with the risk of developing lung cancer. Shamberger and Frost (Shamberger and Frost 1969) were the first to report an inverse relationship between selenium levels in grain, forage crops, human blood and lung cancer mortality in regions of the U.S. Schrauzer (Schrauzer 1976) studied data from 27 countries and showed that dietary intake of selenium was inversely correlated with total cancer mortality as well as with age-adjusted mortality due to lung cancer. These findings were corroborated by population-based epidemiological studies in both the U.S. (Clark 1985) and China (Yu, Chu et al. 1985). A number of case-control studies have examined selenium status in cancer patients compared to controls (Salonen, Alfthan et al. 1984; Nomura, Heilbrun et al. 1987; Knekt, Aromaa et al. 1990; Criqui, Bangdiwala et al. 1991; Kabuto, Imai et al. 1994; Knekt, Marniemi et al. 1998). In most cases, a lower selenium status in cancer patients was reported, although this finding has not been consistent. Methodological issues such as the assessment of selenium exposure and the effects of treatment and disease stage on selenium status may explain some of these apparent inconsistencies. Many prospective studies of serum selenium levels and lung cancer risk have been published. Most of the studies used a nested case-control approach and two studies evaluated prediagnostic concentrations of selenium in toenail clippings and their association with lung cancer (Garland, Morris et al. 1995).

Knekt and coworkers (Knekt, Marniemi et al. 1998) found a significant inverse association between serum selenium and subsequent lung cancer occurrence in men within the cohort studied in the Finnish Mobile Health Examination Survey. However, this study showed no inverse association between reported selenium intake and lung cancer risk (Knekt, Jarvinen et al. 1991). A strong inverse association between toenail selenium and lung cancer in men and women was observed in a longitudinal observational study from the Netherlands (van den Brandt, Goldbohm et al. 1993). Other published studies suggested inverse trends in lung cancer risk with increasing selenium status but were non-significant due to small numbers of cases. Conversely, non-significant positive associations between serum selenium and lung cancer risk have been observed (Menkes, Comstock et al. 1986). Garland and coworkers (Garland, Morris et al. 1995) reported significantly lower toenail selenium levels among lung cancer case patients compared with control subjects; however, control for smoking reversed this association. Methodological issues, including the use of toenail selenium, must be considered.

Northern Italy provided an uncontrolled experiment of selenium exposure and subsequent mortality for cancer in humans. A statistically non-significant lower risk of lung cancer was detected in females residing in the Italian community exposed to selenium through drinking water (Vinceti, Rovesti et al. 1995). Conversely, males exposed through drinking water had a non-significantly increased risk (Vinceti, Rovesti et al. 1995). Overall, observational data tend to show a statistically non-significant inverse association between selenium levels and lung cancer.

Tea and Derivatives

Tea is a beverage made from the leaves of *Camellia sinensis* species of the Theaceae family. This beverage is one of the most ancient and, next to water, the most widely consumed liquid in the world. Tea leaves are primarily manufactured as green or black or oolong, with black tea representing approximately 80% of the tea products consumed. Green tea is the non-oxidized, non-fermented product of the leaves and contains several polyphenolic components, such as epicatechin, epicatechin gallate, epigallocatechin, and epigallocatechin gallate (EGCG). EGCG is the major green tea polyphenol (more than 40% dry weight). The lowest effective dose of 0.016 mmol EGCG/kg/day in rodent cancer models is comparable to the consumption of four cups of green tea or 17.7 mmol/kg/day of EGCG by a 70 kg man (1996).

Tea polyphenols are the major polyphenolic compounds of tea. They scavenge active oxygen radicals (Cheng 1989) and inhibit DNA biosynthesis of the tumor cells (Katiyar, Agarwal et al. 1992) and chemocarcinogen-induced carcinogenesis (Xu, Song et al. 1993). They also block the inhibition effect of carcinogens in intercellular communication (Sigler and Ruch 1993) and induce apoptosis (Zhao, Cao et al. 1997). Tea-derived polyphenols exhibit antimutagenic and genotoxic activities that may be associated with anticarcinogenic activity (Okai and Higashi-Okai 1997). Stich et al. (Stich, Rosin et al. 1982) showed that water-soluble extracts of green and black teas inhibited the mutagenicity in a nitrosation model system.

Because cigarette smoking and tea drinking are very common in many diverse populations, several studies have explored the possible inhibitory effects of tea on lung cancer formation induced by cigarette smoking. Several studies have reported that green tea and black tea inhibit the formation of lung tumors in A/J mice induced by the tobacco-specific nitrosamine 4-(methylnitrosamine)-1-(3-pyridyl)-1-butanone (NNK), the most potent carcinogen found in cigarette smoke (Wang, Hong et al. 1992; Xu, Ho et al. 1992). The effect of tea may be related to the significant inhibitory effects on NNK-induced oncogene expression in mouse lung (Hu, Han et al. 1995).

Tea is a promising agent for the potential chemoprevention of cancer (Yang and Wang 1993; Stoner and Mukhtar 1995). Polyphenolic compounds present in tea afford protection against chemical carcinogen-induced tumor initiation and tumor promotion in lung and forestomach of A/J mice (Wang, Hong et al. 1992; Xu, Ho et al. 1992). A recent study investigated the effects of oral administration of decaffeinated green tea or black tea on NNK-induced lung tumorigenesis (Yang, Yang et al. 1998). Significant protection against lung tumor formation occurred when tea was given either during or after NNK treatment. A study on the bioavailability of radioactive EGCG revealed that radioactivity was widely distributed into various organs of mouse and that 0.16% of total administered radioactivity was observed in lung tissue 24 hours after oral administration (Suganuma, Ohkura et al. 2001).

Ohno et al. (Ohno, Wakai et al. 1995) showed that daily tea consumption significantly decreased the risk of lung squamous cell carcinoma in males and females; the odds ratios were 0.50 and 0.8, respectively. Mendilaharsu et al. (Mendilaharsu, De Stefani et al. 1998) investigated the effect of drinking tea on the lung cancer risk of male cigarette smokers in a case-control study in Uruguay. They found that high intake (two or more cups per day) was associated with a reduced risk of lung cancer in smokers (0.34; 95% CI 0.14–0.84). Flavonoids, including catechins, have been reported to protect against chronic lung disease. Total antioxidant capacity of plasma was significantly increased after taking green tea in amounts of 300 and 450 m and a positive increment according to green tea dosage was also observed (Sung, Nah et al. 2000). A Japanese prospective cohort study revealed that the consumption of 10 cups (120 ml each) of green tea per day delayed cancer onset of both never smokers and current smokers. Green tea showed the strongest protective effects on lung cancer (relative risk, 0.33) (Fujiki, Suganuma et al. 2001). However, results have not been consistent; Tewes and colleagues (Tewes, Koo et al. 1990) reported a tentative increase in lung cancer risk among green tea drinkers. Results were stated as tentative since only 23 cases (11.5%) and 13 controls (6.5%) reported regular tea drinking and the authors did not have data to perform a dose-response analysis.

Investigations into the anticarcinogenic properties of tea (studies of green tea and green tea extracts) have shown growth inhibitory effects in a number cancer cell lines (Ahmad, Feyes et al. 1997; Suganuma, Okabe et al. 1999). Investigation into the mechanism of EGCG-induced apoptosis revealed that treatment with EGCG resulted in DNA fragmentation, induction of caspase-3/CPP32 activity, and cleavage of the death substrate poly(ADP-ribose)polymerase (Islam, Islam et al. 2000). Masuda and co-workers (Masuda, Suzui et al. 2001) examined the molecular effects of EGCG on two human head and neck SCC cell lines, YCU-N861 and YCU-H891, focusing on the EGFR signaling pathway. Treatment with EGCG induced apoptosis and caused a decrease in the Bcl-2 and Bcl-X(L) proteins, an increase in the Bax protein, and activation of caspase 9, suggesting that EGCG induces apoptosis via a mitochondrial pathway. Treatment with EGCG also inhibited phosphorylation of the EGFR and also inhibited basal and transforming growth factor-alpha-stimulated c-fos and cyclin D1 promoter activity. EGCG at 0.1 µg/ml (a concentration found in serum after oral administration) markedly enhanced the growth-inhibitory effects of 5-fluorouracil. Taken together, these findings provide insights into molecular mechanisms of growth inhibition by EGCG.

Conclusion

In the New Millennium, lung cancer continues to exact an extremely large toll in terms of cancer-related morbidity and mortality as well as its effect on health care systems and economies worldwide. This is in spite of public health efforts initiated in the 1960s to educate the public about the dangers of tobacco use and the implementation of smoking cessation programs. While up to 50 to 60% of adults in some countries continue to smoke, formers smokers are growing in number. Unfortunately, this latter population remains at elevated risk for developing lung cancer.

A growing understanding of lung carcinogenesis from the molecular and genetic standpoint has complemented epidemiologic studies that have identified high-risk populations that are most likely to benefit from intervention strategies. Chemoprevention strategies currently employ a wide range of selective chemopreventive approaches that include dietary modification and supplementation using natural products and their derivatives, as well as a range of synthetic agents that may also have utility in treating advanced lung cancer. Complementing chemoprevention efforts is a growing body of research that suggests that state-of-the-art screening techniques for early detection will impact on the morbidity and mortality associated with lung cancer.

References

(1994). "The effect of vitamin E and beta carotene on the incidence of lung cancer and other cancers in male smokers. The Alpha-Tocopherol, Beta Carotene Cancer Prevention Study Group." *N Engl J Med* **330**(15): 1029–1035.

(1996). "Clinical development plan: tea extracts. Green tea polyphenols. Epigallocatechin gallate." *J Cell Biochem Suppl* **26**: 236–257.

(1999). "Tobacco use–United States, 1900–1999." *MMWR Morb Mortal Wkly Rep* **48**(43): 986–993.

(2002). "Cigarette smoking among adults – United States, 2000." *MMWR Morb Mortal Wkly Rep* **51**(29): 642–645.

(2004). "Prevalence of cigarette use among 14 racial/ethnic populations – United States, 1999–2001." *MMWR Morb Mortal Wkly Rep* **53**(3): 49–52.

Ahmad, N., D.K. Feyes, et al. (1997). "Green tea constituent epigallocatechin-3-gallate and induction of apoptosis and cell cycle arrest in human carcinoma cells." *J Natl Cancer Inst* **89**(24): 1881–1886.

Akaike, T., M. Suga, et al. (1998). "Free radicals in viral pathogenesis: molecular mechanisms involving superoxide and NO." *Proc Soc Exp Biol Med* **217**(1): 64–73.

Ames, B.N., L.S. Gold, et al. (1995). "The causes and prevention of cancer." *Proc Natl Acad Sci USA* **92**(12): 5258–5265.

Ames, B.N. and M.K. Shigenaga (1992). DNA damage by endogenous oxidants and mitogenesis as causes of aging and cancer. *Molecular biology of free radical scavenging systems.* J.G. Scandalios. Plainview, N.Y., Cold Spring Harbor Laboratory Press: ix, 284.

Awad, J.A., L.J. Roberts, 2nd, et al. (1996). "Isoprostanes – prostaglandin-like compounds formed in vivo independently of cyclooxygenase: use as clinical indicators of oxidant damage." *Gastroenterol Clin North Am* **25**(2): 409–427.

Belinsky, S.A., K.J. Nikula, et al. (1998). "Aberrant methylation of p16(INK4a) is an early event in lung cancer and a potential biomarker for early diagnosis." *Proc Natl Acad Sci USA* **95**(20): 11891–11896.

Bell, D.A., J.A. Taylor, et al. (1993). "Genetic risk and carcinogen exposure: a common inherited defect of the carcinogen-metabolism gene glutathione S-transferase M1 (GSTM1) that increases susceptibility to bladder cancer." *J Natl Cancer Inst* **85**(14): 1159–1164.

Boffetta, P. and F. Nyberg (2003). "Contribution of environmental factors to cancer risk." *Br Med Bull* **68**: 71–94.

Bohr, V.A., B.G. Taffe, et al. (1995). DNA repair, oxidative stress and aging. *Oxidative stress and aging.* R.G. Cutler. Basel; Boston, Birkhhauser Verlag: 101–110.

Brockmoller, J., R. Kerb, et al. (1993). "Genotype and phenotype of glutathione S-transferase class mu isoenzymes mu and psi in lung cancer patients and controls." *Cancer Res* **53**(5): 1004–1011.

Burns, D. M. (2000). "Primary prevention, smoking, and smoking cessation: implications for future trends in lung cancer prevention." *Cancer* **89**(11 Suppl): 2506–2509.

Chen, Y., M. Sato, et al. (1999). "Expression of Bcl-2, Bax, and p53 proteins in carcinogenesis of squamous cell lung cancer." *Anticancer Res* **19**(2B): 1351–1356.

Cheng, K.C., D.S. Cahill, et al. (1992). "8-Hydroxyguanine, an abundant form of oxidative DNA damage, causes G–T and A–C substitutions." *J Biol Chem* **267**(1): 166–172.

Cheng, S.J. (1989). "[Inhibitory effect of green tea extract on promotion and related action of TPA]." *Zhongguo Yi Xue Ke Xue Yuan Xue Bao* **11**(4): 259–264.

Clark, L.C. (1985). "The epidemiology of selenium and cancer." *Fed Proc* **44**(9): 2584–2589.

Cohen, A.J. (2000). "Outdoor air pollution and lung cancer." *Environ Health Perspect* **108 Suppl 4**: 743–750.

Colby, T.V. (1999). Precursor lesions to pulmonary neoplasia. *Lung tumors: fundamental biology and clinical management.* C. Brambilla and E. Brambilla. New York, Dekker: xxxii, 858.

Combs, G.F., Jr. (1999). "Chemopreventive mechanisms of selenium." *Med Klin (Munich)* **94 Suppl 3**: 18–24.

Criqui, M.H., S. Bangdiwala, et al. (1991). "Selenium, retinol, retinol-binding protein, and uric acid. Associations with cancer mortality in a population-based prospective case-control study." *Ann Epidemiol* **1**(5): 385–393.

Cuendet, M. and J.M. Pezzuto (2000). "The role of cyclooxygenase and lipoxygenase in cancer chemoprevention". *Toxicology* **153**(1–3): 11–26.

Danam, R.P., X.C. Qian, et al. (1999). "Methylation of selected CpGs in the human O6-methylguanine-DNA methyltransferase promoter region as a marker of gene silencing." *Mol Carcinog* **24**(2): 85–89.

Doll, R. (1978). "Atmospheric pollution and lung cancer." *Environ Health Perspect* **22**: 23–31.

Doll, R. and A.B. Hill (1952). "A study of the aetiology of carcinoma of the lung." *Br Med J* **2**(4797): 1271–1286.

Doll, R. and R. Peto (1976). "Mortality in relation to smoking: 20 years' observations on male British doctors." *Br Med J* **2**(6051): 1525–1536.

Doll, R., M.B.Vessey, R.W. Beasley, A.R. Buckley, E.C. Fear, R.E.W. Fisher, E.J. Gammon, W. Gunn, G.O. Hughes, K. Lee, K., et al. (1972). "Mortality of gas workers: final report of a prospective study." *Br J Ind Med* **29**: 394.

Ebbert, J.O., P. Yang, et al. (2003). "Lung cancer risk reduction after smoking cessation: observations from a prospective cohort of women." *J Clin Oncol* **21**(5): 921–926.

El-Bayoumy, K. (2001). "The protective role of selenium on genetic damage and on cancer." *Mutat Res* **475**(1–2): 123–139.

Erhola, M., S. Toyokuni, et al. (1997). "Biomarker evidence of DNA oxidation in lung cancer patients: association of urinary 8-hydroxy-2'-deoxyguanosine excretion with radiotherapy, chemotherapy, and response to treatment." *FEBS Lett* **409**(2): 287–291.

Esteller, M., P.G. Corn, et al. (2001). "A gene hypermethylation profile of human cancer." *Cancer Res* **61**(8): 3225–3229.

Esteller, M., P.G. Corn, et al. (1998). "Inactivation of glutathione S-transferase P1 gene by promoter hypermethylation in human neoplasia." *Cancer Res* **58**(20): 4515–4518.

Esteller, M., S.R. Hamilton, et al. (1999). "Inactivation of the DNA repair gene O6-methylguanine-DNA methyltransferase by promoter hypermethylation is a common event in primary human neoplasia." *Cancer Res* **59**(4): 793–797.

Esteller, M., M. Sanchez-Cespedes, et al. (1999). "Detection of aberrant promoter hypermethylation of tumor suppressor genes in serum DNA from non-small cell lung cancer patients." *Cancer Res* **59**(1): 67–70.

Esteller, M., S. Tortola, et al. (2000). "Hypermethylation-associated inactivation of p14(ARF) is independent of p16(INK4a) methylation and p53 mutational status." *Cancer Res* **60**(1): 129–133.

Etzel, C.J., C.I. Amos, et al. (2003). "Risk for smoking-related cancer among relatives of lung cancer patients." *Cancer Res* **63**(23): 8531–8535.

Farias-Eisner, R., M.P. Sherman, et al. (1994). "Nitric oxide is an important mediator for tumoricidal activity in vivo." *Proc Natl Acad Sci USA* **91**(20): 9407–9411.

Fiala, E.S., M.E. Staretz, et al. (1998). "Inhibition of DNA cytosine methyltransferase by chemopreventive selenium compounds, determined by an improved assay for DNA cytosine methyltransferase and DNA cytosine methylation." *Carcinogenesis* **19**(4): 597–604.

Filep, J.G., C. Baron, et al. (1996). "Involvement of nitric oxide in target-cell lysis and DNA fragmentation induced by murine natural killer cells." *Blood* **87**(12): 5136–5143.

Floyd, R.A. (1990). "The role of 8-hydroxyguanine in carcinogenesis." *Carcinogenesis* **11**(9): 1447–1450.

Floyd, R.A., J.J. Watson, et al. (1986). "Hydroxyl free radical adduct of deoxyguanosine: sensitive detection and mechanisms of formation." *Free Radic Res Commun* **1**(3): 163–172.

Fontana, R.S., D.R. Sanderson, et al. (1984). "Early lung cancer detection: results of the initial (prevalence) radiologic and cytologic screening in the Mayo Clinic study." *Am Rev Respir Dis* **130**(4): 561–565.

Franklin, W.A. (2000). "Pathology of lung cancer." *J Thorac Imaging* **15**(1): 3–12.

Frenkel, K., J.M. Donahue, et al. (1988). Benzo(a)pyrene-induced oxidative DNA damage. A possible mechanism for promotion by complete carcinogens. *Oxy-radicals in molecular biology and pathology: proceedings of an Upjohn-UCLA symposium, held at Park City, Utah, January 24–30, 1988*. P.A. Cerutti, I. Fridovich and J.M. McCord. New York, Liss: xx, 586.

Fujiki, H., M. Suganuma, et al. (2001). "Cancer prevention with green tea and monitoring by a new biomarker, hnRNP B1." *Mutat Res* **480-481**: 299–304.

Garland, M., J.S. Morris, et al. (1995). "Prospective study of toenail selenium levels and cancer among women." *J Natl Cancer Inst* **87**(7): 497–505.

Giovino, G.A., M.W. Schooley, et al. (1994). "Surveillance for selected tobacco-use behaviors – United States, 1900–1994." *MMWR CDC Surveill Summ* **43**(3): 1–43.

Grandis, J.R. and J.C. Sok (2004). "Signaling through the epidermal growth factor receptor during the development of malignancy." *Pharmacol Ther* **102**(1): 37–46.

Gridelli, C., P. Maione, et al. (2000). "Selective cyclooxygenase-2 inhibitors and non-small cell lung cancer." *Drug Metabol Drug Interact* **17**(1–4): 109–157.

Guyton, K.Z. and T.W. Kensler (1993). "Oxidative mechanisms in carcinogenesis." *Br Med Bull* **49**(3): 523–544.

Hahn, S.M., E. Bernhard, et al. (2001). "Farnesyltransferase inhibitors." *Semin Oncol* **28** (5 Suppl 16): 86–93.

Halliwell, B. and O.I. Aruoma (1991). "DNA damage by oxygen-derived species. Its mechanism and measurement in mammalian systems." *FEBS Lett* **281**(1/2): 9–19.

Halpern, M.T., B.W. Gillespie, et al. (1993). "Patterns of absolute risk of lung cancer mortality in former smokers." *J Natl Cancer Inst* **85**(6): 457–464.

Hammond, E.C. (1966). "Smoking in relation to the death rates of one million men and women." *Natl Cancer Inst Monogr* **19**: 127–204.

Hayes, J.D. and D.J. Pulford (1995). "The glutathione S-transferase supergene family: regulation of GST and the contribution of the isoenzymes to cancer chemoprotection and drug resistance." *Crit Rev Biochem Mol Biol* **30**(6): 445–600.

He, X.Z., W. Chen, et al. (1991). "An epidemiological study of lung cancer in Xuan Wei County, China: current progress. Case-control study on lung cancer and cooking fuel." *Environ Health Perspect* **94**: 9–13.

Hecht, S.S. (1999). "Tobacco smoke carcinogens and lung cancer." *J Natl Cancer Inst* **91**(14): 1194–1210.

Henschke, C.I., D.I. McCauley, et al. (1999). "Early Lung Cancer Action Project: overall design and findings from baseline screening." *Lancet* **354**(9173): 99–105.

Hirvonen, A., K. Husgafvel-Pursiainen, et al. (1993). "The GSTM1 null genotype as a potential risk modifier for squamous cell carcinoma of the lung." *Carcinogenesis* **14**(7): 1479–1481.

Hittleman, W.N. (2002). "Effect of tobacco carcinogens on the bronchial epithelium." *American Society of Clinical Oncology*: 18–23.

Hommura, F., H. Dosaka-Akita, et al. (2000). "Prognostic significance of p27KIP1 protein and ki-67 growth fraction in non-small cell lung cancers." *Clin Cancer Res* **6**(10): 4073–4081.

Howard, D.J., L.A. Briggs, et al. (1998). "Oxidative DNA damage in mouse heart, liver, and lung tissue due to acute side-stream tobacco smoke exposure." *Arch Biochem Biophys* **352**(2): 293–297.

Hu, G., C. Han, et al. (1995). "Inhibition of oncogene expression by green tea and (–)-epigallocatechin gallate in mice." *Nutr Cancer* **24**(2): 203–209.

Inoue, M., T. Osaki, et al. (1998). "Lung cancer patients have increased 8-hydroxydeoxyguanosine levels in peripheral lung tissue DNA." *Jpn J Cancer Res* **89**(7): 691–695.

Ip, C., H.J. Thompson, et al. (2000). "Selenium modulation of cell proliferation and cell cycle biomarkers in normal and premalignant cells of the rat mammary gland." *Cancer Epidemiol Biomarkers Prev* **9**(1): 49–54.

Islam, S., N. Islam, et al. (2000). "Involvement of caspase-3 in epigallocatechin-3-gallate-mediated apoptosis of human chondrosarcoma cells." *Biochem Biophys Res Commun* **270**(3): 793–797.

Izzotti, A., R.M. Balansky, et al. (2001). "Modulation of biomarkers by chemopreventive agents in smoke-exposed rats." *Cancer Res* **61**(6): 2472–2479.

Jackson, J.H. (1994). "Potential molecular mechanisms of oxidant-induced carcinogenesis." *Environ Health Perspect* **102 Suppl 10**: 155–157.

Jemal, A., K.C. Chu, et al. (2001). "Recent trends in lung cancer mortality in the United States." *J Natl Cancer Inst* **93**(4): 277–283.

Jemal, A., R.C. Tiwari, et al. (2004). "Cancer statistics, 2004." *CA Cancer J Clin* **54**(1): 8–29.

Kabuto, M., H. Imai, et al. (1994). "Prediagnostic serum selenium and zinc levels and subsequent risk of lung and stomach cancer in Japan." *Cancer Epidemiol Biomarkers Prev* **3**(6): 465–469.

Karch, N.J., M.A. Schneiderman (1981). *Explaining the Urban Factor in Lung Cancer Mortality. A Report of the National Resources Defense Council.* Washington DC, Clement Associates Inc.

Kasai, H. (1998). "Hydroxyguanine in carcinogenesis." *Pathophysiology* **5**(Supplement 1): 140.

Katiyar, S.K., R. Agarwal, et al. (1992). "(–)-Epigallocatechin-3-gallate in Camellia sinensis leaves from Himalayan region of Sikkim: inhibitory effects against biochemical events and tumor initiation in Sencar mouse skin." *Nutr Cancer* **18**(1): 73–83.

Katoh, T., N. Nagata, et al. (1996). "Glutathione S-transferase M1 (GSTM1) and T1 (GSTT1) genetic polymorphism and susceptibility to gastric and colorectal adenocarcinoma." *Carcinogenesis* **17**(9): 1855–1859.

Kawamori, T., K. El-Bayoumy, et al. (1998). "Evaluation of benzyl selenocyanate glutathione conjugate for potential chemopreventive properties in colon carcinogenesis." *Int J Oncol* **13**(1): 29–34.

Keefer, L.K. and D.A. Wink (1996). "DNA damage and nitric oxide." *Adv Exp Med Biol* **387**: 177–185.

Kennedy, T.C., S.P. Proudfoot, et al. (1996). "Cytopathological analysis of sputum in patients with airflow obstruction and significant smoking histories." *Cancer Res* **56**(20): 4673–4678.

Kersting, M., C. Friedl, et al. (2000). "Differential frequencies of p16(INK4a) promoter hypermethylation, p53 mutation, and K-ras mutation in exfoliative material mark the development of lung cancer in symptomatic chronic smokers." *J Clin Oncol* **18**(18): 3221–3229.

Ketterer, B., J.M. Harris, et al. (1992). "The human glutathione S-transferase supergene family, its polymorphism, and its effects on susceptibility to lung cancer." *Environ Health Perspect* **98**: 87–94.

Khuri, F.R., J.S. Lee, et al. (2001). "Modulation of proliferating cell nuclear antigen in the bronchial epithelium of smokers." *Cancer Epidemiol Biomarkers Prev* **10**(4): 311–318.

Khuri, F.R., M.T. Spitz, W.K. Hong (1995). "Lung cancer chemoprevention: targeting former rather than current smokers." *Can Prec Int* **2**: 55.

Kihara, M. and K. Noda (1994). "Lung cancer risk of GSTM1 null genotype is dependent on the extent of tobacco smoke exposure." *Carcinogenesis* **15**(2): 415–418.

Knekt, P., A. Aromaa, et al. (1990). "Serum selenium and subsequent risk of cancer among Finnish men and women." *J Natl Cancer Inst* **82**(10): 864–868.

Knekt, P., R. Jarvinen, et al. (1991). "Dietary antioxidants and the risk of lung cancer." *Am J Epidemiol* **134**(5): 471–479.

Knekt, P., J. Marniemi, et al. (1998). "Is low selenium status a risk factor for lung cancer?" *Am J Epidemiol* **148**(10): 975–982.

Koomagi, R. and M. Volm (2000). "Relationship between the expression of caspase-3 and the clinical outcome of patients with non-small cell lung cancer." *Anticancer Res* **20**(1B): 493–496.

Kurie, J.M., R. Lotan, et al. (2003). "Treatment of former smokers with 9-cis-retinoic acid reverses loss of retinoic acid receptor-beta expression in the bronchial epithelium: results from a randomized placebo-controlled trial." *J Natl Cancer Inst* **95**(3): 206–214.

Kuschner, M. (1968). "The causes of lung cancer." *Am Rev Respir Dis* **98**(4): 573–590.

Lam, S., J.C. leRiche, et al. (1999). "Sex-related differences in bronchial epithelial changes associated with tobacco smoking." *J Natl Cancer Inst* **91**(8): 691–696.

Lane, P. and S.S. Gross (1999). "Cell signaling by nitric oxide." *Semin Nephrol* **19**(3): 215–229.

Le Marchand, L., T. Donlon, et al. (2002). "Association of the hOGG1 Ser326Cys polymorphism with lung cancer risk." *Cancer Epidemiol Biomarkers Prev* **11**(4): 409–412.

Lee, H.Y., J. Chaudhary, et al. (1998). "Suppression of c-Fos gene transcription with malignant transformation of human bronchial epithelial cells." *Oncogene* **16**(23): 3039–3046.

Leo, M.A., S.I. Aleynik, et al. (1997). "F2-isoprostane and 4-hydroxynonenal excretion in human bile of patients with biliary tract and pancreatic disorders." *Am J Gastroenterol* **92**(11): 2069–2072.

Levin, M. L., H. Goldstein, et al. (1950). "Cancer and tobacco smoking; a preliminary report." *J Am Med Assoc* **143**(4): 336–338.

Lippman, S.M., J.J. Lee, et al. (2001). "Randomized phase III intergroup trial of isotretinoin to prevent second primary tumors in stage I non-small-cell lung cancer." *J Natl Cancer Inst* **93**(8): 605–618.

Lubin, J.H. and K. Steindorf (1995). "Cigarette use and the estimation of lung cancer attributable to radon in the United States." *Radiat Res* **141**(1): 79–85.

MacNee, W. (2001). "Oxidants/antioxidants and chronic obstructive pulmonary disease: pathogenesis to therapy." *Novartis Found Symp* **234**: 169–185; discussion 185–188.

Maehira, F., F. Zaha, et al. (2000). "Effects of passive smoking on the regulation of rat aortic cholesteryl ester hydrolases by signal transduction." *Lipids* **35**(5): 503–511.

Mallat, Z., I. Philip, et al. (1998). "Elevated levels of 8-iso-prostaglandin F2alpha in pericardial fluid of patients with heart failure: a potential role for in vivo oxidant stress in ventricular dilatation and progression to heart failure." *Circulation* **97**(16): 1536–1539.

Marks, F., K. Muller-Decker, et al. (2000). "A causal relationship between unscheduled eicosanoid signaling and tumor development: cancer chemoprevention by inhibitors of arachidonic acid metabolism." *Toxicology* **153**(1–3): 11–26.

Masuda, M., M. Suzui, et al. (2001). "Effects of epigallocatechin-3-gallate on growth, epidermal growth factor receptor signaling pathways, gene expression, and chemosensitivity in human head and neck squamous cell carcinoma cell lines." *Clin Cancer Res* **7**(12): 4220–4229.

Mayne, S.T., J. Buenconsejo, et al. (1999). "Familial cancer history and lung cancer risk in United States nonsmoking men and women." *Cancer Epidemiol Biomarkers Prev* **8**(12): 1065–1069.

Melamed, M.R., B.J. Flehinger, et al. (1984). "Screening for early lung cancer. Results of the Memorial Sloan-Kettering study in New York." *Chest* **86**(1): 44–53.

Mendilaharsu, M., E. De Stefani, et al. (1998). "Consumption of tea and coffee and the risk of lung cancer in cigarette-smoking men: a case-control study in Uruguay." *Lung Cancer* **19**(2): 101–107.

Menkes, M.S., G.W. Comstock, et al. (1986). "Serum beta-carotene, vitamins A and E, selenium, and the risk of lung cancer." *N Engl J Med* **315**(20): 1250-1254.

Montine, T.J., M.F. Beal, et al. (1999). "Cerebrospinal fluid F2-isoprostanes are elevated in Huntington's disease." *Neurology* **52**(5): 1104–1105.

Montuschi, P., G. Ciabattoni, et al. (1998). "8-Isoprostane as a biomarker of oxidative stress in interstitial lung diseases." *Am J Respir Crit Care Med* **158**(5 Pt 1): 1524–1527.

Morrow, J.D., T.A. Minton, et al. (1994). "Evidence that the F2-isoprostane, 8-epi-prostaglandin F2 alpha, is formed in vivo." *Biochim Biophys Acta* **1210**(2): 244–248.

Narayanaswami, V. and H. Sies (1990). "Antioxidant activity of ebselen and related selenoorganic compounds in microsomal lipid peroxidation." *Free Radic Res Commun* **10**(4–5): 237–244.

NCI (2004). National Lung Screening Trial Reaches Goal of 50,000 Participants. *http://www.cancer.gov/newscenter/pressreleases/NLSTgoal*, National Cancer Institute Press Release, January 27, 2004.

Nelson, M.A., M. Reid, et al. (2002). "Prostate cancer and selenium." *Urol Clin North Am* **29**(1): 67–70.

Neuberger, J.S. and R.W. Field (2003). "Occupation and lung cancer in nonsmokers." *Rev Environ Health* **18**(4): 251–267.

Nguyen, A., Z. Jing, et al. (2000). "In vivo gene expression profile analysis of metallothionein in renal cell carcinoma." *Cancer Lett* **160**(2): 133–140.

Nigro, J.M., S.J. Baker, et al. (1989). "Mutations in the p53 gene occur in diverse human tumour types." *Nature* **342**(6250): 705–708.

Nomura, A., L.K. Heilbrun, et al. (1987). "Serum selenium and the risk of cancer, by specific sites: case-control analysis of prospective data." *J Natl Cancer Inst* **79**(1): 103–108.

Ohashi, N. and M. Yoshikawa (2000). "Rapid and sensitive quantification of 8-isoprostaglandin F2alpha in human plasma and urine by liquid chromatography-electrospray ionization mass spectrometry." *J Chromatogr B Biomed Sci Appl* **746**(1): 17–24.

Ohno, Y., K. Wakai, et al. (1995). "Tea consumption and lung cancer risk: a case-control study in Okinawa, Japan." *Jpn J Cancer Res* **86**(11): 1027–1034.

Okai, Y. and K. Higashi-Okai (1997). "Potent suppressing activity of the non-polyphenolic fraction of green tea (Camellia sinensis) against genotoxin-induced umu C gene expression in Salmonella typhimurium (TA 1535/pSK 1002)–association with pheophytins a and b." *Cancer Lett* **120**(1): 117–123.

Omenn, G.S., G.E. Goodman, et al. (1996). "Effects of a combination of beta carotene and vitamin A on lung cancer and cardiovascular disease." *N Engl J Med* **334**(18): 1150–1155.

Palmisano, W.A., K.K. Divine, et al. (2000). "Predicting lung cancer by detecting aberrant promoter methylation in sputum." *Cancer Res* **60**(21): 5954–5958.

Park, J.Y., S.Y. Lee, et al. (2002). "Polymorphism of the DNA repair gene XRCC1 and risk of primary lung cancer." *Cancer Epidemiol Biomarkers Prev* **11**(1): 23–27.

Passey, R.D. (1962). "Some problems of lung cancer." *Lancet* **2**: 107–112.

Pemble, S., K.R. Schroeder, et al. (1994). "Human glutathione S-transferase theta (GSTT1): cDNA cloning and the characterization of a genetic polymorphism." *Biochem J* **300 (Pt 1)**: 271–276.

Peterhans, E. (1997). "Reactive oxygen species and nitric oxide in viral diseases." *Biol Trace Elem Res* **56**(1): 107–116.

Petty, W.J., K.H. Dragnev, et al. (2003). "Cyclin D1 as a target for chemoprevention." *Lung Cancer* **41**(1): 155–161.

Phillips, D.H. (2002). "Smoking-related DNA and protein adducts in human tissues." *Carcinogenesis* **23**(12): 1979–2004.

Pratico, D., L. Iuliano, et al. (1998). "Enhanced lipid peroxidation in hepatic cirrhosis." *J Investig Med* **46**(2): 51–57.

Pratico, D., M.Y. L. V, et al. (1998). "Increased F2-isoprostanes in Alzheimer's disease: evidence for enhanced lipid peroxidation in vivo." *Faseb J* **12**(15): 1777–1783.

Prokopczyk, B., J.E. Cox, et al. (1996). "Effects of dietary 1,4-phenylenebis(methylene)seleno-cyanate on 4-(methylnitrosamino)-1-(3-pyridyl)-1-butanone-induced DNA adduct formation in lung and liver of A/J mice and F344 rats." *Carcinogenesis* **17**(4): 749–753.

Rao, C.V., B. Simi, et al. (2000). "Mechanisms in the chemoprevention of colon cancer: modulation of protein kinase C, tyrosine protein kinase and diacylglycerol kinase activities by 1,4-phenylenebis-(methylene)selenocyanate and impact of low-fat diet." *Int J Oncol* **16**(3): 519–527.

Rebbeck, T.R. (1997). "Molecular epidemiology of the human glutathione S-transferase genotypes GSTM1 and GSTT1 in cancer susceptibility." *Cancer Epidemiol Biomarkers Prev* **6**(9): 733–743.

Resnicow, K., G. Kabat, et al. (1991). "Progress in decreasing cigarette smoking." *Important Adv Oncol*: 205–213.

Rogot, E. and J. Murray (1980). "Cancer mortality among nonsmokers in an insured group of U.S. veterans." *J Natl Cancer Inst* **65**(5): 1163–1168.

Ronai, Z., J.K. Tillotson, et al. (1995). "Effects of organic and inorganic selenium compounds on rat mammary tumor cells." *Int J Cancer* **63**(3): 428–434.

Saarikoski, S.T., A. Voho, et al. (1998). "Combined effect of polymorphic GST genes on individual susceptibility to lung cancer." *Int J Cancer* **77**(4): 516–521.

Salonen, J.T., G. Alfthan, et al. (1984). "Association between serum selenium and the risk of cancer." *Am J Epidemiol* **120**(3): 342–349.

Schrauzer, G.N. (1976). "Cancer mortality correlation studies. II. Regional associations of mortalities with the consumptions of foods and other commodities." *Med Hypotheses* **2**(2): 39–49.

Sebti, S.M. (2003). "Blocked pathways: FTIs shut down oncogene signals." *Oncologist* **8**(3): 30–38.

Seidegard, J., W.R. Vorachek, et al. (1988). "Hereditary differences in the expression of the human glutathione transferase active on trans-stilbene oxide are due to a gene deletion." *Proc Natl Acad Sci USA* **85**(19): 7293–7297.

Seow, A., B. Zhao, et al. (2001). "Cytochrome P4501A2 (CYP1A2) activity and lung cancer risk: a preliminary study among Chinese women in Singapore." *Carcinogenesis* **22**(4): 673–677.

Shamberger, R.J. and D.V. Frost (1969). "Possible protective effect of selenium against human cancer." *Can Med Assoc J* **100**(14): 682.

Shen, H.M., C.N. Ong, et al. (1995). "Aflatoxin B1-induced 8-hydroxydeoxyguanosine formation in rat hepatic DNA." *Carcinogenesis* **16**(2): 419–422.

Shopland, D.R. (1995). "Tobacco use and its contribution to early cancer mortality with a special emphasis on cigarette smoking." *Environ Health Perspect* **103**(Suppl 8): 131–142.

Sigler, K. and R.J. Ruch (1993). "Enhancement of gap junctional intercellular communication in tumor promoter-treated cells by components of green tea." *Cancer Lett* **69**(1): 15–19.

Smith, C.A., G. Smith, et al. (1994). "Genetic polymorphisms in xenobiotic metabolism." *Eur J Cancer* **30A**(13): 1921–1935.

Stich, H.F., M.P. Rosin, et al. (1982). "Inhibition of mutagenicity of a model nitrosation reaction by naturally occurring phenolics, coffee and tea." *Mutat Res* **95**(2–3): 119–128.

Stoner, G.D. and H. Mukhtar (1995). "Polyphenols as cancer chemopreventive agents." *J Cell Biochem Suppl* **22**: 169–180.

Strauss, G.M., R.E. Gleason, et al. (1997). "Screening for lung cancer. Another look; a different view." *Chest* **111**(3): 754–768.

Suganuma, M., Y. Ohkura, et al. (2001). "Combination cancer chemoprevention with green tea extract and sulindac shown in intestinal tumor formation in Min mice." *J Cancer Res Clin Oncol* **127**(1): 69–72.

Suganuma, M., S. Okabe, et al. (1999). "Synergistic effects of (–)-epigallocatechin gallate with (–)-epicatechin, sulindac, or tamoxifen on cancer-preventive activity in the human lung cancer cell line PC-9." *Cancer Res* **59**(1): 44–47.

Sung, H., J. Nah, et al. (2000). "In vivo antioxidant effect of green tea." *Eur J Clin Nutr* **54**(7): 527–529.

Takeuchi, T., M. Nakajima, et al. (1994). "Establishment of a human system that generates O2- and induces 8-hydroxydeoxyguanosine, typical of oxidative DNA damage, by a tumor promotor." *Cancer Res* **54**(22): 5837–5840.

Tang, X., F.R. Khuri, et al. (2000). "Hypermethylation of the death-associated protein (DAP) kinase promoter and aggressiveness in stage I non-small-cell lung cancer." *J Natl Cancer Inst* **92**(18): 1511–1516.

Tenkanen, L., T. Hakulinen, et al. (1987). "The joint effect of smoking and respiratory symptoms on risk of lung cancer." *Int J Epidemiol* **16**(4): 509–515.

Tewes, F.J., L.C. Koo, et al. (1990). "Lung cancer risk and mutagenicity of tea." *Environ Res* **52**(1): 23–33.

Tockman, M. (1986). "Survival and mortality from lung cancer in a screened population: the Johns Hopkins Study." *Chest* **89**: 325S–326S.

Tockman, M.S., N.R. Anthonisen, et al. (1987). "Airways obstruction and the risk for lung cancer." *Ann Intern Med* **106**(4): 512–518.

Tokuhata, G.K. and A.M. Lilienfeld (1963). "Familial aggregation of lung cancer in humans." *J Natl Cancer Inst* **30**: 289–312.

Toyokuni, S., K. Okamoto, et al. (1995). "Persistent oxidative stress in cancer." *FEBS Lett* **358**(1): 1–3.

USDDHS (2000). *Healthy People 2010, 2nd Edition*. Washington DC.

USDEW (1964). Smoking and Health. Report of the Advisory Committee to the Surgeon General of the Public Health Service. *DHEW Publication No. 1103*. U.S. Department of Health, Public Health Service, Communicable Disease Center.

USDHHS (1964). Smoking and Health: Report of the Advisory Committee of the Surgeon General of the Public Health Service Source.

USDHHS (1980). The Health Consequences of Smoking for Women. U.S. Department of Health and Human Services, Office on Smoking and Health. Washington.

van den Brandt, P.A., R.A. Goldbohm, et al. (1993). "A prospective cohort study on toenail selenium levels and risk of gastrointestinal cancer." *J Natl Cancer Inst* **85**(3): 224–229.

Vinceti, M., S. Rovesti, et al. (1995). "Cancer mortality in a residential cohort exposed to environmental selenium through drinking water." *J Clin Epidemiol* **48**(9): 1091–1097.

Wagner, H., Jr. and J.C. Ruckdeschel (1995). "Screening, Early Detection, and Early Intervention Strategies for Lung Cancer." *Cancer Control* **2**(6): 493–502.

Wallace, R. (1929). "A 'Lucky' or a sweet – or both!" *Nation* **123**: 305–307.

Wang, X.D. and R.M. Russell (1999). "Procarcinogenic and anticarcinogenic effects of beta-carotene." *Nutr Rev* **57**(9 Pt 1): 263–272.

Wang, Y., Q. Zhou, et al. (2000). "[Transcriptional expression of apoptosis suppression gene bcl-2 in non-small cell lung carcinoma]." *Zhonghua Yi Xue Yi Chuan Xue Za Zhi* **17**(4): 262–265.

Wang, Z.Y., J.Y. Hong, et al. (1992). "Inhibition of N-nitrosodiethylamine- and 4-(methylnitrosamino)-1-(3-pyridyl)-1-butanone-induced tumorigenesis in A/J mice by green tea and black tea." *Cancer Res* **52**(7): 1943–1947.

Wei, L., H. Wei, et al. (1993). "Sensitivity to tumor promotion of SENCAR and C57BL/6J mice correlates with oxidative events and DNA damage." *Carcinogenesis* **14**(5): 841–847.

Wisnivesky, J.P., A.I. Mushlin, et al. (2003). "The cost-effectiveness of low-dose CT screening for lung cancer: preliminary results of baseline screening." *Chest* **124**(2): 614–621.

Wistuba, II, C. Behrens, et al. (1999). "Sequential molecular abnormalities are involved in the multistage development of squamous cell lung carcinoma." *Oncogene* **18**(3): 643–650.

Wood, M.L., M. Dizdaroglu, et al. (1990). "Mechanistic studies of ionizing radiation and oxidative mutagenesis: genetic effects of a single 8-hydroxyguanine (7-hydro-8-oxoguanine) residue inserted at a unique site in a viral genome." *Biochemistry* **29**(30): 7024–7032.

Wu, L., J. Lanfear, et al. (1995). "The selenium metabolite selenodiglutathione induces cell death by a mechanism distinct from H2O2 toxicity." *Carcinogenesis* **16**(7): 1579–1584.

Xu, G.P., P.J. Song, et al. (1993). "Effects of fruit juices, processed vegetable juice, orange peel and green tea on endogenous formation of N-nitrosoproline in subjects from a high-risk area for gastric cancer in Moping County, China." *Eur J Cancer Prev* **2**(4): 327–335.

Xu, Y., C.T. Ho, et al. (1992). "Inhibition of tobacco-specific nitrosamine-induced lung tumorigenesis in A/J mice by green tea and its major polyphenol as antioxidants." *Cancer Res* **52**(14): 3875-3879.

Yamashita, T., T. Uchida, et al. (1997). "Nitric oxide is an effector molecule in inhibition of tumor cell growth by rIFN-gamma-activated rat neutrophils." *Int J Cancer* **71**(2): 223–230.

Yandell, D.W., T.A. Campbell, et al. (1989). "Oncogenic point mutations in the human retinoblastoma gene: their application to genetic counseling." *N Engl J Med* **321**(25): 1689–1695.

Yang, C.S. and Z.Y. Wang (1993). "Tea and cancer." *J Natl Cancer Inst* **85**(13): 1038–1049.

Yang, C.S., G.Y. Yang, et al. (1998). "Tea and tea polyphenols inhibit cell hyperproliferation, lung tumorigenesis, and tumor progression." *Exp Lung Res* **24**(4): 629–639.

Yano, S., K. Kondo, et al. (2003). "Distribution and function of EGFR in human tissue and the effect of EGFR tyrosine kinase inhibition." *Anticancer Res* **23**(5 A): 3639–3650.

Yu, S.Y., Y.J. Chu, et al. (1985). "Regional variation of cancer mortality incidence and its relation to selenium levels in China." *Biological Trace Element Research* **7**: 21–29.

Zhang, J., S. Jiang, et al. (2001). "Antioxidant supplementation prevents oxidation and inflammatory responses induced by sidestream cigarette smoke in old mice." *Environ Health Perspect* **109**(10): 1007–1009.

Zhao, Y., J. Cao, et al. (1997). "Apoptosis induced by tea polyphenols in HL-60 cells." *Cancer Lett* **121**(2): 163–167.

Zhong, S., A.F. Howie, et al. (1991). "Glutathione S-transferase mu locus: use of genotyping and phenotyping assays to assess association with lung cancer susceptibility." *Carcinogenesis* **12**(9): 1533–1537.

Zieba, M., M. Suwalski, et al. (2000). "Comparison of hydrogen peroxide generation and the content of lipid peroxidation products in lung cancer tissue and pulmonary parenchyma." *Respir Med* **94**(8): 800–805.

Zochbauer-Muller, S., K.M. Fong, et al. (2001). "Aberrant promoter methylation of multiple genes in non-small cell lung cancers." *Cancer Res* **61**(1): 249–255.

Breast Cancer Prevention

Patricia A. Thompson, Ana Maria Lopez, and Alison Stopeck

College of Medicine, University of Arizona, Tucson, AZ 85724

Despite advancement in detection and treatment with promising trends in screening over the past three decades, breast cancer remains the most common malignancy and the second cause of cancer death among women. Worldwide, the incidence of breast cancer varies by as much as five-fold based on geographic location. Countries with the highest incidence rates include the United States (U.S.) and the Netherlands (approximately 91 per 100,000). Countries in the far east, such as India and China, have the lowest incidence rates (approximately 20 per 100,000) (Parkin 2004). In the U.S., approximately 217,440 new invasive breast cancers were diagnosed in 2004; an estimated 1,450 of those cancers were diagnosed in men. Approximately 40,580 deaths from breast cancer occurred in 2004 in the U.S. (Jemal, Tiwari et al. 2004). In addition to invasive breast cancers, an additional 59,000 cases of non-invasive *in situ* carcinomas of the breast were diagnosed (Jemal, Tiwari et al. 2004). Breast cancer develops through a series of molecular, genetic and environmental events. As the understanding of the multi-step process of breast cancer tumorigenesis and its underlying molecular events increase, new avenues for breast cancer prevention and early intervention are emerging.

Etiology

The current understanding of breast cancer development suggests that breast tumors arise through the accumulation of a series of molecular alterations that manifest at the cellular level, culminating in an outgrowth of breast epithelial cells demonstrating immortal features and uncontrolled growth (Lacroix, Toillon et al. 2004). There are likely at least three sequential phases of breast tumor development – initiation, promotion and progression. Initiation is widely believed to involve the acquisition of a genetic hit or hits that occur rapidly and that are irreversible. Clonal propagation of cells harboring the initiating events occurs through a prolonged promotion phase. Tumor promotion is determined by growth factors, with estrogen as the major steroid hormone affecting growth in the normal and malignant breast epithelium (Weinstat-Saslow 1995). Dysregulation of cell signaling and cell cycling events associated with promotion are predominantly non-genetic in nature. Since exposure to growth factors in the promotion phase are potentially modifiable, the inhibition of these pathways during this premalignant period, either by suppressing the growth factor itself or blockade of the signaling machinery, may be the most promising targets for preventing development of invasive cancer (Boland, Knox et al. 2002). Entry into the tumor progression phase is coupled with additional irreversible genetic lesions. These additional lesions result in further instability and completion of cellular immortalization and transformation. Progression is associated with the acquisition of invasive characteristics, tumor cell motility, and angiogenic features that define the malignant phenotype. Progression, like the initiation phase, is thought to be largely irreversible and represents the most advanced stage of the disease process and the most difficult to cure. Because it is thought that the process of tumor development encompasses many years or even decades, the development of breast cancer prevention agents is now focused largely on reversing, halting or delaying events in the promotion phase.

Epidemiology

Sporadic breast cancer is relatively uncommon among women younger than 40 years of age but rises significantly thereafter. This is illustrated in the Surveillance, Epidemiology and End Results (SEER) data from 1995 through 2001. During this time period, the incidence rate of invasive breast cancer for all women age 35 to 39 was 30.8 per 100,000 in the U.S. For women age 40 to 44 years of age, this rate doubled to 60.6, and increased to 172.2 per 100,000 by age 55 to 59 (Ries 2004). The lifetime risk of breast cancer is now estimated at 13.4% for all women, 14.2% for non-Hispanic whites and 10.0% for African American women.

The incidence rate continues to rise with advancing age and does not demonstrate a peak or decline among pooled data from the screened and unscreened populations. Among screened populations, incidence rates appear to be highest between 50 to 69 years of age, followed by a leveling off or even decline with age after 70. This suggests that as mammography is universally adopted, the total and age-specific incidence for breast cancer will change to reflect a disease that primarily afflicts women during the sixth and seventh decade of life (Erbas, Amos et al. 2004; Hemminki, Rawal et al. 2004).

With the introduction of screening, a dramatic increase in the incidence of breast cancer has been observed, particularly among women in the targeted population for screening (age 50 to 69 years). The increased incidence initially coincided with a more than doubling of the number of small tumors (less than 2 cm) detected and a reduction in the growth of the incidence rate of advanced disease (Garfinkel, Boring et al. 1994). Despite the slowed increase in the incidence rate of advanced disease, more recent analysis suggests that breast cancer incidence has not yet leveled or declined for most populations. The rate continues to increase among Asian and Pacific Islanders (2.1% per year), Hispanics (1.3% per year) and whites (0.9% per year) with disease among American Indians and Alaska Natives declining by about 3.7% per year (ACS 2004). Rates among African American women appear stable; however, African American women remain more likely than white women to be diagnosed with large tumors (larger than 5 cm). An unexpected increase in large tumors was noted among white women between 1992 and 2000, the cause of which is unknown although hormone use and increasing rates of obesity may be related factors (Ghafoor, Jemal et al. 2003).

The introduction of widespread screening has also resulted in a nearly five-fold increase in the incidence rates of *in situ* or locally-contained disease. The majority of these early-stage lesions are diagnosed as ductal carcinoma *in situ* (DCIS), which are often not clinically appreciated and only detectable by imaging methods (Ernster, Barclay et al. 1996). The increase in incidence rates of DCIS has occurred in all age groups but especially among women over age 50. Detection of DCIS continues to increase annually at a greater rate than detection of invasive cancers of the breast. A second, less common type of *in situ* disease is designated lobular carcinoma in situ (LCIS). LCIS accounts for only 15% of *in situ* lesions and its incidence has increased at about two times the rate of invasive cancers, particularly among postmenopausal women (Li, Anderson et al. 2002).

Risk Factors

There are several risk factors for breast cancer for which sufficient evidence exists to support their use in patient risk assessment (Table 1). Many of these factors form the basis of breast cancer risk assessment tools that will be discussed below.

Age and Gender. Increasing age and female sex are established risk factors for breast cancer. Incidence increases at the time of menopause, with an apparent peak in women between 50 and 69 years of age (Erbas, Amos et al. 2004; Hemminki, Rawal et al. 2004). The significant shift in incidence rates during the years surrounding the menopause has served as the basis for initiating annual mammography screening for all women at age 40. The efficacy of screening among premenopausal women remains unclear in large part due to the reduced sensitivity of current screening methods in younger women (Smith 2000; Buist, Porter et al. 2004). Male breast cancer is rare and distinct from breast cancers that occur among women and is discussed elsewhere (Giordano, Buzdar et al. 2002).

Table 1. Established breast cancer risk factor

Risk Factor	Estimated Relative Risk
Advanced Age	>4
Family History	
Two or more relatives (mother, sister)	>5
One 1st degree relative (mother, sister)	>2
Family history of ovarian cancer <50	>2
Personal History	
Breast cancer	3–4
Positive for BRCA1/BRCA2 mutation	>4
Breast biopsy with atypical hyperplasia	4–5
Breast biopsy with LCIS or DCIS	8–10
Reproductive History	
Early age at menarche (<12)	2
Late age of menopause	1.5–2
Late age of 1st term pregnancy (>30)/nulliparity	2
Use of combined estrogen/progesterone HRT	1.5–2
Current or recent use of OCs	1.5
Lifestyle Factors	
Adult weight gain	1.5–2
Sedentary lifestyle	1.3–1.5
Alcohol consumption	1.5

Family History of Breast Cancer. A positive family history of breast cancer is the most widely recognized risk factor for breast cancer. Risk is approximately five times greater in women with two or more first-degree relatives with breast cancer and is also greater among women with a single first-degree relative, particularly if diagnosed at an early age (age 50 or younger) (Claus, Risch et al. 1991; Olsen, Seersholm et al. 1999; Sakorafas, Krespis et al. 2002). A family history of ovarian cancer in a first-degree relative, especially if the disease occurred at an early age (younger than age 50), has been associated with a doubling of risk of breast cancer. In five to 10% of breast cancer cases, risk is inherited as an autosomal dominant disorder. These hereditary cancers represent a distinct subset of familial breast cancers, which exhibit high penetrance and clustering with ovarian cancers (Antoniou, Pharoah et al. 2003). The *BRCA1* and *BRCA2* gene mutations, discovered as breast cancer causing genes on chromosome 17 and 13, respectively, account for the majority of autosomal dominantly inherited breast cancers (Narod and Foulkes 2004). Women who inherit a mutation in the *BRCA1* or *BRCA2* gene have between a 50 and 80% lifetime risk of developing breast cancer (Antoniou, Pharoah et al. 2003). Three additional genetic conditions are associated with a high risk of breast cancer. These include Li-Fraumeni syndrome, Cowden syndrome and Peutz-Jeghers syndrome. These rare syndromes caused by mutations in known tumor suppressor genes p53, PTEN and LKB1 are all highly associated with increased risk of early onset breast cancer (Hodgson, Morrison et al. 2004). Additional genes are suspect in breast cancer but appear to act in a less dominant fashion. Among some breast cancer families, inheritance of a missense mutation in the ataxia telangiectasia (ATM) gene has been associated with increased risk (Stankovic, Kidd et al. 1998). A variant in the cell-cycle checkpoint kinase (CHEK2) gene that occurs in about 1% of the population has been associated with a two-fold increased risk in carriers and has been described as a moderate effector gene for breast cancer risk (Stankovic, Kidd et al. 1998). Future studies are expected to identify additional moderate effector genes. Adding to the biologic validity of these moderate effector mutations as breast cancer risk genes, both the ATM and CHEK2 proteins have known function in the BRCA1/2 DNA repair pathways.

Reproductive Risk Factors. Late age at first pregnancy, nulliparity, early onset of menses, and late age of menopause have all been consistently associated with an increased risk of breast cancer (Kelsey and Bernstein 1996; Colditz and Rosner 2000; Deligeoroglou, Michailidis et al. 2003; Pike, Pearce et al. 2004). Among the reproductive risk factors, women who experience natural menopause after 55 years of age have about twice the risk of breast cancer compared to women who experience natural menopause before age 45. The observed increased risk among women with early menarche (younger than 12 years of age) appears to be strongest in the premenopausal period, whereas risk of later onset breast cancer appears to be greater among women who experience a late first full-term pregnancy. Women who bear their first child after the age of 30 have twice the risk of developing breast cancer as compared to those who experience first full-term pregnancy before 20 years of age. Nulliparity confers increased risk of postmenopausal breast cancer. At present, the relative effect of these reproductive factors is unclear among mutation carriers and among women with a family history of cancer. There is some limited data to suggest that later age at first pregnancy may be protective in women with hereditary disease (Jernstrom, Lerman et al. 1999; Tryggvadottir, Olafsdottir et al. 2003). Further studies are needed to corroborate early findings regarding the interaction between reproductive risk factors and familial breast cancers.

Prior Breast Health History. A history of breast cancer is associated with a three- to four-fold increased risk of a second primary cancer in the contralateral breast (Kollias, Ellis et al. 1999; Claus, Stowe et al. 2003; Page 2004). In addition to a prior history of breast cancer, a history of breast biopsy that is positive for hyperplasia, fibroadenoma with complex features, sclerosing adenosis and solitary papilloma have been associated with a 1.5- to two-fold increase in risk of breast cancer (Dupont and Page 1985; Page and Jensen 1994; Page 2004; Vogel 2004). In contrast, any diagnosis of atypical hyperplasia that is ductal or lobular in nature has been associated with a four- to five-fold increased risk of breast cancer. A prior history of fibrocystic disease, such as fibrocystic change without proliferative breast disease or fibroadenoma, has not been associated with increased risk (Dupont, Page et al. 1994). A history of premalignant ductal carcinoma *in situ* (DCIS) or lobular carcinoma *in situ* (LCIS) may confer an eight- to 10-fold increase in risk among women who harbor untreated preinvasive lesions (Page 2004).

Lifestyle and Environmental Risk Factors. The wide range of breast cancer incidence rates around the world is largely attributed to differences in dietary intake and reproductive behaviors (Henderson and Bernstein 1991; Kaaks 1996; Stoll 1998; Stoll 1999; Holmes and Willett 2004). As with cancers of the colon and prostate, diets that are enriched in grains, fruits and vegetables, low in saturated fats, and low in energy (calories) and alcohol are thought to be protective against breast cancer (Holmes and Willett 2004). Breast cancer is positively associated with adult weight gain (e.g. perimenopausal and postmenopausal weight gain), a Western diet (high energy content in the form of animal fats and refined carbohydrates), and a sedentary lifestyle. The Western lifestyle (e.g., Western diet and lack of exercise) strongly correlates with the development of obesity, particularly abdominal obesity, and chronic states of hyperinsulinemia. Both of these conditions are associated with an increase in risk of the development of insulin resistance, type 2 diabetes and cardiovascular disease (Stoll 1998; Stoll 1999). Recent studies suggest a link between breast cancer risk and Western lifestyle mediated through chronic exposures to the mitogenic properties of insulin and insulin-like growth factors (IGFs) (Hankinson, Willett et al. 1998; Toniolo, Bruning et al. 2000; Shi, Yu et al. 2004; Sugumar, Liu et al. 2004). Although controversial, circulating IGF-1 levels may be associated with increased risk of breast cancer among premenopausal women and may emerge as targets for modulation in future prevention efforts. Although dietary fat has not emerged as a consistent risk factor for breast cancer, evidence implicating high fat, high energy diets in the shift towards earlier onset of menses in young women in Western cultures, if corroborated, may serve as the basis for future recommendations regarding lifetime breast cancer risk reduction starting with diet modification in childhood (Law 2000). Similar recommendations for reduced sugar intake may also follow to modify risks mediated through insulin and IGF hormones.

Exogenous Hormone Exposure. One of the most widely studied factors in breast cancer etiology has been the use of exogenous hormones in the form of oral contraceptives (OCs) and hormone replacement therapy (HRT) (Garbe, Levesque et al. 2004).

Recent and long-term use of HRT, particularly the use of combined formulations that include both a progesterone and estrogen component, has been associated with an increase in breast cancer risk (Nelson, Humphrey et al. 2002; Rossouw, Anderson et al. 2002). In the Women's Health Initiative (WHI) trial, invasive breast cancer was increased in women randomly assigned to combined HRT as compared to those assigned to placebo (Rossouw, Anderson et al. 2002). In an observational cohort study, risk was also elevated among women with short-term use of synthetic progestin plus estrogen therapy (Fournier, Berrino et al. 2004). A systematic literature review suggests that the long-term use of combined hormones may be associated with later stage at diagnosis and a less favorable outcome (Antoine, Liebens et al. 2004). The estrogen-only arm of the WHI was halted in February 2004 due to safety concerns. After an average 6.8 years of follow up, estrogen alone did not affect the incidence of heart disease, a key endpoint of the study, when compared to placebo. An increased risk of stroke and a decreased risk of hip fractures were identified (Anderson, Limacher et al. 2004). Nevertheless promising results from the estrogen-only arm of the WHI trial (The Women's Health Initiative Steering Committee, 2004) suggest no increase in breast cancer risk among estrogen-only users and suggest there may be benefit. Current recommendations for the use of combined and single-agent HRT are in flux. Studies examining the risks and benefits of alternative hormonal agents and/or doses are planned. When prescribing HRT, a discussion of the most current evidence and an assessment of the potential benefit and harm should be provided to the individual patient. Because estrogen-only formulations pose a known increased risk of the development of endometrial cancer, the use of estrogen and progesterone for the management of menopausal symptoms should be tailored for the individual patient at the lowest effective dose for the shortest time needed to abate symptoms.

Current use of OCs has been inconsistently associated with a slight increased risk of breast cancer. The overall evidence suggests an approximate 25% greater risk of breast cancer among women currently using OCs (1996; Deligeoroglou, Michailidis et al. 2003). The risk appears to diminish with age and time since OC discontinuation. Risk among ever users of OCs declines to the average population risk approximately 10 years after cessation of OC use.

Other Risk Factors. A number of environmental exposures, including cigarette smoking (both active and passive exposure), dietary carcinogens, exposure to pesticides, irradiation and environmental and exogenous estrogens, have been investigated in relation to breast cancer risk in humans (Laden and Hunter 1998; Calle, Frumkin et al. 2002; Coyle 2004; Gammon, Eng et al. 2004). Exposure to high doses of ionizing irradiation to the chest area during puberty has been associated with an increased risk of breast cancer in adulthood (Carmichael, Sami et al. 2003). Because of the strong association between ionizing irradiation and breast cancer risk, care is given in medical diagnostics procedures to minimize exposure to the chest area particularly during adolescence. Women with a prior history of irradiation exposure to the chest area should be examined and counseled on their risk based upon timing and dose of exposure. A patient treated for Hodgkin's lymphoma, particularly at age 30 or earlier, is at very high increased risk of breast cancer (Clemons, Loijens et al. 2000). Current evidence does not support a significant and reproducible link between these environmental exposures and breast cancer risk. Thus, these factors remain suspect but unproven.

Emerging Risk Factors. Emerging evidence suggests that women presenting with radiographically dense breast, particularly in the postmenopausal years, may be at elevated risk of breast cancer (Boyd, Lockwood et al. 1998; Boyd, Martin et al. 2001). Radiographically dense regions have been associated with a higher degree of proliferating epithelium in the breast tissue and may serve as a marker of a susceptible environment for cancer development. Radiographically dense breasts often coincide with increased endogenous or exogenous hormone exposure. The use of mammographic density measures in risk assessment is an area of emerging interest and should be monitored for its future relevance in patient-specific breast cancer risk assessment. For example, HRT use has been associated with increasing mammographic density in the breast. This raises concerns about the effectiveness of screening among women prescribed HRT (Warren 2004). The positive association between HRT and dense breast tissue has been suggested as the explanation for the observed higher incidence of advanced disease among HRT users undergoing regular mammograms (Antoine, Liebens et al. 2004). Thus, screening recommendations for women prescribed HRT and for women with radiographically dense breasts may require modification, particularly in light of the availability of other screening modalities such as ultrasound and magnetic resonance imaging (MRI).

Screening and Early Detection

Early detection remains the primary defense available to patients to prevent the development of life-threatening breast cancer. Detections of breast tumors that are smaller and non-palpable are more likely to be associated with earlier stage disease, which will have a more favorable prognosis than more advanced disease. The efficacy of early detection has been demonstrated in both observation-based studies and in randomized controlled trials. Therefore, early detection is widely endorsed by organizations that issue clinical recommendations for breast cancer care. The most widely endorsed method is annual screening mammography beginning at age 40. For women younger than age 40, monthly breast self-exam practices and clinical breast exams every three years are recommended, beginning at 20 years of age (Smith, Saslow et al. 2003).

Breast Self Exam (BSE) and Clinical Breast Exam (CBE). Though limited to palpable lesions, the rationale for BSE and CBE is similar to that for detection of smaller, non-palpable disease. The earlier the diagnosis, the better the prognosis. Evidence supporting the value of BSE and CBE are limited and largely inferred. Even with appropriate training, BSE has not been found to reduce breast cancer mortality (Thomas, Gao et al. 1997). Evidence suggests that each increase of 5 mm in tumor size is associated with a less favorable outcome (Smith, Saslow et al. 2003). With increasing improvements in treatment regimens for disease that has not metastasized, continued recommendations for BSE and CBE, particularly among women younger than 40 who otherwise have no screening options, are still being developed.

Mammography. Mammography has been demonstrated as an effective tool for the prevention of advanced breast cancer in women at average risk. Mammography is currently the best available population-based method to detect breast cancer in its earliest stages when treatment is most effective (Haffty, Lee et al. 1998). Mammography often detects a lesion before palpable by CBE and, on average, one to two years before noted by BSE.

Recent advances in mammography include the development of digital mammography and the increased use of computer-aided diagnosis (CAD) systems. Digital mammography allows the image to be recorded digitally and stored on the hard drive of a computer. The images are viewed on a computer screen allowing the reviewer to modify the image without making changes in the original image. The digital mammographic image can be magnified and the brightness and contrast modified by the examiner to better elucidate specific areas in question. The ability to manipulate the image may facilitate the identification of breast lesions. Digital images can also be transmitted over phone lines, speeding the transmission to an expert for a second opinion without the risk of losing the film. CAD systems have been developed to help the radiologist identify mammographic abnormalities. Used as an adjunct tool, CAD systems contribute to the earlier diagnosis of breast cancer. The US Preventive Services Task Force estimates the benefit of mammography in women between 50 to 74 years of age to be a 30% reduction in risk of dying from breast cancer. The benefit to women age 40 to 49, the risk of death is decreased by 17% (Humphrey, Helfand et al. 2002). Although mammography guidelines have been in place for over 30 years, many women still do not undergo screening as indicated. The two most significant predictive factors for a woman to undergo mammography are physician recommendation and access to health insurance. Non-white women and those of lower socioeconomic status are less likely to obtain mammography services and more likely to present with life-threatening, advanced stage disease (Ward, Jemal et al. 2004).

Alternative Screening Modalities and Future Directions. Mammography has an approximate false negative rate of 13 to 26% (Warren Burhenne, Wood et al. 2000). This rate is higher among premenopausal women and among those taking HRT due to increased breast density. Therefore, improved imaging modalities would be of great benefit to both those at high risk in cases where breast images are difficult to interpret. Ultrasound has become a widely available and useful adjunct to mammography in the clinical setting. Ultrasound is generally used to assist the clinical exam of a suspicious lesion detected by mammogram or physical examination. As a screening device, the ultrasound is limited by a number of factors but most notably by the failure to detect microcalcifications and a fairly high false positive rate (Smith, Saslow et al. 2003).

In an effort to overcome the limitations of mammography and ultrasound, MRI has been explored as a modality for detecting breast cancer in high-risk populations and in younger women. A combination of T-1, T-2 and 3-D MRI techniques have been found to be diagnostic for malignant changes in the breast (Morris, Liberman et al. 2003). MRI has also been demonstrated to be an important adjunct screening tool for women with *BRCA1* or *BRCA2* mutations; however, methods to address the high rate of false positive findings have yet to be addressed (Fournier, Berrino et al. 2004). A number of studies are ongoing that evaluate molecular changes in tumors as imaging targets. The goal of this work is to develop new molecular imaging techniques with greater specificity. These investigational approaches are based on the discovery that specific cell-surface receptors can be overexpressed in malignant tissue as compared to proximate non-malignant tissue (White, Taetle et al. 1990; Fournier, Berrino et al. 2004). Current studies focus on directly imaging these molecular properties with MRI (Weissleder, Moore et al. 2000). MRI is also being developed to detect angiogenic changes attributed to malignant growth (Louie, Huber et al. 2000). In addition, studies to combine spectroscopy procedures with MRI technology are currently under development to improve the specificity of MRI to detect early malignant changes in the breast (Bolan, Meisamy et al. 2003). Future success in these areas is likely to have a significant impact on the application of MRI for breast imaging; however, high cost of instrumentation and high rate of unnecessary biopsies for false positive findings will likely limit application of these methods to high-risk patients.

Prevention

Pharmacologic and surgical strategies have demonstrated efficacy for lowering the incidence of breast cancer in high-risk women, particularly those responsive to steroid hormones (Smith, Saslow et al. 2003; Calderon-Margalit and Paltiel 2004; Lo and Vogel 2004). The need for primary prevention of breast cancer is clear. In an earlier review by Vogel (Vogel 1991), it was estimated that more than 30 million women in the U.S. were over the age of 50; an estimated two million of these women have a first-degree relative who had been diagnosed with breast cancer. He further estimated that six million women had undergone at least one breast biopsy with one-fourth of those showing evidence of proliferative changes. The continuing maturation of the American

Table 2. Breast cancer early detection guidelines by risk category and age*

Age	Average and Moderate Risk	High Risk
20s and 30s	Monthly Breast Self Exam (BSE) following instruction Clinical Breast Exam (CBE) as part of regular health exams, minimum every three years Awareness to report any change in breast health	BSE and CBE as recommended in average risk women Consideration of earlier initiation of screening methods with shorter screening intervals Consideration of other screening modalities to include ultrasound and magnetic resonance imaging methods Heighten awareness to report any change in breast health
40s through 60s	Continuance of BSE, CBE and introduction of mammography screening Heighten patient awareness to report any change in breast health	Vigilance in patient surveillance and consideration of shorter intervals for screening
Over age 70	Consideration of overall health benefit with mammography in context of health status and expected longevity	Continuance of surveillance vigilance in context of expected patient longevity

* Modified from the ACS Guidelines for Early Breast Cancer Detection, 2003 (Smith, Saslow et al. 2003)

population in combination with an alarming increase in the number of women over age 50 who are overweight or obese (65 and 25%, respectively) and the changes in reproductive patterns suggests the unlikelihood of lowered incidence rates over the next several decades in the absence of active prevention.

Current recommendations for the primary prevention of breast cancer can be divided into those that apply generally to the population and those that can be applied at the individual level based on risk estimates (Table 2).

For the general population, it is now recommended that women maintain healthy body weight, engage in regular physical activity, eat diets enriched in grains, fruits and vegetables, and consume alcoholic beverages in moderation, if at all (Byers, Nestle et al. 2002; Cerhan, Potter et al. 2004; Key, Schatzkin et al. 2004). These recommendations are derived from numerous published case-control studies that consistently demonstrate lower risk among women who maintain their body weight within five pounds of their weight at age 18 and among those who consume a diet rich in fruits and vegetables and consume low amounts of alcoholic beverages. Although the amount of physical activity needed to reduce risk remains unclear, women who engage in some modest physical activity, even walking only two times per week, are afforded a 20% reduction in risk (Chlebowski, Pettinger et al. 2004). Additionally, two recent studies suggest that any intentional weight loss of more than 20 pounds at any time during adult life is associated with a modest reduction in breast cancer risk (Parker and Folsom 2003; Chlebowski, Pettinger et al. 2004; Radimer, Ballard-Barbash et al. 2004). Future recommendations for the general population are likely to include more emphasis on the reduction of simple sugars in the diet and targeted information about the risks associated with abdominal obesity. Further research on the influence of dietary fat on reproductive risk factors, such as age of onset of menarche, is needed. These findings will likely guide future recommendations that may shift the delivery of prevention counseling related to lifestyle factors from adults to children and their parents. It is likely that earlier lifestyle modification will have a greater affect on lifetime risk reduction.

Surgery- and drug-based prevention has proven efficacious for women at high risk for developing breast cancer (Calderon-Margalit and Paltiel 2004; Lo and Vogel 2004). This high-risk population includes women who have tested positive for mutation in the breast cancer-related genes, women with multiple affected relative or relatives with disease presenting at early age, and women with a personal history of breast cancer or history of premalignant disease (DCIS or LCIS). The primary prevention of breast cancer in this population includes intervention options that encompass bilateral mastectomy, oophorectomy or the use of selective estrogen receptor modulators (SERMs).

For women at high risk of breast cancer, bilateral prophylactic mastectomy and oophorectomy are considered highly effective options to reduce risk. In observational studies, premenopausal women with known *BRCA1* or *BRCA2* mutations had a 50% reduction in their age-matched incidence of breast cancer after prophylactic oophorectomy (Rebbeck, Levin et al. 1999). In a retrospective cohort study of women with a moderate to strong family history of breast cancer who underwent subcutaneous rather than total mastectomy (Hartmann, Schaid et al. 1999), the reduction in risk was nearly 95% for women at high risk, and nearly 90% for those at moderate risk. The reduction in risk of death was reported to be approximately 80% for the high-risk woman and 100% for the moderate-risk woman. Though this study clearly shows the relative risk reduction benefit for this population, it is important to recognize that only about 50 women of the 214 in the high-risk group and 37 of the 425 women in the moderate-risk group were expected to develop breast cancers. Thus, the effectiveness of the prevention strategy offered an absolute risk reduction of only 10 to 20% of those at risk. Greater benefit to the individual patient will be gained with future improvements in the accuracy of risk assessment and in the types of prevention that can be offered to women through targeted chemoprevention strategies. In addition, as we gain more information on the types of mutations in the *BRCA* genes and their effects as well as identify additional genetic and environmental components of breast cancer risk, we will see improved stratification of women into risk categories. It is expected that in the future, this type of risk stratification will guide patient and physician decision-making regarding drug based or surgical prophylactic interventions.

Chemoprevention

The use of specific natural or synthetic chemical agents as therapeutic agents to prevent, reverse or suppress carcinogenic events in the breast defines the practice of breast cancer chemoprevention. This definition excludes the use of whole foods in diet. The goal of chemoprevention is to reduce the incidence of breast cancer by inhibiting or delaying the progression of premalignant mammary epithelial cells.

Selective Estrogen Receptor Modulators (SERMs). Having identified estrogen exposure as a risk factor for breast cancer, it was not surprising that adjuvant treatment trials with the selective estrogen receptor modulator, tamoxifen (Nolvadex®, AstraZeneca Pharmaceuticals), showed not only reduced recurrence of breast cancer among women with breast cancers but also a reduction in the number of second primary breast cancers (Nayfield, Karp et al. 1991). Based on these data, a large randomized clinical trial with tamoxifen was initiated by the National Surgical Adjuvant Breast and Bowel Project (NSABP) to test its efficacy as a chemoprevention agent among women at increased risk of breast cancer. There was a 49% reduction in the incidence of invasive breast cancer and a 50% reduction in DCIS among the tamoxifen users compared to those assigned to placebo. The benefit was exclusive for lowering the risk of estrogen receptor (ER)-positive disease, consistent with the known mechanism of action. The greatest benefit was achieved among women with a prior history of LCIS (56%) or atypical hyperplasia (86%). In addition, it was noted that fewer fractures occurred among those treated with tamoxifen. However, a greater number of endometrial cancers, pulmonary thrombosis, stroke and deep vein thrombosis were observed among women taking tamoxifen (Fisher, Costantino et al. 1998). Subsequent analyses demonstrated that the overall health benefit for the patient depended on overall risk of breast cancer, endometrial cancer and for thrombosis (Gail, Costantino et al. 1999). These findings have not been confirmed by other breast cancer chemoprevention trials, such as those conducted in England and Italy (Powles, Eeles et al. 1998). The lack of consistency in findings may be in part due to the differences in study populations. The European studies enrolled patients who were not at increased risk of breast cancer, unlike the NSABP trial. Patients in the European studies were also allowed to remain on hormone replacement therapy, perhaps confounding the potential benefit of tamoxifen.

In addition to the finding that SERMs, such as tamoxifen, demonstrate improved bone health and possible cardioprotection in postmenopausal women, additional

SERMs, such as raloxifene, have been developed. Within the context of a secondary analysis of the Multiple Outcome of Raloxifene Evaluation (MORE) study of osteoporosis, postmenopausal women randomized to raloxifene had a 72% reduction in breast cancer incidence compared to women taking placebo (Cauley, Norton et al. 2001). Greatly encouraged by these data, NSABP investigators sought to compare the effectiveness of raloxifene and tamoxifen in a randomized, double-blind study of postmenopausal women at high-risk of breast cancer. Results from the STAR trial are expected to be reported in the near future.

A subsequent analysis of the tamoxifen data by the US Preventive Services Task Force (USPSTF) resulted in a failure to recommend the routine use of tamoxifen or raloxifene for the primary prevention of breast cancer for women at low or average risk; however, the USPSTF concluded that there was sufficient evidence to recommend the use of these agents in high risk women (2002). In addition, the USPSTF concluded that there was 'good evidence' that these agents increase adverse thromboembolic

Table 3. Current patient management options for women at high risk for breast cancer: benefits and risks

	Surveillance	Bilateral oophorectomy	Risk reduction mastectomy	Tamoxifen
Benefits	Non-invasive, non-toxic Promise of new methods with improved sensitivity (e.g., MRI)	Significant lowering of risk among pre-menopausal women Risk reduction observed in both BRCA1/2 carriers, greatest among BRCA2 carriers undergoing surgery before 35 years	Significant risk reduction (> 90%) in all high risk women including BRCA1/BRCA2 carriers	Approximate 50% reduction in ER+ tumors Greatest benefit for women with history of premalignant disease or family history (high risk women) Effective against only ER+ disease Limited data suggest efficacy in BRCA carriers
Risks	Lack of sensitivity in young women Concerns over low dose irradiation exposure Lack of strong evidence that early detection reduces mortality for all women, particularly in BRCA1/2 carriers	Premature menopause Irreversible Psychological/ quality of life	Extreme Psychological Irreversible	Increased risk of thrombotic events No efficacy for ER negative tumors Efficacy in BRCA carriers not established Data on age of initiation and duration for optimum health benefit unknown Overall health benefit not demonstrated

Table 4. Recommendations for all women to lower the lifetime risk of breast cancer

✓ Maintain healthy body weight
✓ Engage in regular physical activity throughout life
✓ Eat a diet enriched in fruits, vegetables and grains
✓ Eat a diet low in total fats and refined sugars
✓ Substitute saturated fats in diet with unsaturated healthy fats
✓ Drink alcoholic beverages in moderation
✓ Weigh risk and benefits of hormone replacement therapy
✓ Use HRT for shortest interval necessary to manage menopausal symptoms
✓ Follow recommended screening guidelines
✓ Practice monthly self breast exam
✓ Schedule and attend regular health checkups

events and that tamoxifen is associated with increased risk of endometrial cancers. The summary evaluation of the task force resulted in recommendations to clinicians to discuss the benefits and risks of these interventions with patients at high risk of breast cancer. A summary of management options for patients at high risk of breast cancer is presented in Table 3, and a summary of general recommendations for all women is presented in Table 4.

New Agents for Primary Prevention of Breast Cancer

Aromatase Inhibitors. Research on use of aromatase inhibitors in the adjuvant setting for the treatment of breast cancer suggests that this newer class of hormone modulating agents may have greater efficacy than tamoxifen in the primary prevention setting (Tobias 2004). Results from the Arimidex, Tamoxifen, Alone or in Combination (ATAC) trial, though preliminary, suggest that anastrozole (Arimidex®) was better at reducing recurrence, contralateral breast cancers and demonstrated better adverse risk profile with fewer thromboembolic events than tamoxifen (2002). These preliminary findings have served as the impetus for initiating studies to evaluate not only anastrozole but also other aromatase inhibitors, such as letrozole (Femara®) and exemestane (Aromosin®), for efficacy in the primary prevention of breast cancer (Goss and Strasser-Weippl 2004). One such study is a 5,100-participant phase III trial that was initiated in the U.S. in 2004 to evaluate exemestane alone versus exemestane with celecoxib, a cyclooxygenase-2 inhibitor, versus placebo alone for the primary prevention of breast cancer among those at increased risk (Goss and Strasser-Weippl 2004).

Other Agents. There are a number of compounds that do not act through the modulation of estrogen or the estrogen receptor that have demonstrated activity in animal models of breast and other solid tumors. Interest in these agents is strong because of the potential for the broader, estrogen receptor-independent action of these agents. These agents include drugs that target the retinoid receptor, the use of non-steroidal anti-inflammatory drugs (NSAIDs) including aspirin, tyrosine kinase inhibitors and antibodies that target the epidermal growth factor receptor signaling pathway, specific inhibitors of cyclooxygenase-2 (COX-2), inducers of apoptosis, modulators of the IGF signaling pathways and inhibitors of angiogenesis (Shen and Brown 2003). Most of these agents remain in the preclinical or early phase development for use in breast cancer. Agents that modulate the retinoid receptor, and more recently the NSAIDs, have received the most attention and are those for which trial data is likely to emerge over the years 2006 to 2010.

Retinoids. Vitamin A analogs or retinoids have been shown to inhibit the in vitro and in vivo growth of breast tumor cells (Yang, Tin et al. 1999; Serrano, Perego et al. 2004). Two types of nuclear retinoid receptors, the RXR and the RAR, bind to the retinoids to mediate their transcriptional effects on genes involved in controlling cell proliferation, differentiation and apoptosis. The retinoids or vitamin A analogs are highly promising agents for primary breast cancer prevention; however, issues related to their toxicity in vivo pose a challenge for dosing and ultimate efficacy. The development of less toxic synthetic retinoids such as N-4-hydroxyphenyl retinamide (4-HPR, fenretinide) and specific modulators of the RXR receptor hold promise with demonstrated action to prevent tumor development in chemically-induced animal models of mammary tumorigenesis and in the prevention of ER-negative tumors in SV40 T antigen and MMTV-erbB2 mouse models (Costa, Formelli et al. 1994) (Wu, Kim et al. 2002). Results from an early randomized breast cancer trial (Decensi, Serrano et al. 2003) evaluating the efficacy of fenretinide to prevent a second breast malignancy in women with cancer were largely disappointing, with no overall reduction in risk observed. Secondary analyses have raised questions about the interaction of retinoids on the IGF system and potential effects of age and menopausal status. Animal studies have suggested a potential benefit in the less common, but more aggressive, ER-negative tumors; therefore, a phase II clinical (Decensi, Serrano et al. 2003) trial to evaluate the combined effects of 4-HPR and tamoxifen in the primary prevention of breast cancer was developed.

Non-Steroidal Anti-Inflammatory Drugs

Consistent findings across several large epidemiological studies provide strong and compelling evidence for a protective role of NSAIDs to reduce the risk of breast cancer by decreasing the inflammation thought to be related to carcinogenesis (Johnson, Anderson et al. 2002; Davies 2003; Harris, Chlebowski et al. 2003; Moorman, Grubber et al. 2003; Terry, Gammon et al. 2004). In a study of 80,741 postmenopausal women participating in the prospective Women's Health Initiative (WHI) Observational Study, regular NSAID use (largely restricted to ibuprofen or aspirin) of two or more tablets per week was associated with a 21% lower incidence with 5 to 9 years of use and a 28% reduced incidence with 10 years of use (Harris, Chlebowski et al. 2003). There was a statistically significant inverse linear trend of breast cancer incidence with the duration of use. More recent studies report a similar risk reduction in breast cancer incidence (e.g., 20 to 30%). The most recent evidence suggests the risk reduction is limited to ER-positive disease (Terry, Gammon et al. 2004). The use of NSAIDs is not a novel concept for chemoprevention research; however, the results from these studies highlight the need for clinical trials to determine the efficacy of NSAIDs as cancer prevention agents and, ultimately, to determine their specificity for disease subtypes (e.g., ER-positive versus ER-negative).

Phase I and II clinical trials have yet to be conducted to determine target tissue-specific pharmacokinetics and bioavailability. For example, accumulation of long half-life NSAIDs such as naproxen (Naprosyn), sulindac (Clinoril) and piroxicam (Feldene) in breast milk compared to more short-acting agents, such as ibuprofen, provides suggestive evidence that certain agents may be more efficacious for tissue-specific chemoprevention than others (Albert and Gernaat 1984). In addition, there is a particularly strong need to generate clinical data in humans that demonstrate the spectrum of anti-cancer and chemopreventive activity to help prioritize candidate agents for evidence-based testing in clinical trials. Evaluation of drugs in larger trial settings will be conduced when: 1) proof that the candidate agent reaches the breast tissue at an effective dose; and 2) demonstration that the agent modulates key signaling pathways involved in tumor development (apoptosis, proliferation, angiogenesis).

Risk Assessment and Clinical Applications

One of the primary challenges in patient care related to primary breast cancer prevention is the need for accurate assessment and communication of risk to the individual patient (refer to Chapter 4 for a more thorough discussion of this topic). The development of clinical practice guidelines that allow for informed decision making regarding surveillance and the weighing of benefits and risks of prevention options remains hindered by the lack of accuracy of individual patient risk. The subject of breast cancer risk assessment has been extensively reviewed in the literature. Risk assessment practice guidelines are likely to continue to improve as more information on risk factors, molecular biology of premalignancies, and their predictive potential are incorporated into existing models.

Elevated Risk. Elevated risk of breast cancer has been defined as the presence of any factor that is reliably identifiable (i.e., family history, prior history of atypia) and when present has been consistently associated with an increase in risk that nears twice that or greater of the general population. In general, light or mild risk elevation has been associated with factors that confer 1.5- to two-fold increase over the general population. Moderate risk is associated with a three- to five-fold increase in risk, and high risk is associated with factors that confer a greater than five-fold elevated risk. Patients with moderate or high risk of breast cancer should be counseled on the importance of early detection and surveillance methods as well as informed on the benefits and risks of primary prevention and chemoprevention.

Risk Assessment Models. There has been a concerted effort by several groups to develop multivariate methods to use a profile of risk factors (genetic or other) to estimate the risk of breast cancer. Two types of risk models have been employed for use in breast cancer risk assessment – those that estimate the risk of developing breast cancer over time and those that determine the likelihood that an individual is a carrier of a *BRCA1* or *BRCA2* or unknown gene mutation. The first of these models is the original Gail Model 1, which was developed in 1989 based on data derived from the Breast Cancer Detection and Demonstration Project (BCDDP) (Gail, Brinton et al. 1989). This model was developed to estimate the probability of developing breast cancer over a defined age interval and was originally intended to improve screening guidelines. The model was subsequently revised to predict risk of invasive breast cancer and again to include history on first degree affected family members (Vogel 1991). The importance of developing effective risk assessment tools in the breast cancer setting was rapidly elevated in the early 1990s due to the findings that bilateral mastectomy, oopherectomy and new therapeutics, such as SERMs, demonstrated potential efficacy in the breast cancer prevention setting. The ability to stratify women by risk (low, moderate and high) was needed in the clinical and research setting due to the increase in prevention options and new chemoprevention agents. Thus, the modified Gail Model was subsequently used as the basis of eligibility for breast cancer prevention trials (Ruffin, August et al. 1993). The accurate identification of the patient who will benefit from prevention has become a primary motivator for the development of risk assessment models. These models are designed both to improve individual patient care practices and for the selection of participants for chemoprevention trials. At present, the US Food and Drug Administration (FDA) guidelines utilize the NSABP's modified Gail model as the basis for eligibility for the prophylactic use of tamoxifen. Tamoxifen is approved for women 35 years and older who have a five-year risk of breast cancer of 1.67 or greater, based on this model.

Subsequent validations of the utility of the Gail Model 2 (Rockhill, Spiegelman et al. 2001) have shown that it is applicable to the general population. The modified Gail model is accurate in women who receive annual mammograms, but tends to overestimate risk in younger women who do not receive annual mammograms. At the individual level, the model lacks adequate discrimination to predict individual risk. For example, in an evaluation of the Gail model in the Nurses' Health Study, only 3.3% of a total of 1,354 cases of breast cancer that arose in the cohort did so within the age-risk strata defined by the Gail model for which benefit from prophylaxis with tamoxifen would be expected. This lack of discrimination and the outstanding need to develop accurate risk assessment methods has resulted in the development of additional models, such as the Claus model, which relies more heavily on autosomal dominant inheritance of disease, models that are specifically designed to capture genetic risk as methods for individualizing genetic testing, such as BRCAPro, and more recently-developed models that were designed to overcome some of the limitations of previous models. Because of these variations, significant differences exist between existing risk models in terms of their integration of the recognized reproductive, personal history and family history risk factors for breast cancer. To simplify the discussion here we have included a table that compares the variables used in the different models (Table 5).

As can be seen in Table 4, significant differences exist between the five models in terms of their integration of the recognized reproductive, personal history and family history risk factors for breast cancer described above, with the exception of the recently described Tyrer-Cuzick. The Tyrer-Cuzick model based on data obtained from the International Breast Intervention Study (IBIS) and the Manual Model have attempted to integrate family history, reproductive factors associated with endogenous estrogen exposure and breast health history to overcome some of the limitations of prior models. In a recent study (Amir, Evans et al. 2003), five risk models were compared to one another for goodness of fit and discriminatory accuracy using data from a cohort of women participating in a Family-History Evaluation and Screening Program. In this cohort, 52 women developed breast cancer during a mean follow up of 5.3 years. Using a calculated expected to observed event as a measure of performance for each model, the Ford performed the worst, particularly among the screening cohort, the Claus and Gail models performed slightly better but underestimated risk

Table 5. Comparison of risk factors used in risk assessment models in women with no prior history of invasive breast cancer or ductal carcinoma in situ

Gail Model	Claus/Ford[a]	Tyrer-Cuzick/Manual
Age	Age	Age
Reproductive	Reproductive	Reproductive
Age-Menarche	None	Age-Menarche
Age-First live birth	Personal History	Age-Menopause
Personal History	None	Age-First live birth
biopsy	Family History	Personal History
ADH[b]	1st degree relative	Biopsy
Family History	2nd degree relative	Atypical Hyperplasia
1st degree relative	Age of onset	LCIS
Lifestyle	Ovarian cancer (Ford)	Family History
None	Male breast cancer (Ford)	1st degree relative
	Lifestyle	2nd degree relative
	None	Age of onset
		Ovarian cancer
		Male breast cancer (Manual)
		Lifestyle
		BMI[c] (Tyrer-Cuzick)

[a] output BRCAPro software package
[b] Atypical ductal hyperplasia
[c] body mass index as a surrogate for adult weight

across all risk categories with a particular worrisome failure in women with a single first degree relative. Of the models, the Tyrer-Cuzick and the Manual models performed the best in terms of accurately estimating expected cases when compared to what was observed (64 observed versus 69 expected in the Tyrer-Cuzick; 64 observed versus 78 predicted by the Manual model). The Tyrer-Cuzick and the Manual models were designed in an attempt to integrate family history, reproductive factors associated with endogenous estrogen exposure and breast health history to overcome some of the limitations of prior models (Tyrer, Duffy et al. 2004). The Manual model was the only model that accurately predicted risk in the screening program for women with a first-degree affected relative. The further validation of these newer models and their discrimination at the level of the individual will be of particular interest in the clinical and research setting as the field evolves.

Conclusion

The ultimate goal of breast cancer risk assessment is to individualize clinical management for moderate to high-risk women to extend life expectancy. The goals for women at low risk are to minimize cost and adverse effects (Hollingsworth, Singletary et al. 2004). At present, scientific evidence supports the integration of prevention counseling and consideration of prevention options (prophylactic surgery and tamoxifen) for women with strong family history of breast cancer or those with personal history of breast biopsy with proliferative changes (i.e., women with moderate to high risk). Unfortunately, this approach only captures a small number of women who will be affected by a breast cancer diagnosis. Most women who develop breast cancers are often determined to be at low risk. Thus, despite the demonstrated efficacy of tamoxifen to prevent invasive breast cancers, the failure to accurately identify women who would benefit from chemoprevention has prevented the acceptance of tamoxifen as a general preventive recommendation. Practice guidelines and recommendations for the individual patient remain hindered by lack of accuracy of existing risk models, significant adverse effects of current prevention options, and a general gap in the ability to translate advancements made in the field into medical practice in a timely and effective manner. Ongoing and future efforts are being designed to fill these gaps, such as the identification of better discriminators of risk (i.e., waist circumference versus obesity, mammographic density, molecular changes in the breast) and identification of benign prevention strategies (i.e., maintenance of healthy weight, engaging in regular physical activity) that reduce the risk or delay onset of breast cancer. Although the mortality rate due to breast cancer is beginning to decline, the next major breakthrough for breast cancer will come from the application of the knowledge gained on risk factors and tumor biology such that prevention can be efficaciously and safely administered for optimum health benefit for a majority of women in the future.

References

(1996). "Breast cancer and hormonal contraceptives: collaborative reanalysis of individual data on 53,297 women with breast cancer and 100,239 women without breast cancer from 54 epidemiological studies. Collaborative Group on Hormonal Factors in Breast Cancer." *Lancet* **347**(9017): 1713–1727.

(2002). "Anastrozole alone or in combination with tamoxifen versus tamoxifen alone for adjuvant treatment of postmenopausal women with early breast cancer: first results of the ATAC randomised trial." *Lancet* **359**(9324): 2131–2139.

(2002). "Using Medication To Prevent Breast Cancer: Recommendations from the United States Preventive Services Task Force." *Ann Intern Med* **137**(1): I62.

ACS (2004). Breast Cancer Facts and Figures 2003–2004, American Cancer Society: *http://www.cancer.org/downloads/STT/CAFF2003BrFPWSecured.pdf*, accessed 11/20/04.

Albert, K.S. and C.M. Gernaat (1984). "Pharmacokinetics of ibuprofen." *Am J Med* **77**(1A): 40–46.

Amir, E., D.G. Evans, et al. (2003). "Evaluation of breast cancer risk assessment packages in the family history evaluation and screening programme." *J Med Genet* **40**(11): 807–814.

Anderson, G.L., M. Limacher, et al. (2004). "Effects of conjugated equine estrogen in postmenopausal women with hysterectomy: The Women's Health Initiative randomized controlled trial." *JAMA* **291**(14): 1701–1712.

Antoine, C., F. Liebens, et al. (2004). "Influence of HRT on prognostic factors for breast cancer: a systematic review after the Women's Health Initiative trial." *Hum Reprod* **19**(3): 741–756.

Antoniou, A., P.D. Pharoah, et al. (2003). "Average risks of breast and ovarian cancer associated with BRCA1 or BRCA2 mutations detected in case series unselected for family history: a combined analysis of 22 studies." *Am J Hum Genet* **72**(5): 1117–1130.

Bolan, P.J., S. Meisamy, et al. (2003). "In vivo quantification of choline compounds in the breast with 1H MR spectroscopy." *Magn Reson Med* **50**(6): 1134–1143.

Boland, G.P., W.F. Knox, et al. (2002). "Molecular markers and therapeutic targets in ductal carcinoma in situ." *Microsc Res Tech* **59**(1): 3–11.

Boyd, N.F., G.A. Lockwood, et al. (1998). "Mammographic densities and breast cancer risk." *Cancer Epidemiol Biomarkers Prev* **7**(12): 1133–1144.

Boyd, N.F., L.J. Martin, et al. (2001). "Mammographic densities as a marker of human breast cancer risk and their use in chemoprevention." *Curr Oncol Rep* **3**(4): 314–321.

Buist, D.S.M., P.L. Porter, et al. (2004). "Factors Contributing to Mammography Failure in Women Aged 40–49 Years." *J Natl Cancer Inst* **96**(19): 1432–1440.

Byers, T., M. Nestle, et al. (2002). "American Cancer Society Guidelines on Nutrition and Physical Activity for Cancer Prevention: Reducing the Risk of Cancer with Healthy Food Choices and Physical Activity." *CA Cancer J Clin* **52**(2): 92–119.

Calderon-Margalit, R. and O. Paltiel (2004). "Prevention of breast cancer in women who carry BRCA1 or BRCA2 mutations: a critical review of the literature." *Int J Cancer* **112**(3): 357–364.

Calle, E.E., H. Frumkin, et al. (2002). "Organochlorines and Breast Cancer Risk." *CA Cancer J Clin* **52**(5): 301–309.

Carmichael, A., A.S. Sami, et al. (2003). "Breast cancer risk among the survivors of atomic bomb and patients exposed to therapeutic ionising radiation." *European Journal of Surgical Oncology* **29**(5): 475–479.

Cauley, J.A., L. Norton, et al. (2001). "Continued breast cancer risk reduction in postmenopausal women treated with raloxifene: 4-year results from the MORE trial. Multiple outcomes of raloxifene evaluation." *Breast Cancer Res Treat* **65**(2): 125–134.

Cerhan, J.R., J.D. Potter, et al. (2004). "Adherence to the AICR Cancer Prevention Recommendations and Subsequent Morbidity and Mortality in the Iowa Women's Health Study Cohort." *Cancer Epidemiol Biomarkers Prev* **13**(7): 1114–1120.

Chlebowski, R.T., M. Pettinger, et al. (2004). "Insulin, Physical Activity, and Caloric Intake in Postmenopausal Women: Breast Cancer Implications." *J Clin Oncol* **22**(22): 4507–4513.

Claus, E.B., N. Risch, et al. (1991). "Genetic analysis of breast cancer in the cancer and steroid hormone study." *Am J Hum Genet* **48**(2): 232–242.

Claus, E.B., M. Stowe, et al. (2003). "The risk of a contralateral breast cancer among women diagnosed with ductal and lobular breast carcinoma in situ: data from the Connecticut Tumor Registry." *The Breast* **12**(6): 451–456.

Clemons, M., L. Loijens, et al. (2000). "Breast cancer risk following irradiation for Hodgkin's disease." *Cancer Treatment Reviews* **26**(4): 291–302.

Colditz, G.A. and B. Rosner (2000). "Cumulative risk of breast cancer to age 70 years according to risk factor status: data from the Nurses' Health Study." *Am J Epidemiol* **152**(10): 950–964.

Costa, A., F. Formelli, et al. (1994). "Prospects of chemoprevention of human cancers with the synthetic retinoid fenretinide." *Cancer Res* **54**(7 Suppl): 2032s–2037s.

Coyle, Y.M. (2004). "The effect of environment on breast cancer risk." *Breast Cancer Res Treat* **84**(3): 273–288.

Davies, G.L. (2003). "Cyclooxygenase-2 and chemoprevention of breast cancer." *J Steroid Biochem Mol Biol* **86**(3–5): 495–499.

Decensi, A., D. Serrano, et al. (2003). "Breast cancer prevention trials using retinoids." *J Mammary Gland Biol Neoplasia* **8**(1): 19–30.

Deligeoroglou, E., E. Michailidis, et al. (2003). "Oral Contraceptives and Reproductive System Cancer." *Ann NY Acad Sci* **997**(1): 199–208.

Dupont, W.D. and D.L. Page (1985). "Risk factors for breast cancer in women with proliferative breast disease." *N Engl J Med* **312**(3): 146–151.

Dupont, W.D., D.L. Page, et al. (1994). "Long-Term Risk of Breast Cancer in Women with Fibroadenoma." *N Engl J Med* **331**(1): 10–15.

Erbas, B., A. Amos, et al. (2004). "Incidence of Invasive Breast Cancer and Ductal Carcinoma In situ in a Screening Program by Age: Should Older Women Continue Screening?" *Cancer Epidemiol Biomarkers Prev* **13**(10): 1569–1573.

Ernster, V.L., J. Barclay, et al. (1996). "Incidence of and treatment for ductal carcinoma in situ of the breast." *JAMA* **275**(12): 913–918.

Fisher, B., J.P. Costantino, et al. (1998). "Tamoxifen for prevention of breast cancer: report of the National Surgical Adjuvant Breast and Bowel Project P-1 Study." *J Natl Cancer Inst* **90**(18): 1371–1388.

Fournier, A., F. Berrino, et al. (2004). "Breast cancer risk in relation to different types of hormone replacement therapy in the E3N-EPIC cohort." *Int J Cancer* 114(3):448–454.

Gail, M.H., L.A. Brinton, et al. (1989). "Projecting individualized probabilities of developing breast cancer for white females who are being examined annually." *J Natl Cancer Inst* **81**(24): 1879–1886.

Gail, M.H., J.P. Costantino, et al. (1999). "Weighing the risks and benefits of tamoxifen treatment for preventing breast cancer." *J Natl Cancer Inst* **91**(21): 1829–1846.

Gammon, M.D., S.M. Eng, et al. (2004). "Environmental tobacco smoke and breast cancer incidence." *Environmental Research* **96**(2): 176–185.

Garbe, E., L. Levesque, et al. (2004). "Variability of breast cancer risk in observational studies of hormone replacement therapy: a meta-regression analysis." *Maturitas* **47**(3): 175–183.

Garfinkel, L., C. C. Boring, et al. (1994). "Changing trends. An overview of breast cancer incidence and mortality." *Cancer* **74**(1 Suppl): 222–227.

Ghafoor, A., A. Jemal, et al. (2003). "Trends in Breast Cancer by Race and Ethnicity." *CA Cancer J Clin* **53**(6): 342–355.

Giordano, S.H., A.U. Buzdar, et al. (2002). "Breast Cancer in Men." *Ann Intern Med* **137**(8): 678–687.

Goss, P.E. and K. Strasser-Weippl (2004). "Prevention Strategies with Aromatase Inhibitors." *Clin Cancer Res* **10**(1): 372–379.

Haffty, B.G., C. Lee, et al. (1998). "Prognostic significance of mammographic detection in a cohort of conservatively treated breast cancer patients." *Cancer J Sci Am* **4**(1): 35–40.

Hankinson, S.E., W.C. Willett, et al. (1998). "Circulating concentrations of insulin-like growth factor I and risk of breast cancer." *Lancet* **351**(9113): 1393–1396.

Harris, R.E., R.T. Chlebowski, et al. (2003). "Breast cancer and nonsteroidal anti-inflammatory drugs: prospective results from the Women's Health Initiative." *Cancer Res* **63**(18): 6096–6101.

Hartmann, L.C., D.J. Schaid, et al. (1999). "Efficacy of bilateral prophylactic mastectomy in women with a family history of breast cancer." *N Engl J Med* **340**(2): 77–84.

Hemminki, K., R. Rawal, et al. (2004). "Mammographic Screening Is Dramatically Changing Age-Incidence Data for Breast Cancer." *J Clin Oncol* **22**(22): 4652–4653.

Henderson, B.E. and L. Bernstein (1991). "The international variation in breast cancer rates: an epidemiological assessment." *Breast Cancer Res Treat* **18** (Suppl 1): S11–17.

Hodgson, S.V., P.J. Morrison, et al. (2004). "Breast cancer genetics: unsolved questions and open perspectives in an expanding clinical practice." *Am J Med Genet* **129C**(1): 56–64.

Hollingsworth, A.B., S.E. Singletary, et al. (2004). "Current comprehensive assessment and management of women at increased risk for breast cancer." *The American Journal of Surgery* **187**(3): 349–362.

Holmes, M.D. and W.C. Willett (2004). "Does diet affect breast cancer risk?" *Breast Cancer Res* **6**(4): 170–178.

Humphrey, L.L., M. Helfand, et al. (2002). "Breast cancer screening: a summary of the evidence for the U.S. Preventive Services Task Force." *Ann Intern Med* **137**(5 Part 1): 347–360.

Jemal, A., R.C. Tiwari, et al. (2004). "Cancer statistics, 2004." *CA Cancer J Clin* **54**(1): 8–29.

Jernstrom, H., C. Lerman, et al. (1999). "Pregnancy and risk of early breast cancer in carriers of BRCA1 and BRCA2." *The Lancet* **354**(9193): 1846–1850.

Johnson, T.W., K.E. Anderson, et al. (2002). "Association of aspirin and nonsteroidal anti-inflammatory drug use with breast cancer." *Cancer Epidemiol Biomarkers Prev* **11**(12): 1586–1591.

Kaaks, R. (1996). "Nutrition, hormones, and breast cancer: is insulin the missing link?" *Cancer Causes Control* **7**(6): 605–625.

Kelsey, J.L. and L. Bernstein (1996). "Epidemiology and prevention of breast cancer." *Annu Rev Public Health* **17**: 47–67.

Key, T.J., A. Schatzkin, et al. (2004). "Diet, nutrition and the prevention of cancer." *Public Health Nutr* **7**(1A): 187–200.

Kollias, J., I.O. Ellis, et al. (1999). "Clinical and histological predictors of contralateral breast cancer." *Eur J Surg Oncol* **25**(6): 584–589.

Lacroix, M., R.A. Toillon, et al. (2004). "Stable 'portrait' of breast tumors during progression: data from biology, pathology and genetics." *Endocr Relat Cancer* **11**(3): 497–522.

Laden, F. and D.J. Hunter (1998). "Environmental risk factors and female breast cancer." *Annu Rev Public Health* **19**: 101–123.

Law, M. (2000). "Dietary fat and adult diseases and the implications for childhood nutrition: an epidemiologic approach." *Am J Clin Nutr* **72**(5): 1291–1296.

Li, C.I., B.O. Anderson, et al. (2002). "Changing incidence of lobular carcinoma in situ of the breast." *Breast Cancer Res Treat* **75**(3): 259–268.

Lo, S.S. and V.G. Vogel (2004). "Endocrine prevention of breast cancer using selective oestrogen receptor modulators (SORMs)." *Best Practice & Research Clinical Endocrinology & Metabolism* **18**(1): 97–111.

Louie, A.Y., M.M. Huber, et al. (2000). "In vivo visualization of gene expression using magnetic resonance imaging." *Nat Biotechnol* **18**(3): 321–325.

Moorman, P.G., J.M. Grubber, et al. (2003). "Association between non-steroidal anti-inflammatory drugs (NSAIDs) and invasive breast cancer and carcinoma in situ of the breast." *Cancer Causes Control* **14**(10): 915–922.

Morris, E.A., L. Liberman, et al. (2003). "MRI of occult breast carcinoma in a high-risk population." *Am J Roentgenol* **181**(3): 619–626.

Narod, S.A. and W.D. Foulkes (2004). "BRCA1 and BRCA2: 1994 and beyond." *Nature Reviews Cancer* **4**(9): 665–676.

Nayfield, S.G., J.E. Karp, et al. (1991). "Potential role of tamoxifen in prevention of breast cancer." *J Natl Cancer Inst* **83**(20): 1450–1459.

Nelson, H.D., L.L. Humphrey, et al. (2002). "Postmenopausal hormone replacement therapy: scientific review." *JAMA* **288**(7): 872–881.

Olsen, J.H., N. Seersholm, et al. (1999). "Cancer risk in close relatives of women with early-onset breast cancer – a population-based incidence study." *Br J Cancer* **79**(3-4): 673–679.

Page, D.L. (2004). "Breast lesions, pathology and cancer risk." *Breast J* **10** (Suppl 1): S3–4.

Page, D.L. and R.A. Jensen (1994). "Evaluation and management of high risk and premalignant lesions of the breast." *World J Surg* **18**(1): 32–38.

Parker, E.D. and A.R. Folsom (2003). "Intentional weight loss and incidence of obesity-related cancers: the Iowa Women's Health Study." *Int J Obes Relat Metab Disord* **27**(12): 1447–1452.

Parkin, D.M. (2004). "International variation." *Oncogene* **23**(38): 6329–6340.

Pike, M.C., C.L. Pearce, et al. (2004). "Prevention of cancers of the breast, endometrium and ovary." *Oncogene* **23**(38): 6379–6391.

Powles, T., R. Eeles, et al. (1998). "Interim analysis of the incidence of breast cancer in the Royal Marsden Hospital tamoxifen randomised chemoprevention trial." *Lancet* **352**(9122): 98–101.

Radimer, K.L., R. Ballard-Barbash, et al. (2004). "Weight change and the risk of late-onset breast cancer in the original Framingham cohort." *Nutr Cancer* **49**(1): 7–13.

Rebbeck, T.R., A.M. Levin, et al. (1999). "Breast cancer risk after bilateral prophylactic oophorectomy in BRCA1 mutation carriers." *J Natl Cancer Inst* **91**(17): 1475–1479.

Ries, L.A.G., M.P. Eisner, et al. (2004). *SEER Cancer Statistics Review, 1995-2001*. Bethesda, MD, National Cancer Institute.

Rockhill, B., D. Spiegelman, et al. (2001). "Validation of the Gail et al. Model of Breast Cancer Risk Prediction and Implications for Chemoprevention." *J Natl Cancer Inst* **93**(5): 358–366.

Rossouw, J.E., G.L. Anderson, et al. (2002). "Risks and benefits of estrogen plus progestin in healthy postmenopausal women: principal results from the Women's Health Initiative randomized controlled trial." *JAMA* **288**(3): 321–333.

Ruffin, M.T.T., D.A. August, et al. (1993). "Selection criteria for breast cancer chemoprevention subjects." *J Cell Biochem Suppl* **17G**: 234–241.

Sakorafas, G.H., E. Krespis, et al. (2002). "Risk estimation for breast cancer development; a clinical perspective." *Surg Oncol* **10**(4): 183–192.

Serrano, D., E. Perego, et al. (2004). "Progress in chemoprevention of breast cancer." *Critical Reviews in Oncology/Hematology* **49**(2): 109–117.

Shen, Q. and P.H. Brown (2003). "Novel agents for the prevention of breast cancer: targeting transcription factors and signal transduction pathways." *J Mammary Gland Biol Neoplasia* **8**(1): 45–73.

Shi, R., H. Yu, et al. (2004). "IGF-I and breast cancer: a meta-analysis." *Int J Cancer* **111**(3): 418–423.

Smith, R. A. (2000). "Breast cancer screening among women younger than age 50: a current assessment of the issues." *CA Cancer J Clin* **50**(5): 312–336.

Smith, R. A., D. Saslow, et al. (2003). "American Cancer Society guidelines for breast cancer screening: update 2003." *CA Cancer J Clin* **53**(3): 141–169.

Stankovic, T., A. M. Kidd, et al. (1998). "ATM mutations and phenotypes in ataxia-telangiectasia families in the British Isles: expression of mutant ATM and the risk of leukemia, lymphoma, and breast cancer." *Am J Hum Genet* **62**(2): 334–345.

Stoll, B. A. (1998). "Western diet, early puberty, and breast cancer risk." *Breast Cancer Res Treat* **49**(3): 187–193.

Stoll, B. A. (1999). "Western nutrition and the insulin resistance syndrome: a link to breast cancer." *Eur J Clin Nutr* **53**(2): 83–87.

Sugumar, A., Y. C. Liu, et al. (2004). "Insulin-like growth factor (IGF)-I and IGF-binding protein 3 and the risk of premenopausal breast cancer: a meta-analysis of literature." *Int J Cancer* **111**(2): 293–297.

Terry, M. B., M. D. Gammon, et al. (2004). "Association of frequency and duration of aspirin use and hormone receptor status with breast cancer risk." *JAMA* **291**(20): 2433–2440.

The Women's Health Initiative Steering Committee (2004). "Effects of conjugated equine estrogen in postmenopausal women with hysterectomy: The Women's Health Initiative randomized controlled trial." *JAMA* **291**(14): 1701–1712.

Thomas, D. B., D. L. Gao, et al. (1997). "Randomized trial of breast self-examination in Shanghai: methodology and preliminary results." *J Natl Cancer Inst* **89**(5): 355–365.

Tobias, J. S. (2004). "Recent advances in endocrine therapy for postmenopausal women with early breast cancer: implications for treatment and prevention." *Ann Oncol* **15**(12): 1738–1747.

Toniolo, P., P. F. Bruning, et al. (2000). "Serum insulin-like growth factor-I and breast cancer." *Int J Cancer* **88**(5): 828–832.

Tryggvadottir, L., E. J. Olafsdottir, et al. (2003). "BRCA2 mutation carriers, reproductive factors and breast cancer risk." *Breast Cancer Res* **5**(5): R121–128.

Tyrer, J., S. W. Duffy, et al. (2004). "A breast cancer prediction model incorporating familial and personal risk factors." *Stat Med* **23**(7): 1111–1130.

Vogel, V. G. (1991). "High-risk populations as targets for breast cancer prevention trials." *Preventive Medicine* **20**(1): 86–100.

Vogel, V. G. (2004). "Atypia in the assessment of breast cancer risk: implications for management." *Diagn Cytopathol* **30**(3): 151–157.

Ward, E., A. Jemal, et al. (2004). "Cancer disparities by race/ethnicity and socioeconomic status." *CA Cancer J Clin* **54**(2): 78–93.

Warren Burhenne, L. J., S. A. Wood, et al. (2000). "Potential contribution of computer-aided detection to the sensitivity of screening mammography." *Radiology* **215**(2): 554–562.

Warren, R. (2004). "Hormones and mammographic breast density." *Maturitas* **49**(1): 67–78.

Weissleder, R., A. Moore, et al. (2000). "In vivo magnetic resonance imaging of transgene expression." *Nat Med* **6**(3): 351–355.

White, S., R. Taetle, et al. (1990). "Combinations of anti-transferrin receptor monoclonal antibodies inhibit human tumor cell growth in vitro and in vivo: evidence for synergistic antiproliferative effects." *Cancer Res* **50**(19): 6295–6301.

Wu, K., H.-T. Kim, et al. (2002). "Suppression of Mammary Tumorigenesis in Transgenic Mice by the RXR-selective Retinoid, LGD1069." *Cancer Epidemiol Biomarkers Prev* **11**(5): 467–474.

Yang, L. M., U. C. Tin, et al. (1999). "Role of retinoid receptors in the prevention and treatment of breast cancer." *J Mammary Gland Biol Neoplasia* **4**(4): 377–388.

Prostate Cancer Prevention

Suzanne Stratton and Frederick Ahmann

College of Medicine, University of Arizona, Tucson AZ 85724

Research conducted since the 1990s has begun to characterize the molecular pathways involved in carcinogenesis of the prostate. The processes of initiation, cell growth and invasion have begun to be elucidated. In addition, influences of the interactions between cancer cells and their environment that contribute to disease progression are the subject of intense study. Some of these factors include alterations in expression of adhesion molecules that regulate cell-cell and cell-matrix interactions (Mundy 1997; Prasad, Thraves et al. 1998; Mason, Davies et al. 2002; Ross, Sheehan et al. 2002), matrix-metalloproteinase (MMP) expression (Lokeshwar 1999; Zucker, Hymowitz et al. 1999) that contributes to the processes of invasion and metastases, hormone independent growth of prostate cancer cells that have become refractory to androgen ablation therapy (Cronauer, Schulz et al. 2003), and altered expression of proteins that regulate cell proliferation and apoptosis (Johnson and Hamdy 1998; Westin and Bergh 1998).

Prevention of Prostate Carcinogenesis

Prostate cancer, from a prevention perspective, presents several challenges. The rate of occurrence of the steps in carcinogenesis is highly variable. Men begin to develop microscopic foci of prostate cancer in the third decade of life which increase in frequency to such a degree that by a man's 8th decade of life, he has an approximate 67% chance of having microscopic foci of prostate cancer at post mortem exam (Holund 1980). While the vast majority of these microscopic foci do not lead to clinically significant disease, a small percentage of these cancers evolve into aggressive, clinically significant disease that resulted in the diagnoses of 230,110 cases and about 29,900 deaths in 2004 in the United States (U.S.) (Jemal, Tiwari et al. 2004).

Although there has been significant progress that has improved our understanding of the disease, there is still much to be learned about the causes, early diagnostic markers prognostic indicators, therapy and prevention. A large part of the challenge for treatment of prostate cancer is our current inability to differentiate between primary tumors that will result in fatal disease from a tumor that will grow very slowly and hence be clinically insignificant. In order to help overcome this challenge, several areas of research must be approached. First, it is critical that we identify genetic, physiological and environmental factors that contribute to increased risk. Second, molecular and cellular processes contributing to development, invasion and the metastasis of prostate cancer must be examined for development of improved early detection methods and targeted therapies. Third, continuous epidemiological studies must be

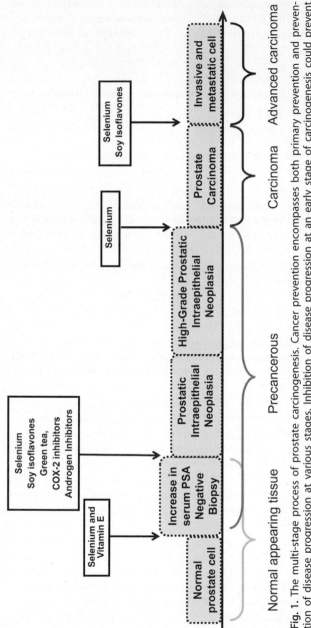
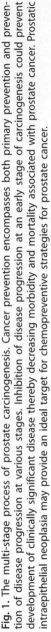

Fig. 1. The multi-stage process of prostate carcinogenesis. Cancer prevention encompasses both primary prevention and prevention of disease progression at various stages. Inhibition of disease progression at an early stage of carcinogenesis could prevent development of clinically significant disease thereby decreasing morbidity and mortality associated with prostate cancer. Prostatic intraepithelial neoplasia may provide an ideal target for chemopreventive strategies for prostate cancer.

ongoing to understand the relationship of incidence and mortality in different populations and within families. Finally, in vitro and in vivo models of prostate cancer must be developed to facilitate preclinical studies that will lead to development of therapeutic and chemopreventive agents. This chapter will discuss prostate cancer screening, molecular mechanisms that regulate prostate carcinogenesis and agents that show promise for prostate cancer chemoprevention.

In considering strategies to prevent prostate cancer it is important to recognize the disease as a continuum with a long, multi-step process in which there are numerous opportunities for intervention (Figure 1). Therefore, the concept of prevention encompasses primary prevention and prevention of progression of disease. Thus, the true idea of prevention is the treatment or inhibition of the process of carcinogenesis.

Part of the challenge in developing prevention strategies is to identify populations within defined risk groups. In prostate cancer, several risk groups can be defined including: average risk, which are normal healthy men with normal prostate specific antigen (PSA) levels; high-risk, which are men who have had either a suspicious digital rectal exam or increased PSA but a normal prostate biopsy; and an even higher-risk group who have had a prostate biopsy negative for cancer, but positive for prostatic intraepithelial neoplasia, a precursor for prostate cancer. Strategies for prevention are being studied in each risk group.

Epidemiology and Risk Factors

Prostate cancer is the second most frequently diagnosed malignancy in men surpassed in incidence only by nonmelanoma skin cancers. In 2004, approximately 230,110 men were diagnosed with prostate cancer and an estimated 29,900 men died from the disease in the U.S. (Jemal, Tiwari et al. 2004). Factors associated with increased risk of developing clinically significant prostate cancer include: advancing age, a positive family history, race (African-American), the presence of high-grade prostatic intraepithelial neoplasia, genetics, hormone levels, a digital rectal exam finding an indurated and/or nodular prostate, and an elevated serum level of PSA (Giovannucci and Platz 2002). These risk associations form the basis for chemoprevention strategies in prostate cancer.

The etiology of prostate cancer remains largely a mystery. Epidemiological studies conducted over the past twenty years have revealed statistically significant differences of clinically apparent prostate carcinoma between several economically developed nations (Table 1). The most recent estimates of worldwide cancer incidence show that prostate cancer is the third most common cancer in men accounting for nearly 10% of male cancers. Because it is a disease of the elderly, the highest incidences are on developed countries with higher proportions of elderly men. In developing countries, prostate cancer accounts for approximately 4% of cancers in men while in developed countries it accounts for 15% of male cancers (Quinn and Babb 2002).

Within the U.S., the incidence of prostate cancer is not evenly distributed among men of different racial background and ethnicity or geographical region. Data describing the epidemiology of prostate cancer from the 1930s to the present document a dramatic racial difference in incidence, survival, and mortality rates in American men. African American men have the highest incidence and mortality rates of prostate cancer in the world (Burks and Littleton 1992; Clegg, Li et al. 2002; Carroll 2003). Survival data

Country	Cases
Australia	53.5
Canada	63.0
Denmark	31.0
Equador	22.4
England & Wales	28.0
France	48.1
Iceland	61.0
India	8.0
Israel	23.9
Japan	6.8
Netherlands	39.6
Norway	48.4
Poland	15.5
Slovakia	22.0
Spain	21.0
Sweden	55.3
USA	118.9

Table 1. Prostate cancer incidence in developed countries (cases per 100,000) (Quinn and Babb 2002)

have been related to access to medical care, genetic and environmental factors, and cultural differences, including diet and social habits. Most reports present conflicting data with no clear positive correlations, and conclusions are often speculative (Burks and Littleton 1992). In addition, while prostate cancer is one of the major malignant diseases in Western countries, in Japan, the incidence and mortality of prostate cancer is remarkably low by comparison; however, it is continuously increasing over time. The increase in incidence within the last ten years in the Japanese population is speculated to be attributed to the growth of the elderly population, a westernized diet in daily life and widespread environmental contamination of carcinogens. Also, the increase in incidence of prostate cancer in Japan has been attributed to the improvement of screening techniques such as the serum PSA test (Imai, Ichinose et al. 1994). This makes the assumption that the low incidence of prostate cancer was always deceivingly low in this population because it was never detected. Epidemiological studies conducted by Imia and colleagues comparing the incidence of prostate cancer in the United States versus Japan suggested that the strikingly large difference in incidence was also skewed because the prostatic cancers diagnosed in men in the United States appeared to be more aggressive than those in men in Japan. The epidemiology of prostate cancer hints that its etiology is both environmental and genetic. Androgenic stimulation over time, perhaps due to a high fat diet, has been suggested as a cause of prostate cancer (Imai, Ichinose et al. 1994; Imai, Hwang et al. 2004).

Risk Factors

Age. The most apparent risk factor of prostatic carcinoma appears to be age. Ninety-five percent of all prostatic cancers occur in men ranging from 45 to 80 years of age. However, before the age of 50, men are at relatively low risk. For men aged 50–54, incidence is approximately 30 cases in 100,000 men. However, beginning at 55 years of age, the potential for developing prostatic carcinoma is heightened dramatically and

Age	Race	Incidence
All ages	All races	176
	Caucasian	168
	African American	277
<65 years	All races	57
	Caucasian	55
	African American	102
≥65 years	All races	975
	Caucasian	947
	African American	1486

Table 2. Prostate cancer incidence per 100,000 by race (1996–2002) (NCI 2004)

can even double with each successive 5-year age increment, or increase 1 percent per year of age resulting in an overall incidence of 1000 cases per 100,000 men aged 85 years and older (Guinan, Gilham et al. 1981; Sharifi, Waters et al. 1981).

Race. The racial disparity observed in prostate cancer incidence and mortality rates among African American and Caucasian males in the United States is the subject of intense investigation. Various reports, including those of the American Cancer Society (ACS) and the Surveillance, Epidemiology, and End Results (SEER) program of the National Cancer Institute (NCI), indicate that African American men are at the highest risk for developing prostate cancer with overall mortality rates up to two-fold higher than white men (Clegg, Li et al. 2002; Sarma and Schottenfeld 2002) (Table 2).

Data adjusted for socioeconomic status and co-morbidities show that African American men are less likely to undergo routine screening for prostate cancer as recommended by the ACS suggesting that greater efforts must be made to advocate screening in this population in order to reduce prostate cancer mortality.

Although these statistics indicate a positive race-association in the high incidence of prostate cancer, race is still a debatable indicator of cancer incidence. Numerous reports have examined variations in dietary factors and biological factors, including genetic susceptibility (Schaid 2004) and testosterone levels (Eastham, May et al. 1998; Winters, Brufsky et al. 2001), however, findings have thus far been inconclusive. Early studies showed promise in identifying candidate regions for prostate cancer susceptibility loci, however replication of the linkage analyses have been challenging (Schaid 2004).

With the intent to reduce the incidence of prostate cancer mortality in African Americans by aggressively increasing the frequency of serum PSA testing, the 2003 ACS report recommends annual serum PSA measurement for African American men aged 45 years and older as opposed to age 50 for men of other races. Unfortunately, adherence of African American men to recommended screening intervals is problematic. In addition, access to PSA screening is a crucial determinant of prostate cancer mortality. Studies conducted by Etzioni and colleagues indicated that African American men were 25% less likely to undergo the recommended routine prostate cancer screening by measurement of serum PSA (Etzioni, Berry et al. 2002). Clearly, methods to educate the population of interest and advocate serum PSA measurement as recommended by the ACS are a great need and could have a profound effect on prostate cancer mortality in African American men and healthcare economics.

Prostatic Intraepithelial Neoplasia (PIN). Prostate cancers are characteristically heterogeneous and multifocal in nature and can have diverse clinical and morphologic manifestations. Although the molecular basis for this heterogeneity has yet to be elucidated, further study of prostatic intraepithelial neoplasia (PIN), a pathologic diagnosis considered to be a precursor lesion for prostate cancer, may help contribute to characterization of specific cancers. Prostate cancer may arise from other types of precursors, however PIN is considered to be the most likely precursor for prostate cancer at present. The strong genetic similarities between PIN and carcinoma of the prostate suggest that evolution and clonal expansion of PIN leads to development of cancer (Alsikafi, Brendler et al. 2001; Fowler, Bigler et al. 2001; Marshall 2001). Data examining age and race as risk factors have revealed that African American men develop more extensive High grade PIN (HGPIN) at a younger age than white men and some studies have shown that patients with PIN will be diagnosed with prostate cancer within 10 years of their original biopsy (Sakr, Grignon et al. 1996; Sakr and Partin 2001). It is of interest that pronounced genetic heterogeneity is characteristic of both PIN and carcinoma. Furthermore multiple foci of PIN and carcinoma can arise independently within the same prostate suggesting a field effect of factors that influence carcinogenesis.

HGPIN lesions and prostatic tumors have been shown to share a broad spectrum of molecular and genetic abnormalities including loss within the chromosome regions 8p, 10q, 16q, 18q, and gain within chromosome regions 7q31, 8q (Sakr and Partin 2001). Other abnormalities that have been identified in both HGPIN lesions and prostatic carcinoma tumors include amplification of the oncogene, c-myc (Sakr and Partin 2001), aberrations in nuclear chromatic pattern (Bartels, Montironi et al. 1998; Bartels, Montironi et al. 1998), altered activity of telomerase (Iczkowski, Pantazis et al. 2002), cell cycle regulators (Henshall, Quinn et al. 2001), proliferative indices, and markers of apoptosis (Johnson, Robinson et al. 1998; Xie, Wong et al. 2000). These data suggest that HGPIN is an intermediate stage between benign prostatic epithelium and prostatic carcinoma and it may be critical in early stages of carcinogenesis and neoplastic progression in the prostate. HGPIN could therefore potentially serve as an ideal target for early diagnosis of prostate cancer and development of agents to prevent progression of early stages of carcinogenesis.

In studying HGPIN as a precursor to prostate cancer, it is important to take into account that endocrine therapy causes alterations in morphology of PIN making it more closely resemble normal prostatic epithelium (Bostwick 2000). Endocrine therapy-induced changes in molecular markers of PIN and induction of resistance to endocrine therapy are currently important areas of study.

Genetic Factors. More recently, genetic factors that contribute to prostate cancer have been examined. Research into the molecular genetics of prostate cancer to date has largely focused on the possible existence of one or several single-locus high-penetrance susceptibility genes and several candidate regions have been identified, but confirmatory studies of these regions have been inconclusive. Increasingly, attention has turned to identification of candidate genes that may increase prostate cancer risk because their products potentially play an important role in possible etiological pathways for prostate cancer (Ostrander and Stanford 2000; Xu, Stolk et al. 2000). Of various such pathways that have been suggested for prostate cancer, the best studied in terms of molecular genetics is the androgen signaling pathway. Two genes in this pathway, the androgen receptor (AR) gene and the steroid 5-alpha reductase type II (SRD5A2) gene, have been under particular scrutiny and polymorphic markers in each of these genes which reproducibly predict prostate cancer risk have been identified (Abate-Shen and Shen 2000).

Abnormalities in Chromosomes 8 and 10 may be associated with development of prostate cancer. Preliminary findings by Kunimi and colleagues in 1991, using restriction fragment length polymorphism analyses (RFLP), showed consistent alterations in genetic information located in chromosomes 8 and 10 in men with prostate cancer (Kunimi, Bergerheim et al. 1991). Subsequent studies of alterations in chromosomes 8 and 10 have been completed. NCI-sponsored studies demonstrated that a deletion in chromosome 8 (8p21) was present in 80% of prostate cancers and approximately 63% of precancerous prostate lesions (Kagan, Stein et al. 1995; Qian, Jenkins et al. 1997; Katoh 2002). Such findings suggest that abnormalities in chromosome 8p21 may be associated with early development of prostate cancer and changes in protein expression associated with this deletion may serve as early diagnostic markers or targets for treatment of early prostate carcinogenesis. Studies conducted by Katoh and colleagues showed downregulation in primary prostate cancer and prostate carcinoma cell cultures, of the SOX7 gene, located on chromosome 8p22 (Katoh 2002; Katoh 2002). This gene is thought to be a tumor suppressor gene for prostate cancer and other solid tumors including kidney and breast. Other genes identified that are potentially involved with the carcinogenesis of prostate cancer include LZTS1 located on chromosome 8p22 (Cabeza-Arvelaiz, Sepulveda et al. 2001) and KLF6 (Narla, Heath et al. 2001), located on chromosome 10p.

Screening

The methods used to detect prostate cancer underwent a dramatic change with the introduction of serum PSA levels as a screening test in the late 1980s. Prior to the late 1980s, men were selected for a prostate biopsy almost entirely on the basis of them having a suspicious feeling prostate on a digital rectal exam (DRE). Beginning in the late 1980s, studies demonstrated the serum levels of PSA had a higher sensitivity and specificity for identifying men who would be found to have prostate cancer on needle biopsies than did the results of DRE (Catalona, Richie et al. 1994). The use of serum PSA levels as a prostate cancer screening test dramatically increased the number of prostate needle biopsies performed in the U.S., and dramatically increased the number of men diagnosed with prostate cancer. Recent mortality figures demonstrate a sharp and continuing decline in prostate cancer mortality since the middle 1990s, approximately six years after screening with serum PSA levels started to be used in clinical practice (Bishop 2000; Quinn and Babb 2002; Stephenson 2002). The most rational explanation for this decline in prostate cancer mortality is the successful use of PSA screening leading to the earlier diagnosis of prostate cancer and the application of potentially curative therapies (radical prostatectomies or radiotherapy).

A second change occurred in how prostate cancers were being diagnosed during this same time period. In the 1980s, the standard prostate needle biopsy technique was accomplished using a digitally guided needle via a transrectal approach. It was recognized in the late 1980s that this biopsy technique was missing prostate cancers

Table 3. Frequency of prostate biopsy following an initial negative prostate biopsy

Reference	Number of 2nd (or more) biopsies	Number (% of total) positive
(Andriole and Catalona 1993)	73	30 (41%)
(Keetch, Catalona et al. 1994)	427	104 (24%)
(Ellis and Brawer 1995)	100	20 (20%)
(Hzyek 1995)	51	8 (16%)
(Lui, Terris et al. 1995)	187	72 (38%)
(Roehrborn, Gregory et al. 1996)	123	30 (24%)
(Rovner, Schanne et al. 1997)	71	17 (24%)
(Perachino, di Ciolo et al. 1997)	148	60 (41%)
(Fleshner, O'Sullivan et al. 1997)	130	39 (30%)
(Ukimura, Durrani et al. 1997)	193	51 (26%)
(Rietbergen and Schroder 1998)	442	49 (11%)
(Letran, Blase et al. 1998)	51	15 (29%)
(Levine, Ittman et al. 1998)	137	43 (31%)
(Durkan and Greene 1999)	48	15 (31%)
(Djavan, Zlotta et al. 2000)	820	83 (10%)
(Borboroglu, Comer et al. 2000)	57	17 (30%)
(Kamoi, Troncoso et al. 2000)	45	10 (22%)
(Fowler, Bigler et al. 2000)	298	80 (27%)
(Stewart, Leibovich et al. 2001)	224	77 (34%)
(Park, Miyake et al. 2003)	104	22 (21%)
Summary	**3729**	**842 (23%)**

that occurred in areas of the gland that were palpably normal (Catalona, Richie et al. 1994). Needle biopsies of the prostate performed under transrectal ultrasound guidance were shown to increase the number of cancers found (Presti 2002). Using this method, the prostate biopsies could now sample the prostate in a reproducible and uniform manner. The technique evolved from a four-quadrant biopsy (two biopsy cores on each side of the prostate) to a standard sextant biopsy (three biopsy cores on each side of the prostate) by the early 1990s. More recently, additional biopsy cores taken from the lateral horns of the prostate have been shown to improve the detection of prostate cancers (Taylor, Gancarczyk et al. 2002).

A dilemma that previously had attracted little attention became recognized as prostate biopsy techniques and screening techniques evolved. Some men had either persistent elevations of serum PSA levels in the face of a negative prostate biopsy or had persistent palpably abnormal prostates despite a negative prostate biopsy. Multiple reports have now been published after performing second biopsies in such men. Table 3 shows 20 studies published since 1993 utilizing sextant (or more) second (or more) biopsies of the prostate in men previously biopsied and having no evidence of prostate cancer. The studies displayed are confined to those conducted in the U.S. and Western Europe to minimize any effect from the well-recognized global variability in the incidence of prostate cancer. The positive second biopsy rate amongst these studies ranges from 10 to 41%. Overall, a total of 3,729 second biopsies were carried out and 842 (23%) were positive. No consistent criteria were utilized in these studies to determine when a second biopsy was done. However, in the vast majority of the series, the reason for a second biopsy was the persistence of an elevated serum PSA level. This correlates well with the usual clinical practice in the United States. Various authors have proposed tools to increase the specificity of a second biopsy including free versus bound PSA ratios, PSA density, age adjusted PSAs, and PSA velocities, but none are definitive.

Molecular Markers of Prostate Carcinogenesis

Elucidation of the molecular mechanisms involved with each stage of carcinogenesis is one of the first steps in identifying targets for chemoprevention strategies; however, the apparent multiplicity of molecular factors in prostate carcinogenesis has proven to be a challenge to decipher. While some genetic abnormalities that result in aberrant gene expression are hereditary, all tumors acquire additional abnormalities in gene expression as the carcinogenesis progresses. Overexpression of genes can be caused by several mechanisms including gene amplification, a mutation within the promoter region or upregulation of an upstream signaling factor. Similarly, decreased expression of tumor suppressor genes can be caused by a promoter region mutation, deletion or by gene silencing due to promoter methylation. Several cell signaling factors have been identified as potential markers for early diagnosis and as possible targets for chemoprevention. These factors include oncogenes, tumor suppressors and proteins involved with inflammation.

Androgens. Testosterone and 5a-dihydrotestosterone are the two most abundant androgens (Figure 2). Both act through one androgen receptor although each androgen plays specific roles during male sexual differentiation. Testosterone is directly involved in the development of structures derived from the wolffian duct (epididymides, vasa deferentia, seminal vesicles and ejaculatory ducts), while 5a-dihydrotestosterone, a metabolite of testosterone, is the active ligand in most androgen-sensitive target tissues including the urogenital sinus and tubercle and their associated structures such as the prostate and urethra. Each isoform interacts with the androgen receptor differently. Testosterone lower affinity for the receptor and a higher dissociation rate compared to 5a-dihydrotestosterone (Schiavi and White 1976; Knol and Egberink-Alink 1989; Vermeulen 1991). This requires that testosterone be present in very high concentration within the tissues in which they act to elicit its downstream signaling.

The biosynthetic conversion of cholesterol to testosterone occurs through several intermediates. The first step entails transfer of cholesterol from the outer to the inner mitochondrial membrane by the steroidogenic acute regulatory protein (StAR) and the subsequent P450scc-mediated side chain cleavage of cholesterol (Aspden, Rodgers et al. 1998). This conversion, resulting in the synthesis of pregnenolone, is a rate-limiting step in testosterone biosynthesis. Subsequent steps require several enzymes including 3β-hydroxysteroid dehydrogenase, 17a-hydroxylase/C17-20-lyase and 17β-hydroxysteroid dehydrogenase (Dessypris 1975; Panaiotov 1978).

Androgen Receptor Polymorphisms. The androgen receptor (AR) is a member of the steroid/nuclear receptor gene superfamily. The encoding gene is located on chromosome loci Xq11.2–q12 and consists of eight exons. There are two domains that are di-

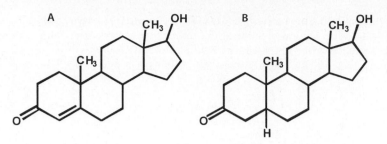

Fig. 2. Structure of (A) testosterone and (B) 5α-dihydrotestosterone

rectly responsible for the transactivation activity of the AR protein. Of these domains, the ligand-independent AF-1 is encoded within exon 1.

There are three known AR gene polymorphisms which may account for variations in risk for prostate cancer. These polymorphisms include the (CAG)n trinucleotide repeat, the (GGC)n trinucleotide repeat, and the R726L single nucleotide polymorphism (Mononen, Syrjakoski et al. 2000). Studies conducted by Irvine et al. suggested that there are 27 observed alleles in various populations with repeats ranging from five to 31. Short CAG repeats (less than or equal to 22 repeats) were found to be more prevalent in African-American males who are at high risk for prostate cancer and less prevalent in Asians who are at lower risk for this disease (Irvine, Yu et al. 1995). These findings suggest that variations in androgen receptor CAG repeat length differs considerably among human populations and may account for variations in risk. African-Americans also had the lowest frequency (20%) of the GGC allele with 16 repeats compared to intermediate-risk whites and low-risk Asians which showed frequency of this sequence 57% and 70%, respectively. In an Australian case control study performed by Beilin and colleagues on studying 545 cases of prostate carcinoma and 456 age-matched controls, the odds ratio of prostate carcinoma for a change of 5 CAG repeats was 0.98 (95% confidence interval, 0.84–1.15); therefore suggesting that the *AR* CAG repeat polymorphism was not a risk factor for prostate carcinoma in this population. However, in this study, a shorter repeat sequence was found to be associated with earlier age at diagnosis (Beilin, Harewood et al. 2001).

In another study conducted in China, Hsing and colleagues showed that Chinese men have longer CAG (equal or longer than 23) repeats compared with US men. It is of interest that this study also suggests that even in a relatively low-risk population, a shorter CAG repeat length is associated with a higher risk of clinically significant prostate cancer. Chinese men with a CAG repeat length shorter than 23 (median length) had a 65% increased risk of prostate cancer (odds ratio [OR] = 1.65; 95% confidence interval [CI]: 1.14–2.39) (Hsing, Gao et al. 2000). In contrast to the previously described studies examining polymorphisms in sporadic prostate cancer, research conducted by study by Miller and colleagues suggest that the (CAG)n and (GGN)n repeats do not play a major role in familial prostate cancer (Miller, Stanford et al. 2001). Clearly, larger studies are needed to evaluate the combined effect of CAG and GGN repeats. Because both genetic and environmental factors contribute to cancer risk, future studies should incorporate biomarkers of environmental exposures as well as AR gene polymorphisms.

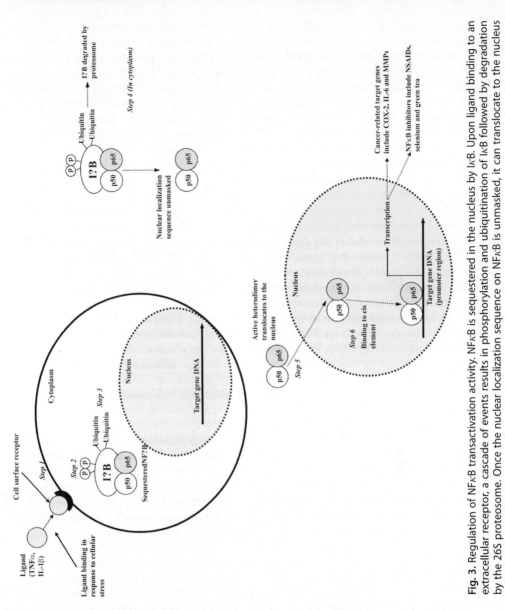

Fig. 3. Regulation of NFκB transactivation activity. NFκB is sequestered in the nucleus by IκB. Upon ligand binding to an extracellular receptor, a cascade of events results in phosphorylation and ubiquitination of IκB followed by degradation by the 26S proteosome. Once the nuclear localization sequence on NFκB is unmasked, it can translocate to the nucleus and bind the promoter region of target genes.

Nuclear Factor Kappa B (NFκB). NFκB is an ideal example of a potential target and biomarker for prostate cancer chemoprevention. The NFκB/Rel family of proteins in mammals consists of five members: c-Rel, NFκB1 (p50/p105), NFκB2 (p52/p100), Rel A (p65), and Rel B, all of which share a matched Rel homology domain (RHD). The NFκB proteins function as a variety of heterodimers, allowing structural and functional versatility (Baldwin 1996). The active form of NFκB, commonly comprised of p50 and p65 subunits of the Rel family of proteins, is known to regulate genes involved in apoptosis, cell cycle arrest and inflammation (Witkamp and Monshouwer 2000; Sun and Andersson 2002). The dimeric protein is sequestered in the nucleus by its inhibitory subunit, IκB. In order to become activated, a cascade of events involving recruitment enzymes and kinases must occur (Figure 3). In response to an NFκB regulatory ligand such as IL-1β or TNFα binding to its respective cell surface receptor, the IκB subunit is phosphorylated at two serine residues and is subsequently ubiquitinated and degraded by the 26S proteosome. This unmasks the nuclear localization sequence located on the p50 subunit of the heterodimer thus allowing the activated NFκB complex to be translocated to the nucleus where it can then bind cis elements within the promoter regions and elicit transactivation of target genes (Sun and Oberley 1996; Mercurio and Manning 1999). This complex mechanism of activation provides several points at which NFκB transactivation activity can be inhibited.

NFκB is frequently overexpressed and constitutively activated in carcinomas and is a key antiapoptotic factor in most mammalian cells (Sellers and Fisher 1999; Bours, Bentires-Alj et al. 2000). Furthermore, NFκB is overexpressed in prostate cancer tissue models derived from metastatic tumors which provides further evidence of its role in cancer progression. Increased activity of NFκB is of particular interest in prostate cancer because some of its downstream genes, including IL-6 and COX-2, play a role in prostate carcinogenesis. Upstream events in the NFκB activation cascade have become of interest as chemotherapeutic and chemopreventive molecular targets. Some agents, including inhibitors of cyclooxygenase (COX) enzymes (Surh, Chun et al. 2001), have been shown to block phosphorylation of IκB causing inhibition of NFκB activation, while other agents, such as the p50 binding peptide produced by Calbiochem (San Diego, CA), block the nuclear localization sequence of the active NFκB heterodimer (Maliner-Stratton, Klein et al. 2001). This mechanism allows dissociation of NFκB from the inhibitory subunit, but blocks nuclear translocation and, therefore, NFκB transactivation activity.

NFκB and Selenium. Several studies have shown that one of the mechanisms by which selenium may elicit anticancer activity may be by inhibition of NFκB transactivation activity. Jiang and colleagues demonstrated that selenium compounds inhibited cell growth and induced apoptosis in human prostate carcinoma cell lines through an NFκB-dependent mechanism (Jiang, Wang et al. 2001; Gasparian, Yao et al. 2002). The effects of methylselenic acid (MSeA), a novel precursor of methylselenol, were compared with sodium selenite on apoptosis, cell cycle arrest and MAP kinase activity on the hormone refractory prostate cancer cell line, DU-145. The agents tested inhibited TNFα-induced NFκB transactivation activity and blocked transcription of several components of the cascade responsible for activation of the NFκB heterodimer. Furthermore, exposure of DU-145 cells to 3 μM MSeA induced cell cycle arrest in G1 after 24 hours; and exposure to higher concentrations resulted in DNA fragmentation and caspase-mediated cleavage of poly(ADP-ribose) polymerase (PARP), two standard hall-marks of apoptosis.

Stable transfection of a prostate carcinoma cell line with a dominant negative IκB caused sensitization to Se-induced apoptosis further suggesting that NFκB may be a primary mechanism for the chemopreventive effects of Se compounds (Gasparian, Yao et al. 2002). Sodium selenite and MSeA, an organic form of Se, have also been shown to block NFκB activation in the prostate carcinoma cell line, JCA1. Both compounds inhibited NFκB transactivation activity in cells transfected with a plasmid construct encoding a luciferase reporter gene driven by a minimal promoter with NFκB *cis* elements (Gasparian, Yao et al. 2002). Clearly, NFκB may serve as an ideal target not only for prostate cancer chemoprevention, but also for treatment of advanced disease.

Interleukin-6. IL-6, which was initially named B cell differentiating factor or hepato-cyte stimulating factor, is produced by many cell types including T cells and B cells (Oleksowicz and Dutcher 1994; O'Shaughnessy, Prosser et al. 1996), macrophages (Bost and Mason 1995), fibroblasts (Carty, Buresh et al. 1991; Raap, Justen et al. 2000) and endothelial cells (Jirik, Podor et al. 1989; Soderquist, Kallman et al. 1998). IL-6 is a pleiotropic cytokine downstream of NFκB. The majority of human cell types are IL-6 responsive, however, it plays a particularly important role in differentiation of B cells to mature antigen presenting cells. In hepatic cells, IL-6 regulates expression of acute immune response phase proteins (Hilbert, Kopf et al. 1995).

Immunohistochemical analyses of frozen tissue sections collected from radical prostatectomies have shown that IL-6 expression is expressed both in the epithelium and stroma, whereas in normal tissue expression is confined to the basal cells of the epithelium (Royuela, Ricote et al. 2004). IL-6 is thought to be involved in progression of prostate cancer at later stages of carcinogenesis and it may therefore be a valuable surrogate marker for androgen-independent prostate cancer. It is of particular interest that several studies have shown that circulating levels of IL-6 are elevated in patients with hormone refractory prostate cancer and that these levels correlate with tumor burden as assessed by PSA or clinically identified metastases (Wise, Marella et al. 2000). In addition, IL-6 signaling is required for bone differentiation which further in-dicates this cytokine as a significant contributor to prostate carcinogenesis due to the propensity of prostate cancer to metastasize to bones of the pelvis and spine. More-over, NFκB-mediated IL-6 signaling is upstream of expression MMPs, which are in-volved with degradation of the extracellular matrix during tumor invasion.

In vitro studies have begun to elucidate the role of IL-6 in prostate carcinogenesis. Cell lines established from androgen-responsive tumors do not endogenously express IL-6 however these cells will become androgen independent when treated with IL-6 (Lee, Lou et al. 2003). Prostate cancer cell lines unresponsive to androgens that are es-tablished from bone and brain metastases express IL-6 and are also androgen inde-pendent (Lee, Pienta et al. 2003). Although hormone-responsive prostate cancer cell lines do not constitutively express IL-6, they can be induced to express IL-6 through an NFκB-dependent mechanism. Studies conducted in our laboratory showed that LNCaP cells secrete IL-6 in response to IL-1β resulting in expression of the MMP, ma-trilysin, which is involved with degradation of the extracellular matrix during invasion and metastases (Maliner-Stratton, Klein et al. 2001). These data suggest that IL-6 may play a role in the point of prostate carcinogenesis at which the cancer cells become androgen independent making it a viable candidate for prevention progression of prostate cancer to an invasive phenotype.

IL-6 Signaling in Prostate Cancer Cells. IL-6 frequently elicits its downstream effects by signaling through the transcription factor, signal transducer and activator of transcription 3 (STAT3). Binding of IL-6 to its receptor leads to activation of Janus kinases as well as two major downstream signaling components, STAT3 and MAPK in the prostate carcinoma cell line, LNCaP (Spiotto and Chung 2000; Spiotto and Chung 2000). STAT3 has been shown to mediate neuroendocrine differentiation of LNCaP cells. In addition, in the differentiated cells showing neurite outgrowth and increased expression of the neuroendocrine markers, neuron specific enolase and chromagranin A that had undergone growth arrest, STAT3 remained active (Spiotto and Chung 2000). Chung and colleagues also demonstrated that STAT3 mediated IL-6-induced growth inhibition in LNCaP cells (Spiotto and Chung 2000). It is of interest that the more progressed and less differentiated prostatic carcinoma cell lines, PC3 and DU-145, express a constitutive level of secreted IL-6, however, those data also showed that the less progressed and hormone responsive LNCaP cells do not secrete any detectable IL-6 (Chung, Yu et al. 1999). In addition, it has been shown that the more progressed prostatic carcinoma cell lines lack a functional STAT3 pathway (Mori, Murakami-Mori et al. 1999). Research conducted by Ni and colleagues demonstrated that cells derived from both rat and human prostate cancers have constitutively activated STAT3; and STAT3 activation was directly correlated with malignant potential. Inhibition of STAT3 transactivation activity by ectopic expression of a dominant-negative STAT3 in human the prostate cancer cells significantly suppresses their growth in vitro and their tumorigenicity in vivo. Furthermore, the Janus kinase inhibitor, tyrphostin AG490, inhibited the constitutive activation of STAT3 and suppressed the growth of human prostate cancer cells in vitro. These results indicate that activation of STAT3 signaling is essential in the progression of prostate cancer cells and suggest that targeting STAT3 signaling may yield a potential early therapeutic intervention for prostate cancer.

Cyclooxygenase-2 (COX-2). The COX enzymes catalyze the rate-limiting steps in the conversion of arachidonic acid to proinflammatory prostaglandins. The COX enzyme exists in two isoforms, COX-1 and COX-2. The COX-1 isoform is constitutively expressed in a majority of human tissues and regulates production of prostaglandins that mediate renal and platelet function, and maintenance of the gastrointestinal mucosa (Oshima, Sugiyama et al. 1993). Conversely, COX-2 isoform is not expressed in normal tissues, but is rapidly induced by inflammatory cytokines, growth factors, oncogenes and tumor promoters (Oshima, Dinchuk et al. 1996; Reddy and Rao 2000). The two isoforms share 60% overall amino acid identity and 75% core sequence identity; and the sizes of the enzymes are comparable (71 kD). However, despite strong similarities in kinetic parameters, binding sites for arachidonic acid, active sites for NSAID binding, and molecular structure (Thun, Namboodiri et al. 1993), the two isoforms differ in substrate affinities due to a single amino acid substitution (isoleucine in COX-1 for valine in COX-2) (Moody, Leyton et al. 1998) in the NSAID binding site resulting in a void volume to the other side of the central active site channel in COX-2. Compounds designed to bind in this additional space are potent and selective inhibitors of COX-2. The advantage of selective COX-2 inhibitors such as celecoxib and rofecoxib is that they are effective in inhibiting inflammation without blocking the COX-1 enzymes that are important for the maintenance of gastrointestinal tract homeostasis and platelet function.

Overexpression of COX-2 in prostate cancer cells is associated with resistance to apoptosis (Tang, Sun et al. 2002). Furthermore, selective inhibition of COX-2 can increase apoptotic index in prostate carcinoma cells in vitro (Fosslien 2001; Kirschenbaum, Liu et al. 2001). These observations concur with data that suggest that COX-2 inhibitors could be effective chemopreventative agents. Lim and colleagues showed that the COX inhibitor sulindac, a NSAID frequently used for chronic inflammatory diseases, was tested for pro-apoptotic activity in the prostate cancer cell lines, PC3 and LNCaP, and a normal prostate epithelial cells line, PrEC, in vitro. Apoptosis was quantified following treatment with either sulindac or an active sulindac metabolite, Exisilund (sulindac sulfide). After 48 hours, 50% of PC3 cells and 40% of LNCaP cells underwent apoptosis while PrEC cells showed no indication of apoptosis at similar concentrations of drug (Lim, Piazza et al. 1999).

Studies evaluating the effects of COX-2 specific inhibitors on angiogenesis in prostate carcinoma cell lines have also been performed. The prostate carcinoma cell lines, LNCaP and PC3 and a normal prostate stroma cell line, PrEC were treated with two COX-2 specific inhibitors, Edolac and NS398. Both compounds decreased cell proliferation in the carcinoma cell lines, but not in the normal prostate stromal cell line. A DNA fragmentation assay revealed that both compounds also induced apoptosis in the two carcinoma cell lines and not the normal stromal cell line (Liu, Yao et al. 1998).

B-Cell Lymphoma/Leukemia 2 (Bcl-2). Bcl-2 is a member of the bcl-2 family of apoptotic regulatory gene products of the proto-oncogene, b-cell lymphoma/leukemia. bcl-2 family members have been characterized as exhibiting both pro-apoptotic and anti-apoptotic properties (Tsujimoto and Croce 1986). Numerous studies have suggested that bcl-2 mediated decrease in apoptotic index plays a role in prostate carcinogenesis (Reed, Miyashita et al. 1996; Gross, McDonnell et al. 1999); and increased expression of bcl-2 and related apoptotic pathways appear to affect the sensitivity of prostate cancer cells to several therapeutic modalities including androgen ablation and radiation. The increase in cell survival following treatment is thought to contribute to development of the androgen-independent phenotype (Apakama, Robinson et al. 1996; Rosser, Reyes et al. 2003). Immunohistochemical analyses of prostate tissue have shown overexpression of bcl-2 in androgen-independent carcinoma tissue, but not in androgen-responsive cancers tissue and HGPIN suggesting that bcl-2 is involved in disease progression and not in the early stages of carcinogenesis (McDonnell, Troncoso et al. 1992; Raffo, Perlman et al. 1995; Apakama, Robinson et al. 1996). Retrospective studies of prostate cancer patient survival following radiation therapy have shown that overexpression of bcl-2 was correlative to poor prognosis (Pollack, Cowen et al. 2003). Additional investigation of bcl-2 in cancerous growth in the peripheral and transitional zones of the prostate have shown a higher incidence of bcl-2 in the highly proliferative peripheral zone when compared to the less proliferative transitional zone in the prostate (Erbersdobler, Fritz et al. 2002).

The emergence of novel and sensitive techniques such as tissue microarray (TMA) has presented both supportive and negating evidence for bcl-2 as an effective biomarker of prostate cancer progression (Merseburger, Kuczyk et al. 2003; Zellweger, Ninck et al. 2003). Elevated levels of bcl-2 have been observed in prostate cancer tissue following both androgen ablation and radiotherapy. This correlates with in vitro studies demonstrating that bcl-2 elicits a protective effect on cancer cells in response to radiation. The role of bcl-2 in the prevention of apoptosis is critical in the development of prostate cancer recurrence and androgen-independent survival. In this sense, bcl-2 is an encouraging prognostic molecular biomarker.

Prevention Strategies

Androgen Inhibitors

In the early 1990s, a prostate cancer prevention clinical trial was designed to test whether the 5 alpha reductase inhibitor finasteride could reduce the number of prostate cancers found in men over the age of 55. The rationale for this strategy was straight forward. Prostate cancer is the leading cause of cancer-related deaths in men over the age of 50 and at the time the trial was designed over 40,000 men were dying each year of prostate cancer. Hormonal factors were targeted for prevention because the only major risk factors identified for prostate cancer development are being male and having normal testosterone production. In the trial planning, various hormonal interventions were considered even including surgical or medical castration but the morbidity of such interventions precluded their use in a prevention study. The debate finally centered on either the use of an antiandrogen which acts via binding to the androgen receptor or the use of finasteride which blocks the conversion of testosterone to another androgen, dihydrotestosterone, which is the most physiologic active androgen acting on the prostate. Finasteride was selected for trial based on its lower toxicity potential. The main potential toxicities known for finasteride were a reduction semen volume, erectile dysfunction, reduced libido and gynecomastia.

The study design was a placebo-controlled randomization of approximately 25,000 men to receive either finasteride 5 mg each day orally or a placebo finasteride pill. Treatment was for seven years with yearly digital rectal exams and serum PSA levels and quarterly contacts for documentation of medical events and/or toxicities. The identification of a suspicious digital rectal examination or an elevated serum PSA level resulted in a recommendation to have a prostate biopsy. At the end of the seven years, all men were to be biopsied. It was anticipated that the placebo group would be found to have a 6% incidence of prostate cancer.

Enrollment was completed by May 1997 and the results of the trial were published in (Thompson, Goodman et al. (2003). The results were perplexing. The first result was expected and was that the finasteride was reasonably well tolerated with less than 15% of men experiencing the anticipated sexual side effects. The second finding was a significant reduction in the number of cancers found on the end of biopsy study for the men who had been randomized to finasteride. Of those receiving placebo, 24.4% were found to have prostate cancer on the biopsy versus only 18.4 percent of the men taking the finasteride ($p < 0.001$). This 24.8% reduction in the prevalence of prostate cancer marked only the second prevention trial where a pharmacologic intervention reduced the incidence of a cancer (the other being tamoxifen in breast cancer prevention).

There were two other findings of note. First, the histologic grade (the Gleason score) of the cancers found in the men who were taking finasteride were significantly more likely to be a higher grade (Gleason score of 7, 8, 9 or 10) and hence of poorer prognosis than the men who took the finasteride placebo (37% versus 22.2%, $p < 0.001$). Since the end point of the study was the incidence of cancer found and not survival, how these conflicting findings (a lower incidence versus a higher histologic grade) effected outcome is not known. The other unexplained finding was an overall incidence of cancer in the placebo group that was 4 times the anticipated incidence of prostate cancer that the study design called for. The significance of this unanticipated finding is also not known.

Overall, the study demonstrated the potential of chemoprevention in prostate cancer. However, the conflicting and unexplained findings are such that the routine use of finasteride as a chemopreventive agent in prostate cancer is not recommended.

Selenium and Vitamin E

Epidemiologic studies have suggested an inverse relationship between intake of dietary selenium and incidence of cancer (Clark and Jacobs 1998; Overvad 1998; Nelson, Reid et al. 2002). Numerous animal studies have demonstrated that dietary supplementation with selenium reduces cancer incidence in animal models including melanoma and cancers of the colon, breast, liver, esophagus, head and neck, pancreas, kidney and lung. One of the central findings of the Nutritional Prevention of Cancer study conducted at the University of Arizona, was a greater than 60% reduction in the incidence of prostate cancer in participants randomized to 200 µg per day of selenium compared to a placebo-treated group (Clark, Combs et al. 1996; Duffield-Lillico, Dalkin et al. 2003). An analysis of an additional three years of the blinded phase of this study showed a continued significant decrease in prostate cancer incidence in participants within the lowest two tertiles of baseline plasma selenium levels. In these groups, the prostate cancer incidence after 13 years of follow-up was decreased by 86% and 67%, respectively, in the treatment group versus placebo (Duffield-Lillico, Dalkin et al. 2003). These findings led to the development of additional, randomized, blinded, placebo-controlled clinical studies testing the effects of selenium on prevention of primary and secondary prostate cancer. Selenium is an ideal example of a potential chemopreventive agent being tested for efficacy in all risk groups and in every stage of prostate carcinogenesis (Figure 4).

Selenium and Prostate Cancer Prevention in Normal Healthy Men (the SELECT Trial). The Selenium and Vitamin E Cancer Prevention Trial (SELECT) is an NCI-sponsored randomized, prospective, double-blind study designed to determine whether selenium and/or vitamin E decrease the risk of prostate cancer in healthy men. SELECT is being coordinated by the Southwest Oncology Group (SWOG) and plans to enroll a total of 32,400 normal, healthy men at over 400 clinical study sites in the United States, Puerto Rico and Canada (Klein, Thompson et al. 2000; Klein, Thompson et al. 2001). Preclinical, epidemiological and phase III data imply that selenium and vitamin E have potential efficacy for prostate cancer prevention. The four arms of this study include: (1) selenium+vitamin E; (2) selenium+placebo; (3) placebo+vitamin E; and (4) placebo+placebo. Enrollment began in July 2001. The trial is expected to be completed in 2013. The dose levels of selenium and vitamin E are 200 µg and 400 mg, respectively (Figure 5a). In addition to primary and prespecified secondary endpoints, including develop-

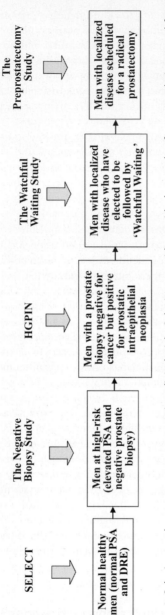

Fig. 4. Selenium and prostate cancer prevention clinical trials. Selenium provides an ideal example of an agent being tested for chemopreventive activity in all stages of prostate carcinogenesis.

ment of biopsy-proven prostate cancer and PSA velocity, additional tertiary/ancillary endpoints, including dietary/nutrient assessments, pathology and molecular/cellular biomarkers, quality of life, and molecular epidemiology will be evaluated.

Selenium and Prostate Cancer Prevention in High-Risk Men (The Negative Biopsy Study). In addition to recruiting participants to SELECT, the Arizona Cancer Center at the University of Arizona is conducting four clinical studies examining the effects of selenium on primary and secondary prevention of prostate cancer in several populations (Stratton, Reid et al. 2003). The "Negative Biopsy Study" is an NCI-sponsored study in which 700 men, who have had at least one negative prostate biopsy within one year of study enrollment, are randomized to receive either 200 µg or 400 µg per day of selenium versus placebo (Figure 5b). Endpoints include PSA velocity, development of biopsy-proven prostate cancer and serum markers including alkaline phosphatase and chromagranin A. Changes in prostate tissue biomarkers are also being examined.

Selenium and Prostate Cancer Prevention in Men with Prostatic Intraepithelial Neoplasia (The HGPIN Study). While the recognized risk factors for prostate cancer (male gender, a positive family history, age, and the presence of androgens) pose targets for prevention efforts, another potential target would be premalignant lesions. While somewhat controversial, high grade prostatic intraepithelial neoplasia (HGPIN) is generally accepted to be a premalignant lesion for prostate cancer when found on a prostate biopsy that does not otherwise have evidence of cancer. At the very least, the presence of HGPIN is associated with a high risk of the subsequent documentation of prostate cancer in an individual (Alsikafi, Brendler et al. 2001; Fowler, Bigler et al. 2001).

Prostatic intraepithelial neoplasia (PIN) is used to describe normal prostate glands and ducts that are lined with atypical cells. These cells have atypia in the nuclei as well as cellular morphologic changes. The degree of change can be categorized into 3 grades. Grade 3 PIN is HGPIN and is the only grade of PIN which is associated with prostate cancer risk. The following evidence supports the association of HGPIN with prostate cancer: HGPIN incidence increases with age at a rate paralleling prostate cancer; HGPIN-like prostate cancer occurs more frequently in African-American men; prostate cancer is more likely to be found in prostates which contain HGPIN; and within the prostate HGPIN and cancer when found together are physically close to each other.

These findings support a conclusion that HGPIN is a premalignant lesion and hence identifies a group of men at significant risk of subsequently being diagnosed with prostate cancer (up to 50%). HGPIN is consequently a reasonable target for a chemoprevention trial. Such a study has been designed and is enrolling patients in a Southwest Oncology Group (SWOG) trial, SWOG 9917 (Marshall 2001). In this study, 466 men with HGPIN but no cancer on a biopsy will be enrolled and randomized to 200 µg of L-selenomethionine or placebo orally daily for three years. If at any time with follow-up every six months for three years a digital rectal exam is suspicious for cancer or the PSA is elevated, a recommendation for a transrectal ultrasound-guided prostate biopsy is made. After the completion of three years of selenomethionine, every participant undergoes a prostate biopsy. The end point is the incidence of prostate cancer on biopsy.

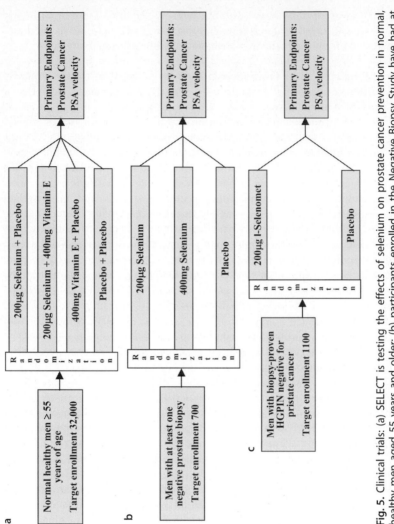

Fig. 5. Clinical trials: (a) SELECT is testing the effects of selenium on prostate cancer prevention in normal, healthy men aged 55 years and older; (b) participants enrolled in the Negative Biopsy Study have had at least one prostate biopsy negative for HGPIN and cancer; the HGPIN study is enrolling men with a prostate biopsy negative for cancer but positive for HGPIN

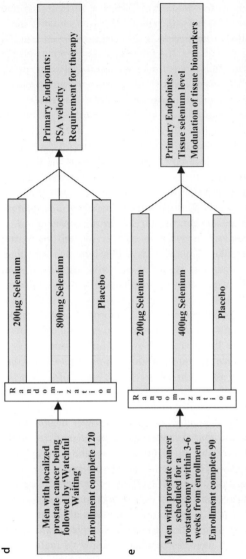

Fig. 5. (d) the Watchful Waiting Study is enrolling men with biopsy-proven prostate cancer who have elected to forgo therapy and be followed by 'watchful waiting' and (e) the Preprostatectomy Study is examining the effects of short-term selenium supplementation on prostate cancer tissue in men with prostate cancer scheduled for a radical prostatectomy.

Selenium and Prostate Cancer Prevention in Men With Localized Prostate Cancer (The Watchful Waiting Study). The "Watchful Waiting" study, which is also NCI-sponsored, is randomizing 220 men with biopsy-proven prostate cancer who have elected not to undergo surgery, radiation, hormone therapy, or any other type of therapy, and are under the age of 85 (Stratton, Reid et al. 2003). Treatment groups include 200 µg or 800 µg of selenium per day or placebo. End points include PSA velocity, time to progression, time to treatment, alkaline phosphatase and chromagranin A levels. Statistical analyses performed in this study will be stratified by Gleason score (Figure 5 d).

Selenium and Modulation of Biomarkers in Prostate Tissue (The Preprostatectomy Study). The "Preprostatectomy Study" is sponsored by the Department of Defense. This study is enrolling men who have been recently diagnosed with prostate cancer and are scheduled for a radical prostatectomy between three and six weeks from the time of enrollment (Stratton and Ahmann 2003). During that time they are randomized to receive 200 µg or 400 µg of selenium per day or placebo. In this study selenium levels in prostate tissue will be measured from the time of the original diagnostic biopsy and from the radical prostatectomy. This will determine whether selenium taken orally can affect selenium levels in prostate tissue. Tissue will also be analyzed for markers of cell growth and apoptosis using immunohistochemistry (Figure 5 e).

Soy Isoflavones

Epidemiologic studies have suggested that a diet rich in soy compounds may reduce the risk of prostate cancer (Cassidy 2003; Lee, Gomez et al. 2003). Soybeans and other soy products contain isoflavones, which show promise as prostate cancer chemopreventive agents. Preclinical data suggest that soy isoflavones, such as genistein and diadzien, may play a role in the hormonal regulation of prostate cancer by inhibiting the enzyme 5α-reductase (Barqawi, Thompson et al. 2004). Early studies on soy isoflavones have also shown inhibition of cell growth and induction of apoptosis in prostate cancer cell lines. In a comparison of various dietary compounds used for chemoprevention, Agarwal and colleagues showed that the soy isoflavone, genistein, induced apoptosis in 30–40% of DU145 prostate cancer cells (Agarwal 2000). This study also provides evidence that genistein induces CDKI-mediated cell cycle arrest.

While this evidence sounds promising in favor of genistein as a prostate cancer chemopreventive agent, some studies have known DNA damage resulting from treating cells with this compound in vitro. DNA strand breaks were noted for high doses of genistein (100 µmol/L or more) in cultured cancer cells of mice and Chinese hamsters, as well as in human lymphoblastoid and blood lymphocyte cells (Miltyk, Craciunescu et al. 2003). These data prompted Miltyk and colleagues to conduct a study on the genetic safety of soy isoflavones in men with prostate cancer. Their results indicated that participants taking as much as 600 mg/day never achieved a blood plasma genistein concentration above 27 µmol/L. DNA strand breaks in peripheral lymphocytes were measured by COMET assay, and no significant increase was found for any participant, suggesting that genistein does not lead to DNA damage within the dosages given in this study and may be safe to study in future clinical trials. However, this does raise a question regarding bioavailability of this agent.

Table 4. Studies testing soy isoflavones for prostate cancer chemoprevention

Research group	Phase	Population	Treatment
H. Lee Moffit Cancer Center	Pilot Study	Patients with stage I or II prostate cancer	Oral isoflavones twice daily and a multivitamin once daily vs. oral placebo twice daily and multivitamin once daily
H. Lee Moffit Cancer Center	Pilot Study	Stage I and II prostate cancer patients pre-prostatectomy	Oral isoflavones (3 dose groups) twice daily or oral lycopene (3 dose groups) twice daily or oral placebo twice daily
Cancer and Leukemia Group B	II	Patients who have an elevated PSA (5–10 ng/ml) and a negative biopsy	Oral soy protein once daily vs. oral placebo once daily
National Cancer Institute of Canada	II	Patients with high grade prostatic intraepithelial neoplasia	Combination of soy, vitamin E and selenium twice daily vs. placebo twice daily
Barbara Ann Karmanos Cancer Institute	II	Stage I and II prostate cancer patients pre-prostatectomy	One of three different dosage levels of soy isoflavones (amounts not specified) daily vs. placebo daily

Several studies on the use of soy isoflavones in prostate cancer prevention and treatment are underway. The H. Lee Moffit Cancer Center and Research Institute in Tampa, Florida, is currently conducting two studies, one on the effect of soy isoflavones versus placebo on hormone levels of stage II and III prostate cancer patients and the other on isoflavones versus lycopene in prostate cancer patients prior to radical prostatectomy. Phase II studies are also being conducted on patients with a negative biopsy and medial PSA levels (5 to 10 ng/ml) and cancer patients prior to radical prostatectomy, with an emphasis on apoptosis levels and cell proliferation rates. Examples of studies on soy isoflavones is presented in Table 4.

Clearly, soy isoflavones are of significant interest to the research community, and the results of these trials will provide important information regarding the efficacy of these compounds as a chemoprevention agent.

COX-2 Inhibitors

COX-2 overexpression stimulates the production of prostanoids including PGE2, which induces angiogenesis in cancer tissue which thereby contributes to tumor blood supply (Banerjee, Liu et al. 2003). Prostate cancer cells containing high levels of COX-2 also display decreased levels of apoptosis (Fosslien 2001; Kirschenbaum, Liu et al. 2001). Inhibition of COX-2 in prostate cancer cell lines has been shown prevent PGE2-mediated expression of vascular endothelial growth factor (VEGF) (Liu, Kirschenbaum

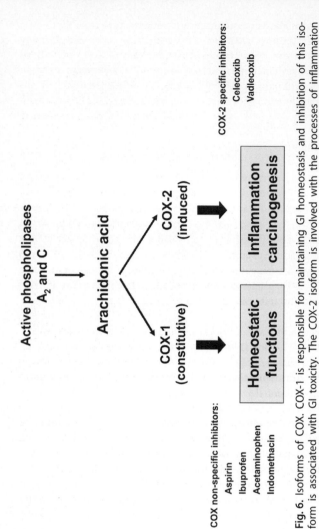

Fig. 6. Isoforms of COX. COX-1 is responsible for maintaining GI homeostasis and inhibition of this isoform is associated with GI toxicity. The COX-2 isoform is involved with the processes of inflammation and carcinogenesis and is a target for cancer chemoprevention. Numerous agents are in clinical development testing efficacy of COX-2 inhibition on carcinogenesis in a variety of tumor types.

et al. 2000) and induce apoptosis in prostate cancer cell lines (Godbey and Atala 2003). These data led to initiation of clinical studies testing effectiveness of COX-2 inhibitors for prostate cancer therapy and prevention. Currently, COX-2 research in prostate cancer falls into one of two categories, which include non-steroidal anti-inflammatory drugs (NSAIDs) that inhibit both the COX-1 and -2 isoforms; and selective COX-2 inhibitors. The androgen inhibitor finasteride has also been shown to block COX-1 and -2 expression. Examples of compounds that have been under investigation are shown in Figure 6.

Several COX-2 specific inhibitors are currently being tested in clinical trials, such as celecoxib (Celebrex) and Etodolac. Celecoxib has been shown to induce apoptosis in both PC-3 and LNCaP cell lines in a dose- and time-dependent manner (Hsu, Ching et al. 2000; Fosslien 2001). In addition, Pruthi and colleagues showed a decrease in prostate specific antigen (PSA) levels and doubling time in response to treatment with celecoxib in men who have recently undergone radiation therapy or radical prostatectomy (Pruthi, Derksen et al. 2004). Johnson and colleagues conducted a study comparing several COX-2 specific inhibitors in vitro, including celecoxib (Johnson, Song et al. 2001). Etodolac was investigated by Kamijo and colleagues in comparison to NS-398. Etodolac decreased cell proliferation in PC-3 and LNCaP prostate cell lines but not in normal prostate epithelial cells (Kamijo, Sato et al. 2001).

In vitro and preclinical animal data suggest that the COX-1 and -2 inhibitor, sulindac sulfone, exhibits anti-tumor activity against prostate cancer contributed to the development of several phase I/II clinical trials examining PSA response as well as measurable disease response rate as a single agent or in combination with taxotere. The secondary objectives include determination of time to disease progression and duration of response in patients with prostate carcinoma (NCI 2004).

The COX-2 specific inhibitor, celecoxib, is also undergoing clinical development for prevention/treatment of prostate cancer. In one NCI-sponsored phase I/II study ongoing at the Johns Hopkins Oncology Center in Maryland, patients are randomized to receive either celecoxib or placebo prior to radical prostatectomy (NCI 2004). The objectives of this study are: (1) to compare biomarker modulation (prostaglandin levels) in tissue samples of patients with localized prostate cancer treated with neoadjuvant celecoxib versus placebo followed by prostatectomy, (2) to compare the effect of these regimens on angiogenic factors within the prostate in these patients, and (3) to determine the pharmacokinetic and pharmacodynamic effects of celecoxib in these patients.

Milk Thistle

Milk thistle extract comes from the seed of the *Silybum marianum* plant and is used clinically for a variety of indications, including neural stimulation, immunostimulation (Wilasrusmee, Kittur et al. 2002) and as a clinical treatment for certain liver diseases (Zi and Agarwal 1999; Singh, Dhanalakshmi et al. 2002). With respect to prostate cancer prevention, preclinical data on DU145 xenografts in nude mice suggests that silibinin (a primary component of milk thistle extract) inhibits cell growth in a dose- and time-dependent manner, and that excessive cell proliferation does not recur after the cessation of treatment. Recent studies have shown cell growth inhibition by milk thistle products occurs at the G1 phase (Shamberger and Frost 1969; Agarwal 2000; Dhanalakshmi, Agarwal et al. 2003) and provides a moderate induction of apoptosis in prostate cancer cell lines. This effect is particularly apparent when silibinin is coupled with other cytotoxic drugs (Tyagi, Singh et al. 2002).

Dhanalakshmi and colleagues observed silibinin combined with cytotoxic platinum compounds cisplatin and carboplatin for inhibition of cell growth in DU145 prostate cancer cell lines. They found that the combination of silibinin and carboplatin inhibited growth in 80 to 90% of cells, while the silibinin and cisplatin pairing caused 63 to 80% inhibition (Dhanalakshmi, Agarwal et al. 2003). These findings were significantly greater than the growth inhibition experienced by cells treated with either platinum compound alone (36 to 65% inhibition). Tyagi and colleagues conducted a similar study doxorubicin, and found that growth inhibition occurred in 88% of DU145 cells treated with a combination of the drug and silibinin, as opposed to 41% in cells treated only with doxorubicin. This study also noted an increase in apoptosis with the combination treatment as opposed to either agent alone (Tyagi, Singh et al. 2002). These data indicate that silibinin may be used in conjunction with cytotoxic drug treatments to inhibit cell growth. Clinically, this is significant due to the danger of toxicity and negative side effects that may occur with both platinum-based treatments and doxorubicin.

Authors Zi and Agarwal chose a different course of study by looking at the effect of silibinin. They noted that intracellular PSA levels decreased upon treatment with silibinin in LNCaP prostate cancer cell lines (Zi, Zhang et al. 2000). As a secondary endpoint to their original study on PSA, Zi and Agarwal also observed growth arrest in the G1 in cells treated with silibinin, but specified that this was not followed by increased apoptosis, which indicates that the ability of silibinin to induce cell death may be questionable when not combined with another substance (Zi and Agarwal 1999).

Overall, milk thistle byproducts appear to be more effective at reducing growth in prostate cancer cell lines, and may increase the effect of other chemopreventive drugs that are currently in clinical use.

Saw Palmetto

Serenoa repens, commonly known as saw palmetto, is often utilized as an herbal treatment option for men diagnosed with benign prostatic hyperplasia (BPH), the non-malignant enlargement of the prostate gland often exhibited in aging men typically associated with voiding symptoms resulting from increased pressure on the urethra (Knaus 2002). Despite the minimal clinical evidence of the therapeutic efficacy and safety of saw palmetto in the United States, the herbal supplement is frequently prescribed as an alternative therapy for BPH. The role of saw palmetto in cancer chemoprevention is speculative and the chemopreventive effects of saw palmetto will require extensive clinical and molecular based research.

An analysis of 18 clinical trials testing safety and efficacy of saw palmetto in patients with BPH showed some therapeutic benefit in urinary symptoms in patients with BPH. However there was considerable commentary on limitations in the analyses regarding the variation in clinical study design and duration of treatment (Wilt, Ishani et al. 1998). Additional review of clinical studies conducted by Gerber and colleagues also implicated the significant positive effects of saw palmetto on urinary tract symptoms in BPH patients (Gerber 2000). Subsequently, Gerber and colleagues conducted a 6 month, randomized, placebo-controlled clinical trial that confirmed that saw palmetto was effective in reducing urinary tract symptoms in BPH (Gerber, Kuznetsov et al. 2001).

Some preliminary in vitro assessment of saw palmetto activity has been performed in prostate cancer cells. The primary therapeutic action is to inhibit 5-alpha reductase in forming DHT and, to a lesser extent, 3-alpha reductase, and to block the action of DHT to receptors on prostate cells via 3-ketosteroid reductase. Saw palmetto was shown to inhibit prostate tumor promotion by 12-O-tetradecanoylphorbol-13-acetate (TPA), demonstrating potential chemopreventive activity (Kapadia, Azuine et al. 2002). Additional in vitro assessment of saw palmetto in prostate cancer cell lines identified a correlation with saw palmetto and a decrease in COX-2 expression (Goldmann, Sharma et al. 2001). In addition, Veltri and colleagues observed epithelial prostate cell chromatin restructuring following 6 months of saw palmetto treatment in a randomized placebo-controlled trial (Veltri, Marks et al. 2002). While some data suggest that saw palmetto shows promise as a prostate cancer-chemopreventive agent, extensive clinical studies will be required to test efficacy.

Resveratrol

Resveratrol is a polyphenolic compound abundant in grapes, red wine, and several types of nuts and berries. Considerable evidence suggests that resveratrol may have inhibitory effects in tumor proliferation, invasion and metastasis; and enhanced tumor cell apoptosis has been documented in studies targeting prostate, breast (Nakagawa, Kiyozuka et al. 2001; Scarlatti, Sala et al. 2003), colon (Wolter, Akoglu et al. 2001; Delmas, Rebe et al. 2003), hepatic (Yu, Sun et al. 2003), and skin cancer (Niles, McFarland et al. 2003). The seminal report by Pezzuto and colleagues showed that resveratrol elicits inhibitory action at each stage of carcinogenesis and that it has multiple targets including kinases, steroid hormone receptors and reactive oxygen species (Jang, Cai et al. 1997). In addition, resveratrol has been shown to impede activation of carcinogens by inhibition of phase I metabolic enzymes such as cytochrome P450 1A1 (Chun, Kim et al. 1999).

Studies in an in vivo rat model showed that resveratrol exerts potent anti-inflammatory effects by inhibition of COX-1 and -2 (Jang, Cai et al. 1997; Subbaramaiah, Chung et al. 1998). It is of interest that inhibition of both COX isoforms is by direct interaction with the enzyme in addition to blocking transcription of COX-2 by inhibition of NFκB transactivation activity. Also relevant to resveratrol's profile as a cancer-chemopreventive agent is its capacity to induce cell cycle arrest in G1, and to trigger caspase-dependent, p53-mediated and bcl-2-sensitive apoptotic responses (Stewart, Christman et al. 2000). Other in vitro studies showed that resveratrol differentially inhibits members of the protein kinase C family (Stewart, Ward et al. 1999; Slater, Seiz et al. 2003). Perhaps the most important mechanism elicited by resveratrol on prostate cancer cells is its ability to modulate the androgen receptor. Mitchell and colleagues showed that resveratrol exerts anti-androgenic effects on the hormone-responsive prostate cancer cell line, LNCaP (Mitchell, Zhu et al. 1999). The inhibitory mechanism involves inhibition of expression of the androgen receptor, the androgen receptor co-activator ARA70 and androgen-mediated genes, including PSA. These data suggest that resveratrol may be a prime candidate for prostate cancer chemoprevention and as a neoadjuvant therapy for prostate cancer.

Table 5. Examples of prostate cancer prevention trials sponsored by the National Cancer Institute (NCI 2004)

Title	Primary Endpoint(s)
Phase III Randomized Study of Selenium and Vitamin E for the Prevention of Prostate Cancer (SELECT)	■ Compare the effect of selenium and vitamin E administered alone vs in combination on the clinical incidence of prostate cancer.
Phase III Randomized Study of Selenium as Chemoprevention of Prostate Cancer in Patients with HGPIN	■ Compare the effects of selenium versus placebo on the 3-year incidence rate of prostate cancer in patients with high-grade prostatic intraepithelial neoplasia.
Phase II Randomized Study of Dietary Soy in Patients With Elevated PSA Levels	■ Compare the reduction in the rate of prostatic cellular proliferation in patients with an elevated PSA (5 to 10 ng/mL) and a negative biopsy for prostate cancer when treated with daily soy protein supplements vs placebo. ■ Compare the effect of these regimens on additional biomarkers of prostate cancer (PSA, high-grade prostate intraepithelial neoplasia, induction of apoptosis, sex steroid receptor expression, and loss of glutathione S-transferase-pi) in these patients.
Phase II Randomized Study of Vitamin E, Selenium, and Soy Protein Isolate in Patients with High-Grade Prostatic Intraepithelial Neoplasia	■ Determine whether nutritional supplementation with soy protein isolate, vitamin E, and selenium can delay the time to development of invasive prostate cancer (disease-free survival) in patients with high-grade prostatic intraepithelial neoplasia. ■ Determine the effect of this supplementation on intermediate endpoints that may reflect a lessened risk of invasive prostate cancer (e.g., serum PSA levels, hormone levels, lycopene, malondialdehyde, vitamin E, and reduced thiol groups) in these patients.
Phase II Randomized Study of Vitamin E, Selenium, and Soy Protein Isolate in Patients with High-Grade Prostatic Intraepithelial Neoplasia	■ Determine whether nutritional supplementation with soy protein isolate, vitamin E, and selenium can delay the time to development of invasive prostate cancer (disease-free survival) in patients with high-grade prostatic intraepithelial neoplasia. ■ Determine the effect of this supplementation on intermediate endpoints that may reflect a lessened risk of invasive prostate cancer (e.g., serum PSA levels, hormone levels, lycopene, malondialdehyde, vitamin E, and reduced thiol groups) in these patients.
A Chemoprevention Study of an Investigational Drug in Men with High Grade Prostate Intraepithelial Neoplasia (PIN)	■ This is a study of an investigational medication that may reduce high-grade PIN and prevent the occurrence of prostate cancer.
Phase II Randomized Study of Toremifene Followed by Radical Prostatectomy in Patients with Stage I or II Adenocarcinoma of the Prostate	■ Compare the percent of high-grade prostatic intraepithelial neoplasia (HGPIN) present in the radical prostatectomy tissue (excluding the luminal area) of patients with stage I or II adenocarcinoma of the prostate treated with toremifene vs observation alone followed by radical prostatectomy. ■ Compare the absolute and relative changes in HGPIN in patients treated with toremifene vs observation alone.

Table 5 (continued)

Title	Primary Endpoint(s)
Phase IIB Randomized Chemoprevention Study of DFMO in Patients at High Genetic Risk for Prostate Cancer	■ Compare the levels of polyamines (putrescine, spermidine, and spermine) and progression-related genes in the prostate tissue of patients at high genetic risk for prostate cancer treated with eflornithine (DFMO) vs placebo.
Phase I Study of Lycopene for the Chemoprevention of Prostate Cancer	■ Determine any dose-limiting toxicities and the maximum tolerated dose of lycopene administered orally as a food-based delivery system in healthy male subjects 18–45 years of age for the chemoprevention of prostate cancer.
Evaluation of Risk Factors which Predict the Transformation of Early Stage to Clinically Aggressive Prostate Cancer	■ Evaluate risk factors which predict the transformation of early stage to clinically aggressive disease.
Randomized Pilot Study of Isoflavones versus Lycopene Prior to Radical Prostatectomy in Patients with Localized Prostate Cancer	■ Compare the effect of isoflavones vs lycopene prior to radical prostatectomy on intermediate biomarkers (e.g., indices of cell proliferation and apoptosis) in patients with localized prostate cancer. ■ Compare the effects of these nutritional supplements on increases in plasma levels and tissue levels of these agents in these patients.

Conclusion

Prostate cancer is a major health problem and is the most commonly diagnosed cancer in North American males. Although incidence has increased in the past decade, probably due to improved screening, mortality has decreased because disease is diagnosed at an earlier stage and treatment strategies have improved. Prevention of prostate cancer and impediment of disease progression at an early stage would have a significant impact on healthcare for men and healthcare economics. The paradigm of prostate cancer prevention is shifting from primary prevention to treatment of the process of carcinogenesis. Successful prostate cancer prevention strategies will be achieved not only by preclusion, inhibition of reversal of early stages of carcinogenesis that lead to tumor development, but also by eradication of incipient populations of more aggressive malignant cells. The latter strategy, which includes immune surveillance, would arrest the process of carcinogenesis prior to development of clinically significant neoplastic disease.

The significant advances in molecular biology techniques including microarray and proteomics within the past decade are allowing us to now identify potential surrogate endpoint biomarkers for prostate cancer prevention trials and recognize risk categories for development of prostate cancer. Currently, several agents in clinical development show promise for effective prostate cancer prevention and numerous clinical studies are ongoing (Table 5). In the majority of ongoing studies, development of biopsy-proven prostate cancer is the primary endpoint. Validation of early markers of carcinogenesis will have a profound impact of chemoprevention studies with regards to time and costs.

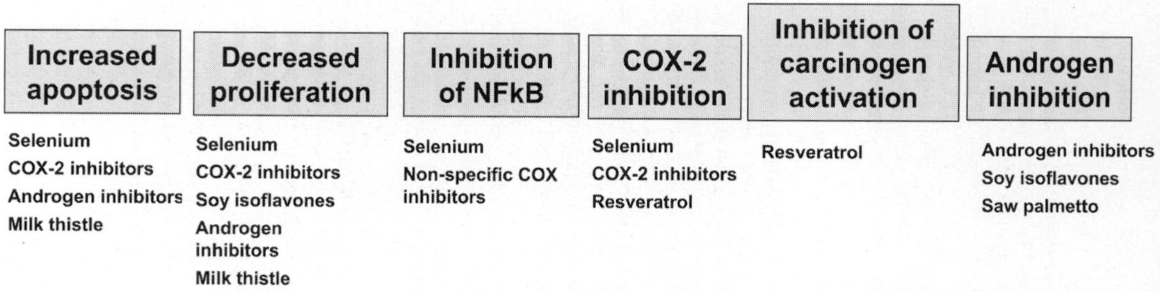

Increased apoptosis	Decreased proliferation	Inhibition of NFkB	COX-2 inhibition	Inhibition of carcinogen activation	Androgen inhibition
Selenium	Selenium	Selenium	Selenium	Resveratrol	Androgen inhibitors
COX-2 inhibitors	COX-2 inhibitors	Non-specific COX inhibitors	COX-2 inhibitors		Soy isoflavones
Androgen inhibitors	Soy isoflavones		Resveratrol		Saw palmetto
Milk thistle	Androgen inhibitors				
	Milk thistle				

Fig. 7. Mechanisms of inhibition of carcinogenesis. Successful cancer-preventive agents may have a variety of molecular mechanisms including increased apoptosis, decreased proliferation, inhibition of proteins that regulate inflammation, inhibition of activation of carcinogens and androgen inhibition. Agents currently in preclinical and clinical development for prostate cancer prevention elicit more than one of these mechanisms on prostate cancer cells.

Several molecular chemopreventive mechanisms have been proposed for each agent being studied (Figure 7). These include inhibition of apoptosis, induction of cell cycle arrest, blockage of androgen activity, inhibition of COX-2 and inhibition of activation of carcinogens. While many agents are in preclinical development and clinical trials, none have been proven to be effective. Further study of potential mechanisms of action will help development of more targeted preventive agents.

References

Abate-Shen, C. and M.M. Shen (2000). "Molecular genetics of prostate cancer." *Genes Dev* **14**(19): 2410–2434.

Agarwal, R. (2000). "Cell signaling and regulators of cell cycle as molecular targets for prostate cancer prevention by dietary agents." *Biochem Pharmacol* **60**(8): 1051–1059.

Alsikafi, N.F., C.B. Brendler, et al. (2001). "High-grade prostatic intraepithelial neoplasia with adjacent atypia is associated with a higher incidence of cancer on subsequent needle biopsy than high-grade prostatic intraepithelial neoplasia alone." *Urology* **57**(2): 296–300.

Andriole, G.L. and W.J. Catalona (1993). "Using PSA to screen for prostate cancer. The Washington University experience." *Urol Clin North Am* **20**(4): 647–651.

Apakama, I., M.C. Robinson, et al. (1996). "bcl-2 overexpression combined with p53 protein accumulation correlates with hormone-refractory prostate cancer." *Br J Cancer* **74**(8): 1258–1262.

Aspden, W.J., R.J. Rodgers, et al. (1998). "Changes in testicular steroidogenic acute regulatory (STAR) protein, steroidogenic enzymes and testicular morphology associated with increased testosterone secretion in bulls receiving the luteinizing hormone releasing hormone agonist deslorelin." *Domest Anim Endocrinol* **15**(4): 227–238.

Baldwin, A.S., Jr. (1996). "The NF-kappa B and I kappa B proteins: new discoveries and insights." *Annu Rev Immunol* **14**: 649–683.

Banerjee, A.G., J. Liu, et al. (2003). "Expression of biomarkers modulating prostate cancer angiogenesis: Differential expression of annexin II in prostate carcinomas from India and USA." *Mol Cancer* **2**(1): 34.

Barqawi, A., I.M. Thompson, et al. (2004). "Prostate cancer chemoprevention: an overview of United States trials." *J Urol* **171**(2 Pt 2): S5–8; discussion S9.

Bartels, P.H., R. Montironi, et al. (1998). "Nuclear chromatin texture in prostatic lesions. I. PIN and adenocarcinoma." *Anal Quant Cytol Histol* **20**(5): 389–396.

Bartels, P.H., R. Montironi, et al. (1998). "Nuclear chromatin texture in prostatic lesions. II. PIN and malignancy associated changes." *Anal Quant Cytol Histol* **20**(5): 397–406.

Beilin, J., L. Harewood, et al. (2001). "A case-control study of the androgen receptor gene CAG repeat polymorphism in Australian prostate carcinoma subjects." *Cancer* **92**(4): 941–949.

Bishop, M.C. (2000). "Trends in prostate cancer mortality in England, Wales, and the USA." *Lancet Oncol* **1**(1): 14.

Borboroglu, P.G., S.W. Comer, et al. (2000). "Extensive repeat transrectal ultrasound guided prostate biopsy in patients with previous benign sextant biopsies." *J Urol* **163**(1): 158–162.

Bost, K.L. and M.J. Mason (1995). "Thapsigargin and cyclopiazonic acid initiate rapid and dramatic increases of IL-6 mRNA expression and IL-6 secretion in murine peritoneal macrophages." *J Immunol* **155**(1): 285–296.

Bostwick, D.G. (2000). "Prostatic intraepithelial neoplasia." *Curr Urol Rep* **1**(1): 65–70.

Bours, V., M. Bentires-Alj, et al. (2000). "Nuclear factor-kappa B, cancer, and apoptosis." *Biochem Pharmacol* **60**(8): 1085–1089.

Burks, D.A. and R.H. Littleton (1992). "The epidemiology of prostate cancer in black men." *Henry Ford Hosp Med J* **40**(1–2): 89–92.

Cabeza-Arvelaiz, Y., J.L. Sepulveda, et al. (2001). "Functional identification of LZTS1 as a candidate prostate tumor suppressor gene on human chromosome 8p22." *Oncogene* **20**(31): 4169–4179.

Carroll, P.R. (2003). "Trends in prostate cancer mortality among black men and white men in the United States. Chu KC, Tarone RE, Freeman HP, Center to Reduce Cancer Health Disparities, National Cancer Institute, Bethesda, MD. Cancer 2003;97:1507–1516." *Urol Oncol* **21**(6): 483–484.

Carty, S.E., C.M. Buresh, et al. (1991). "Decreased IL-6 secretion by fibroblasts following repeated doses of TNF alpha or IL-1 alpha: post-transcriptional gene regulation." *J Surg Res* **51**(1): 24–32.

Cassidy, A. (2003). "Potential risks and benefits of phytoestrogen-rich diets." *Int J Vitam Nutr Res* **73**(2): 120–126.

Catalona, W.J., J.P. Richie, et al. (1994). "Comparison of prostate specific antigen concentration versus prostate specific antigen density in the early detection of prostate cancer: receiver operating characteristic curves." *J Urol* **152**(6 Pt 1): 2031–2036.

Chun, Y.J., M.Y. Kim, et al. (1999). "Resveratrol is a selective human cytochrome P450 1A1 inhibitor." *Biochem Biophys Res Commun* **262**(1): 20–24.

Chung, T.D., J.J. Yu, et al. (1999). "Characterization of the role of IL-6 in the progression of prostate cancer." *Prostate* **38**(3): 199–207.

Clark, L.C., G.F. Combs, Jr., et al. (1996). "Effects of selenium supplementation for cancer prevention in patients with carcinoma of the skin. A randomized controlled trial. Nutritional Prevention of Cancer Study Group." *JAMA* **276**(24): 1957–1963.

Clark, L.C. and E.T. Jacobs (1998). "Environmental selenium and cancer: risk or protection?" *Cancer Epidemiol Biomarkers Prev* **7**(10): 847–848; discussion 851–852.

Clegg, L.X., F.P. Li, et al. (2002). "Cancer survival among US whites and minorities: a SEER (Surveillance, Epidemiology, and End Results) Program population-based study." *Arch Intern Med* **162**(17): 1985–1993.

Cronauer, M.V., W.A. Schulz, et al. (2003). "The androgen receptor in hormone-refractory prostate cancer: relevance of different mechanisms of androgen receptor signaling (Review)." *Int J Oncol* **23**(4): 1095–1102.

Delmas, D., C. Rebe, et al. (2003). "Resveratrol-induced apoptosis is associated with Fas redistribution in the rafts and the formation of a death-inducing signaling complex in colon cancer cells." *J Biol Chem* **278**(42): 41482–41490.

Dessypris, A.G. (1975). "Testosterone sulphate, its biosynthesis, metabolism, measurement, functions and properties." *J Steroid Biochem* **6**(8): 1287–1298.

Dhanalakshmi, S., P. Agarwal, et al. (2003). "Silibinin sensitizes human prostate carcinoma DU145 cells to cisplatin- and carboplatin-induced growth inhibition and apoptotic death." *Int J Cancer* **106**(5): 699–705.

Djavan, B., A. Zlotta, et al. (2000). "Optimal predictors of prostate cancer on repeat prostate biopsy: a prospective study of 1,051 men." *J Urol* **163**(4): 1144–1148; discussion 1148–1149.

Duffield-Lillico, A.J., B.L. Dalkin, et al. (2003). "Selenium supplementation, baseline plasma selenium status and incidence of prostate cancer: an analysis of the complete treatment period of the Nutritional Prevention of Cancer Trial." *BJU Int* **91**(7): 608–612.

Durkan, G.C. and D.R. Greene (1999). "Elevated serum prostate specific antigen levels in conjunction with an initial prostatic biopsy negative for carcinoma: who should undergo a repeat biopsy?" *BJU Int* **83**(1): 34–38.

Eastham, J.A., R.A. May, et al. (1998). "Clinical characteristics and biopsy specimen features in African-American and white men without prostate cancer." *J Natl Cancer Inst* **90**(10): 756–760.

Ellis, W.J. and M.K. Brawer (1995). "Repeat prostate needle biopsy: who needs it?" *J Urol* **153**(5): 1496–1498.

Erbersdobler, A., H. Fritz, et al. (2002). "Tumour grade, proliferation, apoptosis, microvessel density, p53, and bcl-2 in prostate cancers: differences between tumours located in the transition zone and in the peripheral zone." *Eur Urol* **41**(1): 40–46.

Etzioni, R., K.M. Berry, et al. (2002). "Prostate-specific antigen testing in black and white men: an analysis of medicare claims from 1991–1998." *Urology* **59**(2): 251–255.

Fleshner, N.E., M. O'Sullivan, et al. (1997). "Prevalence and predictors of a positive repeat transrectal ultrasound guided needle biopsy of the prostate." *J Urol* **158**(2): 505–508; discussion 508–509.

Fosslien, E. (2001). "Review: molecular pathology of cyclooxygenase-2 in cancer-induced angiogenesis." *Ann Clin Lab Sci* **31**(4): 325–348.

Fowler, J.E., Jr., S.A. Bigler, et al. (2001). "Prospective study of correlations between biopsy-detected high grade prostatic intraepithelial neoplasia, serum prostate specific antigen concentration, and race." *Cancer* **91**(7): 1291–1296.

Fowler, J.E., Jr., S.A. Bigler, et al. (2000). "Predictors of first repeat biopsy cancer detection with suspected local stage prostate cancer." *J Urol* **163**(3): 813–818.

Gasparian, A.V., Y.J. Yao, et al. (2002). "Selenium compounds inhibit I kappa B kinase (IKK) and nuclear factor-kappa B (NF-kappa B) in prostate cancer cells." *Mol Cancer Ther* **1**(12): 1079–1087.

Gerber, G.S. (2000). "Saw palmetto for the treatment of men with lower urinary tract symptoms." *J Urol* **163**(5): 1408–1412.

Gerber, G.S., D. Kuznetsov, et al. (2001). "Randomized, double-blind, placebo-controlled trial of saw palmetto in men with lower urinary tract symptoms." *Urology* **58**(6): 960–964; discussion 964–965.

Giovannucci, E. and E. Platz (2002). Nutritional and Environmental Epidemiology of Prostate Cancer. *Prostate Cancer Principles and Practice*, Lippincott Williams & Wilkins, 8th Edition: 117–139.

Godbey, W.T. and A. Atala (2003). "Directed apoptosis in Cox-2-overexpressing cancer cells through expression-targeted gene delivery." *Gene Ther* **10**(17): 1519–1527.

Goldmann, W.H., A.L. Sharma, et al. (2001). "Saw palmetto berry extract inhibits cell growth and Cox-2 expression in prostatic cancer cells." *Cell Biol Int* **25**(11): 1117–1124.

Gross, A., J.M. McDonnell, et al. (1999). "BCL-2 family members and the mitochondria in apoptosis." *Genes Dev* **13**(15): 1899–1911.

Guinan, P., N. Gilham, et al. (1981). "What is the best test to detect prostate cancer?" *CA Cancer J Clin* **31**(3): 141–145.

Henshall, S.M., D.I. Quinn, et al. (2001). "Overexpression of the cell cycle inhibitor p16INK4A in high-grade prostatic intraepithelial neoplasia predicts early relapse in prostate cancer patients." *Clin Cancer Res* **7**(3): 544–550.

Hilbert, D.M., M. Kopf, et al. (1995). "Interleukin 6 is essential for in vivo development of B lineage neoplasms." *J Exp Med* **182**(1): 243–248.

Holund, B. (1980). "Latent prostatic cancer in a consecutive autopsy series." *Scand J Urol Nephrol* **14**(1): 29–35.

Hsing, A.W., Y.T. Gao, et al. (2000). "Polymorphic CAG and GGN repeat lengths in the androgen receptor gene and prostate cancer risk: a population-based case-control study in China." *Cancer Res* **60**(18): 5111–5116.

Hsu, A.L., T.T. Ching, et al. (2000). "The cyclooxygenase-2 inhibitor celecoxib induces apoptosis by blocking Akt activation in human prostate cancer cells independently of Bcl-2." *J Biol Chem* **275**(15): 11397–11403.

Hzyek (1995). "Prostate Biopsy Rates." *Curr Opinion in Urology* **9**(371).

Iczkowski, K.A., C.G. Pantazis, et al. (2002). "Telomerase reverse transcriptase subunit immunoreactivity: a marker for high-grade prostate carcinoma." *Cancer* **95**(12): 2487–2493.

Imai, K., Y. Ichinose, et al. (1994). "Clinical significance of prostate specific antigen for early stage prostate cancer detection." *Jpn J Clin Oncol* **24**(3): 160–165.

Imai, M., H.Y. Hwang, et al. (2004). "The effect of dexamethasone on human mucin 1 expression and antibody-dependent complement sensitivity in a prostate cancer cell line in vitro and in vivo." *Immunology* **111**(3): 291–297.

Irvine, R.A., M.C. Yu, et al. (1995). "The CAG and GGC microsatellites of the androgen receptor gene are in linkage disequilibrium in men with prostate cancer." *Cancer Res* **55**(9): 1937–1940.

Jang, M., L. Cai, et al. (1997). "Cancer chemopreventive activity of resveratrol, a natural product derived from grapes." *Science* **275**(5297): 218–220.

Jemal, A., R.C. Tiwari, et al. (2004). "Cancer statistics, 2004." *CA Cancer J Clin* **54**(1): 8–29.

Jiang, C., Z. Wang, et al. (2001). "Caspases as key executors of methyl selenium-induced apoptosis (anoikis) of DU-145 prostate cancer cells." *Cancer Res* **61**(7): 3062–3070.

Jirik, F.R., T.J. Podor, et al. (1989). "Bacterial lipopolysaccharide and inflammatory mediators augment IL-6 secretion by human endothelial cells." *J Immunol* **142**(1): 144–147.

Johnson, A.J., X. Song, et al. (2001). "Apoptosis signaling pathways mediated by cyclooxygenase-2 inhibitors in prostate cancer cells." *Adv Enzyme Regul* **41**: 221–235.

Johnson, M.I. and F.C. Hamdy (1998). "Apoptosis regulating genes in prostate cancer (review)." *Oncol Rep* **5**(3): 553–557.

Johnson, M.I., M.C. Robinson, et al. (1998). "Expression of Bcl-2, Bax, and p53 in high-grade prostatic intraepithelial neoplasia and localized prostate cancer: relationship with apoptosis and proliferation." *Prostate* **37**(4): 223–229.

Kagan, J., J. Stein, et al. (1995). "Homozygous deletions at 8p22 and 8p21 in prostate cancer implicate these regions as the sites for candidate tumor suppressor genes." *Oncogene* **11**(10): 2121–2126.

Kamijo, T., T. Sato, et al. (2001). "Induction of apoptosis by cyclooxygenase-2 inhibitors in prostate cancer cell lines." *Int J Urol* **8**(7): S35–39.

Kamoi, K., P. Troncoso, et al. (2000). "Strategy for repeat biopsy in patients with high grade prostatic intraepithelial neoplasia." *J Urol* **163**(3): 819–823.

Kapadia, G.J., M.A. Azuine, et al. (2002). "Inhibitory effect of herbal remedies on 12-O-tetradecanoylphorbol-13-acetate-promoted Epstein-Barr virus early antigen activation." *Pharmacol Res* **45**(3): 213–220.

Katoh, M. (2002). "Expression of human SOX7 in normal tissues and tumors." *Int J Mol Med* **9**(4): 363–368.

Katoh, M. (2002). "Molecular cloning and characterization of human SOX17." *Int J Mol Med* **9**(2): 153–157.

Keetch, D.W., W.J. Catalona, et al. (1994). "Serial prostatic biopsies in men with persistently elevated serum prostate specific antigen values." *J Urol* **151**(6): 1571–1574.

Kirschenbaum, A., X. Liu, et al. (2001). "The role of cyclooxygenase-2 in prostate cancer." *Urology* **58**(2 Suppl 1): 127–131.

Klein, E.A., I.M. Thompson, et al. (2000). "SELECT: the Selenium and Vitamin E Cancer Prevention Trial: rationale and design." *Prostate Cancer Prostatic Dis* **3**(3): 145–151.

Klein, E.A., I.M. Thompson, et al. (2001). "SELECT: the next prostate cancer prevention trial. Selenium and Vitamin E Cancer Prevention Trial." *J Urol* **166**(4): 1311–1315.

Knaus, J. (2002). "Saw palmetto for BPH symptoms." *Adv Nurse Pract* **10**(6): 26–27.

Knol, B.W. and S.T. Egberink-Alink (1989). "Androgens, progestagens and agonistic behaviour: a review." *Vet Q* **11**(2): 94–101.

Kunimi, K., U.S. Bergerheim, et al. (1991). "Allelotyping of human prostatic adenocarcinoma." *Genomics* **11**(3): 530–536.

Lee, H.L., K.J. Pienta, et al. (2003). "The effect of bone-associated growth factors and cytokines on the growth of prostate cancer cells derived from soft tissue versus bone metastases in vitro." *Int J Oncol* **22**(4): 921–926.

Lee, M.M., S.L. Gomez, et al. (2003). "Soy and isoflavone consumption in relation to prostate cancer risk in China." *Cancer Epidemiol Biomarkers Prev* **12**(7): 665–668.

Lee, S.O., W. Lou, et al. (2003). "Interleukin-6 promotes androgen-independent growth in LNCaP human prostate cancer cells." *Clin Cancer Res* **9**(1): 370–376.

Letran, J.L., A.B. Blase, et al. (1998). "Repeat ultrasound guided prostate needle biopsy: use of free-to-total prostate specific antigen ratio in predicting prostatic carcinoma." *J Urol* **160**(2): 426–429.

Levine, M.A., M. Ittman, et al. (1998). "Two consecutive sets of transrectal ultrasound guided sextant biopsies of the prostate for the detection of prostate cancer." *J Urol* **159**(2): 471–475; discussion 475–476.

Lim, J.T., G.A. Piazza, et al. (1999). "Sulindac derivatives inhibit growth and induce apoptosis in human prostate cancer cell lines." *Biochem Pharmacol* **58**(7): 1097–1107.

Liu, X.H., A. Kirschenbaum, et al. (2000). "Inhibition of cyclooxygenase-2 suppresses angiogenesis and the growth of prostate cancer in vivo." *J Urol* **164**(3 Pt 1): 820–825.

Liu, X.H., S. Yao, et al. (1998). "NS398, a selective cyclooxygenase-2 inhibitor, induces apoptosis and down-regulates bcl-2 expression in LNCaP cells." *Cancer Res* **58**(19): 4245–4249.

Lokeshwar, B.L. (1999). "MMP inhibition in prostate cancer." *Ann NY Acad Sci* **878**: 271–289.

Lui, P.D., M.K. Terris, et al. (1995). "Indications for ultrasound guided transition zone biopsies in the detection of prostate cancer." *J Urol* **153**(3 Pt 2): 1000–1003.

Maliner-Stratton, M.S., R.D. Klein, et al. (2001). "Interleukin-1beta-induced promatrilysin expression is mediated by NFkappaB-regulated synthesis of interleukin-6 in the prostate carcinoma cell line, LNCaP." *Neoplasia* **3**(6): 509–520.

Marshall, J.R. (2001). "High-grade prostatic intraepithelial neoplasia as an exposure biomarker for prostate cancer chemoprevention research." *IARC Sci Publ* **154**: 191–198.

Mason, M.D., G. Davies, et al. (2002). "Cell adhesion molecules and adhesion abnormalities in prostate cancer." *Crit Rev Oncol Hematol* **41**(1): 11–28.

McDonnell, T.J., P. Troncoso, et al. (1992). "Expression of the protooncogene bcl-2 in the prostate and its association with emergence of androgen-independent prostate cancer." *Cancer Res* **52**(24): 6940–6944.

Mercurio, F. and A.M. Manning (1999). "NF-kappaB as a primary regulator of the stress response." *Oncogene* **18**(45): 6163–6171.

Merseburger, A.S., M.A. Kuczyk, et al. (2003). "Limitations of tissue microarrays in the evaluation of focal alterations of bcl-2 and p53 in whole mount derived prostate tissues." *Oncol Rep* **10**(1): 223–228.

Miller, E.A., J.L. Stanford, et al. (2001). "Polymorphic repeats in the androgen receptor gene in high-risk sibships." *Prostate* **48**(3): 200–205.

Miltyk, W., C.N. Craciunescu, et al. (2003). "Lack of significant genotoxicity of purified soy isoflavones (genistein, daidzein, and glycitein) in 20 patients with prostate cancer." *Am J Clin Nutr* **77**(4): 875–882.

Mitchell, S.H., W. Zhu, et al. (1999). "Resveratrol inhibits the expression and function of the androgen receptor in LNCaP prostate cancer cells." *Cancer Res* **59**(23): 5892–5895.

Mononen, N., K. Syrjakoski, et al. (2000). "Two percent of Finnish prostate cancer patients have a germ-line mutation in the hormone-binding domain of the androgen receptor gene." *Cancer Res* **60**(22): 6479–6481.

Moody, T.W., J. Leyton, et al. (1998). "Lipoxygenase inhibitors prevent lung carcinogenesis and inhibit non-small cell lung cancer growth." *Exp Lung Res* **24**(4): 617–628.

Mori, S., K. Murakami-Mori, et al. (1999). "Oncostatin M (OM) promotes the growth of DU 145 human prostate cancer cells, but not PC-3 or LNCaP, through the signaling of the OM specific receptor." *Anticancer Res* **19**(2A): 1011–1015.

Mundy, G.R. (1997). "Mechanisms of bone metastasis." *Cancer* **80**(8 Suppl): 1546–1556.

Nakagawa, H., Y. Kiyozuka, et al. (2001). "Resveratrol inhibits human breast cancer cell growth and may mitigate the effect of linoleic acid, a potent breast cancer cell stimulator." *J Cancer Res Clin Oncol* **127**(4): 258–264.

Narla, G., K.E. Heath, et al. (2001). "KLF6, a candidate tumor suppressor gene mutated in prostate cancer." *Science* **294**(5551): 2563–2566.

NCI (2004). PDQ® Clinical Trials Database, National Cancer Institute. http://www.cancer.gov/search/clinical_trails/, Accessed Feb 8, 2005.

NCI (2004). SEER Database. http://seer.cancer.gov, Accessed Feb 8, 2005.

Nelson, M.A., M. Reid, et al. (2002). "Prostate cancer and selenium." *Urol Clin North Am* **29**(1): 67–70.

Niles, R.M., M. McFarland, et al. (2003). "Resveratrol is a potent inducer of apoptosis in human melanoma cells." *Cancer Lett* **190**(2): 157–163.

Oleksowicz, L. and J.P. Dutcher (1994). "A Review of the New Cytokines: IL-4, IL-6, IL-11, and IL-12." *Am J Ther* **1**(2): 107–115.

O'Shaughnessy, C., E. Prosser, et al. (1996). "Differential stimulation of IL-6 secretion following apical and basolateral presentation of IL-1 on epithelial cell lines." *Biochem Soc Trans* **24**(1): 83S.

Oshima, M., J.E. Dinchuk, et al. (1996). "Suppression of intestinal polyposis in Apc delta716 knockout mice by inhibition of cyclooxygenase 2 (COX-2)." *Cell* **87**(5): 803–809.

Oshima, M., H. Sugiyama, et al. (1993). "APC gene messenger RNA: novel isoforms that lack exon 7." *Cancer Res* **53**(23): 5589–5591.

Ostrander, E.A. and J.L. Stanford (2000). "Genetics of prostate cancer: too many loci, too few genes." *Am J Hum Genet* **67**(6): 1367–1375.

Overvad, K. (1998). "Selenium and cancer." *Bibl Nutr Dieta*(54): 141–149.

Panaiotov, D. (1978). "[Testosterone, its biosynthesis, transport and metabolism]." *Vutr Boles* **17**(4): 15–21.

Park, S.J., H. Miyake, et al. (2003). "Predictors of prostate cancer on repeat transrectal ultrasound-guided systematic prostate biopsy." *Int J Urol* **10**(2): 68–71.

Perachino, M., L. di Ciolo, et al. (1997). "Results of rebiopsy for suspected prostate cancer in symptomatic men with elevated PSA levels." *Eur Urol* **32**(2): 155–159.

Pollack, A., D. Cowen, et al. (2003). "Molecular markers of outcome after radiotherapy in patients with prostate carcinoma: Ki-67, bcl-2, bax, and bcl-x." *Cancer* **97**(7): 1630–1638.

Prasad, S., P. Thraves, et al. (1998). "Cytoskeletal and adhesion protein changes during neoplastic progression of human prostate epithelial cells." *Crit Rev Oncol Hematol* **27**(1): 69–79.

Presti, J.C. (2002). Systemic Biopsy of the Prostate: Applications for Detection, Staging and Risk Assessment. *Prostate Cancer Principles and Practice*, Lippencott Williams & Wilkins, **16**: 225–231.

Pruthi, R.S., J.E. Derksen, et al. (2004). "A pilot study of use of the cyclooxygenase-2 inhibitor celecoxib in recurrent prostate cancer after definitive radiation therapy or radical prostatectomy." *BJU Int* **93**(3): 275–278.

Qian, J., R.B. Jenkins, et al. (1997). "Detection of chromosomal anomalies and c-myc gene amplification in the cribriform pattern of prostatic intraepithelial neoplasia and carcinoma by fluorescence in situ hybridization." *Mod Pathol* **10**(11): 1113–1119.

Quinn, M. and P. Babb (2002). "Patterns and trends in prostate cancer incidence, survival, prevalence and mortality. Part II: individual countries." *BJU Int* **90**(2): 174–184.

Raap, T., H.P. Justen, et al. (2000). "Neurotransmitter modulation of interleukin 6 (IL-6) and IL-8 secretion of synovial fibroblasts in patients with rheumatoid arthritis compared to osteoarthritis." *J Rheumatol* **27**(11): 2558–2565.

Raffo, A.J., H. Perlman, et al. (1995). "Overexpression of bcl-2 protects prostate cancer cells from apoptosis in vitro and confers resistance to androgen depletion in vivo." *Cancer Res* **55**(19): 4438–4445.

Reddy, B.S. and C.V. Rao (2000). "Colon cancer: a role for cyclo-oxygenase-2-specific nonsteroidal anti-inflammatory drugs." *Drugs Aging* **16**(5): 329–334.

Reed, J.C., T. Miyashita, et al. (1996). "BCL-2 family proteins: regulators of cell death involved in the pathogenesis of cancer and resistance to therapy." *J Cell Biochem* **60**(1): 23–32.

Rietbergen, J.B. and F.H. Schroder (1998). "Screening for prostate cancer – more questions than answers." *Acta Oncol* **37**(6): 515–532.

Roehrborn, C.G., A. Gregory, et al. (1996). "Comparison of three assays for total serum prostate-specific antigen and percentage of free prostate-specific antigen in predicting prostate histology." *Urology* **48**(6A Suppl): 23–32.

Ross, J.S., C.E. Sheehan, et al. (2002). "Prognostic markers in prostate cancer." *Expert Rev Mol Diagn* **2**(2): 129–142.

Rosser, C.J., A.O. Reyes, et al. (2003). "Bcl-2 is significantly overexpressed in localized radio-recurrent prostate carcinoma, compared with localized radio-naive prostate carcinoma." *Int J Radiat Oncol Biol Phys* **56**(1): 1–6.

Rovner, E.S., F.J. Schanne, et al. (1997). "Transurethral biopsy of the prostate for persistently elevated or increasing prostate specific antigen following multiple negative transrectal biopsies." *J Urol* **158**(1): 138–141; discussion 141–142.

Royuela, M., M. Ricote, et al. (2004). "Immunohistochemical analysis of the IL-6 family of cytokines and their receptors in benign, hyperplasic, and malignant human prostate." *J Pathol* **202**(1): 41–49.

Sakr, W.A., D.J. Grignon, et al. (1996). "Age and racial distribution of prostatic intraepithelial neoplasia." *Eur Urol* **30**(2): 138–144.

Sakr, W.A. and A.W. Partin (2001). "Histological markers of risk and the role of high-grade prostatic intraepithelial neoplasia." *Urology* **57**(4 Suppl 1): 115–120.

Sarma, A.V. and D. Schottenfeld (2002). "Prostate cancer incidence, mortality, and survival trends in the United States: 1981–2001." *Semin Urol Oncol* **20**(1): 3–9.

Scarlatti, F., G. Sala, et al. (2003). "Resveratrol induces growth inhibition and apoptosis in metastatic breast cancer cells via de novo ceramide signaling." *Faseb J* **17**(15): 2339–2341.

Schaid, D.J. (2004). "The Complex Genetic Epidemiology of Prostate Cancer." *Hum Mol Genet.*

Schiavi, R.C. and D. White (1976). "Androgens and male sexual function: a review of human studies." *J Sex Marital Ther* **2**(3): 214–228.

Sellers, W.R. and D.E. Fisher (1999). "Apoptosis and cancer drug targeting." *J Clin Invest* **104**(12): 1655–1661.

Shamberger, R.J. and D.V. Frost (1969). "Possible protective effect of selenium against human cancer." *Can Med Assoc J* **100**(14): 682.

Sharifi, R., W.B. Waters, et al. (1981). "Diagnosis of cancer of the prostate." *Curr Surg* **38**(5): 297–299.

Singh, R.P., S. Dhanalakshmi, et al. (2002). "Dietary feeding of silibinin inhibits advance human prostate carcinoma growth in athymic nude mice and increases plasma insulin-like growth factor-binding protein-3 levels." *Cancer Res* **62**(11): 3063–3069.

Slater, S.J., J.L. Seiz, et al. (2003). "Inhibition of protein kinase C by resveratrol." *Biochim Biophys Acta* **1637**(1): 59–69.

Soderquist, B., J. Kallman, et al. (1998). "Secretion of IL-6, IL-8 and G-CSF by human endothelial cells in vitro in response to Staphylococcus aureus and staphylococcal exotoxins." *Apmis* **106**(12): 1157–1164.

Spiotto, M.T. and T.D. Chung (2000). "STAT3 mediates IL-6-induced growth inhibition in the human prostate cancer cell line LNCaP." *Prostate* **42**(2): 88–98.

Spiotto, M.T. and T.D. Chung (2000). "STAT3 mediates IL-6-induced neuroendocrine differentiation in prostate cancer cells." *Prostate* **42**(3): 186–195.

Stephenson, R.A. (2002). "Prostate cancer trends in the era of prostate-specific antigen. An update of incidence, mortality, and clinical factors from the SEER database." *Urol Clin North Am* **29**(1): 173–181.

Stewart, C.S., B.C. Leibovich, et al. (2001). "Prostate cancer diagnosis using a saturation needle biopsy technique after previous negative sextant biopsies." *J Urol* **166**(1): 86–91; discussion 91–92.

Stewart, J.R., K.L. Christman, et al. (2000). "Effects of resveratrol on the autophosphorylation of phorbol ester-responsive protein kinases: inhibition of protein kinase D but not protein kinase C isozyme autophosphorylation." *Biochem Pharmacol* **60**(9): 1355–1359.

Stewart, J.R., N.E. Ward, et al. (1999). "Resveratrol preferentially inhibits protein kinase C-catalyzed phosphorylation of a cofactor-independent, arginine-rich protein substrate by a novel mechanism." *Biochemistry* **38**(40): 13244–13251.

Stratton, M.S. and F.R. Ahmann (2003). Molecular Mechanisms of Selenium and Prostate Cancer Chemoprevention. *National Biotechnology in the Feed and Food Industry.* P. Lyons. London, Nottingham Press. **1**: 31–51.

Stratton, M.S., M.E. Reid, et al. (2003). "Selenium and inhibition of disease progression in men diagnosed with prostate carcinoma: study design and baseline characteristics of the 'Watchful Waiting' Study." *Anticancer Drugs* **14**(8): 595–600.

Stratton, M.S., M.E. Reid, et al. (2003). "Selenium and prevention of prostate cancer in high-risk men: the Negative Biopsy Study." *Anticancer Drugs* **14**(8): 589–594.

Subbaramaiah, K., W.J. Chung, et al. (1998). "Resveratrol inhibits cyclooxygenase-2 transcription and activity in phorbol ester-treated human mammary epithelial cells." *J Biol Chem* **273**(34): 21875–21882.

Sun, Y. and L.W. Oberley (1996). "Redox regulation of transcriptional activators." *Free Radic Biol Med* **21**(3): 335–348.

Sun, Z. and R. Andersson (2002). "NF-kappaB activation and inhibition: a review." *Shock* **18**(2): 99–106.

Surh, Y.J., K.S. Chun, et al. (2001). "Molecular mechanisms underlying chemopreventive activities of anti-inflammatory phytochemicals: down-regulation of COX-2 and iNOS through suppression of NF-kappa B activation." *Mutat Res* **480-481**: 243–268.

Tang, X., Y.J. Sun, et al. (2002). "Cyclooxygenase-2 overexpression inhibits death receptor 5 expression and confers resistance to tumor necrosis factor-related apoptosis-inducing ligand-induced apoptosis in human colon cancer cells." *Cancer Res* **62**(17): 4903–4908.

Taylor, J.A., 3rd, K.J. Gancarczyk, et al. (2002). "Increasing the number of core samples taken at prostate needle biopsy enhances the detection of clinically significant prostate cancer." *Urology* **60**(5): 841–845.

Thompson, I.M., P.J. Goodman, et al. (2003). "The influence of finasteride on the development of prostate cancer." *N Engl J Med* **349**(3): 215–224.

Thun, M.J., M.M. Namboodiri, et al. (1993). "Aspirin use and risk of fatal cancer." *Cancer Res* **53**(6): 1322–1327.

Tsujimoto, Y. and C. M. Croce (1986). "Analysis of the structure, transcripts, and protein products of bcl-2, the gene involved in human follicular lymphoma." *Proc Natl Acad Sci USA* **83**(14): 5214–5218.

Tyagi, A.K., R.P. Singh, et al. (2002). "Silibinin strongly synergizes human prostate carcinoma DU145 cells to doxorubicin-induced growth Inhibition, G2-M arrest, and apoptosis." *Clin Cancer Res* **8**(11): 3512–3519.

Ukimura, O., O. Durrani, et al. (1997). "Role of PSA and its indices in determining the need for repeat prostate biopsies." *Urology* **50**(1): 66–72.

Veltri, R.W., L.S. Marks, et al. (2002). "Saw palmetto alters nuclear measurements reflecting DNA content in men with symptomatic BPH: evidence for a possible molecular mechanism." *Urology* **60**(4): 617–622.

Vermeulen, A. (1991). "Clinical review 24: Androgens in the aging male." *J Clin Endocrinol Metab* **73**(2): 221–224.

Westin, P. and A. Bergh (1998). "Apoptosis and other mechanisms in androgen ablation treatment and androgen independent progression of prostate cancer: a review." *Cancer Detect Prev* **22**(5): 476–484.

Wilasrusmee, C., S. Kittur, et al. (2002). "Immunostimulatory effect of Silybum Marianum (milk thistle) extract." *Med Sci Monit* **8**(11): BR439–443.

Wilt, T.J., A. Ishani, et al. (1998). "Saw palmetto extracts for treatment of benign prostatic hyperplasia: a systematic review." *JAMA* **280**(18): 1604–1609.

Winters, S.J., A. Brufsky, et al. (2001). "Testosterone, sex hormone-binding globulin, and body composition in young adult African American and Caucasian men." *Metabolism* **50**(10): 1242–1247.

Wise, G.J., V.K. Marella, et al. (2000). "Cytokine variations in patients with hormone treated prostate cancer." *J Urol* **164**(3 Pt 1): 722–725.

Witkamp, R. and M. Monshouwer (2000). "Signal transduction in inflammatory processes, current and future therapeutic targets: a mini review." *Vet Q* **22**(1): 11–16.

Wolter, F., B. Akoglu, et al. (2001). "Downregulation of the cyclin D1/Cdk4 complex occurs during resveratrol-induced cell cycle arrest in colon cancer cell lines." *J Nutr* **131**(8): 2197–2203.

Xie, W., Y.C. Wong, et al. (2000). "Correlation of increased apoptosis and proliferation with development of prostatic intraepithelial neoplasia (PIN) in ventral prostate of the Noble rat." *Prostate* **44**(1): 31–39.

Xu, J., J.A. Stolk, et al. (2000). "Identification of differentially expressed genes in human prostate cancer using subtraction and microarray." *Cancer Res* **60**(6): 1677–1682.

Yu, L., Z.J. Sun, et al. (2003). "Effect of resveratrol on cell cycle proteins in murine transplantable liver cancer." *World J Gastroenterol* **9**(10): 2341–2343.

Zellweger, T., C. Ninck, et al. (2003). "Tissue microarray analysis reveals prognostic significance of syndecan-1 expression in prostate cancer." *Prostate* **55**(1): 20–29.

Zi, X. and R. Agarwal (1999). "Silibinin decreases prostate-specific antigen with cell growth inhibition via G1 arrest, leading to differentiation of prostate carcinoma cells: implications for prostate cancer intervention." *Proc Natl Acad Sci USA* **96**(13): 7490–7495.

Zi, X., J. Zhang, et al. (2000). "Silibinin up-regulates insulin-like growth factor-binding protein 3 expression and inhibits proliferation of androgen-independent prostate cancer cells." *Cancer Res* **60**(20): 5617–5620.

Zucker, S., M. Hymowitz, et al. (1999). "Measurement of matrix metalloproteinases and tissue inhibitors of metalloproteinases in blood and tissues. Clinical and experimental applications." *Ann NY Acad Sci* **878**: 212–227.

Cervical and Endometrial Cancer Prevention

Francisco Garcia, J. Newton, and Susie Baldwin

College of Medicine, Department of Obstetrics and Gynecology, University of Arizona, Tucson, AZ 85724

Cervical cancer prevention

Incidence and Mortality of Cervical Cancer

Cervical cancer is the most common gynecologic malignancy world wide, accounting for about 371,200 cases each year (Parkin, Pisani et al. 1999). Most of these cases (77.5%) occur in the developing world where it is the second most common malignancy in women after breast cancer (Parkin, Pisani et al. 1999). By contrast, in the United States (U.S.) cervical cancer has decreased dramatically since the introduction of cytologic screening (Pap smear), and is now a relatively infrequent neoplasm, especially among well-screened majority populations with access to health care services. In the U.S., an individual woman's lifetime risk of developing cervical cancer is estimated to be 1 in 117 (2002). In 2004, there were approximately 10,520 new cases of cervical cancer, and 3,900 deaths in the U.S. (Jemal, Tiwari et al. 2004).

In the developed world, cervical cancer disproportionately affects poor and minority women without adequate access to cervical cancer screening. It is estimated that nearly 50% of U.S. cervical cancer cases occur in women who have never been screened, and an additional 10% in women who have been under-screened (NIH, 1996). Significant racial and ethnic disparities exist with regard to screening, incidence, mortality, and survival associated with the diagnosis of cervical cancer in this country (Table 1) (2003). Notably, the gap in incidence and mortality between white women and other racial/ethnic groups increases with age (2001). Although disparities in incidence and mortality have decreased in recent years, cervical cancer incidence remains about 50% higher among black women (11.2/100,000) compared to white women (7.3/100,000) (Miller 1996; Ries 1999), and cervical cancer mortality among black women which is the highest (6.7/100,000) of any racial or ethnic group (Miller 1996). Black women are less likely to present with localized disease (44% compared to 56% of white women) and are twice as likely to die of their disease (Ries 2001). Additionally, black women are less likely to receive surgery (33.5% compared to 48.2% in

Table 1. Racial/ethnic disparities in cervical cancer (Jemal, Clegg, et al. 2004)

	White	Black	Hispanic*
Incidence (per 100,000)	9.2	12.4	16.8
Mortality (per 100,000)	2.7	5.9	3.7
5-year survival (%)	11%	10%	81%

* The category Hispanic is not mutually exclusive from Black or White

white women) and more likely to receive radiation (35.3% compared to 25.2%) (Howell, Chen et al. 1999). Women of Vietnamese origin have the highest age-adjusted incidence rate (43/100,000) and Japanese origin individuals have the lowest (5.8/100,000) (Miller 1996). Surveillance, epidemiology and end results (SEER) data for 1992 through 1998 continue to demonstrate a disproportionately higher incidence (14.4/100,000) and mortality (3.3/100,000) for Hispanic compared to non-Hispanic whites (6.9/100,000 and 2.3/100,000 incidence and mortality rates, respectively) (Ries 2001). Hispanics are also more likely to present with advanced stages of invasive disease (Napoles-Springer, Perez-Stable et al. 1996; Mitchell and McCormack 1997; Howe, Delfino et al. 1998). Not surprisingly, higher rates of precursor lesions have been documented for both African-American and Hispanic women (Howe, Delfino et al. 1998; Liu, Wang et al. 1998).

Etiology of Cervical Cancer

Prior to the definitive identification of human papillomavirus (HPV) infection as a necessary agent in cervical carcinogenesis, observational studies had already suggested that a sexually transmitted agent was involved in the disease and that male sexual behavior could affected the risk of cancer in the female partners. Specifically, research demonstrated geographic clustering of cervical and penile cancers, the low prevalence of disease among non-sexually active women, and increased risk in partners of men whose first wives had died of cervical cancer. More sophisticated and recent molecular epidemiology work has further clarified this relationship (Buckley, Harris et al. 1981; Zunzunegui, King et al. 1986; Agarwal, Sehgal et al. 1993; Thomas, Ray et al. 1996) and has highlighted the role of a potential "male factor" (Castellsague, Bosch et al. 2002).

In the mid 1970s, Zur Hausen first suggested a relationship between HPV infection and cervical cancer (zur Hausen 1977); by the early 1980s, electron-micrography work had identified the presence of the virus in cervical intraepithelial neoplasia (CIN) (Meisels, Morin et al. 1983). Since that time, cervical carcinoma and its precursor lesion, CIN, have been consistently causally linked to sexually transmission of human papillomavirus (HPV) infection (Schiffman, Bauer et al. 1993; Palefsky and Holly 1995; 1996; Morris, Tortolero-Luna et al. 1996).

HPV infection is ubiquitous and widespread across many species; more than one hundred different types can infect humans. Transmission of this small icosohedral double-stranded DNA virus occurs through direct contact with epithelial surfaces. Lower genital tract HPV infection is common during the second and third decade of life, and is a marker of human sexual activity (Fig. 1). The vast majority of immunocompetent women appear to clear the infection without sequelae. By comparison, cervical cancer is a relatively rare event that peaks in the fourth and fifth decade. Infections with HPV are classified as high-risk (oncogenic) or low-risk (non-oncogenic) genotypes, based on the association with cervical cancer. High-risk HPV infection with types 16 and 18 has the highest prevalence and is associated with approximately three quarters of all cancer and high-grade precursor lesions. Additional high-risk types include 31, 33, 35, 39, 45, 51, 52, 56, 58, 59, 68, 73, 82, and possibly 26, 53, and 66. By contrast, HPV 6 and 11, the etiologic agents of genital warts, and types 42, 43, 44, 54, 61, 70, 72, and 81 are infrequently associated with advanced cervical lesions and are considered low-risk (Palefsky and Holly 1995; Franco 1996; Munoz, Bosch et al. 2003). Beyond viral type dif-

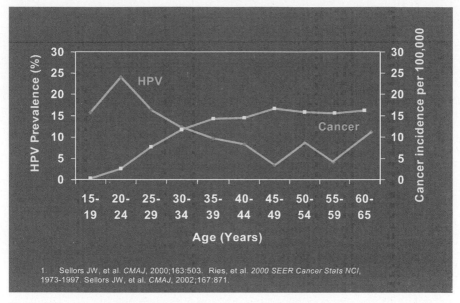

Fig. 1. HPV point prevalence and cervical cancer incidence by age

ferences, there are significant differences in genetic variation, viral load (van Duin, Snijders et al. 2002), and persistence which may confer increased risk for cervical neoplasia. In total, the strength of the association between high-risk HPV infection and cervical cancer is such that all squamous cell cervical malignancies are now thought to be related to HPV infection. It is clear that HPV infection is a necessary prerequisite, but by itself an insufficient cause for cervical cancer.

Natural History of Cervical Cancer

HPV enters the basal layer of the genital tract through micro-tears that occur in the squamous epithelium during the course of sexual activity. The mitotically active transformation zone is particularly vulnerable, especially early in adolescence when it covers a relatively broad surface area of the cervix. The viral DNA enters the cellular nucleus where it exists as a circular episome composed of three distinct regions. In general, the long control region (LCR) regulates early viral transcription, while the late (L) region encodes structural proteins involved in the assembly and production of the viral capsid. The early (E) region encodes proteins necessary for viral replication. The E6 and E7 gene products bind p53 and retinoblastoma proteins respectively, and interfere with their tumor suppressor function leading ultimately to cellular transformation (Shirodkar, Ewen et al. 1992; Scheffner, Huibregtse et al. 1993; Jones, Alani et al. 1997; Denk, Butz et al. 2001). Precursor lesions and cervical carcinoma require the non-random integration of extra chromosomal viral DNA into the host genome (Thorland, Myers et al. 2000). This integration of viral DNA into the host genome results in disruption of the E2 region of the viral episome (Choo, Pan et al. 1987), which is responsible for down regulation of E6 and E7, and ultimately to cellular transformation.

Natural History of HPV & Cervical Cancer

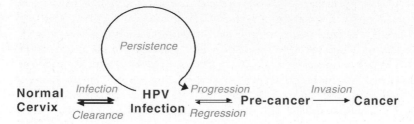

Fig. 2. Natural history of HPV and cervical cancer, adapted (Alberts 2004; Schiffman and Kjaer 2003)

As the cells of the basal layer of the squamous epithelium mature, they are pushed out to the epithelial surface where replication of the viral genome takes place. Eventually the viral DNA copies are packaged in the protein capsid. These viral particles are released through the normal process of epithelial desquamation and cell death, and upon shedding, are available for transmission of the infection.

Generally, HPV infection is transient, asymptomatic, clinically insignificant, and occasionally associated with temporary cytologic and/or histologic abnormalities (Fig. 2). The median duration of infection has been estimated to be about eight months for young sexually active women (Ho, Bierman et al. 1998). This time period may be longer for women infected with oncogenic viral types (Richardson, Kelsall et al. 2003). Although older individuals may be less likely to clear the virus, in general, about 90% of infected women will have undetectable evidence of infection at 24 months (Moscicki, Shiboski et al. 1998).

In some cases, infection leads to characteristic cellular abnormalities beginning at the basal layer and involving increasingly more layers of cervical epithelium. These are described histologically as cervical intraepithelial neoplasia (CIN) (Wright 1994). CIN is generally divided into low-grade (CIN 1) and high-grade (CIN 2 and CIN 3) disease. This grading generally reflects the underlying risk for progression to malignancy (highest for CIN3) and decreasing likelihood of spontaneous regression (highest for CIN 1) (Ostor 1993; Barker, Garcia et al. 2001). Low-grade CIN occurs most frequently in younger women (Jones and Novis 2000) and is more likely to spontaneously regress in that age group. Viral persistence is required for progression from high-grade CIN and invasive carcinoma, and is related not only to viral type, but also to viral load and increasing age (Koutsky, Holmes et al. 1992; Londesborough, Ho et al. 1996; Ho, Bierman et al. 1998). The protracted process of progression (estimated at more than 10 years) from CIN 3 to invasive disease provides an ideal time frame that permits screening, identification and treatment of these precursor lesions.

Co-factors for Cervical Cancer

The largely endemic nature of HPV infection and the relative rarity of cervical cancer argue for an important role of co-factors that may affect progression or regression of cervical cancer precursors (Table 1). Historically, parity has been identified consistently as an important risk factor in cervical cancer (Brinton, Reeves et al. 1989; Parkin, Vizcaino et al. 1994; Yoo, Kang et al. 1997; Munoz, Franceschi et al. 2002). It is unlikely that the effect of parity is simply related to childbirth itself; instead parity may be a surrogate for a spectrum of high-risk sexual behavior including total lifetime number of male sexual partners, early age at sexual intercourse, co-morbid sexually transmitted infections (STI), and potentially even smoking and hormonal contraceptive use with regard to smoking, nicotine metabolites can be recovered in the cervical and vaginal secretions of women who smoke or those exposed passively (McCann, Irwin et al. 1992; Prokopczyk, Cox et al. 1997). In particular, the use of tobacco products may be associated with a 2 to 4 fold increased risk for cervical cancer and its precursors (McCann, Irwin et al. 1992; de Vet, Sturmans et al. 1994; Prokopczyk, Cox et al. 1997; Deacon, Evans et al. 2000). Likewise, there may be a role for other STIs that infect the female lower genital tract, and may potentiate the oncogenicity of high-risk HPV. This may be mediated through the cellular-mediated immune mechanism (Konya and Dillner 2001) and/or a localized inflammatory effect on the cervico-vaginal epithelium (van Duin, Snijders et al. 2002; Garcia, Mendez de Galaz et al. 2003). Long-term use of combined oral contraceptive pills is also associated with cervical cancer risk in the presence of HPV infection (Moreno, Bosch et al. 2002). These findings are particularly difficult to interpret given the complex nature of sexual behavior and the adverse effect of multiparity on the risk for cervical cancer. It is possible that the effects of tobacco and contraceptive use are mediated by promoting persistence of the viral infection.

Risk Factors Associated with HPV Infection, Cervical Intraepithelial Neoplasia, and Cancer

- Smoking
- Lower genital tract infection (chlamydia, HSV, bacterial vaginosis)
- Sexual behavior (number of partners, age at first intercourse, partner's sexual behavior)
- Parity
- Impaired immune function (HIV/AIDS, post transplantation, chronic steroid, collagen vascular disease, pregnancy)
- Hormonal combined oral contraceptive use
- Nutrition
- Poverty (low socio-economic status)
- Lack of access of healthcare/screening

Viral Persistence

Numerous studies consistently demonstrate that persistent, as compared to transient, high-risk HPV infection is required for the development of cervical cancer precursor lesions (Koutsky, Holmes et al. 1992; Ho, Burk et al. 1995; Coker and Bond 1999; Hernandez and Goodman 1999; ter Harmsel, Smedts et al. 1999). It has also been shown that persistent high risk HPV infection is a prerequisite for development and maintenance of CIN 3 (Meijer, Nobbenhuis et al. 1999), while low-risk type infections have very high rates of regression (Moscicki, Shiboski et al. 1998).

Clearance of HPV from the genital tract requires an active cell-mediated immune response. Cellular immune response is characterized by an interaction between antigen presenting cells (APCs), T-helper cells, and cytotoxic T cells. Activated natural killer (NK) cells may also play a role. Cell-mediated viral clearance and control of tumor growth were identified in studies of CIN in HIV-positive women. The observation that CIN occurs with disproportionate frequency among immuno-compromised women (e.g., AIDS, transplantion), suggests that CD4 lymphocytes (T-helper cells) are involved in prevention or limitation of HPV-associated lesions (Maiman 1998). Studies of immunocyte counts in HPV lesions have confirmed the role of the cellular immune system in controlling viral infection. Significantly, greater numbers of T-lymphocytes and macrophages are found within the stroma and epithelium of HPV lesions that regress as compared to non-regressing lesions (Coleman, Birley et al. 1994).

Cytotoxic responses against HPV are mediated by T helper cells (CD4 cells) and antigen presenting cells such as Langerhans cells (LCs), whose interactions result in the stimulation of cytotoxic T cells (CD8 cells). Immune response is generated and maintained through the release of cytokines, intracellular chemical signals, from these different cell types. Cytokines secreted by CD4 cells include type 1 cytokines such as interleukin 2 (IL-2) and interferon gamma (IFN), and type 2 cytokines, including IL-4, IL-6, and IL-10. Type 1 cytokines are immuno-stimulatory for cell-mediated immune response; they promote CD8 responses, activate natural killer cell (NK) functions, and have been shown to be capable of limiting tumor growth. Interleukin 12 (IL-12) is a type 1 cytokine which is secreted by dendritic cells, including LCs, and which has been demonstrated to induce differentiation of naive T cells, to up-regulate IFN gamma production in T cells and NK cells, and to have anti-tumor activity (Nastala, Edington et al. 1994; Zola, Roberts-Tompson et al. 1995; Clerici, Shearer et al. 1998; Giannini, Al-Saleh et al. 1998).

Cytokine expression in cervical tissue has been variously associated with cervical intraepithelial neoplasia. Investigators have found a significant increase in the density of IL-4 positive cells in low grade and high grade SILs, compared with histologically normal tissues from adjacent ectocervical regions (al-Saleh, Delvenne et al. 1995). Another study showed that expression of IL-10 increased continuously from a relatively low level in normal ectocervix to a high level in HSIL, and that IL-12 expression was higher in LSIL than in HSIL (Giannini, Al-Saleh et al. 1998). In women with CIN 3, in vitro production of IL-2 by peripheral mononuclear blood cells (PMBCs) was found to be decreased, and production of type 2 cytokines IL-4 and IL-10 increased, in women with more extensive HPV infection (Clerici, Merola et al. 1997).

Screening and Early Detection of Cervical Cancer

Cytologic Screening. Exfoliative cytology has been the mainstay of cervical cancer prevention since its description by Papanicolau in the 1940s, and its large-scale adoption is frequently credited for the drop in cervical cancer incidence and mortality in North America and Western Europe (Anttila, Pukkala et al. 1999). This technique takes advantage of the prolonged pre-invasive nature of CIN, and samples the transformation zone of the uterine cervix where the process of metaplasia turns the columnar epithelium of the endocervical canal into the more robust mature squamous epithelium of the ectocervix and vagina. It is these metaplastic cells that are the most vulnerable to oncogenic HPV infection; the most invasive and precursor lesions arise from this area. Detailed evidence-based screening recommendations (Table 2), and triage algorithms for the management of abnormal cervical cytology are published elsewhere (Saslow, Runowicz et al. 2002; Wright, Cox et al. 2002; Wright, Cox et al. 2003).

Although in widespread use there have never been, nor would it now be ethical to conduct, large randomized control trials of cervical cytology (Table 3). Nonetheless, prolonged clinical experience with this technique has permitted the characterization of the test performance qualities. The sensitivity of cytologic screening is estimated to range between 50 and 70%, with specificity in the 70% range (Fahey, Irwig et al. 1995, 1999).

More recent technologic advances in cytologic processing and technology aim to improve the performance characteristics of this screening technique. One important advance has been improvement of the quality of the specimen submitted for analysis, with thin-layer cytologic slides prepared from specimens collected in a liquid fixative. This technique appears to reduce false positive rates by improving the interpretability of the slide, by decreasing the presence of cells and debris associated with bleeding and inflammation. The thin layer also slightly improves the sensitivity of cytology (Lee, Ashfaq et al. 1997; Hutchinson, Zahniser et al. 1999; Vassilakos, Saurel et al. 1999; Belinson, Qiao et al. 2001; Clavel, Masure et al. 2001) by providing a more evenly distributed cellular sampling which may lead to more accurate interpretation. The sum of the evidence is sufficiently compelling to recommend that with the use of thin layer cytology cervical cancer screening intervals may be lengthened to every two years (after three consecutive normal screens) in women at least 30 years of age (Saslow, Runowicz et al. 2002).

A variety of computerized cytologic screening devices have entered clinical use. The automated image-analysis, algorithm-based screening devices generate a score in-

Table 2. Comparison of Screening Guidelines (1999; Saslow, Runowicz et al. 2002, 2003)

	Start Age	Stop Age	Interval (years)	Post Hysterectomy	HPV Adjunct
USPTF (1996)	21*	≥65	3	No	No
ACS (2002)	21*	≥70	1–2**	No***	Yes
ACOG (2003)	21*		1	No***	Yes

USPSTF-US Preventive Services Task Force
ACS-American Cancer Society
ACOG-American College of Obstetricians & Gynecologists
* Or within 3 years of onset of sexual activity
** Yearly for conventional cytology, every 2 years for liquid-based
***Continue screening for history of CIN2/3 or cancer

dicative of the risk for significant disease and identifies high-risk fields for pathologic review (Patten, Lee et al. 1997; Howell, Belk et al. 1999). Such devices have made their way into large laboratories where they are used largely to comply with federally mandated re-screening of 10% of negative cytologies, and increasingly for primary screening. Such technology specifically addresses the contribution of human misclassification to cytologic inaccuracy, which results from fatigue and human error.

Bethesda System Pap Smear Result Terminology (Abridged) (NCI 2001)
- Negative for intraepithelial lesion or malignancy (NILM)
- Atypical squamous cells
  - Of undetermined significance (ASC-US)
  - Can not exclude HSIL (ASC-H)
- Low-grade squamous intraepithelial lesion (LSIL)
- High-grade squamous intraepithelial lesion (HSIL)
- Squamous cell carcinoma
  - Atypical glandular cells
  - Identified by site of origin (endocervical, endometrial, not otherwise specified) (AGC)
  - Favor neoplastic
  - Adenocarcinoma in situ
  - Adenocarcinoma

HPV Testing

The etiologic role of HPV in cervical cancer has lead to incorporation of HPV testing into a variety of screening and management algorithms for cervical disease. Oncogenic HPV testing has been proposed as a primary screening modality for screening for cervical cancer and its precursors (Cuzick, Szarewski et al. 2003). While in some settings HPV testing is more sensitive than cervical cytology, the endemic nature of high-risk oncogenic HPV infection, especially among young reproductive age populations, would lead to low specificity of screening with predictably high false positive rates (Cuzick, Sasieni et al. 2000).

More recent guidelines have opened the door to the use of HPV testing as an adjunct to cytology, in an effort to safely extend screening intervals (Fig. 3) (Saslow, Runowicz et al. 2002; Wright, Schiffman et al. 2004). In general the test performance characteristics of combined HPV and cytology screening (sensitivity of about 92 to 100% and specificity of 70 to 96%) exceed that of cytology alone (Wright, Schiffman et al. 2004). Current evidence suggests that co-testing with HPV and cytology, if it is performed, should be limited to women 30 years of age and older and should be performed no more frequently than every three years (Wright, Schiffman et al. 2004).

High-risk HPV testing has come into clinical use as one of three evidence based management strategies for the triage of ASC-US cytology (along with repeat cytology and colposcopy). The sensitivity of HPV DNA hybrid capture testing for the detection of CIN 2 and CIN 3 is estimated to be between 80 and 100% (Wright, Lorincz et al. 1998; Sherman, Schiffman et al. 2002); women with negative testing in this setting have an extremely low likelihood of having clinically significant disease. When testing is available from liquid-based cytology specimen or when viral specimens are co-col-

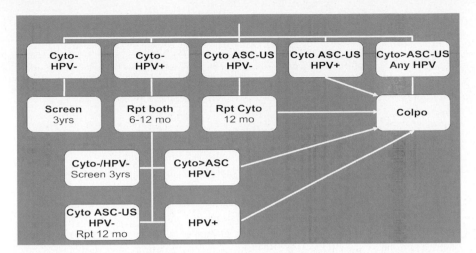

Fig. 3. Management of Cytology/HPV Results

lected at the time of screening cytology, this is the preferred triage for the ASC-US pap (Wright, Cox et al. 2002).

Therapeutic Approach to Precursor Lesions of Cervical Cancer

The foundation of cervical cancer precursor therapy involves access to definitive colposcopic evaluation and histologic diagnosis. Treatment has been divided into ablative and excisional modalities. Excisional therapy has generally been reserved for high-grade lesions (CIN 2 and 3) with true malignant potential. Loop electrosurgical excision procedure (LEEP) requires an experienced operator but may be performed in the office setting. It is the most common approach to treatment of high-grade lesions in the U.S., is well tolerated by patients, and results in a histologic specimen that is evaluable for evidence of invasion. Bleeding and infection are potential complications of LEEP procedures and may occur in about 2% of cases (compared to 10% for cold knife conizations) (Montz 2000). While cervical stenosis and impaired fertility are rare complications, women who undergo LEEP may be at increased risk for pre-term delivery and low birth weight infants in subsequent pregnancies (Samson 2005).

Cryotherapy, by comparison, is used most commonly for low-grade lesions (CIN 1), which should be treated only when they are persistent (24 months or more) (Wright, Cox et al. 2003), because 90% of these lesions will regress spontaneously within 2 years (Ostor 1993). The regression rate is generally lower for women after their mid thirties and among those who smoke. Cryotherapy is safe, effective, and economical; typically requiring less operator experience than excisional modalities. It does not, however, produce a histologic specimen and should never be used when there is any question of potential microinvasive disease. In general the resolution rates for both these therapies is in the 90% range (Martin-Hirsch, Paraskevaidis et al. 2000), and a recent randomized trial of cryotherapy, laser vaporization, and LEEP found comparable cure rates for CIN 2/3 (Mitchell, Tortolero-Luna et al. 1998). This trial also found that failure rates were highest for women with large lesion (3 or 4 quadrants). Previously treated patients, those over 30, and women with oncogenic HPV infection were also at significantly higher risk for treatment failure. Outpatient therapeutic modalities may lend themselves well for single visit and "see-and-treat" therapy that obviate the need for biopsy and even colposcopic examination, and may promote compliance among poor or underserved women.

Novel Agents for Cervical Cancer Prevention

Chemopreventive Agents. The search for chemopreventive agents for use in cervical cancer prevention is logical given the well characterized, protracted preinvasive character of CIN, encouraging preclinical laboratory data, and epidemiologic findings that suggest a protective role for a variety of nutritional agents. These chemoprevention studies, however, have been largely disappointing and plagued by a variety of methodological challenges. Problems include a lack of concensus as to the appropriate grade of disease to be studied (CIN 1, 2 or 3), the appropriate definition of response (histologic regression, viral clearance) given significant rates of spontaneous regression, the selection of appropriate endpoint biomarkers, as well as ethical and safety considerations (withholding treatment for potentially preinvasive disease). Despite these challenges a significant number of trials have been conducted in this area (Table 3). The most thorough review of cervical chemoprevention trials to date was recently published by Mitchell and colleagues (Follen, Meyskens et al. 2003).

Topical and oral retinoids are a group of agents that have been well characterized and that have significant promise in this tissue type. These agents may decrease the expression of E6/E7, tumor growth factors, and telomerase activity associated with carcinogenesis (Sizemore, Choo et al. 1998; Ding, Green et al. 2002). They have generally good toxicity and tolerability profiles and early phase I data suggest significant chemopreventive activity (Surwit, Graham et al. 1982; Meyskens, Graham et al. 1983; Weiner, Surwit et al. 1986). One clinical trial of cervical all-trans retinoic (0.327%) acid application demonstrated significant activity for CIN 2 (43% compared to 27% in the placebo group), but not for CIN 3 (Meyskens, Surwit et al. 1994). Likewise, trials of an oral synthetic retinoid (4-HPR) and cis retinoic acid have been negative (Follen, Atkinson et al. 2001; Alvarez, Conner et al. 2003). Indole carbinol is another promising agent, that may in part explain the cancer protective effect of cruciferous vegetable intake in some epidemiologic studies. This compound has been demonstrated to induce the protective effective cytochrome p-450 (Wattenberg and Loub 1978; Grubbs, Steele et al. 1995). A phase II study, of two different doses of this agent for 90 days in subjects with CIN 2/3, reported a consistent response rate of 44 to 50% (compared to no responders in the control group) (Bell, Crowley-Nowick et al. 2000). Randomized trials of imiquimod, a topical cellular immune response modulator, used for HPV related genital condyloma, have been performed although not yet reported for cervical disease endpoints. Clinical trials are planned for di-indolylmethane, selective cycloxygenase-2 inhibitors, and green tea related compounds.

Prophylactic Vaccines. Animal models have established that antibodies to epitopes on the viral capsid can prevent HPV infection (Breitburd, Kirnbauer et al. 1995). This observation has led to the development of virus like particles (VLPs) spontaneously as-

Table 3. Published chemopreventive clinical trials for cervical intraepithelial neoplasia (CIN)

Agent	Published Trials	Spectrum of CIN	References
Retinoids			
Retinyl acetate topical gel	1	1–2	(Romney, Dwyer et al. 1985)
All-trans retinoic acid topical*	7	1–3	(Surwit, Graham et al. 1982;
4-HPR	1	2–3	Meyskens, Graham et al. 1983;
9-cis retinoic acid	1	2–3	Graham, Surwit et al. 1986;
			Weiner, Surwit et al. 1986;
			Meyskens, Surwit et al. 1994)
			(Follen, Atkinson et al. 2001)
			(Alvarez, Conner et al. 2003)
Micro-nutrients			
Beta carotene	6	1–3	(de Vet, Knipschild et al. 1991;
Folate	3	1–2	Fairley, Tabrizi et al. 1996; Ma-
Vitamin C	2	1–2	netta, Schubbert et al. 1996;
			Romney, Ho et al. 1997; Mack-
			erras, Irwig et al. 1999; Keefe,
			Schell et al. 2001)
			(Butterworth, Hatch et al. 1992;
			Butterworth, Hatch et al. 1992;
			Childers, Chu et al. 1995)
			(Romney, Basu et al. 1987;
			Mackerras, Irwig et al. 1999)
Dietary Supplements			
Indole 3-carbinole*	1	2–3	(Bell, Crowley-Nowick et al. 2000)
Green tea compounds	1	1–3	(Ahn, Yoo et al. 2003)
Diflouromethylornithine (DFMO)	1	3	(Mitchell, Tortolero-Luna et al. 1998)
Other 2YC101	2	2–3	(Garcia 2004)

* Positive phase 2 trial results

sembled from capsid proteins. Early clinical trial results confirm the safety, tolerability, and immunogenicity of the agents (Evans, Bonnez et al. 2001; Harro, Pang et al. 2001). A large randomized, double blind, placebo controlled trial to test the efficacy of HPV 16 VLP was conducted in a population of 16 to 23 year old patients (Koutsky, Ault et al. 2002). Subjects were evaluated for evidence of persistent HPV infection and were followed for 48 months. One hundred eleven women among 750 in the placebo group developed persistent HPV 16 infection compared with 7 of 755 in the vaccine group, yielding a vaccine efficacy of 94% for the prevention of HPV persistence. Twelve women in the placebo group, and none in the vaccine group, developed HPV 16-related CIN 2-3, making the vaccine 100% effective at preventing high-grade disease during the study period (Moyer 2004). These very encouraging results open the door for further vaccine development with broader viral coverage. It is unclear at this time if the duration of protective effect will be long term, whether broad cross reactivity to other viral types is conferred, and whether the immune response will translate into lower long-term rates of high-grade precursor lesions.

Other preclinical efforts have focused on the development of chimeric VLPs. These agents are intended to elicit a T-cell response against HPV-infected cells in addition to eliciting the production of neutralizing antibodies (Muller, Zhou et al. 1997). A variety of other prophylactic vaccine concepts are currently in preclinical development.

Therapeutic Vaccines. An alternative therapeutic approach has targeted the elimination of high-grade precursor and even invasive lesions in individuals with established HPV infection. Such a strategy is dependent on cellular immune response, rather than antibody development. In general, this involves the stimulation of a cytotoxic T-lymphocyte response to the E6 and E7 oncoproteins. HPV peptide trials that have used this approach have shown modest promise. A small trial of a preparation using E7 epitope peptides in subjects with cervical and vulvar squamous intraepithelial lesions demonstrated T-lymphocyte response in 10 of 18 subjects, with three demonstrating a complete response (Muderspach, Wilczynski et al. 2000). Another trial using a longer E7 peptide with a palmitic acid adjuvant in 12 cervical cancer patients resulted in a 25% T-lymphocyte response rate and a single complete response (Zwaveling, Ferreira Mota et al. 2002). An alternate promising approach involves the use of a non-integrating, non-replicating plasmid encoding multiple HPV 16 and 18 E6 and E7 epitopes, formulated in small biodegradable polymer microparticles with a good profile of safety and tolerability (zyc 101) (Klencke, Matijevic et al. 2002; Sheets, Urban et al. 2003). A recent large multicenter randomized placebo controlled trial tested the safety and efficacy of this agent in subjects with histologically confirmed CIN 2 or 3 (Garcia, Petry et al. 2004). Of 127 randomized participants for whom cervical conization specimens were available, there was a trend toward higher rates of regression in the active drug group, 43% compared to 27%. More significantly 70% of subjects less than 25 years of age demonstrated histologically confirmed regression (compared to 23% in the placebo group). Additional encouraging data from an early phase E7 heat shock protein vaccine have not reached publication.

The search for therapeutic medical modalities to address cervical and endometrial intraepithelial neoplasias is particularly important within the larger framework for cervical cancer prevention (Table 4). Chemopreventive and immune therapies open the door for potentially non-surgical, fertility sparing, minimally morbid interventions especially for young women who are increasingly burdened by these diseases. These efforts also provide a vehicle for an even more profound understanding of HPV infection, which will serve future generations of women.

Endometrial Cancer Prevention

Epidemiology of Endometrial Cancer

There are 180,000 new cases of endometrial cancer diagnosed worldwide each year leading to 44,000 deaths (Parkin, Pisani et al. 1999; Greenlee, Hill-Harmon et al. 2001; Parkin, Bray et al. 2001). In the U.S., endometrial cancer is the most common malignancy of the lower female genital tract with an incidence of 40,320 per year, affecting nearly four times as many women as cervical cancer (Jemal, Tiwari et al. 2004). Despite the relatively high incidence of endometrial cancer, the prognosis for endometrial cancer is better than for other gynecologic malignancies. Even though endometrial cancer is nearly 1.6 times more common than ovarian cancer, the disease kills less than half as many women. Approximately 7,090 deaths occur due to endometrial cancer each year, compared to 16,090 deaths annually from ovarian cancer (Jemal, Tiwari et al. 2004).

Endometrial cancer can occur in a wide age range, with the median age of diagnosis at 61 years (Plaxe and Saltzstein 1997; Sherman and Devesa 2003). Three quarters of the women diagnosed with endometrial cancer are post-menopausal. In addition to age, race and country of origin also appear to be factors. For example, Japan has incidence rates four to five times lower than Western countries (Parkin, Pisani et al. 1999). The lowest incidence rates worldwide are found in Southern Asia and Africa. In the U.S., black women have a 40% lower risk of developing endometrial cancer compared to other populations. However, black women with endometrial cancer are often diagnosed later in the course of disease and have a 54% greater risk of dying from the disease (Parazzini, La Vecchia et al. 1991; Plaxe and Saltzstein 1997; Madison, Schottenfeld et al. 1998; Sherman and Devesa 2003).

Using the California Cancer Registry data, Plaxe and Saltzstein (Plaxe and Saltzstein 1997) found that approximately three quarters of endometrial cancers present as low-grade disease in whites, Hispanics, and Asians. However, only 56% of endometrial cancers in black women are low grade at the time of diagnosis. Age-specific rate analysis confirms that white women present with lower grades and at younger ages than do black, Hispanic, or Asian women. Survival is also different between racial and ethnic groups. Ninety percent of white endometrial cancer patients can expect to survive three years, while only 62% of blacks survive three years. This data is consistent with that of Liu et al. (Liu, Conaway et al. 1995) who also found a survival disadvantage among black patients. More recent data demonstrates that the survival disparity has not improved much in the past decade and cannot be explained by treatment differences between blacks and whites (Sherman and Devesa 2003). One explanation for this disparity is that endometrial cancer types differ between blacks and whites.

There are several types of malignant neoplasms in the uterine corpus. Ninety-seven percent are limited to the endometrium, and the remaining 3% are sarcomas. Endometrial carcinomas are divided into various histologically defined types. These include estrogen-dependent endometrial adenocarcinoma (type I) and non-estrogen-dependent (type II) forms of serous, mucinous, and squamous carcinomas (Bokhman 1983). The endometrioid variant accounts for greater than 90% of endometrial cancers. The type II carcinomas are much more aggressive and less predictable. Description of racial disparities by Sherman and Devesa (Sherman and Devesa 2003) document significantly higher rates of aggressive cancers such as serous adenocarcinoma and clear cell adenocarcinoma (as well as sarcomas) among black women. Survival rates are universally low with aggressive forms (50 versus 36% for whites and blacks, with serous or clear cell adenocarcinoma) but survival rates are lower for blacks even with the less aggressive endometrioid adenocarcinoma.

The Hispanic population is the most rapidly growing ethnic group in the United States (del Pinal 1996). The incidence and survival curves for Hispanic women with endometrial cancer are similar to their white counterparts. One potential racial difference is that high-grade disease may have a peak incidence slightly earlier in Hispanics compared to whites and blacks (late sixties versus mid-to-late seventies) (Plaxe and Saltzstein 1997). In contrast to cervical cancer, which is relatively prevalent in Hispanics, endometrial cancer rates are comparable in the Hispanic population and other non-black groups. The increasing incidence of obesity among Hispanics may be a harbinger of future disparities in type I carcinoma.

Risk Factors for Endometrial Cancer

The risk of developing endometrial adenocarcinoma is based largely on the fact that it is an estrogen-dependent cancer. Factors that increase estrogen levels tend to be associated with increased risk and factors that either lower estrogen levels or balance estrogen with progesterone tend to lower risk (Liu, Conaway et al. 1995). Conditions that may increase risk are obesity, diabetes, polycystic ovary syndrome, feminizing ovarian tumors, nulliparity, menopause after age 52, unopposed estrogen replacement, and tamoxifen treatment lasting longer than two years. By contrast, factors that may reduce relative risk include normal weight, regular ovulation, combination estrogen-progesterone oral contraceptive pills, multiparity, menopause before age 49, and progestin therapy. Several of the factors on both side of the risk profile are related physiologically such as obesity, insulin resistance, and the resultant hyperinsulinemia and chronic anovulation that are all associated with polycystic ovarian syndrome (Salehi, Bravo-Vera et al. 2004).

Obesity is a major risk factor for endometrial cancer. An early study demonstrated a clear relationship between obesity and endometrial cancer (Swanson, Potischman et al. 1994). The study included 403 cases and 297 controls and found that those in the top quartile of body weight had a 2.3-fold increased risk of developing endometrial cancer. Interestingly, fat distribution was found to be an independent risk factor. Increasing upper body obesity (determined by waist-to-hip circumference ratio, WHR) is associated with increasing endometrial cancer risk. This data has been supported by a slightly smaller retrospective study which found a positive correlation between body mass index (BMI) in the highest quartile and endometrial cancer (Goodman, Hankin et al. 1997). This later study also began to address the influence that diet may have on endometrial cancer. Based on dietary recall data, cases consumed a higher percentage of their calories from fat than did controls. However, the odds ratio was reduced if dietary history was correlated with BMI at the time of interview. This suggests that obesity itself may be more important than dietary fat intake and that a healthy diet is more protective because it reduces the risk of obesity.

Data obtained through the Iowa Women's Health Study have demonstrated that women with diabetes mellitus may be at increased risk of developing endometrial cancer (Anderson, Anderson et al. 2001). A positive correlation between increasing BMI or WHR and endometrial cancer was also found. The association with diabetes was attenuated when BMI was accounted for in the analysis, but consideration of BMI did not completely remove the added risk of diabetes in the population studied. The mechanism by which diabetes may contribute to risk of endometrial cancer is not understood. Higher circulating insulin levels in type II diabetics may result in insulin-mediated activation of IGF-1 receptors in the endometrium (Corocleanu 1993; Ordener, Cypriani et al. 1993; Murphy 1994; Thiet, Osathanondh et al. 1994; Irwin, Suen et al. 2001). However, this hypothesis was not supported by data that found no difference between C-peptide levels in endometrial cancer cases compared to controls (Troisi, Potischman et al. 1997; Weiderpass, Brismar et al. 2003). Diabetes itself may be an additional risk factor, but is probably much less important than the obesity itself that often precedes type II diabetes.

The major impact of obesity on endometrial cancer is thought to be largely mediated by increased circulating estrogens. Several important correlations support the association between estrogen and endometrial cancer. Epidemiologic studies reviewed by Akhmedkhanov et al. (Akhmedkhanov, Zeleniuch-Jacquotte et al. 2001) point very clearly to conditions of relative physiologic hyperestrogenism or prolonged estrogen exposure to the endometrium. Conditions that lower the estrogen to progesterone ratio such as the use of oral contraceptive pills or parity are found to be protective. The role of progesterone is highlighted by increased endometrial cancer risk following exposure to unopposed estrogen in post-menopausal hormone replacement therapy and the use of Tamoxifen in the treatment of breast cancer.

Unopposed estrogen as the mechanism in endometrial carcinogenesis is also supported by the observation of a correlation between age-adjusted endometrial cancer incidence data and menopausal status. Endometrioid adenocarcinoma, the most common histologic variant, is relatively rare prior to menopause (Kosary 1994; Plaxe and Saltzstein 1997). The incidence rises sharply after menopause when the ovaries are no longer producing estrogen and progesterone. After cessation of ovarian function, estrogens are still produced in the body by peripheral conversion of andostenedione to estrone by the enzyme aromatase. Aromatase is expressed in adipose tissue providing a very plausible link between obesity and endometrial cancer. A positive correlation has been found between obesity and circulating estrone and estradiol (Judd, Lucas et al. 1976; MacDonald, Edman et al. 1978). Without a similar mechanism for post-menopausal production of progesterone, the post-menopausal state is one of relative increase in the ratio of estrogen to progesterone.

Prolonged exposure to physiologic estrogen, through early menarche, late menopause, nulliparity, or ovarian dysfunction, increases the risk of endometrial carcinoma (MacDonald, Edman et al. 1978; La Vecchia, Franceschi et al. 1984; Dahlgren, Friberg et al. 1991; Brinton, Berman et al. 1992). Polycystic ovary syndrome is one form of ovarian dysfunction in which there is increased circulating andostenedione and increased peripheral conversion to estrone. Polycystic ovary syndrome is also an interesting entity in relation to endometrial cancer because of its characteristic association with obesity, hyperinsulinemia, and anovulation. Chronic anovulation is an important mechanism by which prolonged estrogen exposure occurs without the benefit of progesterone secreted by the corpus luteum. Persistent estrogen stimulation of the endometrium is also seen in ovarian tumors that secrete estrogen (granulosa cell or theca cell).

Yet another risk factor associated with increased lifetime estrogen exposure is nulliparity. Nulliparity increases lifetime exposure to estrogen because pregnancy is a progesterone-dominant state, despite increased circulating levels of both estrogen and progesterone. In addition to the presence of progesterone, pregnancy is thought to be protective due to its association with relatively fewer ovulatory cycles and the related endometrial proliferation. Prevention of nulliparity is not a focus of public health efforts. However, nulliparity is a reality in a growing percentage of the female population as women choose to delay childbirth.

The use of exogenous estrogens has provided even stronger evidence for the unopposed estrogen mechanism of endometrial carcinogenesis. Estrogen therapy for postmenopausal women is associated with a 2.3-fold risk of endometrial cancer (Akhmedkhanov, Zeleniuch-Jacquotte et al. 2001). The longer the duration of use, the higher the risk. However, menopausal hormonal therapy is not associated with increased risk if both estrogen and progesterone are combined (Rossouw, Anderson et al. 2002). Although the use of combined estrogen and progesterone does not increase the risk of endometrial cancer, the combination has not been demonstrated to be protective (Pike, Peters et al. 1997). A more recent study supports this conclusion in that addition of progesterone to the estrogen replacement regimen simply negated the increased risk of endometrial cancer conferred by estrogen alone (Archer 2001).

The concept of combined estrogen and progesterone therapy raises the issue of oral contraceptives (OCs), which are thought to be protective against endometrial cancer. A large meta-analysis suggests that the protective effect is very modest and increases the probability of remaining free of endometrial cancer until age 74 from 97.6 to 98.6% (Schlesselman 1997). A more recent review of the data (Deligeoroglou, Michailidis et al. 2003) confirmed this modest degree of protection. Furthermore, the protective benefit was not realized unless OCs were used for five years. Interestingly, the protective benefit appears to persist even twenty years after discontinuation of OC use.

An important exogenous estrogen source in endometrial cancer has turned out to be tamoxifen. The use of tamoxifen has been shown to be effective in reducing tumor recurrence and prolonging survival for women when used as adjuvant therapy after surgical treatment for stage I and II breast cancer (Fisher, Costantino et al. 1998). In analysis of data demonstrating the effectiveness of tamoxifen treatment for breast cancer, it was found that the incidence of endometrial cancer was 2.53 times greater in the treatment group compared with the placebo group. In this study, all of the participants were part of a study design that included appropriate follow up. Close patient monitoring partially

Table 4. TNM and FIGO staging of endometrial cancer (Greene 2002)

TNM Category	FIGO Stage	
TX		Primary tumor cannot be assessed
T0		No evidence of primary tumor
Tis	0	Carcinoma *in situ*
T1	I	Tumor confined to corpus uteri
T1a	IA	Tumor limited to endometrium
T1c	IB	Tumor invades less than one-half of the myometrium
T1c	IC	Tumor invades one-half or more of the myometrium
T2	II	Tumor invades cervix but does not extend beyond uterus
T2a	IIA	Tumor limited to the glandular epithelium of the endocervix. There is no evidence of connective tissue stromal invasion
T2b	IIB	Invasion of the stromal connective tissue of the cervix
T3	III	Local and/or regional spread as defined below
T3a	IIIA	Tumor involves serosa and/or adnexa (direct extension or metastatis) and/or cancer cells in ascites or peritoneal washings
T3b	IIIB	Vaginal involvement (direct extension or metastasis)
T4	IVA	Tumor involves bladder mucosa and/or bowel mucosa (bullous edema is not sufficient to classify a tumor as T4)

explains why the endometrial cancers that did occur were almost entirely FIGO stage I or endometrial intraepithelial neoplasia (EIN) (Table 4). Because of these observations, patients receiving tamoxifen without a prior hysterectomy require careful and regular gynecologic follow up and aggressive evaluation of abnormal uterine bleeding.

More effort has been focused lately on the role dietary factors play is cancer prevention. Dietary influences related to endometrial cancer have thus far focused on phytoestrogens, total calorie intake, dietary fat intake, glycemic index, food sources, and micronutrients. Data suggest that positive risk factors for endometrial cancer include a high glycemic index (Folsom, Demissie et al. 2003) and dietary fat consumption (Littman, Beresford et al. 2001). Some dietary influences that may reduce risk include fatty fish consumption (Terry, Wolk et al. 2002), nuts and seeds (Petridou, Kedikoglou et al. 2002), beta-carotene, vitamin C (Negri, La Vecchia et al. 1996), and soy (Goodman, Wilkens et al. 1997; Lian, Niwa et al. 2001; Horn-Ross, John et al. 2003). Phytoestrogens are natural products present in soy beans and soy food products. There are many types of phytoestrogens but the most important ones appear to be genestein and diadzen. These compounds bind to estrogen receptors and have partial agonist or partial antagonist activities. A more specific look at phytoestrogens was provided by Horn-Ross and colleagues (Horn-Ross, John et al. 2003). In this study it was found that the phytoestrogen isoflavones (including genistein and diadzen) and lignans are associated with a reduced risk of endometrial cancer. Importantly, the intake required to reach this protective effect was not greater than that found in the typical American diet.

Smoking has been shown to lower the incidence of endometrial cancer. In a review of the literature (Terry, Rohan et al. 2002) it was found that smokers have a reduced risk of cancer. This may be explained by an anti-estrogen effect, an idea supported by the higher incidence of osteoporosis in smokers (Baron 1984; Jensen, Christiansen et al. 1985; Jensen and Christiansen 1988; Baron, La Vecchia et al. 1990). Other possibilities include the association between earlier age of menopause and chronic tobacco use, as well as a negative association between smoking and obesity. Given the injurious nature of tobacco use and its role as major cancer risk factor in other organ sites, the protective effect of smoking is unlikely to have any application to endometrial cancer prevention.

In addition to the risk factors discussed above, the characteristics of the endometrium itself determine a level of risk for developing endometrial cancer. A continuum of progression from normal to carcinoma exists in the endometrium in an analogous fashion to that described for carcinoma of the colon (Vogelstein, Fearon et al. 1988) or uterine cervix (O'Shaughnessy, Kelloff et al. 2002). The healthy, cycling, pre-menopausal endometrium will vary between the physiologic states of the menstrual cycle. A very early change along the progression toward cancer is simple hyperplasia of the endometrium. In simple hyperplasia the endometrium is stimulated by estrogen to proliferate but fails to shed completely, leaving behind tissue upon which the next level of proliferation builds. Over time this can lead to abnormal uterine bleeding. Histologic evaluation at this early condition is characterized by normal appearing glands and stroma with increased endothelial cellularity but without cytologic atypia. Hyperplasia with abnormal, crowded glands is termed complex hyperplasia. As with simple hyperplasia, the increased cellularity can exist with or without cytologic atypia in complex hyperplasia. In both simple and complex hyperplasias, the presence of nuclear atypia is the risk factor for progression to endometrial adenocarcinoma. The vast majority of hyperplastic states occur in post-menopausal women who may not shed atypical cells in the course of normal menses. In addition, hyperplasia in older women is associated with increased risk of progression (Zaino, Kurman et al. 1996). The details underlying the specific changes that occur along the continuum are still poorly understood. Future work in this area is likely to provide objective prognostic criteria for women who present within this continuum of disease.

Genetic Factors in Endometrial Cancer

Endometrial adenocarcinoma is an estrogen-driven cancer. Several of the risk factors, as discussed, are related to hyperestrogenic states within the body and possibly locally within the endometrium as well. In addition, there are underlying genetic factors that play a role in endometrial carcinogenesis.

Only a few genes have been implicated in the development of endometrial cancer. Some of these include receptors for estrogen, progesterone, and androgens. Other genes that may be associated include the oncogenes K-ras and HER-2/neu, tumor suppressor genes p53, p21, p16, and PTEN, as well as DNA repair genes hMLH2, hMSH2, and hMSH6. Recently, genes that affect estrogen metabolism have also been implicated.

The ras proto-oncogene functions in the intracellular signaling cascade from receptor tyrosine kinases. Constitutive ras activity leads to unregulated cell growth and duplication via the mitogen-activated protein kinase cascade. Analysis of 58 endometrial carcinomas and 22 endometrial hyperplasias identified K-ras mutations in 18.9% of carcinomas (Lagarda, Catasus et al. 2001). All mutations were found in carcinomas; no K-ras mutations were found in hyperplastic endometria negative for carcinoma. Several earlier studies have suggested K-ras mutations occur early in the course of endometrial adenocarcinoma because somatic mutations can be found in samples of hyperplastic endometrium (Enomoto, Inoue et al. 1990; Sasaki, Nishii et al. 1993; Duggan, Felix et al. 1994; Tsuda, Jiko et al. 1995; Ito, Watanabe et al. 1996). However, a complete survey of all endometrial tissue is very difficult and some hyperplasias in earlier studies may have contained only a small foci of carcinoma.

The oncogene HER-2/neu has been implicated in type II cancers. Overexpression of HER-2/neu has been demonstrated in 10 to 30% of all endometrial cancers, but nearly 80% of serous papillary forms (Oehler, Brand et al. 2003). The human epidermal growth factor-2 receptor (HER-2) is one member of a family of tyrosine kinases in which HER-1 is the bona fide epidermal growth factor receptor. No ligand has yet been identified for HER-2. Overexpression of the HER-2/neu variant is associated with increased growth via activation of the PI3K/AKT pathway (Di Fiore, Pierce et al. 1987; Liu, el-Ashry et al. 1995; Karunagaran, Tzahar et al. 1996; Waterman, Alroy et al. 1999; Muthuswamy, Li et al. 2001; Menard, Pupa et al. 2003). Using various methods (e.g. FISH), HER-2/neu has been found to be overexpressed in high-grade, advanced type II cancers (Lukes, Kohler et al. 1994; Rolitsky, Theil et al. 1999). Positive HER-2/neu overexpression is thereby associated with a poor prognosis.

p53, an essential protein used by cells to signal DNA damage, is a well-studied tumor suppressor gene known to be altered in a variety of cancers. It can function to delay cell-cycle progression until the damage is repaired or it can induce apoptosis

(Vousden and Lu 2002). Mutations in the p53 gene (TP53) are found in approximately 20% of endometrioid carcinomas (Lax, Kendall et al. 2000) and up to 90% of serous papillary forms (Inoue 2001). p53 mutations are readily found in endometrial carcinoma, but rarely in endometrial hyperplasia suggesting that p53's role in pathogenesis occurs rather late in the carcinogenesis process (Salvesen and Akslen 2002). p21 is a downstream target of p53 activity (el-Deiry, Tokino et al. 1993) and functions through interaction with cyclin-dependent kinases. Decreased p21 has been found in many tumor types including endometrial carcinoma (Palazzo, Mercer et al. 1997). The p16INK4 protein also interacts with the cyclin-dependent kinases. p16 binds to CDK4 and thereby inhibits progression through the cell cycle by inhibiting the CDK4-cyclin D complex (Kamb, Gruis et al. 1994). Like p21, decreased p16 expression has been demonstrated in endometrial carcinoma (Hatta, Hirama et al. 1995; Shiozawa, Nikaido et al. 1997; Milde-Langosch, Riethdorf et al. 1999; Nakashima, Fujita et al. 1999). Tumor suppressor genes, such as p53, p21 and p16, are found to be altered in many tumor types and are a necessary step along the path to cancer. By their very nature and integral role in all cell types, they are fundamental to cancer progression but are not tissue specific. Their broad expression makes them excellent targets for therapy aimed at mutant forms; however, they provide little insight into mechanisms of specific cancer varieties. More can be gained from knowledge of genetic alterations with more limited expression. PTEN is one such tumor suppressor involved in endometrial carcinoma.

PTEN is a tumor suppressor with tyrosine phosphatase activity and sequence homology to tensin, a matrix protein (Li, Yen et al. 1997; Steck, Pershouse et al. 1997). Growth factor receptors signal through tyrosine kinase cascades and often involve phosphatidylinositol-3-kinase activity and the generation of the intracellular signaling molecule phosphatidylinositol-(3,4,5)-triphosphate (PIP$_3$) (Risinger, Hayes et al. 1997; Tashiro, Blazes et al. 1997; Latta and Chapman 2002). PTEN removes the 3-phosphate from PIP$_3$ and thus negatively regulates AKT. Negative regulation of the survival-associated Ser/Thr kinase AKT prevents abnormal cell growth. Another key point regarding PTEN is its differential expression in the endometrium during the menstrual cycle (Mutter, Lin et al. 2000; Mutter, Lin et al. 2000; Mutter, Baak et al. 2001). It is highly expressed during the proliferative phase and has been proposed to function in preventing hyperstimulation by estrogen. Estrogen promotes PIP$_3$ production and may induce PTEN expression concurrently as a balance. Loss of PTEN function could then lead to increased PIP$_3$ signaling for survival and growth. Endometrial carcinomas show loss of heterozygosity for PTEN in approximately 40% of cases, and somatic mutations of PTEN have been found in up to 60% of endometrial carcinoma in some studies (Peiffer, Herzog et al. 1995; Kong, Suzuki et al. 1997; Risinger, Hayes et al. 1997; Tashiro, Blazes et al. 1997). PTEN mutations are most common in type I, estrogen-dependent, endometrial carcinomas but can also be identified in endometrial hyperplasias. This is consistent with an early role for PTEN in the pathogenesis of endometrial cancer (Mutter, Lin et al. 2000).

All cancers have an element of DNA damage. This means that alterations in the activity of DNA repair systems must be considered. One well studied DNA repair system comes from investigations into the hereditary nonpolyposis colorectal cancer syndrome (HNPCC) (Dunlop, Farrington et al. 1997). This is an autosomal dominant cancer syndrome in which many tissues are affected, including the endometrium. The genes identified in HNPCC function in the mismatch repair system. The most frequently involved genes include hMLH2, hMSH2, and hMSH6. Although females with HNPCC are at risk for developing cancers in many organs, endometrial carcinoma is the most frequently identified cancer in these patients (Watson, Vasen et al. 1994). Like the tumor suppressor genes, the mismatch repair system is of obvious importance in carcinogenesis, but does not shed light on the mechanisms of specific cancer types.

More recent studies regarding genetic loci involved in endometrial cancer have begun to look more closely at the role of estrogen metabolism and the activity of estrogen metabolites. Estrogen is synthesized mainly in the ovary but estrogen compounds are also produced by peripheral conversion of precursors via aromatase found in adipose tissue. Subsequently, several metabolites of estrogen are created by the activity of numerous members of the CYP family of enzymes. CYP enzymes are predominantly expressed by the liver where they function in the metabolism of a bewildering array of compounds. However, some CYP enzymes are also expressed outside the liver where they can create a local environment of a given metabolite. Relevant for estrogen metabolism, CYP17A1, CYP1A1, CYP11A1, CYP1B1, and CYP3A7 have all been implicated in endometrial cancer (Vadlamuri, Glover et al. 1998; Haiman, Hankinson et al. 2001; McKean-Cowdin, Feigelson et al. 2001; Berstein, Imyanitov et al. 2002; Lee, Cai et al. 2003; Sarkar, Vadlamuri et al. 2003; Sasaki, Kaneuchi et al. 2003). Interestingly, the pregnane X receptor, a new steroid receptor, has been proposed to regulate CYP3A expression in response to estrogen stimulation (Masuyama, Hiramatsu et al. 2003). Estrogen-dependent expression of CYP3A7 is consistent with the demonstrated variation of CYP expression during the menstrual cycle (Sarkar, Vadlamuri et al. 2003). A local environment of estrogen metabolites may provide a mechanism for estrogen-stimulated progression toward endometrial carcinoma.

Screening and Early Detection of Endometrial Cancer

Although endometrial cancer is the most common malignancy in the female genital tract, it accounts for a relatively low percentage of cancer deaths. The main reason that this is the case is that most patients present with locally confined disease (i.e. FIGO stages I or II). Most patients present with complaints of post-menopausal bleeding or abnormal uterine bleeding (AUB) if still pre-menopausal. When presented with AUB, the appropriate work-up includes a detailed history and physical examination, as well a transvaginal sonography and assessment of the endometrium by blind endometrial aspiration biopsy, hysteroscopy and/or dilation and curettage.

It is likely that in the future evaluation for AUB will include genetic profiling. Compared to other cancer types, the molecular genetics of endometrial cancer is still relatively under-studied. However, there are several research groups using microarray technology to characterize gene expression profiles in endometrial cancer (Mutter, Lin et al. 2000; Mutter, Baak et al. 2001; Smid-Koopman, Blok et al. 2004). It is thought that such profiling will identify additional targets for therapy, better characterization of individual tumors, and more specific treatments. One study found that genetic expression profiling with cluster analysis accurately places samples into separate clusters that contain either normal or cancer profiles (Smid-Koopman, Blok et al. 2004). This result argues that expression profiles are useful. However, this small study of only 12 endometrial cancers and six controls failed to find clusters that correlated with differing grade or stage. A large study may be required to determine if such a prognostic result can be obtained from genetic profiling.

Until the cancer genetics field catches up with current tests, evaluation of AUB will continue to rely on histopathologic studies. An argument for management of these women by a gynecologic oncologist was recently put forth (Roland, Kelly et al. 2004). Early screening and diagnosis, however, can easily be accomplished by general gynecologist. The role of transvaginal ultrasound is clear because determination of the endometrial thickness has good negative predictive value among post menopausal women. Endometrial stripes (thickness on ultrasound) less than 5 mm essentially rule out endometrial cancer. Stripes greater than 5 mm require additional follow up because the thickened stripe may be due to a variety of benign endometrial conditions, including polyps or hyperplasias of different grades, or cancer.

A second or concurrent step to ultrasound is endometrial sampling. Endometrial sampling may be performed in conjunction with hysteroscopy. However, hysteroscopy is a more invasive procedure that does not appear to provide much useful additional information for the plan of treatment (Bain, Parkin et al. 2002). Biopsy results taken by whatever means place the endometrium into a category along the continuum between normal cycling endometrium, hyperplasia, hyperplasia with cytologic atypia, or endometrial cancer. Treatment depends on histologic type. Simple hyperplasia in women wishing to preserve fertility can be treated with oral progestational agent therapy (Eichner and Abellera 1971; Bokhman, Chepick et al. 1985; Wentz 1985; Hunter, Tritz et al. 1994; Kim, Holschneider et al. 1997; Randall and Kurman 1997; Perez-Medina, Bajo et al. 1999). When fertility preservation is not a concern or among menopausal patients, the spectrum of management may include hysterectomy. An alternative to hysterectomy is dilation and curettage. Dilation and curettage removes only a fraction of the total endometrium and may require repeated future procedures. Endometrial ablation is generally not recommended due in part to the theoretical concern of burying potential neoplastic lesions. Surgery is recommended for patients found to have hyperplasia with atypia due to the increased risk for co-existing cancer and progression to cancer. When hysterectomies are performed the uterus should be bi-valved and inspected for myometrial invasion. Tumors found to have invaded more than one third the depth of the myometrium warrant lymph node sampling (Peters, Andersen et al. 1983; Goff and Rice 1990; Bloss, Berman et al. 1991; Kilgore, Partridge et al. 1995; Mohan, Samuels et al. 1998).

A small percentage of post-menopausal women may have endometrial malignancy identified incidentally on screening cervical cytology (Papanicolaou smear). This finding requires thorough evaluation of the endometrium to establish a diagnosis. However, cervicovaginal cytology should not be mistaken for a screening test for this malignancy. Endometrial cytology has been described previously and proposed as a potential screening test (Garcia, Barker et al. 2003) but its utility is limited by its difficult interpretation and problems with reproducibility.

The prevention of any cancer at the primary level can occur by reducing risk factors. In endometrial cancer the risk factors essentially all involve reducing the lifetime exposure to estrogens. These estrogens can come from endogenous production or from exogenous sources. Often the exogenous source is in the form of post-menopausal unopposed estrogen therapy. To minimize the risks associated with exogenous estrogen, it is important that estrogen therapy always occur in combination with progesterone in women with intact uteri.

Prevention of endometrial cancer through reduction of endogenous estrogen levels is aimed at reducing obesity. Many risk factors and modifying factors have been mentioned in this chapter, the majority of which are directly impacted by obesity. For example, early menarche, polycystic ovary syndrome, and diabetes are all associated with obesity. High fat, low fiber diets are associated with endometrial cancer independently (Littman, Beresford et al. 2001) even though their relative impact is small when the BMI of the patient is factored into the risk analysis. A similar argument is made for diabetes as a risk factor. The most powerful prevention is likely to come from promotion of balanced, low fat, high fiber diets, exercise, and appropriate surveillance for disease in women with abnormal uterine bleeding. This approach aims to prevent the main risk factor of obesity and diagnose cancers early in their course so as to allow for successful treatment and recovery. Such health promotion needs to start early in life and be reinforced at home, school, as well as in the physician's office.

Conclusion

Cervical and endometrial cancers are devastating diseases with major emotional and economic implications for women and their families. Cervical cancer is perhaps the best understood of any malignancy, and its etiologic agent, although ubiquitous, is well characterized and typically innocuous. Moreover, a cost effective screening intervention is generally available for the detection of pre-invasive disease. At least theoretically, cervical cancer is entirely preventable given the tools available to practitioners today (Table 5). Efforts should therefore be aimed at bringing the significant numbers of under and unscreened women into the screening pool and providing clinical services that facilitate their accurate diagnosis and adequate treatment prior to the point of developing invasive disease. Such women are in general medically underserved and uninsured, and bringing them into the health care system presents challenges that are at least as formidable as vaccine development.

Table 5. Theoretical framework for cervical cancer prevention

Primary Prevention – HPV infection prevention	Secondary Prevention – CIN detection & treatment	Tertiary Prevention – Cervical cancer treatment and control
Behavioral modification Sexual practices Tobacco cessation	Behavioral modification Sexual practices Tobacco cessation	Behavioral modification Tobacco cessation
Prophylactic vaccine	Screening programs HPV cytology	Medical therapeutics Radical surgery Radiation therapy Chemotherapy Therapeutic vaccines
Nutrition	Medical therapeutics Excisional therapy Therapeutic vaccines Chemo-preventive agents Retinoids Indole carbinol Immune response modulators	Surveillance

References

(1996). "National Institutes of Health Consensus Development Conference statement on cervical cancer. April 1–3, 1996." *J Womens Health* **1**: 1–38.

(1999). Evaluation of Cervical Cytology. *Evidence Report/Technology Assessment No. 5*. Rockville, MD, Agency of Health Care Policy and Researh.

(2001). Surveillance, Epidemiology, End Results Program, End Results Program 1975–2000. Atlanta, American Cancer Society.

(2002). Cancer Facts and Figures 2002. Atlanta, American Cancer Society.

(2003). "ACOG Practice Bulletin #45: Cervical Cytology Screening." *Obstet Gynecol* **102**(2): 417–428.

(2003). Cancer Facts & Figures for Hispanics/Latinos 2003–2005. Atlanta, American Cancer Society.

Agarwal, S.S., A. Sehgal, et al. (1993). "Role of male behavior in cervical carcinogenesis among women with one lifetime sexual partner." *Cancer* **72**(5): 1666–1669.

Akhmedkhanov, A., A. Zeleniuch-Jacquotte, et al. (2001). "Role of exogenous and endogenous hormones in endometrial cancer: review of the evidence and research perspectives." *Ann N Y Acad Sci* **943**: 296–315.

Alberts, D.S., R.R. Barakat, et al. (2004). Prevention of gynecologic malignancies. In: *Gynecologic Cancer: Controversies in Management*. D.M. Gershenson, W.P. McGuire, M. Gore, M.A. Quinn, G. Thomas (Eds.), Philadelphia, Elsevier Ltd.

al-Saleh, W., P. Delvenne, et al. (1995). "Inverse modulation of intraepithelial Langerhans' cells and stromal macrophage/dendrocyte populations in human papillomavirus-associated squamous intraepithelial lesions of the cervix." *Virchows Arch* **427**(1): 41–48.

Alvarez, R.D., M.G. Conner, et al. (2003). "The efficacy of 9-cis-retinoic acid (aliretinoin) as a chemopreventive agent for cervical dysplasia: results of a randomized double-blind clinical trial." *Cancer Epidemiol Biomarkers Prev* **12**(2): 114–119.

Anderson, K.E., E. Anderson, et al. (2001). "Diabetes and endometrial cancer in the Iowa women's health study." *Cancer Epidemiol Biomarkers Prev* **10**(6): 611–616.

Anttila, A., E. Pukkala, et al. (1999). "Effect of organised screening on cervical cancer incidence and mortality in Finland, 1963–1995: recent increase in cervical cancer incidence." *Int J Cancer* **83**(1): 59–65.

Archer, D.F. (2001). "The effect of the duration of progestin use on the occurrence of endometrial cancer in postmenopausal women." *Menopause* **8**(4): 245–251.

Bain, C., D.E. Parkin, et al. (2002). "Is outpatient diagnostic hysteroscopy more useful than endometrial biopsy alone for the investigation of abnormal uterine bleeding in unselected premenopausal women? A randomised comparison." *BJOG* **109**(7): 805–811.

Barker, B., F. Garcia, et al. (2001). "The correlation between colposcopically directed cervical biopsy and loop electrosurgical excision procedure pathology and the effect of time on that agreement." *Gynecol Oncol* **82**(1): 22–26.

Baron, J.A. (1984). "Smoking and estrogen-related disease." *Am J Epidemiol* **119**(1): 9–22.

Baron, J.A., C. La Vecchia, et al. (1990). "The antiestrogenic effect of cigarette smoking in women." *Am J Obstet Gynecol* **162**(2): 502–514.

Belinson, J., Y.L. Qiao, et al. (2001). "Shanxi Province Cervical Cancer Screening Study: a cross-sectional comparative trial of multiple techniques to detect cervical neoplasia." *Gynecol Oncol* **83**(2): 439–444.

Bell, M.C., P. Crowley-Nowick, et al. (2000). "Placebo-controlled trial of indole-3-carbinol in the treatment of CIN." *Gynecol Oncol* **78**(2): 123–129.

Berstein, L.M., E.N. Imyanitov, et al. (2002). "CYP17 genetic polymorphism in endometrial cancer: are only steroids involved?" *Cancer Lett* **180**(1): 47–53.

Bloss, J.D., M.L. Berman, et al. (1991). "Use of vaginal hysterectomy for the management of stage I endometrial cancer in the medically compromised patient." *Gynecol Oncol* **40**(1): 74–77.

Bokhman, J.V. (1983). "Two pathogenetic types of endometrial carcinoma." *Gynecol Oncol* **15**(1): 10–17.

Bokhman, J.V., O.F. Chepick, et al. (1985). "Can primary endometrial carcinoma stage I be cured without surgery and radiation therapy?" *Gynecol Oncol* **20**(2): 139–155.

Breitburd, F., R. Kirnbauer, et al. (1995). "Immunization with viruslike particles from cotton-tail rabbit papillomavirus (CRPV) can protect against experimental CRPV infection." *J Virol* **69**(6): 3959–3963.

Brinton, L.A., M.L. Berman, et al. (1992). "Reproductive, menstrual, and medical risk factors for endometrial cancer: results from a case-control study." *Am J Obstet Gynecol* **167**(5): 1317–1325.

Brinton, L.A., W.C. Reeves, et al. (1989). "Parity as a risk factor for cervical cancer." *Am J Epidemiol* **130**(3): 486–496.

Buckley, J.D., R.W. Harris, et al. (1981). "Case-control study of the husbands of women with dysplasia or carcinoma of the cervix uteri." *Lancet* **2**(8254): 1010–1015.

Butterworth, C.E., Jr., K.D. Hatch, et al. (1992). "Folate deficiency and cervical dysplasia." *JAMA* **267**(4): 528–533.

Butterworth, C.E., Jr., K.D. Hatch, et al. (1992). "Oral folic acid supplementation for cervical dysplasia: a clinical intervention trial." *Am J Obstet Gynecol* **166**(3): 803–809.

Castellsague, X., F.X. Bosch, et al. (2002). "Male circumcision, penile human papillomavirus infection, and cervical cancer in female partners." *N Engl J Med* **346**(15): 1105–1112.

Childers, J.M., J. Chu, et al. (1995). "Chemoprevention of cervical cancer with folic acid: a phase III Southwest Oncology Group Intergroup study." *Cancer Epidemiol Biomarkers Prev* **4**(2): 155–159.

Choo, K.B., C.C. Pan, et al. (1987). "Integration of human papillomavirus type 16 into cellular DNA of cervical carcinoma: preferential deletion of the E2 gene and invariable retention of the long control region and the E6/E7 open reading frames." *Virology* **161**(1): 259–261.

Clavel, C., M. Masure, et al. (2001). "Human papillomavirus testing in primary screening for the detection of high-grade cervical lesions: a study of 7932 women." *Br J Cancer* **84**(12): 1616–1623.

Clerici, M., M. Merola, et al. (1997). "Cytokine production patterns in cervical intraepithelial neoplasia: association with human papillomavirus infection." *J Natl Cancer Inst* **89**(3): 245–250.

Clerici, M., G.M. Shearer, et al. (1998). "Cytokine dysregulation in invasive cervical carcinoma and other human neoplasias: time to consider the TH1/TH2 paradigm." *J Natl Cancer Inst* **90**(4): 261–263.

Coker, A. and S. Bond (1999). *Persistent oncogenic HPV and risk of SIL progression and LSIL maintenance.* 18th International Human Papillomavirus conference, Charleston, SC.

Coleman, N., H.D. Birley, et al. (1994). "Immunological events in regressing genital warts." *Am J Clin Pathol* **102**(6): 768–774.

Corocleanu, M. (1993). "Hypothesis for endometrial carcinoma carcinogenesis. Preventive prospects." *Clin Exp Obstet Gynecol* **20**(4): 254–258.

Cuzick, J., P. Sasieni, et al. (2000). "Asystematic review of the role of human papillomavirus (HPV) testing within a cervical screening programme: summary and conclusions." *Br J Cancer* **83**: 561–565.

Cuzick, J., A. Szarewski, et al. (2003). "Management of women who test positive for high-risk types of human papillomavirus: the HART study." *Lancet* **362**(9399): 1871–1876.

Dahlgren, E., L.G. Friberg, et al. (1991). "Endometrial carcinoma; ovarian dysfunction – a risk factor in young women." *Eur J Obstet Gynecol Reprod Biol* **41**(2): 143–150.

de Vet, H.C., P.G. Knipschild, et al. (1991). "The effect of beta-carotene on the regression and progression of cervical dysplasia: a clinical experiment." *J Clin Epidemiol* **44**(3): 273–283.

de Vet, H.C., F. Sturmans, et al. (1994). "The role of cigarette smoking in the etiology of cervical dysplasia." *Epidemiology* **5**(6): 631–633.

Deacon, J.M., C.D. Evans, et al. (2000). "Sexual behaviour and smoking as determinants of cervical HPV infection and of CIN3 among those infected: a case-control study nested within the Manchester cohort." *Br J Cancer* **83**(11): 1565–1572.

del Pinal, J.H. (1996). "Hispanic Americans in the United States: Young, dynamic and diverse." *Stat Bull Metrop Insur Co* **77**(4): 2–13.

Deligeoroglou, E., E. Michailidis, et al. (2003). "Oral contraceptives and reproductive system cancer." *Ann N Y Acad Sci* **997**: 199–208.

Denk, C., K. Butz, et al. (2001). "p53 mutations are rare events in recurrent cervical cancer." *J Mol Med* **79**(5–6): 283–288.

Di Fiore, P.P., J.H. Pierce, et al. (1987). "erbB-2 is a potent oncogene when overexpressed in NIH/3T3 cells." *Science* **237**(4811): 178–182.

Ding, Z., A.G. Green, et al. (2002). "Retinoic acid inhibits telomerase activity and downregulates expression but does not affect splicing of hTERT: correlation with cell growth rate inhibition in an in vitro cervical carcinogenesis/multidrug-resistance model." *Exp Cell Res* **272**(2): 185–191.

Duggan, B.D., J.C. Felix, et al. (1994). "Early mutational activation of the c-Ki-ras oncogene in endometrial carcinoma." *Cancer Res* **54**(6): 1604–1607.

Dunlop, M.G., S.M. Farrington, et al. (1997). "Cancer risk associated with germline DNA mismatch repair gene mutations." *Hum Mol Genet* **6**(1): 105–110.

Eichner, E. and M. Abellera (1971). "Endometrial hyperplasia treated by progestins." *Obstet Gynecol* **38**(5): 739–742.

el-Deiry, W.S., T. Tokino, et al. (1993). "WAF1, a potential mediator of p53 tumor suppression." *Cell* **75**(4): 817–825.

Enomoto, T., M. Inoue, et al. (1990). "K-ras activation in neoplasms of the human female reproductive tract." *Cancer Res* **50**(19): 6139–6145.

Evans, T.G., W. Bonnez, et al. (2001). "A Phase 1 study of a recombinant viruslike particle vaccine against human papillomavirus type 11 in healthy adult volunteers." *J Infect Dis* **183**(10): 1485–1493.

Fahey, M.T., L. Irwig, et al. (1995). "Meta-analysis of Pap test accuracy." *Am J Epidemiol* **141**(7): 680–689.

Fairley, C., S. Tabrizi, et al. (1996). "A randomized clinical trial of beta carotene vs. placebo for the treatment of cervical HPV infection." *Int J Gynecol Cancer* **6**: 225–230.

Fisher, B., J.P. Costantino, et al. (1998). "Tamoxifen for prevention of breast cancer: report of the National Surgical Adjuvant Breast and Bowel Project P-1 Study." *J Natl Cancer Inst* **90**(18): 1371–1388.

Follen, M., E.N. Atkinson, et al. (2001). "A randomized clinical trial of 4-hydroxyphenylretinamide for high-grade squamous intraepithelial lesions of the cervix." *Clin Cancer Res* **7**(11): 3356–3365.

Follen, M., F.L. Meyskens, Jr., et al. (2003). "Cervical cancer chemoprevention, vaccines, and surrogate endpoint biomarkers." *Cancer* **98**(9 Suppl): 2044–2051.

Folsom, A.R., Z. Demissie, et al. (2003). "Glycemic index, glycemic load, and incidence of endometrial cancer: the Iowa women's health study." *Nutr Cancer* **46**(2): 119–124.

Franco, E.L. (1996). "Epidemiology of anogenital warts and cancer." *Obstet Gynecol Clin North Am* **23**(3): 597–623.

Fraser, I.S. and G.T. Kovacs (2003). "The efficacy of non-contraceptive uses for hormonal contraceptives." *Med J Aust* **178**(12): 621–623.

Garcia, F., B. Barker, et al. (2003). "Thin-layer cytology and histopathology in the evaluation of abnormal uterine bleeding." *J Reprod Med* **48**(11): 882–888.

Garcia, F., E. Mendez de Galaz, et al. (2003). "Factors that affect the quality of cytologic cervical cancer screening along the Mexico-United States border." *Am J Obstet Gynecol* **189**(2): 467–472.

Garcia, F., K.U. Petry, et al. (2004). "ZYC101a for Treatment of High-Grade Cervical Intraepithelial Neoplasia: A Randomized Controlled Trial." *Obstet Gynecol* **103**(2): 317–326.

Giannini, S.L., W. Al-Saleh, et al. (1998). "Cytokine expression in squamous intraepithelial lesions of the uterine cervix: implications for the generation of local immunosuppression." *Clin Exp Immunol* **113**(2): 183–189.

Goff, B.A. and L.W. Rice (1990). "Assessment of depth of myometrial invasion in endometrial adenocarcinoma." *Gynecol Oncol* **38**(1): 46–48.

Goodman, M.T., J.H. Hankin, et al. (1997). "Diet, body size, physical activity, and the risk of endometrial cancer." *Cancer Res* **57**(22): 5077–5085.

Goodman, M.T., L.R. Wilkens, et al. (1997). "Association of soy and fiber consumption with the risk of endometrial cancer." *Am J Epidemiol* **146**(4): 294–306.

Graham, V., E.S. Surwit, et al. (1986). "Phase II trial of beta-all-trans-retinoic acid for cervical intraepithelial neoplasia delivered via a collagen sponge and cervical cap." *West J Med* **145**(2): 192–195.

Greene, F.L., D.L. Page, et al. (2002). *AJCC Cancer Staging Manual, Sixth Edition*. Chicago, American Joint Committee on Cancer.

Greenlee, R.T., M.B. Hill-Harmon, et al. (2001). "Cancer statistics, 2001." *CA Cancer J Clin* **51**(1): 15–36.

Grubbs, C.J., V.E. Steele, et al. (1995). "Chemoprevention of chemically-induced mammary carcinogenesis by indole-3-carbinol." *Anticancer Res* **15**(3): 709–716.

Haiman, C.A., S.E. Hankinson, et al. (2001). "A polymorphism in CYP17 and endometrial cancer risk." *Cancer Res* **61**(10): 3955–3960.

Harro, C.D., Y.Y. Pang, et al. (2001). "Safety and immunogenicity trial in adult volunteers of a human papillomavirus 16 L1 virus-like particle vaccine." *J Natl Cancer Inst* **93**(4): 284–292.

Hatta, Y., T. Hirama, et al. (1995). "Alterations of the p16 (MTS1) gene in testicular, ovarian, and endometrial malignancies." *J Urol* **154**(5): 1954–1957.

Hernandez, B. and M. Goodman (1999). *Association of HPV viral load and risk of cervical squamous intraepithelial neoplasia (SIL) among multi-ethnic women in Hawaii*. 18th International Human Papillomavirus conference, Charleston, SC.

Ho, G.Y., R. Bierman, et al. (1998). "Natural history of cervicovaginal papillomavirus infection in young women." *N Engl J Med* **338**(7): 423–428.

Ho, G.Y., R.D. Burk, et al. (1995). "Persistent genital human papillomavirus infection as a risk factor for persistent cervical dysplasia." *J Natl Cancer Inst* **87**(18): 1365–1371.

Horn-Ross, P.L., E.M. John, et al. (2003). "Phytoestrogen intake and endometrial cancer risk." *J Natl Cancer Inst* **95**(15): 1158–1164.

Howe, S.L., R.J. Delfino, et al. (1998). "The risk of invasive cervical cancer among Hispanics: evidence for targeted preventive interventions." *Prev Med* **27**(5 Pt 1): 674–680.

Howell, E.A., Y.T. Chen, et al. (1999). "Differences in cervical cancer mortality among black and white women." *Obstet Gynecol* **94**(4): 509–515.

Howell, L.P., T. Belk, et al. (1999). "AutoCyte interactive screening system. Experience at a university hospital cytology laboratory." *Acta Cytol* **43**: 58–64.

Hunter, J.E., D.E. Tritz, et al. (1994). "The prognostic and therapeutic implications of cytologic atypia in patients with endometrial hyperplasia." *Gynecol Oncol* **55**(1): 66–71.

Hutchinson, M.L., D.J. Zahniser, et al. (1999). "Utility of liquid-based cytology for cervical carcinoma screening: results of a population-based study conducted in a region of Costa Rica with a high incidence of cervical carcinoma." *Cancer* **87**(2): 48–55.

Inoue, M. (2001). "Current molecular aspects of the carcinogenesis of the uterine endometrium." *Int J Gynecol Cancer* **11**(5): 339–348.

Irwin, J.C., L.F. Suen, et al. (2001). "Insulin-like growth factor (IGF)-II inhibition of endometrial stromal cell tissue inhibitor of metalloproteinase-3 and IGF-binding protein-1 suggests paracrine interactions at the decidua:trophoblast interface during human implantation." *J Clin Endocrinol Metab* **86**(5): 2060–2064.

Ito, K., K. Watanabe, et al. (1996). "K-ras point mutations in endometrial carcinoma: effect on outcome is dependent on age of patient." *Gynecol Oncol* **63**(2): 238–246.

Jemal, A., L.X. Clegg, et al. (2004). "Annual report to the nation on the status of cancer, 1995–2001." *Cancer* **101**: 3–27.

Jemal, A., R.C. Tiwari, et al. (2004). "Cancer statistics, 2004." *CA Cancer J Clin* **54**(1): 8–29.

Jensen, J. and C. Christiansen (1988). "Effects of smoking on serum lipoproteins and bone mineral content during postmenopausal hormone replacement therapy." *Am J Obstet Gynecol* **159**(4): 820–825.

Jensen, J., C. Christiansen, et al. (1985). "Cigarette smoking, serum estrogens, and bone loss during hormone-replacement therapy early after menopause." *N Engl J Med* **313**(16): 973–975.

Jones, B.A. and D.A. Novis (2000). "Follow-up of abnormal gynecologic cytology: a college of American pathologists Q-probes study of 16132 cases from 306 laboratories." *Arch Pathol Lab Med* **124**(5): 665–671.

Jones, D.L., R.M. Alani, et al. (1997). "The human papillomavirus E7 oncoprotein can uncouple cellular differentiation and proliferation in human keratinocytes by abrogating p21Cip1-mediated inhibition of cdk2." *Genes Dev* **11**(16): 2101–2111.

Judd, H.L., W.E. Lucas, et al. (1976). "Serum 17 beta-estradiol and estrone levels in postmenopausal women with and without endometrial cancer." *J Clin Endocrinol Metab* **43**(2): 272–278.

Kamb, A., N.A. Gruis, et al. (1994). "A cell cycle regulator potentially involved in genesis of many tumor types." *Science* **264**(5157): 436–440.

Karunagaran, D., E. Tzahar, et al. (1996). "ErbB-2 is a common auxiliary subunit of NDF and EGF receptors: implications for breast cancer." *Embo J* **15**(2): 254–264.

Keefe, K.A., M.J. Schell, et al. (2001). "A randomized, double blind, Phase III trial using oral beta-carotene supplementation for women with high-grade cervical intraepithelial neoplasia." *Cancer Epidemiol Biomarkers Prev* **10**(10): 1029–1035.

Kilgore, L.C., E.E. Partridge, et al. (1995). "Adenocarcinoma of the endometrium: survival comparisons of patients with and without pelvic node sampling." *Gynecol Oncol* **56**(1): 29–33.

Kim, Y.B., C.H. Holschneider, et al. (1997). "Progestin alone as primary treatment of endometrial carcinoma in premenopausal women. Report of seven cases and review of the literature." *Cancer* **79**(2): 320–327.

Klencke, B., M. Matijevic, et al. (2002). "Encapsulated plasmid DNA treatment for human papillomavirus 16-associated anal dysplasia: a Phase I study of ZYC101." *Clin Cancer Res* **8**(5): 1028–1037.

Kong, D., A. Suzuki, et al. (1997). "PTEN1 is frequently mutated in primary endometrial carcinomas." *Nat Genet* **17**(2): 143–144.

Konya, J. and J. Dillner (2001). "Immunity to oncogenic human papillomaviruses." *Adv Cancer Res* **82**: 205–238.

Kosary, C.L. (1994). "FIGO stage, histology, histologic grade, age and race as prognostic factors in determining survival for cancers of the female gynecological system: an analysis of 1973-87 SEER cases of cancers of the endometrium, cervix, ovary, vulva, and vagina." *Semin Surg Oncol* **10**(1): 31–46.

Koutsky, L.A., K.A. Ault, et al. (2002). "A controlled trial of a human papillomavirus type 16 vaccine." *N Engl J Med* **347**(21): 1645–1651.

Koutsky, L.A., K.K. Holmes, et al. (1992). "A cohort study of the risk of cervical intraepithelial neoplasia grade 2 or 3 in relation to papillomavirus infection." *N Engl J Med* **327**(18): 1272–1278.

La Vecchia, C., S. Franceschi, et al. (1984). "Risk factors for endometrial cancer at different ages." *J Natl Cancer Inst* **73**(3): 667–671.

Lagarda, H., L. Catasus, et al. (2001). "K-ras mutations in endometrial carcinomas with microsatellite instability." *J Pathol* **193**(2): 193–199.

Latta, E. and W.B. Chapman (2002). "PTEN mutations and evolving concepts in endometrial neoplasia." *Curr Opin Obstet Gynecol* **14**(1): 59–65.

Lax, S.F., B. Kendall, et al. (2000). "The frequency of p53, K-ras mutations, and microsatellite instability differs in uterine endometrioid and serous carcinoma: evidence of distinct molecular genetic pathways." *Cancer* **88**(4): 814–824.

Lee, A.J., M.X. Cai, et al. (2003). "Characterization of the oxidative metabolites of 17beta-estradiol and estrone formed by 15 selectively expressed human cytochrome p450 isoforms." *Endocrinology* **144**(8): 3382–3398.

Lee, K.R., R. Ashfaq, et al. (1997). "Comparison of conventional Papanicolaou smears and a fluid-based, thin-layer system for cervical cancer screening." *Obstet Gynecol* **90**(2): 278–284.

Li, J., C. Yen, et al. (1997). "PTEN, a putative protein tyrosine phosphatase gene mutated in human brain, breast, and prostate cancer." *Science* **275**(5308): 1943–1947.

Lian, Z., K. Niwa, et al. (2001). "Preventive effects of isoflavones, genistein and daidzein, on estradiol-17beta-related endometrial carcinogenesis in mice." *Jpn J Cancer Res* **92**(7): 726–734.

Littman, A.J., S.A. Beresford, et al. (2001). "The association of dietary fat and plant foods with endometrial cancer (United States)." *Cancer Causes Control* **12**(8): 691–702.

Liu, J.R., M. Conaway, et al. (1995). "Relationship between race and interval to treatment in endometrial cancer." *Obstet Gynecol* **86**(4 Pt 1): 486–490.

Liu, T., X. Wang, et al. (1998). "Relationships between socioeconomic status and race-specific cervical cancer incidence in the United States, 1973–1992." *J Health Care Poor Underserved* **9**(4): 420–432.

Liu, Y., D. el-Ashry, et al. (1995). "MCF-7 breast cancer cells overexpressing transfected c-erbB-2 have an in vitro growth advantage in estrogen-depleted conditions and reduced estrogen-dependence and tamoxifen-sensitivity in vivo." *Breast Cancer Res Treat* **34**(2): 97–117.

Londesborough, P., L. Ho, et al. (1996). "Human papillomavirus genotype as a predictor of persistence and development of high-grade lesions in women with minor cervical abnormalities." *Int J Cancer* **69**(5): 364–368.

Lukes, A.S., M.F. Kohler, et al. (1994). "Multivariable analysis of DNA ploidy, p53, and HER-2/neu as prognostic factors in endometrial cancer." *Cancer* **73**(9): 2380–2385.

MacDonald, P.C., C.D. Edman, et al. (1978). "Effect of obesity on conversion of plasma androstenedione to estrone in postmenopausal women with and without endometrial cancer." *Am J Obstet Gynecol* **130**(4): 448–455.

Mackerras, D., L. Irwig, et al. (1999). "Randomized double-blind trial of beta-carotene and vitamin C in women with minor cervical abnormalities." *Br J Cancer* **79**(9–10): 1448–1453.

Madison, T., D. Schottenfeld, et al. (1998). "Cancer of the corpus uteri in white and black women in Michigan, 1985–1994: an analysis of trends in incidence and mortality and their relation to histologic subtype and stage." *Cancer* **83**(8): 1546–1554.

Maiman, M. (1998). "Management of cervical neoplasia in human immunodeficiency virus-infected women." *J Natl Cancer Inst Monogr* (23): 43–49.

Manetta, A., T. Schubbert, et al. (1996). "beta-Carotene treatment of cervical intraepithelial neoplasia: a phase II study." *Cancer Epidemiol Biomarkers Prev* **5**(11): 929–932.

Martin-Hirsch, P., E. Paraskevaidis, et al. (2000). Surgery for cervical intraepithelial neoplasia. *Cochrane Database Syst Rev* (2): CD001318.

Masuyama, H., Y. Hiramatsu, et al. (2003). "Expression and potential roles of pregnane X receptor in endometrial cancer." *J Clin Endocrinol Metab* **88**(9): 4446–4454.

McCann, M.F., D.E. Irwin, et al. (1992). "Nicotine and cotinine in the cervical mucus of smokers, passive smokers, and nonsmokers." *Cancer Epidemiol Biomarkers Prev* **1**(2): 125–129.

McKean-Cowdin, R., H.S. Feigelson, et al. (2001). "Risk of endometrial cancer and estrogen replacement therapy history by CYP17 genotype." *Cancer Res* **61**(3): 848–849.

Meijer, C.J., M.A. Nobbenhuis, et al. (1999). *Human papillomavirus and cervical lesions in a prospective study of 353 women with abnormal cytology.* 18th International Human Papillomavirus Conference, Charleston, SC.

Meisels, A., C. Morin, et al. (1983). "Human papillomavirus (HPV) venereal infections and gynecologic cancer." *Pathol Annu* **18 Pt 2**: 277–293.

Menard, S., S.M. Pupa, et al. (2003). "Biologic and therapeutic role of HER2 in cancer." *Oncogene* **22**(42): 6570–6578.

Meyskens, F.L., Jr., V. Graham, et al. (1983). "A phase I trial of beta-all-trans-retinoic acid delivered via a collagen sponge and a cervical cap for mild or moderate intraepithelial cervical neoplasia." *J Natl Cancer Inst* **71**(5): 921–925.

Meyskens, F.L., Jr., E. Surwit, et al. (1994). "Enhancement of regression of cervical intraepithelial neoplasia II (moderate dysplasia) with topically applied all-trans-retinoic acid: a randomized trial." *J Natl Cancer Inst* **86**(7): 539–543.

Milde-Langosch, K., L. Riethdorf, et al. (1999). "P16/MTS1 and pRB expression in endometrial carcinomas." *Virchows Arch* **434**(1): 23–28.

Miller, B.A., L.N. Kolonel, et al., editors (1996). Racial/ethnic patterns of cancer in the United States 1988–1992. Bethesda, National Cancer Institute.

Mitchell, J.B. and L.A. McCormack (1997). "Time trends in late-stage diagnosis of cervical cancer. Differences by race/ethnicity and income." *Med Care* **35**(12): 1220–1224.

Mitchell, M.F., G. Tortolero-Luna, et al. (1998). "A randomized clinical trial of cryotherapy, laser vaporization, and loop electrosurgical excision for treatment of squamous intraepithelial lesions of the cervix." *Obstet Gynecol* **92**(5): 737–744.

Mitchell, M.F., G. Tortolero-Luna, et al. (1998). "Phase I dose de-escalation trial of alpha-di-fluoromethylornithine in patients with grade 3 cervical intraepithelial neoplasia." *Clin Cancer Res* **4**(2): 303–310.

Mohan, D.S., M.A. Samuels, et al. (1998). "Long-term outcomes of therapeutic pelvic lymphadenectomy for stage I endometrial adenocarcinoma." *Gynecol Oncol* **70**(2): 165–171.

Montz, F.J. (2000). "Management of high-grade cervical intraepithelial neoplasia and low-grade squamous intraepithelial lesion and potential complications." *Clin Obstet Gynecol* **43**(2): 394–409.

Moreno, V., F.X. Bosch, et al. (2002). "Effect of oral contraceptives on risk of cervical cancer in women with human papillomavirus infection: the IARC multicentric case-control study." *Lancet* **359**(9312): 1085–1092.

Morris, M., G. Tortolero-Luna, et al. (1996). "Cervical intraepithelial neoplasia and cervical cancer." *Obstet Gynecol Clin North Am* **23**(2): 347–410.

Moscicki, A.B., S. Shiboski, et al. (1998). "The natural history of human papillomavirus infection as measured by repeated DNA testing in adolescent and young women." *J Pediatr* **132**(2): 277–284.

Moyer, P. (2004). "Vaccine against HPV strain protects against high-grade cervical neoplasia." *Medscape Medical News* Report on 44th Interscience Conference on Antimicrobial Agents and Chemotherapy, Abstract 3741. *http://www.medscape.com*, Accessed Feb 8, 2005.

Muderspach, L., S. Wilczynski, et al. (2000). "A phase I trial of a human papillomavirus (HPV) peptide vaccine for women with high-grade cervical and vulvar intraepithelial neoplasia who are HPV 16 positive." Clin Cancer Res **6**(9): 3406–3416.

Muller, M., J. Zhou, et al. (1997). "Chimeric papillomavirus-like particles." *Virology* **234**(1): 93–111.

Munoz, N., F.X. Bosch, et al. (2003). "Epidemiologic classification of human papillomavirus types associated with cervical cancer." *N Engl J Med* **348**(6): 518–527.

Munoz, N., S. Franceschi, et al. (2002). "Role of parity and human papillomavirus in cervical cancer: the IARC multicentric case-control study. [see comments.]." *Lancet* **359**(9312): 1093–1101.

Murphy, L.J. (1994). "Growth factors and steroid hormone action in endometrial cancer." *J Steroid Biochem Mol Biol* **48**(5–6): 419–423.

Muthuswamy, S.K., D. Li, et al. (2001). "ErbB2, but not ErbB1, reinitiates proliferation and induces luminal repopulation in epithelial acini." *Nat Cell Biol* **3**(9): 785–792.

Mutter, G.L., J.P. Baak, et al. (2001). "Global expression changes of constitutive and hormonally regulated genes during endometrial neoplastic transformation." *Gynecol Oncol* **83**(2): 177–185.

Mutter, G.L., M.C. Lin, et al. (2000). "Altered PTEN expression as a diagnostic marker for the earliest endometrial precancers." *J Natl Cancer Inst* **92**(11): 924–930.

Mutter, G.L., M.C. Lin, et al. (2000). "Changes in endometrial PTEN expression throughout the human menstrual cycle." *J Clin Endocrinol Metab* **85**(6): 2334–2338.

Nakashima, R., M. Fujita, et al. (1999). "Alteration of p16 and p15 genes in human uterine tumours." *Br J Cancer* **80**(3–4): 458–467.

Napoles-Springer, A., E.J. Perez-Stable, et al. (1996). "Risk factors for invasive cervical cancer in Latino women." *J Med Syst* **20**(5): 277–293.

Nastala, C.L., H.D. Edington, et al. (1994). "Recombinant IL-12 administration induces tumor regression in association with IFN-gamma production." *J Immunol* **153**(4): 1697–1706.

NCI (2001). NCI Bethesda System 2001, National Cancer Institute, *http://www.bethesda2001.cancer.gov/*, Accessed Feb 8, 2005.

Negri, E., C. La Vecchia, et al. (1996). "Intake of selected micronutrients and the risk of endometrial carcinoma." *Cancer* **77**(5): 917–923.

NIH (1996). Cervical Cancer: NIH Consensus Statement. **14:** 1–38.

Oehler, M.K., A. Brand, et al. (2003). "Molecular genetics and endometrial cancer." *J Br Menopause Soc* **9**(1): 27–31.

Ordener, C., B. Cypriani, et al. (1993). "Epidermal growth factor and insulin induce the proliferation of guinea pig endometrial stromal cells in serum-free culture, whereas estradiol and progesterone do not." *Biol Reprod* **49**(5): 1032–1044.

O'Shaughnessy, J.A., G.J. Kelloff, et al. (2002). "Treatment and prevention of intraepithelial neoplasia: an important target for accelerated new agent development." *Clin Cancer Res* **8**(2): 314–346.

Ostor, A.G. (1993). "Natural history of cervical intraepithelial neoplasia: a critical review." *Int J Gynecol Pathol* **12**(2): 186–192.

Palazzo, J.P., W.E. Mercer, et al. (1997). "Immunohistochemical localization of p21(WAF1/CIP1) in normal, hyperplastic, and neoplastic uterine tissues." *Hum Pathol* **28**(1): 60–66.

Palefsky, J.M. and E.A. Holly (1995). "Molecular virology and epidemiology of human papillomavirus and cervical cancer." *Cancer Epidemiol Biomarkers Prev* **4**(4): 415–428.

Parazzini, F., C. La Vecchia, et al. (1991). "The epidemiology of endometrial cancer." *Gynecol Oncol* **41**(1): 1–16.

Parkin, D.M., F. Bray, et al. (2001). "Estimating the world cancer burden: Globocan 2000." *Int J Cancer* **94**(2): 153–156.

Parkin, D.M., P. Pisani, et al. (1999). "Estimates of the worldwide incidence of 25 major cancers in 1990." *Int J Cancer* **80**(6): 827–841.

Parkin, D.M., P. Pisani, et al. (1999). "Global cancer statistics." *CA Cancer J Clin* **49**(1): 33–64, 1.

Parkin, D.M., A.P. Vizcaino, et al. (1994). "Cancer patterns and risk factors in the African population of southwestern Zimbabwe, 1963–1977." *Cancer Epidemiol Biomarkers Prev* **3**(7): 537–547.

Patten, S.F., J.S.J. Lee, et al. (1997). "The AutoPap 300 QC system multicenter clinicaltials for use in quality control rescreening of cervical smears. I. A prospective intended use study." *Cancer Cytopathol* **81**: 337–342.

Peiffer, S.L., T.J. Herzog, et al. (1995). "Allelic loss of sequences from the long arm of chromosome 10 and replication errors in endometrial cancers." *Cancer Res* **55**(9): 1922–1926.

Perez-Medina, T., J. Bajo, et al. (1999). "Atypical endometrial hyperplasia treatment with progestogens and gonadotropin-releasing hormone analogues: long-term follow-up." *Gynecol Oncol* **73**(2): 299–304.

Peters, W.A., 3rd, W.A. Andersen, et al. (1983). "The selective use of vaginal hysterectomy in the management of adenocarcinoma of the endometrium." *Am J Obstet Gynecol* **146**(3): 285–289.

Petridou, E., S. Kedikoglou, et al. (2002). "Diet in relation to endometrial cancer risk: a case-control study in Greece." *Nutr Cancer* **44**(1): 16–22.

Pike, M.C., R.K. Peters, et al. (1997). "Estrogen-progestin replacement therapy and endometrial cancer." *J Natl Cancer Inst* **89**(15): 1110–1116.

Plaxe, S.C. and S.L. Saltzstein (1997). "Impact of ethnicity on the incidence of high-risk endometrial carcinoma." *Gynecol Oncol* **65**(1): 8–12.

Prokopczyk, B., J.E. Cox, et al. (1997). "Identification of tobacco-specific carcinogen in the cervical mucus of smokers and nonsmokers." *J Natl Cancer Inst* **89**(12): 868–873.

Randall, T.C. and R.J. Kurman (1997). "Progestin treatment of atypical hyperplasia and well-differentiated carcinoma of the endometrium in women under age 40." *Obstet Gynecol* **90**(3): 434–440.

Richardson, H., G. Kelsall, et al. (2003). "The natural history of type-specific human papillomavirus infections in female university students." *Cancer Epidemiol Biomarkers Prev* **12**(6): 485–490.

Ries, L.A.G., M.P. Eisner, et al., editors (2001). SEER Cancer Statistics Review, 1973–1998. Bethesda, National Cancer Institute.

Ries, L.A.G., L.N. Kosary, et al., editors (1999). SEER Cancer Statistics Review, 1973–1996. Bethesda, National Cancer Institute.

Risinger, J.I., A.K. Hayes, et al. (1997). "PTEN/MMAC1 mutations in endometrial cancers." *Cancer Res* **57**(21): 4736–4738.

Roland, P.Y., F.J. Kelly, et al. (2004). "The benefits of a gynecologic oncologist: a pattern of care study for endometrial cancer treatment." *Gynecol Oncol* **93**(1): 125–130.

Rolitsky, C.D., K.S. Theil, et al. (1999). "HER-2/neu amplification and overexpression in endometrial carcinoma." *Int J Gynecol Pathol* **18**(2): 138–143.

Romney, S.L., J. Basu, et al. (1987). "Plasma reduced and total ascorbic acid in human uterine cervix dysplasias and cancer." *Ann N Y Acad Sci* **498**: 132–143.

Romney, S.L., A. Dwyer, et al. (1985). "Chemoprevention of cervix cancer: Phase I–II: A feasibility study involving the topical vaginal administration of retinyl acetate gel." *Gynecol Oncol* **20**(1): 109–119.

Romney, S.L., G.Y. Ho, et al. (1997). "Effects of beta-carotene and other factors on outcome of cervical dysplasia and human papillomavirus infection." *Gynecol Oncol* **65**(3): 483–492.

Rossouw, J.E., G.L. Anderson, et al. (2002). "Risks and benefits of estrogen plus progestin in healthy postmenopausal women: principal results From the Women's Health Initiative randomized controlled trial." *JAMA* **288**(3): 321–333.

Salehi, M., R. Bravo-Vera, et al. (2004). "Pathogenesis of polycystic ovary syndrome: what is the role of obesity?" *Metabolism* **53**(3): 358–376.

Salvesen, H.B. and L.A. Akslen (2002). "Molecular pathogenesis and prognostic factors in endometrial carcinoma." *Apmis* **110**(10): 673–689.

Samson, S.-L.A., J.R. Bentley, et al. (2005). "The effect of LEEP electrosurgical excision procedure on future pregnancy outcome." *Obstet Gynecol* **105**(2): 325–332.

Sarkar, M.A., V. Vadlamuri, et al. (2003). "Expression and cyclic variability of CYP3A4 and CYP3A7 isoforms in human endometrium and cervix during the menstrual cycle." *Drug Metab Dispos* **31**(1): 1–6.

Sasaki, H., H. Nishii, et al. (1993). "Mutation of the Ki-ras protooncogene in human endometrial hyperplasia and carcinoma." *Cancer Res* **53**(8): 1906–1910.

Sasaki, M., M. Kaneuchi, et al. (2003). "CYP1B1 gene in endometrial cancer." *Mol Cell Endocrinol* **202**(1–2): 171–176.

Saslow, D., C.D. Runowicz, et al. (2002). "American Cancer Society guideline for the early detection of cervical neoplasia and cancer." *CA Cancer J Clin* **52**(6): 342–362.

Scheffner, M., J.M. Huibregtse, et al. (1993). "The HPV-16 E6 and E6-AP complex functions as a ubiquitin-protein ligase in the ubiquitination of p53." *Cell* **75**(3): 495–505.

Schiffman, M.H., H.M. Bauer, et al. (1993). "Epidemiologic evidence showing that human papillomavirus infection causes most cervical intraepithelial neoplasia." *J Natl Cancer Inst* **85**(12): 958–964.

Schiffman, M.H. and S.K. Kjaer (2003). "Natural history of anogenital human papillomavirus infection and neoplasia." *J Natl Cancer Inst Monogr* **31**: 14–19.

Schlesselman, J.J. (1997). "Risk of endometrial cancer in relation to use of combined oral contraceptives. A practitioner's guide to meta-analysis." *Hum Reprod* **12**(9): 1851–1863.

Sheets, E.E., R.G. Urban, et al. (2003). "Immunotherapy of human cervical high-grade cervical intraepithelial neoplasia with microparticle-delivered human papillomavirus 16 E7 plasmid DNA." *Am J Obstet Gynecol* **188**(4): 916–926.

Sherman, M.E. and S.S. Devesa (2003). "Analysis of racial differences in incidence, survival, and mortality for malignant tumors of the uterine corpus." *Cancer* **98**(1): 176–186.

Sherman, M.E., M. Schiffman, et al. (2002). "Effects of age and human papilloma viral load on colposcopy triage: data from the randomized Atypical Squamous Cells of Undetermined Significance/Low-Grade Squamous Intraepithelial Lesion Triage Study (ALTS)." *J Natl Cancer Inst* **94**(2): 102–107.

Shiozawa, T., T. Nikaido, et al. (1997). "Immunohistochemical analysis of the expression of cdk4 and p16INK4 in human endometrioid-type endometrial carcinoma." *Cancer* **80**(12): 2250–2256.

Shirodkar, S., M. Ewen, et al. (1992). "The transcription factor E2F interacts with the retinoblastoma product and a p107-cyclin A complex in a cell cycle-regulated manner." *Cell* **68**(1): 157–166.

Sizemore, N., C.K. Choo, et al. (1998). "Transcriptional regulation of the EGF receptor promoter by HPV16 and retinoic acid in human ectocervical epithelial cells." *Exp Cell Res* **244**(1): 349–356.

Smid-Koopman, E., L.J. Blok, et al. (2004). "Gene expression profiling in human endometrial cancer tissue samples: utility and diagnostic value." *Gynecol Oncol* **93**(2): 292–300.

Steck, P.A., M.A. Pershouse, et al. (1997). "Identification of a candidate tumour suppressor gene, MMAC1, at chromosome 10q23.3 that is mutated in multiple advanced cancers." *Nat Genet* **15**(4): 356–362.

Surwit, E.A., V. Graham, et al. (1982). "Evaluation of topically applied trans-retinoic acid in the treatment of cervical intraepithelial lesions." *Am J Obstet Gynecol* **143**(7): 821–823.

Swanson, C.A., N. Potischman, et al. (1994). "Endometrial cancer risk in relation to serum lipids and lipoprotein levels." *Cancer Epidemiol Biomarkers Prev* **3**(7): 575–581.

Tashiro, H., M.S. Blazes, et al. (1997). "Mutations in PTEN are frequent in endometrial carcinoma but rare in other common gynecological malignancies." *Cancer Res* **57**(18): 3935–3940.

ter Harmsel, B., F. Smedts, et al. (1999). "Relationship between human papillomavirus type 16 in the cervix and intraepithelial neoplasia." *Obstet Gynecol* **93**(1): 46–50.

Terry, P., A. Wolk, et al. (2002). "Fatty fish consumption lowers the risk of endometrial cancer: a nationwide case-control study in Sweden." *Cancer Epidemiol Biomarkers Prev* **11**(1): 143–145.

Terry, P.D., T.E. Rohan, et al. (2002). "Cigarette smoking and the risk of endometrial cancer." *Lancet Oncol* **3**(8): 470–480.

Thiet, M.P., R. Osathanondh, et al. (1994). "Localization and timing of appearance of insulin, insulin-like growth factor-I, and their receptors in the human fetal mullerian tract." *Am J Obstet Gynecol* **170**(1 Pt 1): 152–156.

Thomas, D.B., R.M. Ray, et al. (1996). "Prostitution, condom use, and invasive squamous cell cervical cancer in Thailand." *Am J Epidemiol* **143**(8): 779–786.

Thorland, E.C., S.L. Myers, et al. (2000). "Human papillomavirus type 16 integrations in cervical tumors frequently occur in common fragile sites." *Cancer Res* **60**(21): 5916–5921.

Troisi, R., N. Potischman, et al. (1997). "Insulin and endometrial cancer." *Am J Epidemiol* **146**(6): 476–482.

Tsuda, H., K. Jiko, et al. (1995). "Frequent occurrence of c-Ki-ras gene mutations in well differentiated endometrial adenocarcinoma showing infiltrative local growth with fibrosing stromal response." *Int J Gynecol Pathol* **14**(3): 255–259.

Vadlamuri, S.V., D.D. Glover, et al. (1998). "Regiospecific expression of cytochrome P4501A1 and 1B1 in human uterine tissue." *Cancer Lett* **122**(1–2): 143–150.

van Duin, M., P.J. Snijders, et al. (2002). "Human papillomavirus 16 load in normal and abnormal cervical scrapes: an indicator of CIN II/III and viral clearance." *Int J Cancer* **98**(4): 590–595.

Vassilakos, P., J. Saurel, et al. (1999). "Direct-to-vial use of the AutoCyte PREP liquid-based preparation for cervical-vaginal specimens in three European laboratories." *Acta Cytol* **43**(1): 65–68.

Vogelstein, B., E.R. Fearon, et al. (1988). "Genetic alterations during colorectal-tumor development." *N Engl J Med* **319**(9): 525–532.

Vousden, K.H. and X. Lu (2002). "Live or let die: the cell's response to p53." *Nat Rev Cancer* **2**(8): 594–604.

Waterman, H., I. Alroy, et al. (1999). "The C-terminus of the kinase-defective neuregulin receptor ErbB-3 confers mitogenic superiority and dictates endocytic routing." *Embo J* **18**(12): 3348–3358.

Watson, P., H.F. Vasen, et al. (1994). "The risk of endometrial cancer in hereditary nonpolyposis colorectal cancer." *Am J Med* **96**(6): 516–520.

Wattenberg, L.W. and W.D. Loub (1978). "Inhibition of polycyclic aromatic hydrocarbon-induced neoplasia by naturally occurring indoles." *Cancer Res* **38**(5): 1410–1413.

Weiderpass, E., K. Brismar, et al. (2003). "Serum levels of insulin-like growth factor-I, IGF-binding protein 1 and 3, and insulin and endometrial cancer risk." *Br J Cancer* **89**(9): 1697–1704.

Weiner, S.A., E.A. Surwit, et al. (1986). "A phase I trial of topically applied trans-retinoic acid in cervical dysplasia-clinical efficacy." *Invest New Drugs* **4**(3): 241–244.

Wentz, W.B. (1985). "Progestin therapy in lesions of the endometrium." *Semin Oncol* **12**(1 Suppl 1): 23–27.

Wright, T.C., J.T. Cox, et al. (2002). "2001 consensus guidelines for the management of women with cervical cytological abnormalities." *JAMA* **287**: 2120–2129.

Wright, T.C., Jr. (1994). Precancerous lesions of the cervix. In: *Blaustein's Pathology of the Female Genital Tract*. R. Kurman (Ed.), Springer Verlag: 229–278.

Wright, T.C., Jr., J.T. Cox, et al. (2003). "2001 consensus guidelines for the management of women with cervical intraepithelial neoplasia." *Am J Obstet Gynecol* **189**(1): 295–304.

Wright, T.C., Jr., A. Lorincz, et al. (1998). "Reflex human papillomavirus deoxyribonucleic acid testing in women with abnormal Papanicolaou smears." *Am J Obstet Gynecol* **178**(5): 962–966.

Wright, T.C., Jr., M. Schiffman, et al. (2004). "Interim guidance for the use of human papillomavirus DNA testing as an adjunct to cervical cytology for screening." *Obstet Gynecol* **103**(2): 304–309.

Yoo, K.Y., D. Kang, et al. (1997). "Risk factors associated with uterine cervical cancer in Korea: a case- control study with special reference to sexual behavior." *J Epidemiol* **7**(3): 117–123.

Zaino, R.J., R.J. Kurman, et al. (1996). "Pathologic models to predict outcome for women with endometrial adenocarcinoma: the importance of the distinction between surgical stage and clinical stage – a Gynecologic Oncology Group study." *Cancer* **77**(6): 1115–1121.

Zola, H., P. Roberts-Tompson, et al. (1995). *Diagnostic Immunopathology*, Cambridge.

Zunzunegui, M.V., M.C. King, et al. (1986). "Male influences on cervical cancer risk." *Am J Epidemiol* **123**(2): 302–307.

zur Hausen, H. (1977). "Human papillomaviruses and their possible role in squamous cell carcinomas." *Curr Top Microbiol Immunol* **78**: 1–30.

Zwaveling, S., S.C. Ferreira Mota, et al. (2002). "Established human papillomavirus type 16-expressing tumors are effectively eradicated following vaccination with long peptides." *J Immunol* **169**(1): 350–358.

Ovarian Cancer Prevention

Kathryn Coe, Ana Maria Lopez, and Lisa M. Hess

College of Medicine, University of Arizona, Tucson, AZ 85724

Ovarian cancer is the fifth most commonly diagnosed cancer in women in the United States (U.S.) excluding non-melanoma skin cancers. It accounts for about 25,800 cancer diagnoses each year. The average lifetime risk for developing ovarian cancer in the U.S. is about 1 in 59. Although most cases may be sporadic, the most clinically significant risk factors include *BRCA1/2* mutations, aging, a previous diagnosis of breast cancer, and having a first-degree relative (mother, sister, or daughter) who has been diagnosed with ovarian cancer. Some factors that may protect women from ovarian cancer are modifiable (e.g. oral contraceptive use, regular intake of aspirin), while other possible protective factors are not (e.g. race, multiparity).

Ovarian cancer is not a single disease; there are 30 types and subtypes of ovarian malignancies, each with its own histopathologic appearance, biologic behavior and possible etiology (Hildreth, Kelsey et al. 1981). Ovarian malignancies are categorized into three major groups: epithelial; germ cell; and sex cord-stromal tumors.

Ovarian cancer that begins on the surface of the ovary (epithelial ovarian carcinoma) is the most common type; 85 to 90% of ovarian cancers originate in the ovarian surface epithelium (Bai, Oliveros-Saunders et al. 2000). Malignant germ cell tumors and sex cord-stromal tumors are less common. Carcinosarcoma of the ovary, defined by the presence of malignant epithelial and mesenchymal elements, accounts for fewer than 1% of ovarian malignancies. Occasionally, the site of origin is in the peritoneum. Ovarian and peritoneal cancers are similar in terms of their tissue of origin, clinical and pathologic presentation, and response to standard treatment regimens. Most often, it is impossible to make a clear distinction between an ovarian and peritoneal carcinoma and peritoneal carcinoma may be a variant, or subset, of ovarian cancer (Barda, Menczer et al. 2004).

In 2004, approximately 25,800 women were diagnosed with ovarian cancer and 16,090 died from the disease in the U.S. (Jemal, Tiwari et al. 2004). While a number of prognostic factors influence ovarian cancer survival (e.g. stage of disease at diagnosis, age at diagnosis), if diagnosed in its early stages, ovarian cancer is curable in a high percentage of patients (McGuire, Herrinton et al. 2002). However, as ovarian cancer is often asymptomatic in early stages, most patients (roughly 75%) have metastatic disease at the time of diagnosis (Goodman, Correa et al. 2003).

The overall five-year survival rate of ovarian cancer is 53% for all stages, a rate which drops to 28.8% in women age 65 and older (Ries 2004). Over the past 20 years, ovarian cancer mortality has remained more or less constant despite the introduction of new chemotherapy agents. It is likely that these mortality data will not change until there are effective screening technologies to detect early stage disease.

Risk Factors for Ovarian Cancer

The incidence rate of ovarian cancer varies internationally, with lower incidence in Japan and higher rates among women of North America and northern Europe (Holschneider and Berek 2000; Bray, Loos et al. 2005). Data from cancer registries indicate that epithelial ovarian cancer rates are generally higher in industrialized nations, with the exception of Japan, and lower in non-industrialized parts of the world, such as Sub-Saharan Africa and China (Katchy and Briggs 1992; Holschneider and Berek 2000). The first step in understanding the risk factors for ovarian cancer involves the process of repeated, uninterrupted ovulation, which is a trigger for potential malignant transformation of ovarian epithelial cells.

Ovarian cancer is a disease of aging (Yancik 1993). Incidence begins to rise in the late teenage years and gradually increases with age. After age 40, incidence and mortality rise sharply and the highest incidence occurs among women from 80 to 84 years of age (61.8 per 100,000 women) (Edmondson and Monaghan 2001). While certain reproductive factors, such as multiparity and breastfeeding, may offer protection against ovarian cancer, others, including early onset of menstruation, nulliparity, and having a first child after age 30, may increase risk. Thus, factors that reduce the total number of ovulations reduce ovarian cancer risk and those that increase the number of ovulations tend to increase risk.

Family History. A family history of ovarian cancer, especially if two or more first- or second-degree relatives have been affected, is associated with an increased risk of ovarian cancer. Ovarian cancers tend to occur at an early age among cancer family members (e.g., before age 50) and tend to be advanced serous epithelial cancers.

Approximately 10% of all ovarian cancers are associated with family history and inherited genetic factors, such as *BRCA1/2* mutations (Claus, Schildkraut et al. 1996). *BRCA1* and *BRCA2* are genes that normally work together to prevent breast and ovarian cancer; however, in some cases a mutated or altered form of *BRCA1* or *BRCA2* is inherited. This mutation interferes with the normal activity of the gene, making individuals more susceptible to both breast and ovarian cancer. Individuals with one of these gene mutations have a higher risk of developing breast and ovarian cancers and may also pass that gene mutation on to his or her children. Researchers have identified three ways in which ovarian cancer can be inherited (Fig. 1). The syndromes include the Site-Specific Ovarian Cancer Syndrome, the Breast/Ovarian Cancer Syndromes (involving mutation in either the *BRCA1* or *BRCA2* genes) and the Lynch Syndrome II, which applies to women with female or male relatives who have had nonpolyposis-related colorectal or endometrial cancer (Murdoch and McDonnel 2002). Mutations at other loci, such as p53, may explain other inherited ovarian cancer cases (Sellers, Gapstur et al. 1993).

The *BRCA* genes seem to work differently in different environments; a number of factors (e.g. reproductive history, hormone therapy, diet, and the presence of other genes which, for example, control the metabolism of hormones) modify the effect of any gene in determining the final outcome. For women with a *BRCA1* mutation, the lifetime risk of ovarian cancer is approximately 54% and for women with *BRCA2* mutations, it is about 23% (Couzin 2003) (Table 1). All cancers are ultimately determined by a combination of genetic and environmental factors.

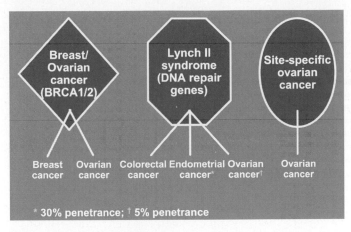

Fig. 1. Ovarian cancer syndromes

Endogenous Hormones. Women who give birth to their first child at age 25 or younger have a decreased risk of ovarian cancer (Daly and Obrams 1998). Higher risk of ovarian cancer is associated with first childbirth after age 35 (Negri, Franceschi et al. 1991). Nulliparous women experience a higher risk of ovarian cancer (Negri, Franceschi et al. 1991). In a prospective cohort study of 31,377 Iowa women, age 55 to 69, nulliparous women with a family history of ovarian cancer were at much higher risk than were their parous counterparts (relative risk = 2.7, 95% confidence interval [CI]: 1.1–6.6) (Vachon, Mink et al. 2002). There was an increased risk for nulliparous women when family history included first- and second-degree relatives with breast or ovarian cancer.

An analysis of pooled interview data on infertility and fertility drug use from eight case-control studies conducted in the U.S., Denmark, Canada and Australia found that nulligravid women who attempted to become pregnant for more than five years, compared with nulligravid women who attempted to become pregnant for less than one year, experienced a 2.7-fold increased risk of ovarian cancer (Ness, Cramer et al. 2002). Significant controversy surrounds the relationships among infertility, fertility drug use and the risk of ovarian cancer (Sit, Modugno et al. 2002). These pooled interview data on infertility and fertility drug use found that among nulliparous, subfertile women, neither use of any fertility drug nor use of fertility drug for more than 12 months were associated with ovarian cancer risk (Ness, Cramer et al. 2002). These

Table 1. Lifetime risk of ovarian cancer

Family history of ovarian cancer	Lifetime risk
None	1.5%
One first degree relative	5%
Two first degree relatives	7%
Hereditary ovarian cancer syndrome	40%
Known *BRCA1/2* germline mutation	35–65%

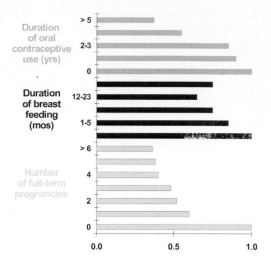

Fig. 2. Protective effects of oral contraceptives, breastfeeding and multiparity (Whittemore, Harris et al. 1992)

data suggest that specific biological causes of infertility, and not the use of fertility drugs, may play a role in overall risk for ovarian cancer.

Multiparity appears to decrease the risk of ovarian cancer (Daly and Obrams 1998). The Nurses Cohort Study of 121,700 women found that parity reduced ovarian cancer risk (odds ratio [OR] = 0.84; 95% CI: 0.77–0.91 for each pregnancy) (Hankinson, Colditz et al. 1995). A summary of seven case-control studies found that one full-term pregnancy had a significant reduction on ovarian cancer risk (OR = 0.47) (John, Whittemore et al. 1993). Risk decreased as the number of pregnancies increased; after six full-term pregnancies, the odds ratio was 0.29, with a 95% confidence interval of 0.20–0.42. Risk declined by about 15% for each additional full-term pregnancy (Risch, Marrett et al. 1994). As shown in Figure 2, data collected by Whittemore et al. (Whittemore, Harris et al. 1992) demonstrate the protective effects of oral contraceptive (OC) use, breastfeeding and multiparity.

Early menarche has been associated with increased risk of ovarian cancer in a number of studies conducted in the U.S. and elsewhere (Wu, Whittemore et al. 1988). Late menopause has been associated with a higher risk of ovarian cancer (Hildreth, Kelsey et al. 1981; Malik 2002). The lifetime cumulative duration of ovulation may play a role in the risk of ovarian cancer, which is demonstrated by the protective effects of ovulation inhibition, such as by hysterectomy or oral contraceptive use.

Epidemiologic studies suggest that tubal ligation and prior hysterectomy may decrease the risk of ovarian cancer. In a case-control study, Rosenblatt and Thomas (Rosenblatt and Thomas 1996) found that the possible protective effect of tubal ligation was greatest in women of parity less than four and that the protective effect was only for clear cell and endometrioid tumors. When Cramer and Xu (Cramer and Xu 1995) combined data from two case-control studies, they found that both tubal ligation and prior hysterectomy were protective.

Exogenous Hormones. Estrogens may act as promoters in the carcinogenic process and occasionally their metabolites may act as antihormones or have other physiologic effects (Lipsett 1979). As oral contraceptives (OCs) suppress ovulation, they have demonstrated the potential to reduce risk of ovarian cancer. In a follow-up analysis of the Norwegian Women and Cancer Cohort Study, there were 171 cases of ovarian cancer diagnosed in the 96,355-woman cohort. The risk of ovarian cancer decreased with the use of oral contraceptives (p for trend <0.0001) (Kumle, Alsaker et al. 2003). In Australia, a case-control study examined the effects of oral contraceptive use (Siskind, Green et al. 2000). After controlling for estimated number of ovulatory cycles, the protective effect of oral contraceptive use appeared to be multiplicative. There was a 7% decrease in relative risk per year that persisted beyond 15 years of exposure (95% CI: 4.0–9.0%). Even short-term use, up to one year, may have an effect (OR=0.57; 95% CI: 0.40–0.82) (Siskind, Green et al. 2000).

Women with pathogenic mutations in the *BRCA1* and *BRCA2* genes may also experience a reduced risk of ovarian cancer with OC use (Narod, Risch et al. 1998). Any history of OC use was associated with a 0.5 odds ratio (95% CI: 0.3–0.8). OC use was protective for both *BRCA1* (OR=0.5; 95% CI: 0.3–0.9) and *BRCA2* mutation carriers (OR= 0.4; 95% CI: 0.2–1.1) (Narod, Risch et al. 1998). A population-based case-control study of 767 women also found that four to eight years of OC use may reduce the risk of ovarian cancer by approximately 50% in women with a family history of the disease (Walker, Schlesselman et al. 2002).

Hormone replacement therapy (HRT) and estrogen replacement therapy (ERT) may also be related to ovarian cancer risk. While the data associating ovarian cancer to HRT have been inconsistent (Sit, Modugno et al. 2002), this inconsistency may be related to the fact that estrogen formulations in HRT vary in their effects on estrogen-sensitive target tissues, such as the ovary. A prospective study of 211,581 healthy post-menopausal women in the U.S. evaluated women who had taken oral HRT or ERT after age 35 to compare ovarian cancer mortality with the effect of HRT (Rodriguez, Patel et al. 2001). Risk of ovarian cancer mortality was reported to be higher in HRT users at baseline and slightly higher for previous users than never users. Risk doubled with ten years or more duration of use; however, only 66 of the 944 women who died of ovarian cancer had used HRT for at least 10 years. Furthermore, most of these 66 women took unopposed estrogen (ERT) during the 1970s and early 1980s, when the use of higher doses of synthetic estrogen was common.

Others have also found that long-term, high-dose unopposed ERT may increase the risk of ovarian cancer (Drew 2001). A study of 44,241 postmenopausal women found that those who used ERT, particularly use for ten years or more, were at significantly increased risk of ovarian cancer (Lacey, Mink et al. 2002). Women who used short-term HRT did not experience increased risk. A study of 655 histologically-verified epithelial ovarian cancer cases and 3,899 randomly selected controls found that risk of ovarian cancer was elevated among ever users as compared with never users of both ERT and HRT (Riman, Dickman et al. 2002). Ever users of ERT and HRT-sequentially added progestins, but not HRT-continuously added progestins, may increase risk of ovarian cancer (Riman, Dickman et al. 2002).

Sociodemographic Factors. In 2004, the incidence rates of ovarian cancer in U.S. Latina, American Indian and African American women were lower than those for white women; however, the lower incidence does not correspond to a lower mortality rate from ovarian cancer among these populations (Jemal, Tiwari et al. 2004; Ries 2004). The difference in incidence rates among racial/ethnic groups can be at least partially explained by reproductive histories, which in turn are influenced by culture (Daly 1992). Women of Ashkenazi Jewish ancestry are reported to be at greater risk for ovarian cancer because they are more likely to have inherited and to carry a mutation in BRCA1 or BRCA2 (Daly and Obrams 1998; Steinberg, Pernarelli et al. 1998; Koifman and Jorge Koifman 2001).

Poverty, which is associated with ethnicity in the U.S. as well as various parts of the world, may be a risk factor for a number of chronic diseases, including ovarian cancer. This risk may be conferred through an association with smoking, nutrition, alcohol consumption or exposure to certain infectious agents. Ethnicity, when associated with poverty, also may be related to increases in ovarian cancer mortality (Averette, Janicek et al. 1995; McGuire, Herrinton et al. 2002), although this relationship has not been consistent (Polednak 1992; Brewster, Thomson et al. 2001).

Diet. A number of studies have proposed that high dietary fat intake is associated with increased risk of epithelial ovarian cancer; this conclusion, however, remains speculative in part due to the fact that the mechanism by which dietary fat, or even stored fat, increases risk is unknown. The effect of dietary fat may be independent or may act primarily though an influence on hormonal status. Dietary fat consumption appears to impact enteric reabsorption of steroid hormones mediated by the intestinal flora (Mansfield 1993). A meta-analysis of the association between high as compared to low dietary fat intake and risk of ovarian cancer found that high dietary fat intake appeared to represent a significant risk factor in the development of ovarian cancer (Huncharek and Kupelnick 2001). A case-control study in China investigated whether dietary factors had an etiological association with ovarian cancer (Zhang, Yang et al. 2002). Controlling for demographic, lifestyle, familial factors, hormonal status, family history and total energy intake, ovarian cancer risk decreased with a high consumption of vegetables and fruits and increased with high intake of animal fat and salted vegetables. Risk appeared to increase among women who consumed high fat, fried, cured and smoked foods (Zhang, Yang et al. 2002).

Dietary sugar consumption may be related to increased risk of ovarian cancer based on evidence that galactose may be toxic to ovarian germ cells (Cramer, Harlow et al. 1998). In populations with a high dietary intake of lactose and in which individuals lack the enzyme galactose-1-phosphate uridyltransferase (GALT), galactose and its metabolites accumulate in the ovary. If galactose raises gonadotropin levels, the ovarian epithelium may proliferate. Preliminary evidence suggests that certain genetic or biochemical features of galactose metabolism may influence the risk for particular types of ovarian cancer (Cramer, Greenberg et al. 2000).

Tea, which is consumed on a daily basis in many parts of the world, may decrease risk for ovarian cancer. One case-control study found that the risk of ovarian cancer declined with increasing frequency and duration of overall tea consumption (Zhang, Binns et al. 2002). The mechanism for this reduced risk is unclear and this finding has yet to be thoroughly evaluated.

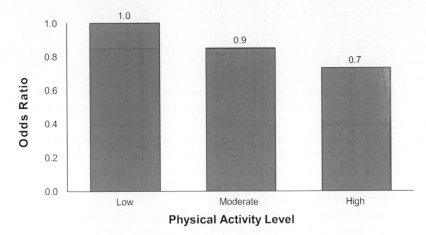

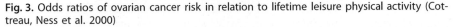

Fig. 3. Odds ratios of ovarian cancer risk in relation to lifetime leisure physical activity (Cottreau, Ness et al. 2000)

Obesity and Physical Activity. While obesity is more common in westernized than non-westernized societies, women in some ethnic groups are more likely to be obese. In the U.S., over 30% of all adults are obese, according to analyses of the National Health and Nutrition Examination Survey (1999–2000) (Flegal, Carroll et al. 2002). In this study, there were higher rates of obesity in certain racial groups; more than half of adult African American women over the age of 40 were obese. Obesity and body fat distribution may increase risk for ovarian cancer, perhaps due to the effect of obesity on estrogen levels. Further, where the body fat is stored and the age at which obesity occurs may also be important in ovarian cancer risk. Women who have a high waist-to-hip ratio and a family history of ovarian cancer experience a 4.83-fold increased risk (95% CI: 1.55–15.1) (Sellers, Gapstur et al. 1993). An analysis of data from 109,445 women who participated in the Nurses' Health Study found that women who were overweight as teenagers may be more likely to develop premenopausal ovarian cancer (Fairfield, Willett et al. 2002).

Physical activity has demonstrated a protective effect against ovarian cancer. A case-control study (767 cases and 1367 controls) found that leisure-time physical activity was associated with a reduction in the incidence of ovarian cancer ($p=0.01$) (Cottreau, Ness et al. 2000). This association remained statistically significant even after controlling for tubal ligation, age, body mass index, family history, and OC use (OR = 0.73; 95% CI: 0.56–0.94) (Fig. 3).

Early Detection and Prevention of Ovarian Cancer

Ovarian cancer is the leading cause of gynecologic cancer death. Most patients are diagnosed with advanced disease (stage III or IV) (Ries 2004) because there are few early warning symptoms or signs to alert the patient or the clinician to its presence. Tumors that are identified and treated when the disease has not progressed beyond stage I result in a 5-year survival rate of over 80% (Rosenthal and Jacobs 1998).

Screening. Screening for ovarian cancer is difficult because the disease is not highly prevalent in the general population (only 0.075% of the U.S. female population has been diagnosed with ovarian cancer) (Ries 2004). A woman's lifetime risk of developing ovarian cancer is 1 in 59 (Gloeckler Ries, Reichman et al. 2003). An effective screening test for ovarian cancer would have a sensitivity of at least 80% for early-stage, curable disease, a positive predictive value of at least 10% and consequently, a specificity of over 99% (Jacobs 1998). To date, there are no screening methods for ovarian cancer available to the general population.

The CA-125 antigen is a reliable marker for disease progression or regression in most women who have been diagnosed with ovarian cancer (Gladstone 1994). Despite its reliability in the ovarian cancer patient, it is not a useful screening marker due to its lack of specificity. CA-125 levels vary with the menstrual cycle and are elevated in approximately 20 other benign conditions (Buamah 2000). When used as a screening tool in the general population, it has only a 21–33% positive detection rate (Hakama, Stenman et al. 1996).

Most imaging technologies currently available are not well suited for the detection of ovarian cancer. Computed tomography (CT) scans and magnetic resonance imaging (MRI) are not sensitive enough for early detection (generally cannot detect lesions less than one centimeter in diameter, especially in the pelvis) and as a result, they tend to have a high rate of false negative results even among women undergoing evaluation for recurrence (van der Burg, Lammes et al. 1993; De Rosa, Mangoni di Stefano et al. 1995). Although cost prohibitive, positron emission tomography (PET) scans are more sensitive than a CT scan for the evaluation of lesions. The PET scan, like a CT scan, has more value in the setting of evaluation for recurrent disease or for ruling out/confirming the growth of an existing tumor than for general screening purposes. A better option for patients with indications of ovarian cancer or other diseases (e.g. fibroid tumor, pelvic inflammatory disease) is ultrasound since it can generally detect the presence of a mass.

Improved technologies, such as a transvaginal ultrasound (TVUS) or transvaginal sonography (TVS) have a calculated specificity and sensitivity of 98.9 and 81%, respectively (van Nagell, DePriest et al. 2000). This improvement is due to the fact that with transvaginal procedures, the transducer is closer to the ovaries as compared to standard ultrasound procedures. Unfortunately, the positive predictive value is low (9.3%), as it is unable to differentiate benign conditions. Furthermore, TVS is unable to detect peritoneal cancers or cancers that do not affect ovary size.

At this time, these methods are generally only used when there is substantial risk of ovarian cancer and surgery is not a reasonable or preferred option. Despite their limitations, a combined strategy of CA-125 evaluations plus TVUS is currently the recommended screening option for women at high risk who no not elect to undergo surgery (DHHS 1996). This strategy is not recommended for population-based screening.

Prior to implementing an ovarian cancer prevention program, the at-risk population needs to be defined. This can only be accomplished currently by questioning the patient about her family history. Since only 10% of women with ovarian cancer have a positive family history for ovarian cancer (Schildkraut and Thompson 1988), additional methodology to identify women who may be at risk must be developed. Research to better understand the development and progression of premalignant changes in the ovary is ongoing.

Prevention. Women at high risk of ovarian cancer (e.g. *BRCA1/2* mutation, family history) frequently choose to undergo surgical removal of the ovaries and fallopian tubes (risk-reducing oophorectomy) in an attempt to reduce the risk of developing ovarian cancer, as it is currently the most effective method to reduce risk and to identify early cancers (Rebbeck 2000). Risk-reducing surgery results in a significant reduction of the lifetime risk of developing ovarian cancer (Nguyen, Averette et al. 1994). The true effectiveness of surgery to successfully prevent ovarian cancer is unknown at this time, although preliminary evidence suggests that there is a 90% reduction in the risk of ovarian cancer among *BRCA1* mutation carriers following prophylactic oophorectomy, as well as a 50% reduction in the risk of breast cancer (Rebbeck, Levin et al. 1999; Rebbeck 2000). Two to 10 percent of patients who undergo oophorectomy will still be diagnosed with ovarian or peritoneal cancer at some point following surgery (Tobacman, Greene et al. 1982; Piver, Jishi et al. 1993). Among women who are at high risk and select surgery, reports demonstrate that nine to 17% of women have had ovarian cancer detected incidentally during this surgical procedure (Morice, Pautier et al. 1999; Leeper, Garcia et al. 2002). Furthermore, future breast cancer risk is lowered among women who are at high risk and undergo prophylactic oophorectomy (Rebbeck, Levin et al. 1999). Despite its effectiveness in early detection and prevention of future cancers, surgery is not without risk. In addition to the general risks associated with abdominal surgery, removal of the reproductive organs in the pre-menopausal woman is associated with loss of fertility, induced menopause and its symptoms and adverse effects (e.g. bone loss, hormonal changes), and the need for long-term hormone replacement therapy. The potential benefits of surgery need to be weighed against the emotional stress of losing the ovaries and the physical consequences of premature menopause.

Early Detection. Although often called a clinically 'silent' disease, ovarian cancer is associated with symptoms that are consistent with those of menstruation, but are frequently more severe and persist longer than would be expected. Furthermore, woman will generally experience a greater number of these same symptoms (Goff, Mandel et al. 2004). Since approximately 80% of all cancers occur in the absence of family or genetic risk factors, the need to be alert to new onset, persistent symptomology cannot be understated. Symptoms of ovarian cancer include cramping, pelvic or abdominal pain, bloating, indigestion, increased abdominal size, urinary urgency, menstrual irregularities, or vaginal bleeding after menopause (Goff, Mandel et al. 2004; Yawn, Barrette et al. 2004).

Chemoprevention of Ovarian Cancer

The first step in understanding ovarian carcinogenesis involves the observation that nulliparous women are at higher risk for ovarian cancer. This hypothesis asserts that the process of repeated, uninterrupted ovulation is a trigger for potential malignant transformation of these cells. The ability of OCs to prevent ovulation has resulted in their study as an ovarian cancer preventive agent. It is currently estimated that over 50% of ovarian cancers could be prevented by the use of estrogen and progestin-containing OCs for at least five years (Stanford 1991; Ness, Grisso et al. 2000). An additional benefit of OC use may be an increased rate of progestin-induced apoptosis of aberrant epithelial cells as demonstrated in animal models (Rodriguez, Walmer et al. 1998). Although OC use may be effective as ovarian cancer prevention agents by preventing ovulation in the premenopausal woman, postmenopausal targets are also necessary since most ovarian cancers present after the age of 50.

Due to the hormone receptors on the ovarian epithelium, a number of potential chemotherapeutic agents are under investigation for their role in ovarian cancer prevention. Progestin therapy in the postmenopausal woman is one such agent under consideration. In animal models, progestins have been shown to induce apoptosis, inhibit proliferation and to upregulate TGF-β (transforming growth factor-beta) (Rodriguez, Walmer et al. 1998). As compared to control and ethinyl estradiol-treated monkeys, a statistically significant increase in apoptosis (six-fold) was noted in the ovarian epithelium of monkeys treated with levonorgestrel alone. The degree of apoptosis was not different between ethinyl estradiol-treated monkeys and controls. This demonstrated that exposure to the progestin component of oral contraceptives induced apoptosis in the ovarian epithelium (Rodriguez, Walmer et al. 1998). Apoptosis is the mechanism by which the body eliminates cells that have undergone DNA damage. Damaged cells that persist could lead to the development of a malignancy (Canman, Chen et al. 1994). The induction of apoptosis may also be the primary mechanism of action for a number of other chemopreventive agents, such as the retinoids (Delia, Aiello et al. 1993; Ponzoni, Bocca et al. 1995; Toma, Isnardi et al. 1997), anti-inflammatory drugs (Thompson, Jiang et al. 1997), and selenium (Thompson, Wilson et al. 1994; el-Bayoumy, Upadhyaya et al. 1995).

Vitamin A and its derivatives (retinoids) are under investigation as potential chemopreventive agents because of their ability to induce differentiation and inhibit cellular proliferation. Naturally-occurring retinoids often require high doses and are associated with significant side effects; therefore, vitamin A analogs have been developed. Fenretinide, N-(4-hydroxyphenyl)retinamide or 4-HPR, has been demonstrated to have antitumor activity in human ovarian cancer cell lines (Formelli and Cleris 1993). Further studies have demonstrated the antiproliferative and apoptotic effects of fenretinide (Supino, Crosti et al. 1996). Clinical trial data from a chemopreventive study of women with early-stage breast cancer revealed a statistically significant decreased incidence of ovarian cancer in the fenretinide treatment group (De Palo, Veronesi et al. 1995).

Nonsteroidal anti-inflammatory agents (NSAIDs), specifically COX-2 inhibitors [due to the high COX-2 positivity among ovarian cancer patients who do not respond to chemotherapy (Ferrandina, Ranelletti et al. 2002)], may have a potential role in the chemoprevention of ovarian cancer. The biologic mechanisms may be related to immune enhancement, inhibition of cyclooxygenase (COX) and inhibition of apoptosis associated with NSAID treatment (Rodriguez-Burford, Barnes et al. 2002). In preclinical models, aspirin induced inhibition of tumor cell growth (Drake and Becker 2002). Aspirin may work by reducing levels of cyclooxygenase or by blocking the HER-2/neu proto-oncogene, which is sometimes overexpressed in ovarian cancer. However, research to date has been inconclusive, with some preclinical studies demonstrating a possible protective effect, while case-control and cohort trials have not consistently seen a protective effect (Tavani, Gallus et al. 2000; Fairfield, Hunter et al. 2002). Much work has yet to be done to understand the mechanisms by which these agents may work and to identify the target population for clinical research trials.

References

Averette, H.E., M.F. Janicek, et al. (1995). "The National Cancer Data Base report on ovarian cancer. American College of Surgeons Commission on Cancer and the American Cancer Society." *Cancer* **76**(6): 1096–1103.

Bai, W., B. Oliveros-Saunders, et al. (2000). "Estrogen stimulation of ovarian surface epithelial cell proliferation." *In Vitro Cell Dev Biol Anim* **36**(10): 657–666.

Barda, G., J. Menczer, et al. (2004). "Comparison between primary peritoneal and epithelial ovarian carcinoma: a population-based study." *Am J Obstet Gynecol* **190**(4): 1039–1045.

Bray, F., A.H. Loos, et al. (2005). "Ovarian cancer in Europe: Cross-sectional trends in incidence and mortality in 28 countries, 1953–2000." *Int J Cancer* **113**(6): 977–990.

Brewster, D.H., C.S. Thomson, et al. (2001). "Relation between socioeconomic status and tumour stage in patients with breast, colorectal, ovarian, and lung cancer: results from four national, population based studies." *BMJ* **322**(7290): 830–831.

Buamah, P. (2000). "Benign conditions associated with raised serum CA-125 concentration." *J Surg Oncol* **75**(4): 264–265.

Canman, C.E., C.Y. Chen, et al. (1994). "DNA damage responses: p53 induction, cell cycle perturbations, and apoptosis." *Cold Spring Harb Symp Quant Biol* **59**: 277–286.

Claus, E.B., J.M. Schildkraut, et al. (1996). "The genetic attributable risk of breast and ovarian cancer." *Cancer* **77**(11): 2318–2324.

Cottreau, C.M., R.B. Ness, et al. (2000). "Physical activity and reduced risk of ovarian cancer." *Obstet Gynecol* **96**(4): 609–614.

Couzin, J. (2003). "Choices – and uncertainties – for women with BRCA mutations." *Science* **302**(5645): 592.

Cramer, D.W., E.R. Greenberg, et al. (2000). "A case-control study of galactose consumption and metabolism in relation to ovarian cancer." *Cancer Epidemiol Biomarkers Prev* **9**(1): 95–101.

Cramer, D.W., B.L. Harlow, et al. (1998). "Over-the-counter analgesics and risk of ovarian cancer." *Lancet* **351**(9096): 104–107.

Cramer, D.W. and H. Xu (1995). "Epidemiologic evidence for uterine growth factors in the pathogenesis of ovarian cancer." *Ann Epidemiol* **5**(4): 310–314.

Daly, M. and G.I. Obrams (1998). "Epidemiology and risk assessment for ovarian cancer." *Semin Oncol* **25**(3): 255–264.

Daly, M.B. (1992). "The epidemiology of ovarian cancer." *Hematol Oncol Clin North Am* **6**(4): 729–738.

De Palo, G., U. Veronesi, et al. (1995). "Can fenretinide protect women against ovarian cancer?" *J Natl Cancer Inst* **87**(2): 146–147.

De Rosa, V., M.L. Mangoni di Stefano, et al. (1995). "Computed tomography and second-look surgery in ovarian cancer patients. Correlation, actual role and limitations of CT scan." *Eur J Gynaecol Oncol* **16**(2): 123–129.

Delia, D., A. Aiello, et al. (1993). "N-(4-hydroxyphenyl)retinamide induces apoptosis of malignant hemopoietic cell lines including those unresponsive to retinoic acid." *Cancer Res* **53**(24): 6036–6041.

DHHS (1996). "Ovarian Cancer: Screening, Treatment and Followup." *NIH Consensus Statement* **12**(3): April 5–7.

Drake, J.G. and J.L. Becker (2002). "Aspirin-induced inhibition of ovarian tumor cell growth." *Obstet Gynecol* **100**(4): 677–682.

Drew, S.V. (2001). "Oestrogen replacement therapy and ovarian cancer." *Lancet* **358**(9296): 1910.

Edmondson, R.J. and J.M. Monaghan (2001). "The epidemiology of ovarian cancer." *Int J Gynecol Cancer* **11**(6): 423–429.

el-Bayoumy, K., P. Upadhyaya, et al. (1995). "Chemoprevention of cancer by organoselenium compounds." *J Cell Biochem Suppl* **22**: 92–100.

Fairfield, K.M., D.J. Hunter, et al. (2002). "Aspirin, other NSAIDs, and ovarian cancer risk (United States)." *Cancer Causes Control* **13**(6): 535–542.

Fairfield, K.M., W.C. Willett, et al. (2002). "Obesity, weight gain, and ovarian cancer." *Obstet Gynecol* **100**(2): 288–296.

Ferrandina, G., F.O. Ranelletti, et al. (2002). "Cyclooxygenase-2 (COX-2), epidermal growth factor receptor (EGFR), and Her-2/neu expression in ovarian cancer." *Gynecol Oncol* **85**(2): 305–310.

Flegal, K. M., M. D. Carroll, et al. (2002). "Prevalence and trends in obesity among US adults, 1999–2000." *JAMA* **288**(14): 1723–1727.

Formelli, F. and L. Cleris (1993). "Synthetic retinoid fenretinide is effective against a human ovarian carcinoma xenograft and potentiates cisplatin activity." *Cancer Res* **53**(22): 5374–5376.

Gladstone, C.Q. (1994). Screening for ovarian cancer. *In: Canadian Task Force on the Periodic Health Examination. Canadian Guide to Clinical Preventive Health Care*. Ottawa, Health Canada: 870–881.

Gloeckler Ries, L.A., M.E. Reichman, et al. (2003). "Cancer survival and incidence from the Surveillance, Epidemiology, and End Results (SEER) program." *Oncologist* **8**(6): 541–552.

Goff, B.A., L.S. Mandel, et al. (2004). "Frequency of symptoms of ovarian cancer in women presenting to primary care clinics." *JAMA* **291**(22): 2705–2712.

Goodman, M.T., C.N. Correa, et al. (2003). "Stage at diagnosis of ovarian cancer in the United States, 1992–1997." *Cancer* **97**(10 Suppl): 2648–2659.

Hakama, M., U.H. Stenman, et al. (1996). "CA 125 as a screening test for ovarian cancer." *J Med Screen* **3**(1): 40–42.

Hankinson, S.E., G.A. Colditz, et al. (1995). "A prospective study of reproductive factors and risk of epithelial ovarian cancer." *Cancer* **76**(2): 284–290.

Hildreth, N.G., J.L. Kelsey, et al. (1981). "An epidemiologic study of epithelial carcinoma of the ovary." *Am J Epidemiol* **114**(3): 398–405.

Holschneider, C.H. and J.S. Berek (2000). "Ovarian cancer: epidemiology, biology, and prognostic factors." *Semin Surg Oncol* **19**(1): 3–10.

Huncharek, M. and B. Kupelnick (2001). "Dietary fat intake and risk of epithelial ovarian cancer: a meta-analysis of 6,689 subjects from 8 observational studies." *Nutr Cancer* **40**(2): 87–91.

Jacobs, I. (1998). Overview-progress in screening for ovarian cancer. In: *Ovarian Cancer*. F. Sharp, A. Blackett, et al. (Eds.). Oxford, Isis Medical Media.

Jemal, A., R.C. Tiwari, et al. (2004). "Cancer statistics, 2004." *CA Cancer J Clin* **54**(1): 8–29.

John, E.M., A.S. Whittemore, et al. (1993). "Characteristics relating to ovarian cancer risk: collaborative analysis of seven U.S. case-control studies. Epithelial ovarian cancer in black women. Collaborative Ovarian Cancer Group." *J Natl Cancer Inst* **85**(2): 142–147.

Katchy, K.C. and N.D. Briggs (1992). "Clinical and pathological features of ovarian tumours in Rivers state of Nigeria." *East Afr Med J* **69**(8): 456–459.

Koifman, S. and R. Jorge Koifman (2001). "Breast cancer mortality among Ashkenazi Jewish women in Sao Paulo and Porto Alegre, Brazil." *Breast Cancer Res* **3**(4): 270–275.

Kumle, M., E. Alsaker, et al. (2003). "[Use of oral contraceptives and risk of cancer, a cohort study]." *Tidsskr Nor Laegeforen* **123**(12): 1653–1656.

Lacey, J.V., Jr., P.J. Mink, et al. (2002). "Menopausal hormone replacement therapy and risk of ovarian cancer." *JAMA* **288**(3): 334–341.

Leeper, K., R. Garcia, et al. (2002). "Pathologic findings in prophylactic oophorectomy specimens in high-risk women." *Gynecol Oncol* **87**(1): 52–56.

Lipsett, M.B. (1979). "Interaction of drugs, hormones, and nutrition in the causes of cancer." *Cancer* **43**(5 Suppl): 1967–1981.

Malik, I.A. (2002). "A prospective study of clinico-pathological features of epithelial ovarian cancer in Pakistan." *J Pak Med Assoc* **52**(4): 155–158.

Mansfield, C.M. (1993). "A review of the etiology of breast cancer." *J Natl Med Assoc* **85**(3): 217–221.

McGuire, V., L. Herrinton, et al. (2002). "Race, epithelial ovarian cancer survival, and membership in a large health maintenance organization." *Epidemiology* **13**(2): 231–234.

Morice, P., P. Pautier, et al. (1999). "Laparoscopic prophylactic oophorectomy in women with inherited risk of ovarian cancer." *Eur J Gynaecol Oncol* **20**(3): 202–204.

Murdoch, W.J. and A.C. McDonnel (2002). "Roles of the ovarian surface epithelium in ovulation and carcinogenesis." *Reproduction* **123**(6): 743–750.

Narod, S.A., H. Risch, et al. (1998). "Oral contraceptives and the risk of hereditary ovarian cancer. Hereditary Ovarian Cancer Clinical Study Group." *N Engl J Med* **339**(7): 424–428.

Negri, E., S. Franceschi, et al. (1991). "Pooled analysis of 3 European case-control studies: I. Reproductive factors and risk of epithelial ovarian cancer." *Int J Cancer* **49**(1): 50–56.

Ness, R.B., D.W. Cramer, et al. (2002). "Infertility, fertility drugs, and ovarian cancer: a pooled analysis of case-control studies." *Am J Epidemiol* **155**(3): 217–224.

Ness, R.B., J.A. Grisso, et al. (2000). "Risk of ovarian cancer in relation to estrogen and progestin dose and use characteristics of oral contraceptives. SHARE Study Group. Steroid Hormones and Reproductions." *Am J Epidemiol* **152**(3): 233–241.

Nguyen, H.N., H.E. Averette, et al. (1994). "Ovarian carcinoma. A review of the significance of familial risk factors and the role of prophylactic oophorectomy in cancer prevention." *Cancer* **74**(2): 545–555.

Piver, M.S., M.F. Jishi, et al. (1993). "Primary peritoneal carcinoma after prophylactic oophorectomy in women with a family history of ovarian cancer. A report of the Gilda Radner Familial Ovarian Cancer Registry." *Cancer* **71**(9): 2751–2755.

Polednak, A.P. (1992). "Cancer incidence in the Puerto Rican-born population of Connecticut." *Cancer* **70**(5): 1172–1176.

Ponzoni, M., P. Bocca, et al. (1995). "Differential effects of N-(4-hydroxyphenyl)retinamide and retinoic acid on neuroblastoma cells: apoptosis versus differentiation." *Cancer Res* **55**(4): 853–861.

Rebbeck, T.R. (2000). "Prophylactic oophorectomy in BRCA1 and BRCA2 mutation carriers." *J Clin Oncol* **18**(21 Suppl): 100S–103S.

Rebbeck, T.R., A.M. Levin, et al. (1999). "Breast cancer risk after bilateral prophylactic oophorectomy in BRCA1 mutation carriers." *J Natl Cancer Inst* **91**(17): 1475–1479.

Ries, L.A.G., M.P. Eisner, et al. (2004). *SEER Cancer Statistics Review, 1995–2001.* Bethesda, MD, National Cancer Institute.

Riman, T., P.W. Dickman, et al. (2002). "Risk factors for invasive epithelial ovarian cancer: results from a Swedish case-control study." *Am J Epidemiol* **156**(4): 363–373.

Risch, H.A., L.D. Marrett, et al. (1994). "Parity, contraception, infertility, and the risk of epithelial ovarian cancer." *Am J Epidemiol* **140**(7): 585–597.

Rodriguez, C., A.V. Patel, et al. (2001). "Estrogen replacement therapy and ovarian cancer mortality in a large prospective study of US women." *Jama* **285**(11): 1460–1465.

Rodriguez, G.C., D.K. Walmer, et al. (1998). "Effect of progestin on the ovarian epithelium of macaques: cancer prevention through apoptosis?" *J Soc Gynecol Investig* **5**(5): 271–276.

Rodriguez-Burford, C., M.N. Barnes, et al. (2002). "Effects of nonsteroidal anti-inflammatory agents (NSAIDs) on ovarian carcinoma cell lines: preclinical evaluation of NSAIDs as chemopreventive agents." *Clin Cancer Res* **8**(1): 202–209.

Rosenblatt, K.A. and D.B. Thomas (1996). "Reduced risk of ovarian cancer in women with a tubal ligation or hysterectomy. The World Health Organization Collaborative Study of Neoplasia and Steroid Contraceptives." *Cancer Epidemiol Biomarkers Prev* **5**(11): 933–935.

Rosenthal, A. and I. Jacobs (1998). "Ovarian cancer screening." *Semin Oncol* **25**(3): 315–325.

Schildkraut, J.M. and W.D. Thompson (1988). "Familial ovarian cancer: a population-based case-control study." *Am J Epidemiol* **128**(3): 456–466.

Sellers, T.A., S.M. Gapstur, et al. (1993). "Association of body fat distribution and family histories of breast and ovarian cancer with risk of postmenopausal breast cancer." *Am J Epidemiol* **138**(10): 799–803.

Siskind, V., A. Green, et al. (2000). "Beyond ovulation: oral contraceptives and epithelial ovarian cancer." *Epidemiology* **11**(2): 106–110.

Sit, A.S., F. Modugno, et al. (2002). "Hormone replacement therapy formulations and risk of epithelial ovarian carcinoma." *Gynecol Oncol* **86**(2): 118–123.

Stanford, J.L. (1991). "Oral contraceptives and neoplasia of the ovary." *Contraception* **43**(6): 543–556.

Steinberg, K.K., J.M. Pernarelli, et al. (1998). "Increased risk for familial ovarian cancer among Jewish women: a population-based case-control study." *Genet Epidemiol* **15**(1): 51–59.

Supino, R., M. Crosti, et al. (1996). "Induction of apoptosis by fenretinide (4HPR) in human ovarian carcinoma cells and its association with retinoic acid receptor expression." *Int J Cancer* **65**(4): 491–497.

Tavani, A., S. Gallus, et al. (2000). "Aspirin and ovarian cancer: an Italian case-control study." *Ann Oncol* **11**(9): 1171–1173.

Thompson, H.J., C. Jiang, et al. (1997). "Sulfone metabolite of sulindac inhibits mammary carcinogenesis." *Cancer Res* **57**(2): 267–271.

Thompson, H.J., A. Wilson, et al. (1994). "Comparison of the effects of an organic and an inorganic form of selenium on a mammary carcinoma cell line." *Carcinogenesis* **15**(2): 183–186.

Tobacman, J.K., M.H. Greene, et al. (1982). "Intra-abdominal carcinomatosis after prophylactic oophorectomy in ovarian-cancer-prone families." *Lancet* **2**(8302): 795–797.

Toma, S., L. Isnardi, et al. (1997). "Effects of all-trans-retinoic acid and 13-cis-retinoic acid on breast-cancer cell lines: growth inhibition and apoptosis induction." *Int J Cancer* **70**(5): 619–627.

Vachon, C.M., P.J. Mink, et al. (2002). "Association of parity and ovarian cancer risk by family history of breast or ovarian cancer in a population-based study of postmenopausal women." *Epidemiology* **13**(1): 66–71.

van der Burg, M.E., F.B. Lammes, et al. (1993). "The role of CA 125 and conventional examinations in diagnosing progressive carcinoma of the ovary." *Surg Gynecol Obstet* **176**(4): 310–314.

van Nagell, J.R., Jr., P.D. DePriest, et al. (2000). "The efficacy of transvaginal sonographic screening in asymptomatic women at risk for ovarian cancer." *Gynecol Oncol* **77**(3): 350–356.

Walker, G.R., J.J. Schlesselman, et al. (2002). "Family history of cancer, oral contraceptive use, and ovarian cancer risk." *Am J Obstet Gynecol* **186**(1): 8–14.

Whittemore, A.S., R. Harris, et al. (1992). "Characteristics relating to ovarian cancer risk: collaborative analysis of 12 US case-control studies. IV. The pathogenesis of epithelial ovarian cancer. Collaborative Ovarian Cancer Group." *Am J Epidemiol* **136**(10): 1212–1220.

Wu, M.L., A.S. Whittemore, et al. (1988). "Personal and environmental characteristics related to epithelial ovarian cancer. I. Reproductive and menstrual events and oral contraceptive use." *Am J Epidemiol* **128**(6): 1216–1227.

Yancik, R. (1993). "Ovarian cancer. Age contrasts in incidence, histology, disease stage at diagnosis, and mortality." *Cancer* **71**(2 Suppl): 517–523.

Yawn, B.P., B.A. Barrette, et al. (2004). "Ovarian cancer: the neglected diagnosis." *Mayo Clin Proc* **79**(10): 1277–1282.

Zhang, M., C.W. Binns, et al. (2002). "Tea consumption and ovarian cancer risk: a case-control study in China." *Cancer Epidemiol Biomarkers Prev* **11**(8): 713–718.

Zhang, M., Z.Y. Yang, et al. (2002). "Diet and ovarian cancer risk: a case-control study in China." *Br J Cancer* **86**(5): 712–717.

Cancer Survivorship

Robert Krouse[1] and Noreen M. Aziz[2]

[1] College of Medicine, University of Arizona, Tucson, AZ 85724
[2] Division of Cancer Control & Population Science, National Cancer Institute, Bethesda, MD 20892

Survival from cancer has improved quite dramatically over the past three decades as a result of advances in early detection, adjuvant and other aggressive therapeutic strategies, and the widespread use of combined modality therapy (surgery, chemotherapy, and radiotherapy). Cancers such as testicular, childhood leukemia, and Hodgkin's lymphoma are now considered amenable to cure, patients with common cancers such as breast or colorectal can look forward to a vastly improved disease free and overall survival, and patients with potentially incurable disease can look forward to living for extended periods of time as a result of better disease control (Meadows 1980; Ganz 1998; Schwartz 1999; Aziz 2002; Aziz and Rowland 2003). However, the therapeutic modalities mentioned are associated with a spectrum of late complications ranging from minor and treatable to serious or, occasionally, potentially lethal. One-fourth of late deaths occurring among survivors during the extended survivorship period, when the chances of primary disease recurrence are negligible, can be attributed to a treatment-related effect such as a second cancer or cardiac dysfunction. Most frequently observed sequelae include endocrine complications, growth hormone deficiency, primary hypothyroidism, and primary ovarian failure (Sklar 1999). Also included within the rubric of late effects are second malignant neoplasms arising as a result of genetic predisposition (e.g., familial cancer syndromes) or the mutagenic effects of therapy. These factors may act independently or synergistically. Synergistic effects of mutagenic agents such as cigarette smoke or toxins such as alcohol are largely unknown.

There is today a greater recognition of symptoms that persist following completion of treatment and those that arise years after primary therapy. Both acute organ toxicities, such as radiation pneumonitis, and chronic toxicities, such as congestive cardiac failure, neurocognitive deficits, infertility, and second malignancies, are being described as the price of cure or prolonged survival.

Generally, long-term cancer survivors are defined as those individuals who are five or more years beyond the diagnosis of their primary disease. *Long-term effects* refer to any side effects or complications of treatment for which a cancer patient must compensate; also known as persistent effects, they begin during treatment and continue beyond the end of treatment. *Late effects*, in contrast, appear months to years after the completion of treatment. Since tissue damage noted during or at the end of therapy may remain stable or become progressive, late effects refer specifically to these unrecognized toxicities that are absent or subclinical at the end of therapy but manifest later as a result of growth, development, increased demand, or aging. These can be due to any of the following factors: developmental processes; the failure of compensatory mechanisms with the passage of time; or organ senescence. Compensatory mechanisms that initially maintain the function of injured organs may fail over time or with organ senescence. Persistent symptoms differ from late effects of treatment because they begin during treatment and continue following treatment rather than appearing months to years after the completion of treatment (Kolb and Poetscher 1997). Some researchers classify cognitive problems, fatigue, lymphedema, and peripheral neuropathy as persistent symptoms. Patients demonstrating signs or symptoms of late or long-term effects may have to undergo major adjustments to a lifestyle for which they are unprepared (Loescher, Welch-McCaffrey et al. 1989; Welch-McCaffrey, Hoffman et al. 1989; Herold and Roetzheim 1992; Marina 1997; Aziz 2002).

Late effects of cancer treatment occur because effects of therapy on maturing organs may become manifest only with time or with the unmasking of hitherto unseen injury to immature organs by developmental processes (Schwartz 1999; Aziz 2002). The study of late effects, originally within the realm of pediatric cancer, is now germaine to cancer survivors at all ages as concerns may continue to surface throughout the life cycle. These concerns underscore the need to follow up and screen survivors of cancer for toxicities in order to prevent or ameliorate these problems (Aziz 2002; Aziz and Rowland 2003).

Prevalence

The number of cancer survivors in the United States has risen steadily over the past three decades for all cancers combined. In 1971, only 3.0 million people were living with cancer, representing approximately 1.5% of the population. Recent estimates suggest that there are now 9.8 million cancer survivors in the United States, representing approximately 3.5% of the population. In the absence of other competing causes of death, current figures indicate that for adults whose cancer is diagnosed today, 64% can expect to be alive in 5 years; this is up from 50% estimated for those with a cancer diagnosis during 1974 through 1976. Among children, 79% of childhood cancer survivors will be alive at 5 years and nearly 75% at 10 years, compared with 56% alive 5 years after diagnosis during 1974 through 1976. Of child and adult survivors, 14% had a cancer diagnosis 20 or more years ago. More women than men are survivors, even though more males than females receive a cancer diagnosis annually. Men have a higher proportion of lung cancer, for which survival is poor, whereas women have higher proportions of readily detectable and treatable cancers (e.g., breast, gynecologic). Additionally, women generally have a lower all-cause mortality rate than men. Of the prevalent cancer population, the largest constituent group is breast cancer survivors (22%), followed by survivors of prostate cancer (17%), colorectal cancer (11%) and gynecologic cancer (10%). Cancer is a disease associated with aging. Sixty percent of all newly diagnosed cancers occur among people aged 65 or older, and most survivors (61%) are aged 65 or older. Researchers currently estimate that one of every six persons over the age of 65 is living with a history of cancer. Thirty-three percent of cancer survivors are between the ages of 40 and 64, 5% are 20 to 39 years of age, and less than 1% are 19 or younger (Aziz 2002; Aziz and Rowland 2003; Rowland 2004).

Fitzhugh Mullan, a physician diagnosed with and treated for cancer himself, first described cancer survivorship as a concept (Mullan 1985). Definitional issues for cancer survivorship encompass three related aspects. First, who is a cancer survivor? Philosophically, anyone who has been diagnosed with cancer is a survivor, from the time of diagnosis to the end of life (Aziz 2002; Aziz and Rowland 2003). Caregivers and family members are also included within this definition as secondary survivors. Second, what is cancer survivorship? Mullan described the survivorship experience as similar to the seasons of the year. He recognized three seasons or phases of survival: *acute* (extending from diagnosis to the completion of initial treatment, encompassing issues dominated by treatment and its side effects), *extended* (beginning with the completion of initial treatment for the primary disease, remission of disease, or both; dominated by watchful waiting, regular follow-up examinations and, perhaps, intermittent therapy) and *permanent* survival (not a single moment; evolves from extended disease-free survival when the likelihood of recurrence is sufficiently low). An understanding of these phases of survival is important for facilitating an optimal transition into and management of survivorship. Third, what is cancer survivorship research? Cancer survivorship research seeks to identify, examine, prevent, and control adverse cancer diagnosis and treatment-related outcomes (such as late effects of treatment, second cancers and quality of life), to provide a knowledge base regarding optimal follow-up care and surveillance of cancer survivors, and to optimize health after cancer treatment (Aziz 2002; Aziz and Rowland 2003).

Consistent with the shift in our perceptions of cancer as a chronic disease, new perspectives and an emerging body of scientific knowledge must now be incorporated into Mullan's original description of the survivorship experience (Aziz and Rowland 2003). Mullan's comparison of cancer survivorship with "seasons of the year" had implied that the availability and widespread use of curative and effective treatments would lead to a low likelihood of recurrence and longer survival times. However, the potential impact of late and long-term adverse physiologic and psychosocial effects of treatment was not described. In addition, further advances in survivorship research over the past few years have necessitated the incorporation of other emerging concepts into the evolving paradigm of cancer survivorship research (Aziz 2002; Aziz and Rowland 2003). These include: the key role of lifestyle and health promotion in ameliorating adverse treatment and disease-related consequences; the impact of comorbidities on a survivor's health status and their possible interaction with risk for or severity of late effects; the effect of cancer on the family; and the need for incorporating a developmental and life-stage perspective in order to facilitate optimally a cancer patient's journey into the survivorship phase. A developmental or life-stage perspective is particularly important as it carries the potential to affect and modify treatment decisions, the intensity of post-treatment follow-up care, the risk and severity of adverse sequelae of treatment, and the need for or use of technology (e.g., sperm banking) depending on the survivor's age at diagnosis and treatment) (Aziz 2002; Aziz and Rowland 2003).

Survivorship as a Scientific Discipline

The creation of the Office of Cancer Survivorship Program at the U.S. National Cancer Institute (NCI) in 1996 helped to highlight the key importance of cancer survivorship as a research area in its own right, and an integral part of the cancer prevention and control spectrum. Research related to cancer survivors, pertaining to the amelioration or management of adverse late or long-term sequelae of cancer and its treatment, the prevention, control, or management of sources of morbidity, and enhanced length and quality of survival, is a burgeoning area of interest among investigators, practitioners, survivor advocacy groups, and policy makers. Several highly successful research initiatives have been released over the past eight years by the Office of Cancer Survivorship in order to lay the foundation for and stimulate growth in key areas of cancer survivorship research. The large numbers of successful investigator-initiated grant submissions addressing cancer survivorship relevant research questions who pass through the same stringent scientific criteria for peer review as other grants at the National Institutes of Health (NIH) bear testament to the continued evolution and growth of this scientific discipline, as do the increasing numbers of peer reviewed manuscripts in leading national and international oncologic, medical, psychosocial, and health-related journals.

Prevention

The study of cancer prevention focuses on populations who are most at risk of a potential malignancy. Some populations are at such high risk of cancer that more aggressive treatment interventions may be advocated. Examples include patients with the familial polyposis syndromes or who carry BRCA-1 or BRCA-2 genes. In these instances, early surgical intervention or intense follow up is warranted.

The risk of colorectal cancer approaches 100% in those that suffer from familial polyposis syndromes. Therefore, it is the standard of care to recommend a total proctocolectomy, leaving the patient with either a permanent ileostomy or an ileal pouch anastamosis to the anus. There are many quality of life (QOL) considerations for each approach, such as the multifaceted problems associated with an intestinal stoma, or the risk of multiple bowel movements a day or pouchitis that is associated with an ileal pouch anastamosis. In addition, if the patient opts to leave part or the entire rectum in place, the patient must endure frequent proctoscopic examinations throughout life and will suffer inherent discomfort, along with the psychological stress of potential rectal cancer in the future. These patients must also face the possibility that there is also the chance for tumor occurring somewhere else in the alimentary tract, most notably the duodenum, and upper endoscopy is frequently recommended.

Hereditary breast or ovarian cancer is a second common example wherein a negative cancer survivorship outcome may be manifested in a setting that has generally been considered part of cancer prevention. Patients who are at higher risk must weigh the risks of BRCA-1 and BRCA-2 testing. If positive, patients may opt for prophylactic bilateral mastectomies, with or without reconstruction. Women must also consider bilateral oophorectomy related to the high risk of ovarian cancer (10–60% increased risk). Adverse medical, physiological, or psychological outcomes may be observed. For example, the impact of knowing that one is at a higher risk of cancer, the potential surgical procedure and its effect on self-image, the effect of suffering from possible lymphedema even without a lymph node dissection, and finally, the outcomes associated with undergoing early menopause, infertility, and concern for future generations.

Acute Effects of Treatment

Acute effects of treatment are those that occur during and soon after treatment. Patients suffer many side effects that need to be addressed throughout their course of therapy. Supportive care in the acute setting is focused on known side effects of treatments and, if possible, pre-emptively treating these problems. Surgical, radiation therapy, and chemotherapy techniques continue to make significant improvements that lead to better QOL for cancer survivors. For example, minimally invasive surgical techniques may reduce pain and post operative rehabilitation. Use of high dose brachytherapy for some sarcoma patients can simplify therapy such that patients are less isolated during these treatments. Finally, oral agents (e.g., 5-FU) enable a much simpler and less uncomfortable administation of chemotherapy for colorectal cancer patients.

Chemotherapy

There are many acute systemic effects related to chemotherapy. Presently, many of these can be adequately treated with medications to reduce the toxicity associated with current chemotherapy regimens. Gastrointestinal complications, such as nausea, vomiting, and diarrhea have historically been a major difficulty related to chemotherapy, as well as immunotherapy. They may be effectively treated with multiple medical strategies.

Nausea and Vomiting. Certain chemotherapeutics carry higher risks of nausea and vomiting, including doxirubicin, cisplatin, iphosphamide, and dacarbazube. Other risk factors may include chronic alcohol use, female gender, and a history of poor control of nausea and vomiting (Bartlett and Koczwara 2002). While persistent difficulties throughout therapy can lead to altering chemotherapy dosing or discontinuing treatments, initiating antiemetics with treaments can frequently control symptoms. In fact, the use of dexamethasone along with 5-HT$_3$ antagonists has been shown to completely control acute emesis in approximately 85 to 90% of patients (Bartlett and Koczwara 2002). For patients at moderate risk, dexamethasone alone can control emesis in 90% of patients. Other anti-emetics that can be useful in this setting are metoclopromide, prochorperazine, and benzodiazepines.

Asthenia is a problem with multiple potential etiologies (Von Hoff 1998). If related to anemia, multiple strategies can be attempted, the most straighforward being transfusional therapy. This is most useful for patients who have extremely low hemoglobin or those that are unresponsive to other treatments. Treatment with recombinant human erythropoietin, three times a week or weekly, has been shown to have response rates of 50 to 60% (Gordon 2002). Darbepoetin alfa, a newer erythropoiesis-stimulating protein, can be dosed weekly or every other week, and may show improved response rates (Gordon 2002). Increased hemoglobin levels are correlated with an improvement in symptoms of fatigue. While there are other mechanisms related to fatigue (i.e., other medical problems such as congestive heart failure, depression, homonal abnormalities, or cytokine production), future studies will help to discern other approaches to this problem.

Anorexia and Cachexia are frequently mentioned along with asthenia based on potentially similar pathophysiologies (Von Hoff 1998). Poor appetite and wasting frequently co-exist in a patient, either causally or due to similar etiologic mechanisms. Anorexia and cachexita are problems not only for patients, but are also stressful for families that watch loved ones become thinner and less energetic. Cachexia consists of a constellation of metabolic and symptomatic changes. These include a reduction in lean body tissues and fatty tissues, hypoglycemia, hypercalcemia, as well as asthenia and anorexia. Progressive weight loss is a common problem faced by cancer patients and is responsible not only for a reduced QOL and poor response to chemotherapy, but also a shorter survival time as compared to patients with comparable tumors who do not suffer from weight loss (Tisdale 1999). Medications such as megastrol acetate (Splinter 1992; Downer, Joel et al. 1993; Mantovani 1995; Neri, Garosi et al. 1997; De Conno, Martini et al. 1998; Mantovani, Maccio et al. 1998), medroxyprogesterone acetate (Splinter 1992; Downer, Joel et al. 1993; Mantovani 1995; Neri, Garosi et al. 1997; De Conno, Martini et al. 1998; Mantovani, Maccio et al. 1998), and potentially thalidomide (Bruera, Neumann et al. 1999) can be helpful for some patients, but further study is warranted.

Immunosuppression and Risk of Infection play an overwhelming role in a patient's QOL. The risk of infection mandates lifestyle changes for patients and as well as for families to protect their loved ones. This may include minimal contact with people, careful and frequent washing of hands, and the use of masks. Judicious use of antibiotics, along with cytokine therapy to enhance white blood cell counts, lessen infection (ASCO 1994). Granulocyte colony-stimulating factor has also been shown to reduce hospitalization and antibiotic therapy (Garcia-Carbonero, Mayordomo et al. 2001). Patients who maintain or achieve adequate white blood cell counts have an improved QOL and may be better able to tolerate of chemotherapy treatment (Jones, Schottstaedt et al. 1996), although this is not always seen (Steward, von Pawel et al. 1998).

Surgery

Operative therapies is frequently curative and QOL improving in a number of cancers (i.e., breast cancer, colon cancer, and melanoma). Improvement in QOL may be related to the removal of a potentially painful or problematic tumor-related wound (e.g., from a breast or skin cancer), or the removal of a tumor in the colon that had been causing bleeding or obstruction. For a tumor that is unlikely to be cured via an operation, such as esophageal or gastric cancers, surgical approaches have been shown improve the ability to swallow for many patients, which can in turn improve QOL (Branicki, Law et al. 1998). Surgical procedures can also lead to multiple acute morbidities. Risks associated with each surgical procedure must be carefully considered, as complications will still occur even in the most fastidious care, especially if the patient is debilitated related to the cancer or underlying conditions. First, surgical morbidity may include complications unrelated to the surgical site, such as pneumonia, deep venous thrombosis, ileus, and heart failure. With meticulous care, these can often be avoided. Related to the procedure itself, pain is a major issue that occurs in the postoperative setting, and may persist. Epidural, patient controlled analgesia, and local anesthetic pumps may improve pain control and ultimate outcomes. Improved outcomes can be seen as less impariment of pulmonary, bowel, mental functions, nutritional status, co-agulation, immune function, along with an increased risk of chronic pain (Karanikolas and Swarm 2000; Reid 2001; Fotiadis, Badvie et al. 2004). Acceptance of disfigurement and lifestyle changes are most pronounced in the immediate postoperative setting. For example, for many patients undergoing surgery related to colorectal cancer, the shock of a permanent stoma may be overwhelming. In fact, this may be the overwhelming issue of concern for patients with a new cancer, possibly even leading to delay in treatment (Cohen, Minsky et al. 1997). Recent evidence suggests that QOL problems related to ostomies may diminish with time, but nevertheless remain a significant factor in the postoperative setting (Krouse in preparation, 2004).

Wound complications must always be considered in the setting of cancer-related surgical procedures. This is certainly true of lymph node dissections; wound problems have been noted to be 47% for axillary node and 71% after inguinal node dissections (Serpell, Carne et al. 2003). Seromas and infections may take from several weeks to months to heal. Lymphatic leaks may necessitate procedures to isolate the offending lymphatic vessel. Therefore, when considering any surgical procedure, whether for curative or palliative intent, these issues must be discussed prior to the operation. As new innovations are utilized, outcomes will continue to improve for surgical patients.

Radiation Therapy

There are many acute effects of radiation therapy. These are based on the location of the treatment. If treatment is directed into the peritoneal cavity, the most likely problems will be related to cramping, abdominal pain, and diarrhea. Fatigue is also a common problem for patients undergoing radiation therapy (Irvine, Vincent et al. 1998). Radiation of the upper aerodigestive tract may lead to edema and inability to swallow. Localized skin irradiation can lead to painful burns. These symptoms may be very difficult to control initially, but frequently improve with time. Newer treatments are being tested to reduce the acute effects of radiation, such as silver leaf nylon dressings for perineal irradiation (Vuong, Franco et al. 2004). Other promising treatments include glutamine, to protect against radiation-induced injury (Savarese, Savy et al. 2003), and hyperbaric oxygen therapy for radiation-induced osteoradionecrosis, soft tissue necrosis, cystitis, proctitis (Bui, Lieber et al. 2004), or breast skin burns (Borg, Wilkinson et al. 2001). Other treatments for skin damage, such as transparent, hydro-colloid, and hydrogel dressings, have demonstrated some benefit, as have sucralfate cream and corticosteroid cream. Aloe vera may be beneficial and has no known side effects (Wickline 2004).

Long-term and Late Effects of Cancer Treatment

Most cancer treatments carry substantial risk of adverse long-term or late effects, including neurocognitive problems, premature menopause, cardiac dysfunction, sexual impairment, chronic fatigue, pain, and second malignancies for both adult and childhood cancer survivors (Schwartz, Hobbie et al. 1993; Kolb and Poetscher 1997; Aziz 2002; Aziz and Rowland 2003). One fourth to one third of breast and lymphoma survivors who receive chemotherapy may develop detectable neurocognitive deficits (Cimprich 1992; Ganz 1998; Brezden, Phillips et al. 2000; Ahles, Saykin et al. 2002). Late clinical cardiotoxicity, often life threatening, may occur in 5 to 10% of long-term pediatric cancer survivors even 5 to 10 years after therapy (Simbre, Adams et al. 2001).

Late effects of radiotherapy and chemotherapy are related to organ dysfunction and impact a patient's life by altering functional abilities (Table 1). The lifestyle

Table 1. Possible late effects of radiotherapy & chemotherapy

Organ system	Late effect/sequelae of radiotherapy	Late effect/sequelae of chemotherapy	Chemotherapeutic drugs responsible
Bone and soft tissues	Short stature; atrophy, fibrosis, osteonecrosis	Avascular necrosis	Steroids
Cardiovascular	Pericardial effusion; pericarditis; CAD	Cardiomyopathy; CCF	Anthracylines Cyclophosphamide
Pulmonary	Pulmonary fibrosis; decreased lung volume	Pulmonary fibrosis; interstitial pneumo-nitis	Bleomycin BCNU Methotrexate Adriamycin
Central nervous system	Neuropsychological deficits; structural changes; hemorrhage	Neuropsychological deficits, structural changes; hemiplegia; seizure	Methotrexate
Peripheral nervous system		Peripheral neuro-pathy; hearing loss	Cisplatin Vinca alkaloids
Hematological	Cytopenia, myelodysplasia	Myelodysplastic syndromes	Alkylating agents
Renal	Decreased creatinine clearance; hyperten-sion	Dec. creatinine clearance; Inc. creatinine; Renal F Delayed Renal F	Cisplatin Methotrexate Nitrosoureas
Genitourinary	Bladder fibrosis, contractures	Bladder fibrosis; Hemorrhagic cystitis	Cyclophosphamide
Gastrointestinal	Malabsorption; stricture; abnormal LFT	Abnormal LFT; Hepatic fibrosis; cirrhosis	Methotrexate BCNU
Pituitary	Growth hormone deficiency; pituitary deficiency		
Thyroid	Hypothyroidism; nodules		
Gonadal	Men: risk of sterility; Leydig cell dysfunction Women: ovarian failure; early menopause	Men: sterility Women: sterility, premature menopause	Alkylating agents Procarbazine
Dental/oral health	Poor enamel and root formation; dry mouth		
Opthalmological	Cataracts; retinopathy	Cataracts	Steroids

Adapted from Aziz NA (Aziz 2002; Aziz and Rowland 2003) and Ganz PA (Ganz 1998)

changes required by patients are associated with specific drugs used in the treatment regimen, which are frequently prescribed dependent on the location of a solid tumor. Combinations of chemotherapy and radiation therapy have a higher incidence of late effects of treatment (Aziz 2002; Aziz and Rowland 2003). In addition, long-term effects on organ systems may lead to mortality. This has been noted by investigators to account for one-fourth of late deaths of cancer survivors. The most common causes of late deaths among survivors of pediatric cancer incluse secondary cancer or cardiac dysfunction (Sklar 1999).

Late effects can be classified further as: (a) *system specific* (i.e., damage, failure or premature aging of organs, immunosuppression or compromised immune systems, and endocrine damage); (b) *second malignant neoplasms* (i.e., increased risk of a certain cancer associated with the primary cancer and a second cancer associated with cytotoxic or radiological cancer therapies); (c) *functional changes* (lymphedema, incontinence, pain syndromes, neuropathies and fatigue); (d) *cosmetic changes* (i.e., amputations, ostomies and skin and hair alterations); and (e) *associated comorbidities* (i.e., osteoporosis, arthritis, scleroderma and hypertension) (Aziz 2002; Aziz and Rowland 2003). The risk of a recurrence of the primary malignancy, while not a late effect, is also ever present and affects surveillance, monitoring and post-treatment follow-up management decisions.

Generalizations

Certain types of late effects can be anticipated from exposure to specific therapies, age of the survivor at the time of treatment, combinations of treatment modalities and dosage administered (Aziz 2002). Susceptibility differs for children and adults. Generally, chemotherapy results in acute toxicities that can persist, whereas radiation therapy leads to sequelae that are not immediately apparent. Combinations of chemotherapy and radiation therapy are more often associated with late effects. Risk of late death from causes other than recurrence is greatest among survivors treated with a combination of chemotherapy and radiotherapy. Toxicities related to chemotherapy, especially those of an acute but possibly persistent nature, can be related to proliferation kinetics of individual cell populations because these drugs are usually cell-cycle dependent. Organs or tissues most susceptible have high cell proliferation rates and include the skin, bone marrow, gastrointestinal mucosa, liver and testes. The least susceptible organs and tissues replicate very slowly or not at all and include muscle cells, neurons and connective tissue. However, neural damage may be caused by commonly used chemotherapeutic drugs such as methotrexate, vinca alkaloids and cytosine arabinoside, bone injury may be caused by methotrexate, and cardiac sequelae can occur after treatment with adriamycin. Injuries in tissues or organs with low repair potential may be permanent or long lasting.

Issues Unique to Certain Cancer Sites. The examination of late effects for childhood cancers such as leukemia, Hodgkin's lymphoma and brain tumors have provided the foundation for this area of research. A body of knowledge on late effects of radiation and chemotherapy is also now appearing for adult cancer sites such as breast cancer. For example, neurocognitive deficits that may develop after chemotherapy for breast cancer are an example of a late effect that was initially observed among survivors of childhood cancer receiving cranial irradiation, chemotherapy or both (Kreuser, Hetzel et al. 1988; van Dam, Schagen et al. 1998; Ahles, Saykin et al. 2002; Aziz 2002; Aziz and Rowland 2003). Late effects of bone marrow transplantation have been studied for both adult and childhood cancer survivors as have sequelae associated with particular chemotherapeutic regimens for Hodgkin's lymphoma and breast cancer (Sankila, Garwicz et al. 1996; Schwartz 1999; Greendale, Petersen et al. 2001; Aziz 2002). The side effects of radiotherapy, both alone and with chemotherapy, have been reported fairly comprehensively for most childhood cancer sites associated with good survival rates. Most cancer treatment regimens consist of chemotherapy in conjunction with surgery or radiation, and multidrug chemotherapeutic regimens are the rule rather the exception. As such, the risk of late effects must always be considered in light of all other treatment modalities to which the patient has been exposed.

Special Considerations Related to Age at Diagnosis. Long-term cancer survivors are faced with different effects of treatment depending on the age at diagnosis. Children face growth, neurocognitive, and hormonal imbalance related to cancer treatment. Young adults frequently face issues such as reproductive function and risks for second cancers. Middle age patients face problems related to chronic disease due to the effects of treatment and early menopause, and older patients frequently suffer from additional co-morbidities, making long-term complications potentially more deleterious (Aziz 2002; Aziz and Rowland 2003).

Special Considerations when Primary Diagnosis and Treatment Occurs in Childhood. Cancer therapy during childhood may interfere with physical and musculoskeletal development (Blatt, Lee et al. 1988; Furst, Lundell et al. 1989; Sklar, Mertens et al. 1993; Ogilvy-Stuart, Clayton et al. 1994; Didi, Didcock et al. 1995), neurocognitive and intellectual growth (Ochs, Mulhern et al. 1991; Haupt, Fears et al. 1994), and pubertal development (Kreuser, Hetzel et al. 1988). These effects may be most notable during the adolescent growth spurt. Prevention of second cancers is also a key issue (Mullan 1985; Aziz 2002).

Some late effects of chemotherapy may assume special importance depending on the adult patient's age at the time of diagnosis and treatment (Schwartz 1999; Aziz 2002; Aziz and Rowland 2003). Diagnosis and treatment during the young adult or early reproductive years may call for a special cognizance of the importance of maintaining reproductive function and the prevention of second cancers (Shahin and Puscheck 1998). Cancer patients who are diagnosed and treated around age 30 to 50 may need specific attention for premature menopause, issues relating to sexuality and intimacy, the use of estrogen replacement therapy, prevention of neurocognitive, cardiac and other sequelae of chemotherapy, and prevention of coronary artery disease and osteoporosis (Herold and Roetzheim 1992; Marina 1997; Schwartz 1999; Aziz 2002). Sexual dysfunction may persist after breast cancer treatment and may include vaginal discomfort, hot flashes, and alterations in bioavailable testosterone, luteinizing hormone and sex hormone binding globulin (Ganz, Greendale et al. 2000; Greendale, Petersen et al. 2001). Menopausal symptoms such as hot flashes, vaginal dryness and stress urinary incontinence are very common in breast cancer survivors and cannot be managed with standard estrogen replacement therapy in these patients. The normal life expectancy of survivors of early-stage cancers during these years of life underscores the need to address their long-term health and QOL issues (Herold and Roetzheim 1992; Marina 1997; Schwartz 1999).

Although older patients (65 years of age or more) bear a disproportionate burden of cancer, advancing age is also associated with increased vulnerability to other age-related health problems, any of which could affect treatment choice, prognosis and survival. Hence, cancer treatment decisions may have to consider preexisting or concurrent health problems (comorbidities). Measures that can help to evaluate comorbidities reliably in older cancer patients are warranted. Little information is available on how comorbid age-related conditions influence treatment decisions and the subsequent course of cancer or the comorbid condition. It is also not known how already compromised older cancer patients tolerate the stress of cancer and its treatment and how comorbid conditions are managed in light of the cancer diagnosis (Yancik, Ganz et al. 2001; Aziz 2002).

Physiologic Sequalae of Cancer and its Treatment

Second Cancers. Second cancers may account for a substantial number of new cancers. A second primary cancer is associated with the primary malignancy or with certain cancer therapies (e.g., breast cancer after Hodgkin's lymphoma, ovarian cancer after primary breast cancer) (Ho and Frei 1971; Zimm, Collins et al. 1983; Meadows, Baum et al. 1985; Hawkins, Draper et al. 1987; Hildreth, Shore et al. 1989; Sankila, Garwicz et al. 1996). Commonly cited secondary malignancies include: (a) approximate 20% risk of myelodysplasic syndromes, acute leukemia, and non-Hodgkin's lymphoma due to the chemotherapy combinations for Hodgkin's lymphoma (alkylating agents and podophyllotoxins); (b) solid tumors such as breast, bone, and thyroid cancer in the radiation fields in patients treated with radiotherapy; and (c) bladder cancer after cyclophosphamide. Secondary solid malignancies have been associated with chemotherapy treatments Hodgkin's lymphoma up to 20 years after therapy (Foss Abrahamsen, Andersen et al. 2002). Secondary cancers may also include risks of squamous cell cancer of the skin and sarcoma in radiation fields, such as with breast cancer patients. Within 20 years, survivors of childhood cancer have an 8 to 10% risk of developing a second cancer (Draper, Sanders et al. 1986). This can be attributed to the mutagenic risk of both radiotherapy and chemotherapy, which is further compounded in patients with genetic predispositions to malignancy. The risk of a second cancer induced by cytotoxic agents is related to the cumulative dose of drug or radiotherapy (Herold and Roetzheim 1992; Marina 1997; Schwartz 1999; Aziz 2002).

The risk of malignancy with normal aging may be a result of cumulative cellular mutations. The interaction of the normal aging process and exposure to mutagenic cytotoxic therapies may result in an increased risk of second malignancy, particularly after radiotherapy and treatment with alkylating agents and podophyllotoxins. Commonly cited second cancers include leukemia after alkylating agents and podophyllotoxins; solid tumors, including breast, bone and thyroid cancer in radiation fields; and bladder cancer after cyclophosphamide. Second cancers may also occur in the same organ site (e.g., breast, colorectal); thus, there is definite need for continued surveillance (Herold and Roetzheim 1992; Marina 1997; Schwartz 1999; Aziz 2002).

The risk of secondary malignancy can have long-term psychological impact for patients, as well as overwhelming life changes should a second malignancy occur. In efforts to prevent secondary cancers, treatments may be offered that are associated with other risks on patient QOL. For example, oophorectomy in a breast cancer patient may lead to early menopause, and the risks associated with surgery. If anti-hormonal treatments are implemented, such as tamoxifen to prevent another breast cancer, risks include cardiac toxicity, thrombotic events, or endometrial cancer. These risks must be considered by practitioners and patients prior to initiating treatment. Some patients may initiate alternative medical approaches, which frequently carry unknown risks and unclear benefits (Aziz 2002).

Neurocognitive Function. Chemotherapeutics have been associated with long-term neurocognitive deficits. While in adults this has been primarily investigated among breast cancer survivors (Schagen, van Dam et al. 1999; Ahles, Saykin et al. 2002; Schagen, Muller et al. 2002), neurocognitive decline is likely to occur in many patients who have been treated with chemotherapeutics (Ahles, Saykin et al. 2002). Despite the preliminary state of this field of research, studies have consistently demonstrated a decline in verbal memory, executive function, and motor function among cancer patients (Anderson-Hanley, Sherman et al. 2003). Future research efforts should further investigate these problems to better understand these neurocognitive changes so that preventive or treatment strategies can be developed.

Gastrointestinal Dysfunction. Radiation therapy has been found to cause fibrosis and stricturing along the alimentary tract, and is caused by both brachytherapy (Hishikawa, Kamikonya et al. 1986) and external beam (DeCosse, Rhodes et al. 1969; Palmer and Bush 1976). This problem has also been noted with the utilization of photodynamic therapy (McCaughan, Ellison et al. 1996; Overholt and Panjehpour 1996). The alimentary tract is at risk in the primary or adjuvent treatment of esophageal or rectal tumors; small bowel injury may also occur in the treatment of other intraabdominal processes, such as pre- or post-operative radiation therapy for retroperitoneal sarcomas. Large or small bowel strictures can lead to obstruction, the symptoms of which include nausea, vomiting, pain, and bloating. Esophageal strictures can also cause difficulty or inability to swallow. For esophageal or colonic strictures, endoscopic approaches utilizing stents may be beneficial. This approach is not applicable for most of the small bowel, which may necessitate an operative approach, usually either a bypass or resection. Some surgeons utilize minimally invasive laparoscopic techniques, although this may not be possible if there are abundant adhesions. Long-term gastrointestinal function is also common among patients suffering from gynecologic cancers. One common example is related to radiation enteritis in the setting of radiation therapy for cervial cancers. In addition, anywhere from 5 to 51% of ovarian cancers present with a bowel obstruction, either as an initial presention or as a recurrence (Davis and Nouneh 2001). Treatment in both of these settings may be difficult and there is no obvious standard of care.

Pulmonary Dysfunction. Pulmonary dysfunction may be related to major resections, radiation injury, or chemotherapeutic injury. This may be enhanced if the patient has preexisting pulmonary problems. The incidence of lung injury after breast irradiation and after lumpectomy is minimal, but not irrelevant (Kimsey, Mendenhall et al. 1994; Dolsma 1997; Theuws, Seppenwoolde et al. 2000). In the context of the large numbers of women undergoing lumpectomy and radiation therapy as a primary treatment for breast cancer, this problem may be significant, and even more so among women who have underlying lung disease (Theuws, Kwa et al. 1998). There are many chemotherapeutic agents that can cause pulmonary injury. Bleomycin may be the most notorious, although others include cyclophosphamide, mitomycin, carmustine, and methotrexate. Whenever using these medications, this complication should be anticipated. Therefore, it is recommended to assess pulmonary function tests at baseline and every three months while on therapy, and carefully follow patients for signs of impending problems such as dyspnea and hypoxia (Ignoffo 1998). Finally, major resections, such as pneumonectomy, may leave patients debilitated and unable to carry out normal functions.

Cardiac Dysfunction. Injury to the heart from chemotherapy, most notably doxorubicin, or from chest wall irradiation is a known risk of cancer treatment. Clinical manifestation of anthracyclins include reduced cardiac function, arrhythmia, and heart failure (Lipshultz, Colan et al. 1991; Ganz 1998; Lipshultz, Lipsitz et al. 2002). Radiation therapy can lead to valvular damage, pericardial thickening, ischemic heart disease (Lipshultz, Colan et al. 1991; Lipshultz, Lipsitz et al. 2002) and a decreased ejection fraction (Mukherjee, Aston et al. 2003). These may have long-term impact on a patient's QOL and ability to lead a reasonably active life. Protective agents, such as dexrazoxane or amifostine, may be given during chemotherapy to lessen the risk of cardiac damage. Consideration of myocardial injury at the time of radiotherapy and may be lessened by breathing techniques (Sixel, Aznar et al. 2001). Despite these preventive measures, heart damage is not completely avoidable in patients undergoing these treatments, and may cause considerable long-term morbidity.

Endocrine Dysfunction. There are multiple potential endocrine problems related to cancer prevention and treatment (Sklar 1999). One common disorder is related to thyroid cancer, whereby total thyroidectomy will necessitate life-long thyroid replacement therapy. In the case of pancreatic surgery, deficiencies of pancreatic hormones, such as insulin, are treatable, yet they may severely alter a patient's life. This may include the need to control diet, use oral hypoglysurics, or prescribe insulin therapy. Perhaps the most common hormonal difficulty is related to the surgical or medical ablation of estrogen in female patients. This will lead to temporary or permanent menopause symptoms. Hot flashes related to tamoxifen can be debilitating and necessitate discontinuing this medication. Tamoxifen blocks estrogen receptors in most hormonal tissues, but is considered a mixed estrogen antagonist/agonist. Other newer medications that block estrogen, either through production or activity, are aromatase inhibitors, megestrol acetate and fulvestrant, which are great cause for optimism for breast cancer patients (Osipo, Liu et al. 2004). However, control of symptoms does not also compensate for the loss of hormones with regard to bone loss. Future strategies to prevent this side effect must be considered in the future (Coleman 2004).

Another hormone dysfunction that can severely alter a patient's QOL is related to advanced neuroendocrine tumors. These can include the carcinoid syndrome, glucagonoma, and insulinoma. There are multiple techniques that can limit the effects of these tumors. These include somatostatin, alpha-interferon, ablative techniques (e.g., radiofrequency ablation, hepatic artery chemoembolization) and surgical extirpation)

(Krouse 2004). These techniques have shown benefit in multiple instances. The rarity of these tumors makes large prospective studies for these cancers very difficult.

Intestinal Stomas. While intestinal stomas will clearly lead to QOL difficulties as described above, some patients will have long-term problems that may continue to affect daily life. Reasons for this may be due to lack of peri-operative teaching, poor stoma placement, stoma related complications such as hernia or prolapse, or lack of a familial or support group assistance. Multiple studies have examined the QOL difficulties related to ostomies, which might be all-encompassing in a person's quality of life. Research is still needed to better understand the nature and cause of many of these problems so that appropriate interventions may be designed.

Lymphedema. The long-term effects of lymph node dissection are frequently related to disruption of nerves or lymphatics. Nerve disruption may lead to pain syndromes, numbness, or other effects such as parasthesias (Nagel, Bruggink et al. 2003). There is a large spectrum of presentations of lymphedema from axillary dissection, from arm "heaviness" to elephantiasis. Reported lymphedema rates are variable but likely around 27% (Beaulac, McNair et al. 2002; Golshan, Martin et al. 2003; Voogd, Ververs et al. 2003). This rate may be as high as 49% for long-term survivors (Petrek, Senie et al. 2001). Sentinel node mapping decreases this risk (Haid, Kuehn et al. 2002; Golshan, Martin et al. 2003; Schijven, Vingerhoets et al. 2003). It is likely that large numbers of patients (38 to 93%) will also have other arm symptoms such as pain, numbness, poor range of motion, and weakness (Ververs, Roumen et al. 2001; Engel, Kerr et al. 2003; Nagel, Bruggink et al. 2003; Schijven, Vingerhoets et al. 2003). Lymphedema is a risk for patients who have radiation therapy to lymph node basins (Erickson, Pearson et al. 2001; Meric, Buchholz et al. 2002). This is especially accentuated if there is a previous lymph node dissection in the same basin. Lymphedema may occur early or many years from treatments and is especially true if lymph node basins have been irradiated in addition to node dissections (Kissin, Querci della Rovere et al. 1986; Ryttov, Holm et al. 1988). Close observation and prevention must be considered along with treatment approaches, including arm elevation, use of compression stockings, and massage techniques.

Pain. The issue of pain related to cancer and its treatment is quite common and plays an overwhelming role in a patient's life. Nearly 75% of patients with advanced cancer have pain, with most having moderate or greater levels of pain (ACS 2001). Chronic pain may be related to nerve disruption at the time of surgery, tumor-related persistent pain, or other treatment related issues. Frequently, these may not be well described by the patient, or well understood by the medical team. The psychological health of the patient may have a significant role in the perception of pain, and chronic pain may also severely negatively impact a patient's psychological health (ACS 2001). If a patient has a poor prognosis, pain may be accentuated in comparison to a patient who is in remission.

A focus on pain has brought anesthesia pain specialists, palliative care specialists, and others together to study optimal approaches to the myriad of pain syndromes that long-term cancer survivors face. Clearly, there are many approaches to the treatment of pain. The etiology, type, intensity, location, and time course of pain, as well as a patient's tolerance to pain, may all impact the choices of care. For example, bone metastases may be treated with the use of opioids, steroids, radiation therapy, radiofrequency ablation, or nerve blockade. Based on a thorough understanding of the pain experienced by the patient, the optimal approach or approaches can be initiated. The recent use of radiofrequency ablation to treat soft tissue pain (Locklin, Mannes et al. 2004) is a novel attempt to treat pain based on a new technology. The use of complementary non-drug techniques may play an increasing role as they are studied. In addition, techniques that do not help can be debunked through additional reseach in this area.

Cosmesis. Cosmetic problems are noted with many surgical procedures, such as amputations, neck dissections, major facial tumor resections, mastectomies, and placement of intestinal stomas. Scarring can be psychologically debilitating for a patient. Minimally invasive procedures have provided improved cosmetic results. This may include laparoscopic colectomies for colon cancer, with smaller incisions and thus smaller scars and limb-sparing approaches for sarcomas. These approaches are either not applicable or attempted for many surgical procedures due to size of tumor, location of tumor, experience of the surgeon, or inability to achieve surgical objectives such as negative margins.

Cosmetic problems are most notable with head and neck cancers. Surgical treatment, or effects of the tumor itself, may result in facial nerve injury. Major reconstruction may be necessary, and results are most obvious to patients, families, and onlookers. In fact, about 50% of patients who undergo procedures on head and neck cancers feel that this is a moderate to severe problem (List and Bilir 2004). Survival is not diminished with breast-sparing lumpectomies followed by radiation (Fisher, Anderson et al. 1995). Cosmesis is usually quite good; this a standard of care for breast cancer patients. For those who choose to have mastectomy, or those for whom a mastectomy is recommended, reconstruction approaches are available to improve one's body image.

Radiation therapy may leave cosmetic results that can be quite disturbing to the patient and family. Cosmetic damage due to radiation may lead to trismus when treating head and neck cancers, or alterations of the breast. While these problems may improve with time, there may be long-term or even lifetime difficulties.

Phonation. The ability to speak may be impaired with many head and neck cancers and brain tumors (primary and metastatic). This may be due to recurrent layrngeal nerve invasion or injury during a surgical procedure, laryngectomy, or tongue resections. Recurrent laryngeal injury will lead to a hoarse voice and inablility to yell, although this frequently improves with time. Removal of the larynx will leave the patient unable to speak, requiring that a patient communicate by writing or through a device pressed against the submental area. This device gives the patient a robotic voice, which may be unacceptable for many patients. Loss of the tongue will make it difficult or impossible to enunciate words, although many patients will frequently be able to be understood in conversation. The ability to speak and be understood is a human function that is frequently taken for granted until it is no longer possible.

Swallowing. The ability to swallow, imperative for the ability to eat, has significant social impact of a person's QOL (List and Bilir 2004). The inability to swallow and the need for a feeding tube has been noted to be the most important QOL issue among head and neck cancer patients (Terrell, Ronis et al. 2004). The ability to preserve swallowing function is likely the most important outcome of esophageal surgery. Curative surgery is generally unlikely in the setting of esophageal cancer, but maintaining the ability to eat is an attainable goal by removing the tumor and maintaining gastrointestinal continuity via a surgically created neoesophagus (Branicki, Law et al. 1998).

Sexual Dysfunction. Sexual function is important to most people, yet estimates of the prevalence of sexual dysfunction in persons with cancer range from 20 to 90% (Ganz 1998; Varricchio 2000; Ganz 2001; Aziz 2002). Sexuality encompasses a spectrum of issues ranging from how one feels about one's body to the actual ability to function as a sexual being. Sexual dysfunction has been reported as a persistent effect of cancer treatment. Dysfunction may be related to multiple factors, including nerve injury, disfigurement and perceived loss of sexuality, and loss of libido. Pre-existing sexual dysfunction may also be exacerbated by cancer and its treatment (Ganz, Schag et al. 1992).

Emotional response to the diagnosis or treatment of cancer can have dramatic effect on sexuality issues (Varricchio 2000). Loss of perceived sexuality, by either the patient or the partner, can lead to loss of sexual interactions that once were active and fulfilling. These perceptions may be related to bodily changes, such as creation of a stoma or removal of a breast. These perceptions can limit a patient's interest in sex and interfere with sexual arousal and satisfaction. Pain or bodily function problems may not allow the patient to relax and enjoy sex. By learning what cancer means to the patient and their loved ones, the clinician can correct misinformation and facilitate the patient's adjustment to the illness (Ell, Nishimoto et al. 1988).

Gonadal dysfunction or failure can lead to infertility for both male and female cancer survivors (Sklar 1999; Ganz 2001; Aziz 2002). Recovery of gonadal function will depend on type of therapy (such as radiation therapy or alkylating agents) and dosing. Cryopreservation of sperm should always be considered, and ova if possible.

Nerve injury has implications for both males and females, although these issues have been studied much more for males. Without rehabilitation, approximately 85 to 90% of men with prostate cancer suffer erectile impotence secondary to surgery or radiation (Stoudemire, Techman et al. 1985; McKenna 1995). For pelvic cases in males, surgical strategies employing sharp dissection of the mesorectum will allow visualization of the sympathetic and parasympathetic nerves, thus preserving erectile and ejaculatory function in most cases (Meuleman and Mulders 2003). These strategies should also be employed in women to best preserve sexual function. While radiation therapy has less incidence of nerve injury than surgical interventions, it nevertheless carries this risk (Goldstein, Feldman et al. 1984).

Xerastomia. Dry mouth is a common effect of head and neck irradiation including the parotid nodal field. Patients who suffer from xerastomia frequently must have water nearby at all times. This problem is usually a lifetime issue for patients (August, Wang et al. 1996; Liem, Olmos et al. 1996; Kosuda, Satoh et al. 1999; Johansson, Svensson et al. 2002). While it has been shown that many patients adequately adapt to this problem, it remains a serious morbidity of head and neck irradiation. Salivary flow can be stimulated by the use of cholinergic pharmaceutical preparations. Pilocarpine may lead to symptomatic improvement, (Hawthorne and Sullivan 2000) but research is necessary to improve this treatment-related survivorship issue. If these treatments fail, mouthwash and saliva substitutes are secondary options (Nieuw Amerongen and Veerman 2003). Bio-active saliva substitutes and mouthwashes are currently under investigation for application in the clinic. These contain antimicrobial peptides to protect the oral tissues against microbial colonization and to suppress and to cure mucosal and gingival inflammation (Nieuw Amerongen and Veerman 2003).

Asthenia/Anorexia/Cachexia. Overwhelming fatigue, loss of appetite, and wasting are difficult issues that affect the QOL of cancer survivors. Asthenia impacts all phases of life, and therefore must be addressed over time. Severe fatigue is a problem for almost 40% of breast cancer survivors (Servaes, Verhagen et al. 2002). Breast cancer patients who experienced severe fatigue suffered from problems with psychological well-being, functional impairment, sleep disturbance, physical activity, social support, neuropsychological and social functioning as compared with breast cancer survivors who did not have persisant fatigue. Therefore, it is imperative to address all known etiologies, including depression, anemia and drug and alcohol use. For patients who are Hodgkin's lymphoma survivors, one-half of the fatigue cases have psychological distress that may respond to treatment (Loge, Abrahamsen et al. 2000). Related to chronic anorexia, progestational drugs can somewhat stimulate appetite, food intake, and energy level, they promote weight gain in some patients, and often decrease nausea and vomiting severity; however, pharmacologic treatment of cancer cachexia remains disappointing (Body 1999).

Cachexia is the most common paraneoplastic syndrome of malignancy, causing the death in as many as 20% of patients with cancer (Ottery 1994). While frequently considered for patients undergoing treatment or those near the end of life, these problems may persist among cancer survivors (Body 1999). Patients with advanced or chronic disease may live for years and suffer slow wasting over time. There are few current treatment options.

Grading of Late Effects

The assessment and reporting of toxicity, based on the toxicity criteria system, plays a central role in oncology. Grading of late effects can provide valuable information for systematically monitoring the development, progression, or regression of late effects (Trotti 2002). While multiple systems have been developed for grading the adverse effects of cancer treatment (Ganz 1998), there is no current universally-accepted grading system (Aziz 2002; Trotti 2002; Aziz and Rowland 2003). In contrast to the progress made in standardizing the measurement of acute effects, the use of multiple grading systems for late effects hinders the comparability of clinical trials, impedes the development of toxicity interventions, and encumbers the proper recognition and reporting of late effects. The wide adoption of a standardized criteria system can facilitate comparisons between institutions and across clinical trials (Trotti 2002; Aziz and Rowland 2003).

Multiple systems have been developed and have evolved substantially since first introduced more than 20 years ago (Hoeller, Tribius et al. 2003). Garre et al. (Garre, Gandus et al. 1994) developed a set of criteria to grade late effects by degree of toxicity as follows: grade 0 – no late effect; grade 1 – asymptomatic changes not requiring any corrective measures, and not influencing general physical activity; grade 2 – moderate symptomatic changes interfering with activity; grade 3 – severe symptomatic changes that require major corrective measures and strict and prolonged surveillance; and grade 4 – life threatening sequelae. A similar system, he Swiss Pediatric Oncology Group (SPOG) grading system, has not yet been validated. The SPOG system also ranges from 0 to 4: grade 0 – no late effect; grade 1 – asymptomatic patient requiring no therapy; grade 2 – asymptomatic patient, requires continuous therapy, continuous medical follow-up, or symptomatic late effects resulting in reduced school, job, or psychosocial adjustment while remaining fully independent; grade 3 – physical or mental s equelae not likely to be improved by therapy but able to work partially; and grade 4 – severely handicapped, unable to work independently (von der Weid 1996).

The NCI Common Toxicity Criteria (CTC) system was first developed in 1983. The most recent version, Common Terminology Criteria for Adverse Events version 3.0 (CTCAE v3.0) represents the first comprehensive, multi-modality grading system for reporting both acute and late effects of cancer treatment. This new version incorporates psysiologic changes in two areas: (a) application of adverse event criteria (e.g., new guidelines regarding late effects, surgical and pediatric effects, and issues relevant to the impact of multi modal therapies); and (b) reporting of the duration of an effect. This instrument carries the potential to facilitate the standardized reporting of adverse events and a comparison of outcomes between trials and institutions (Trotti 2002).

Tools for grading late effects of cancer treatment are available for validation in larger populations and to examine their utility in survivors of adult cancers. Oncologists, primary care physicians, and ancillary providers should be educated and trained to effectively monitor, evaluate, and optimize the health and well being of a patient who has been treated for cancer. Additional research is needed to provide adequate knowledge about symptoms that persist following cancer treatment or those that arise as late effects especially among survivors diagnosed as adults. Prospective studies that collect data on late effects will provide much needed information regarding the temporal sequence and timing of symptoms related to cancer treatment. It may be clinically relevant to differentiate between onset of symptoms during treatment, immediately following treatment, and months to years later (Aziz 2002; Aziz and Rowland 2003). Continued, systematic follow up of cancer survivors will result in information about the full spectrum of damage caused by cytotoxic or radiation therapy and possible interventions that may mitigate these adverse effects. The role of co-morbidities on the risk for, and development of, late effects of cancer treatment among, especially, adult cancer survivors has yet to be fully understood. Practice guidelines for follow-up care of cancer survivors and evaluation and management of late effects also have yet to be developed so that effects can be mitigated whenever possible (Aziz 2002; Aziz and Rowland 2003).

Advanced Illness

Care for patients with incurable disease has been recognized as an important component of quality care for cancer patients (Foley 2001). Patients with advanced illness face many of the same issues of other survivors, although issues may be magnified. The most common problem for patients with advanced cancer is asthenia (Verger,

Conill et al. 1992). There are many other specific pain and symptom management issues that present for patients with advanced illness that must be better understood so that improved treatments can be developed. Examples include malignant bowel obstruction, malignant ascites, fungating breast tumors, and painful bony metastasis. These are just some of the many problems that cancer patients frequently face with advanced disease. While there are many explanations as to why there is a paucity of data in many of these situations, it is an opportunity for researchers to explore best practices of care in these situations (Krouse, Rosenfeld et al. 2004). Research goals and standards must be equivelent to those for other medical specialties (Casarett 2002).

End of life (EOL) care is a complex subject, and yet simply a focus on QOL of patients and their families is of utmost importance. There are many areas of need for patients and families, and resources are often available. However, EOL care in the U.S. is frequently substandard (2003). Patients too frequently die in the hospital, hospice services are either not available or not consulted until quite late in the patient's course, and too few palliative care specialists are available. The tardiness of hospice consultation may be related to multiple factors, including the poor prognostication of physicians (Lamont and Christakis 2001). Only a minority of hospitals have palliative care services to address the needs of patients and their families in the dying process (Billings and Pantilat 2001), and there are gaps in education of cancer specialists related to EOL care (McCahill, Krouse et al. 2002; Cherny and Catane 2003). This is a specific area of needed focus for researchers and educators. Communication skills, knowledge of resources, planning for death, pain and symptom management, and advanced directives are all factors that must be considered in the optimal care for the patient facing death. There are multiple ethical dilemmas related to EOL care and research in this population, although opportunities are available to expand research in this population (Krouse, Easson et al. 2003; Krouse, Rosenfeld et al. 2004). Care should always be made to involve families in all decision-making processes, as they are frequently ignored or forgotten in the process of dying. The Education for Physicians on End-of-Life Care (EPEC) Project was developed by the American Medical Association (AMA) and funded by a grant from The Robert Wood Johnson Foundation. It is a series of courses concerning EOL issues. These courses are taught around the country, and materials can be obtained from the AMA website (http://www.ama-assn.org).

Future Directions

A large and growing community of cancer survivors is one of the major achievements of cancer research over the past three decades. Both length and quality of survival are important end points. Many cancer survivors are at risk for and develop physiologic and psychosocial late and long-term effects of cancer treatment that may lead to premature mortality and morbidity. As in the past when treatments were modified to decrease the chance of toxicities in childhood cancer survivors, the goal of future research and treatment should also be to evaluate these adverse consequences systematically and further modify toxicities without diminishing cures. Interventions and treatments that can ameliorate or manage effectively both persistent and late medical or psychosocial effects of treatment should be developed and promoted for use in this population. Oncologists, primary care physicians and ancillary providers should be

Table 2. Domains and priority areas for cancer survivorship research

Survivorship research domain	Definition and potential research foci

Descriptive and analytic research	▪ Documenting for diverse cancer sites the prevalence and incidence of physiologic and psychosocial late effects, second cancers and their associated risk factors.
	  – *Physiologic outcomes of interest* include late and long-term medical effects such as cardiac or endocrine dysfunction, premature menopause and the effect of other comorbidities on these adverse outcomes
	  – *Psychosocial outcomes of interest* include the longitudinal evaluation of survivors' quality of life, coping and resilience, spiritual growth

Intervention research	▪ Examining strategies that can prevent or diminish adverse physiologic or psychosocial sequelae of cancer survivorship ▪ Elucidating the impact of specific interventions (psychosocial, behavioral or medical) on subsequent health outcomes or health practices
Examination of survivorship sequelae for understudied cancer sites	▪ Examining the physiologic, psychosocial, and economic outcomes among survivors of colorectal, head and neck, hematologic, lung, or other understudied sites
Follow-up care and surveillance	▪ Examining the impact of high quality follow-up care on early detection or prevention of late effects ▪ Elucidating whether the timely introduction of optimal treatment strategies can prevent or control late effects ▪ Evaluating the effectiveness of follow-up care clinics/programs in preventing or ameliorating long-term effects of cancer and its treatment ▪ Evaluating alternative models of follow-up care for cancer survivors ▪ Developing a consistent, standardized model of service delivery for cancer related follow-up care across cancer centers and community oncology practices ▪ Assessing the optimal quality, content and frequency, setting, and provider of follow-up care for survivors
Economic sequelae	▪ Examining the economic effect of cancer for the survivor and family and the health and quality-of-life outcomes resulting from diverse patterns of care and service delivery settings
Health disparities	▪ Elucidating similarities and differences in the survivorship experience across diverse ethnic groups ▪ Examining the potential role of ethnicity in influencing the quality and length of survival from cancer
Family and caregiver issues	▪ Exploring the impact of cancer diagnosis in a loved one on the family and vice versa

Table 2 (continued)

Survivorship research Domain	Definition and potential research foci
Instrument development	▪ Developing Instruments capable of collecting valid data on survivorship outcomes and developed specifically for survivors beyond the acute cancer treatment period ▪ Developing/testing tools to evaluate long-term survival outcomes; and those that (i) Are sensitive to change, (ii) Include domains of relevance to long-term survivorship, (iii) Will permit comparison of survivors to groups of individuals without a cancer history and/or with other chronic diseases over time ▪ Identifying criteria or cut-off scores for qualifying a change in function as clinically significant (for example improvement or impairment)

Adapted from Aziz NM (Aziz 2002; Aziz and Rowland 2003)

educated and trained to effectively monitor, evaluate and optimize the health and well-being of a patient who has been treated for cancer.

Additional research is required to provide adequate knowledge about symptoms that persist after cancer treatment or arise as late effects and interventions that are effective in preventing or controlling them. Continued, systematic follow-up of survivors will result in information about the full spectrum of damage caused by cytotoxic and radiation therapy and possible interventions that may mitigate the effects. Interventions, both therapeutic and lifestyle, that carry the potential to treat or ameliorate these late effects must be developed, and should be investigated in larger populations of cancer survivors, those with understudied cancer sites, and ethnocultural minority or medically underserved groups.

The relative lack of knowledge that currently exists about the physical health and quality-of-life outcomes of cancer survivors represents a clear area of challenge. It is also one for exciting opportunity and growth. Cancer is expected to become the leading cause of death in the future as a result of our aging population, reduced death rates from cardiovascular disease, and efficacious treatment and screening methodologies. Effective strategies to prevent and delay treatment-related physiologic and psychosocial sequelae must be developed, tested, and disseminated (if found to be effective) to achieve not only the goal of higher cancer cure rates but also a decreased risk of adverse health and social outcomes. As survivorship issues are increasingly explored and mandates are promoted from the survivor community, research in each of the areas described in this chapter should increase in the future (Tables 2 and 3). Ethical dilemmas and barriers to care and research must be addressed so that optimal follow-up and/or supportive care for cancer survivors across the trajectory of their experience post diagnosis continues to be studied and improved as patients live longer with the effects of cancer and its treatments.

Table 3. Future areas of research emphasis in long-term cancer survivorship research

Area of research emphasis	Potential research questions
A) *Research related to specific survivor groups:*	▪ What are the late or persistent effects of cancer and its treatment in *older adult (65 years or older) long term cancer survivors?*
(1) Those treated for previously understudied cancer sites (e.g. colo-rectal, gynecologic, hematologic, head and neck, lung)	▪ What is the health status, functioning, and quality of life of long term cancer survivors belonging to diverse cancer sites? ▪ Which are the most common chronic and late effects among survivors across diverse cancer sites and which may be unique to subsets of different cancer survivor groups?
(2) Those belonging to understudied or under-served populations (adult, elderly, rural, low education/income, and diverse racial and ethnic populations)	▪ What are the characteristics of long-term survivors from rural communities and those from low income and educational backgrounds? ▪ What are the similarities and differences in the survivor-ship experience among underserved cancer survivors and Caucasian survivors?
B) *Research addressing specific gaps in our knowledge:* In particular as related to: (1) *Physiologic late or long-term effects*	(1) *Physiologic late or long-term effects* ▪ Who is at risk for late and long-term effects and can they be protected? Are there specific, modifiable risk factors (other than exposure to treatment) for the development of late effects? ▪ Which sub-groups of adult cancer survivors are at elevated risk for declines in functional status? ▪ What are the most common late physiological sequelae of cancer and its treatment among adults, and their effect on physical and psychosocial health? ▪ To what extent does cancer treatment accelerate age-related changes? ▪ Do co-morbidities affect risk for, development of, severity and timing of late effects of cancer treatment among adult cancer survivors? ▪ What proportion of survivors will experience recurrent or second malignancies?
(2) *Psychosocial effects*	(2) *Psychosocial effects* ▪ What are the psychosocial and behavioral consequences of late and or long-term physiological sequelae for survivors' health and well-being? ▪ Which factors promote resilience and optimal well-being in survivors and their families?
(3) *Interventions*	(3) *Interventions* ▪ Which interventions (medical, educational, psychosocial or behavioral) are most effective in preventing or controlling late or long term physiologic or psychosocial effects? When in the course of illness or recovery should they be delivered and by whom? ▪ Can interventions delivered years after treatment control, reduce, or treat chronic or late cancer related morbidity?

Table 3 (continued)

Area of research emphasis	Potential research questions
(4) *Health behaviors*	(4) *Health behaviors* ■ Does regular physical activity after cancer (or avoidance of weight gain after hormonally dependent cancers) increase length and quality of survival? ■ Does having a cancer history alter cancer risk behaviors among long term survivors (e.g., smoking, alcohol consumption, sunscreen use)?
(5) *Impact of cancer on family members*	(5) *Impact of cancer on family members:* ■ What long-term impact does cancer have on the functioning and well-being of family members of survivors?
(6) *Post treatment follow-up care, surveillance, and health care utilization*	(6) *Post treatment follow-up care, surveillance, and health care utilization* ■ Who is currently following cancer survivors for disease recurrence, and cancer treatment-related late and long-term effects? ■ What is the optimal frequency, content, and setting of post-treatment medical surveillance of cancer survivors, especially for those who are adults, and by whom should it be delivered? ■ How does cancer history affect subsequent health care utilization, both cancer-related and that associated with co-morbidities?
C) *Research that takes advantage of existing survivor cohorts or study populations*	■ Comparison of survivors' functioning over time and/or with other non-cancer populations (e.g., cohort or nested case-control studies)

Adapted from Aziz NM (Aziz and Rowland 2003)

References

(2003). "U.S. end-of-life care gets a (barely) passing grade." *Healthcare Benchmarks Qual Improv* **10**(1): 9–10.

ACS (2001). American Cancer Society's Guide to Pain Control: Powerful Methods to Overcome Cancer Pain. Atlanta, American Cancer Society.

Ahles, T.A., A.J. Saykin, et al. (2002). "Neuropsychologic impact of standard-dose systemic chemotherapy in long-term survivors of breast cancer and lymphoma." *J Clin Oncol* **20**(2): 485–493.

Anderson-Hanley, C., M.L. Sherman, et al. (2003). "Neuropsychological effects of treatments for adults with cancer: a meta-analysis and review of the literature." *Journal of the International Neuropsychological Society* **9**(7): 967–982.

ASCO (1994). "American Society of Clinical Oncology: Recommendations for the use of hematopoietic colony-stimulating factors: evidence-based, clinical practice guidelines." *J Clin Oncol* **12**(11): 2471–2508.

August, M., J. Wang, et al. (1996). "Complications associated with therapeutic neck radiation." *J Oral Maxillofac Surg* **54**(12): 1409–1415; discussion 1415–1416.

Aziz, N.M. (2002). "Cancer survivorship research: challenge and opportunity." *J Nutr* **132**(11 Suppl): 3494S–3503S.

Aziz, N.M. (2002). Long-term survivorship: late effects. *Principles and Practice of Palliative Care and Supportive Oncology.* A.M. Berger, Portenoy, R.K, Weissman, D.E. Philadelphia, Lippincott Williams & Wilkins.

Aziz, N.M. and J.H. Rowland (2003). "Trends and advances in cancer survivorship research: challenge and opportunity." *Semin Radiat Oncol* **13**(3): 248–266.

Bartlett, N. and B. Koczwara (2002). "Control of nausea and vomiting after chemotherapy: what is the evidence?" *Intern Med J* **32**(8): 401–407.

Beaulac, S.M., L.A. McNair, et al. (2002). "Lymphedema and quality of life in survivors of early-stage breast cancer." *Arch Surg* **137**(11): 1253–1257.

Billings, J.A. and S. Pantilat (2001). "Survey of palliative care programs in United States teaching hospitals." *J Palliat Med* **4**(3): 309–314.

Blatt, J., P. Lee, et al. (1988). "Pulsatile growth hormone secretion in children with acute lymphoblastic leukemia after 1800 cGy cranial radiation." *Int J Radiat Oncol Biol Phys* **15**(4): 1001–1006.

Body, J.J. (1999). "The syndrome of anorexia-cachexia." *Curr Opin Oncol* **11**(4): 255–260.

Borg, M., D. Wilkinson, et al. (2001). "Successful treatment of radiation induced breast ulcer with hyperbaric oxygen." *Breast* **10**(4): 336–341.

Branicki, F.J., S.Y. Law, et al. (1998). "Quality of life in patients with cancer of the esophagus and gastric cardia: a case for palliative resection." *Arch Surg* **133**(3): 316–322.

Brezden, C.B., K.A. Phillips, et al. (2000). "Cognitive function in breast cancer patients receiving adjuvant chemotherapy." *J Clin Oncol* **18**(14): 2695–2701.

Bruera, E., C.M. Neumann, et al. (1999). "Thalidomide in patients with cachexia due to terminal cancer: preliminary report." *Ann Oncol* **10**(7): 857–859.

Bui, Q.C., M. Lieber, et al. (2004). "The efficacy of hyperbaric oxygen therapy in the treatment of radiation-induced late side effects." *Int J Radiat Oncol Biol Phys* **60**(3): 871–878.

Casarett, D. (2002). "Randomize the first patient: old advice of a new field." *AAHPM Bull* **2**: 4–5.

Cherny, N.I. and R. Catane (2003). "Attitudes of medical oncologists toward palliative care for patients with advanced and incurable cancer: report on a survery by the European Society of Medical Oncology Taskforce on Palliative and Supportive Care." *Cancer* **98**(11): 2502–2510.

Cimprich, B. (1992). "Attentional fatigue following breast cancer surgery." *Res Nurs Health* **15**(3): 199–207.

Cohen, A.M., B.D. Minsky, et al. (1997). Cancer of the colon. *Cancer : principles & practice of oncology.* V.T. DeVita, S. Hellman and S.A. Rosenberg. Philadelphia, Lippincott-Raven: 2 v. (lxix, 3125, 92).

Coleman, R.E. (2004). "Hormone- and chemotherapy-induced bone loss in breast cancer." *Oncology (Huntingt)* **18**(5 Suppl 3): 16–20.

Davis, M.P. and C. Nouneh (2001). "Modern management of cancer-related intestinal obstruction." *Curr Pain Headache Rep* **5**(3): 257–264.

De Conno, F., C. Martini, et al. (1998). "Megestrol acetate for anorexia in patients with far-advanced cancer: a double-blind controlled clinical trial." *Eur J Cancer* **34**(11): 1705–1709.

DeCosse, J.J., R.S. Rhodes, et al. (1969). "The natural history and management of radiation induced injury of the gastrointestinal tract." *Ann Surg* **170**(3): 369–384.

Didi, M., E. Didcock, et al. (1995). "High incidence of obesity in young adults after treatment of acute lymphoblastic leukemia in childhood." *J Pediatr* **127**(1): 63–67.

Dolsma, W.V., E.G. De Vries, T.W. Van der Mark, D.T. Sleijfer, P.H. Willemse, W.T. Van Der Graaf, P.O. Mulder, B.G. Szabo, N.H. Mulder (1997). "Pulmonary function after high-dose chemotherapy with autologous bone marrow transplantation and radiotherapy in patients with advanced loco-regional breast cancer." *Anticancer Res* **17**(1B): 537–540.

Downer, S., S. Joel, et al. (1993). "A double blind placebo controlled trial of medroxyprogesterone acetate (MPA) in cancer cachexia." *Br J Cancer* **67**(5): 1102–1105.

Draper, G.J., B.M. Sanders, et al. (1986). "Second primary neoplasms in patients with retinoblastoma." *Br J Cancer* **53**(5): 661–671.

Ell, K., R. Nishimoto, et al. (1988). "Longitudinal analysis of psychological adaptation among family members of patients with cancer." *J Psychosom Res* **32**(4–5): 429–438.

Engel, J., J. Kerr, et al. (2003). "Axilla surgery severely affects quality of life: results of a 5-year prospective study in breast cancer patients." *Breast Cancer Res Treat* **79**(1): 47–57.

Erickson, V.S., M.L. Pearson, et al. (2001). "Arm edema in breast cancer patients." *J Natl Cancer Inst* **93**(2): 96–111.

Fisher, B., S. Anderson, et al. (1995). "Reanalysis and results after 12 years of follow-up in a randomized clinical trial comparing total mastectomy with lumpectomy with or without irradiation in the treatment of breast cancer." *N Engl J Med* **333**(22): 1456–1461.

Foley, K.M., H. Gelband (2001). *Improving palliative care for cancer, summary and recommendations.* Washington, DC, National Cancer Policy Board, Institute of Medicine and National Research Council, National Academy Press.

Foss Abrahamsen, A., A. Andersen, et al. (2002). "Long-term risk of second malignancy after treatment of Hodgkin's disease: the influence of treatment, age and follow-up time." *Ann Oncol* **13**(11): 1786–1791.

Fotiadis, R.J., S. Badvie, et al. (2004). "Epidural analgesia in gastrointestinal surgery." *Br J Surg* **91**(7): 828–841.

Furst, C.J., M. Lundell, et al. (1989). "Breast hypoplasia following irradiation of the female breast in infancy and early childhood." *Acta Oncol* **28**(4): 519–523.

Ganz, P.A. (1998). *Cancer survivors: Physiologic and psychosocial outcomes,* American Society of Clinical Oncology Book.

Ganz, P.A. (1998). "Cognitive dysfunction following adjuvant treatment of breast cancer: a new dose-limiting toxic effect?" *J Natl Cancer Inst* **90**(3): 182–183.

Ganz, P.A. (2001). "Late effects of cancer and its treatment." *Semin Oncol Nurs* **17**(4): 241–248.

Ganz, P.A., G.A. Greendale, et al. (2000). "Managing menopausal symptoms in breast cancer survivors: results of a randomized controlled trial." *J Natl Cancer Inst* **92**(13): 1054–1064.

Ganz, P.A., C.A. Schag, et al. (1992). "The CARES: a generic measure of health-related quality of life for patients with cancer." *Qual Life Res* **1**(1): 19–29.

Garcia-Carbonero, R., J.I. Mayordomo, et al. (2001). "Granulocyte colony-stimulating factor in the treatment of high-risk febrile neutropenia: a multicenter randomized trial." *J Natl Cancer Inst* **93**(1): 31–38.

Garre, M.L., S. Gandus, et al. (1994). "Health status of long-term survivors after cancer in childhood. Results of an uniinstitutional study in Italy." *Am J Pediatr Hematol Oncol* **16**(2): 143–152.

Goldstein, I., M.I. Feldman, et al. (1984). "Radiation-associated impotence. A clinical study of its mechanism." *JAMA* **251**(7): 903–910.

Golshan, M., W.J. Martin, et al. (2003). "Sentinel lymph node biopsy lowers the rate of lymphedema when compared with standard axillary lymph node dissection." *Am Surg* **69**(3): 209–211; discussion 212.

Gordon, M.S. (2002). "Managing anemia in the cancer patient: old problems, future solutions." *Oncologist* **7**(4): 331–341.

Greendale, G.A., L. Petersen, et al. (2001). "Factors related to sexual function in postmenopausal women with a history of breast cancer." *Menopause* **8**(2): 111–119.

Haid, A., T. Kuehn, et al. (2002). "Shoulder-arm morbidity following axillary dissection and sentinel node only biopsy for breast cancer." *Eur J Surg Oncol* **28**(7): 705–710.

Haupt, R., T.R. Fears, et al. (1994). "Educational attainment in long-term survivors of childhood acute lymphoblastic leukemia." *Jama* **272**(18): 1427–1432.

Hawkins, M.M., G.J. Draper, et al. (1987). "Incidence of second primary tumours among childhood cancer survivors." *Br J Cancer* **56**(3): 339–347.

Hawthorne, M. and K. Sullivan (2000). "Pilocarpine for radiation-induced xerostomia in head and neck cancer." *Int J Palliat Nurs* **6**(5): 228–232.

Herold, A.H. and R.G. Roetzheim (1992). "Cancer survivors." *Prim Care* **19**(4): 779–791.

Hildreth, N.G., R.E. Shore, et al. (1989). "The risk of breast cancer after irradiation of the thymus in infancy." *N Engl J Med* **321**(19): 1281–1284.

Hishikawa, Y., N. Kamikonya, et al. (1986). "Esophageal stricture following high-dose-rate intracavitary irradiation for esophageal cancer." *Radiology* **159**(3): 715–716.

Ho, D.H. and E. Frei, 3rd (1971). "Clinical pharmacology of 1-beta-d-arabinofuranosyl cytosine." *Clin Pharmacol Ther* **12**(6): 944–954.

Hoeller, U., S. Tribius, et al. (2003). "Increasing the rate of late toxicity by changing the score? A comparison of RTOG/EORTC and LENT/SOMA scores." *Int J Radiat Oncol Biol Phys* **55**(4): 1013–1018.

Ignoffo, R.J., C.S. Viele, L.E. Damon, A. Venook (1998). *Cancer Chemotherapy Pocket Guide*, Lippincott-Raven.

Irvine, D.M., L. Vincent, et al. (1998). "Fatigue in women with breast cancer receiving radiation therapy." *Cancer Nurs* **21**(2): 127–135.

Johansson, S., H. Svensson, et al. (2002). "Dose response and latency for radiation-induced fibrosis, edema, and neuropathy in breast cancer patients." *Int J Radiat Oncol Biol Phys* **52**(5): 1207–1219.

Jones, S.E., M.W. Schottstaedt, et al. (1996). "Randomized double-blind prospective trial to evaluate the effects of sargramostim versus placebo in a moderate-dose fluorouracil, doxorubicin, and cyclophosphamide adjuvant chemotherapy program for stage II and III breast cancer." *J Clin Oncol* **14**(11): 2976–2983.

Karanikolas, M. and R.A. Swarm (2000). "Current trends in perioperative pain management." *Anesthesiol Clin North America* **18**(3): 575–599.

Kimsey, F.C., N.P. Mendenhall, et al. (1994). "Is radiation treatment volume a predictor for acute or late effect on pulmonary function? A prospective study of patients treated with breast-conserving surgery and postoperative irradiation." *Cancer* **73**(10): 2549–2555.

Kissin, M.W., G. Querci della Rovere, et al. (1986). "Risk of lymphoedema following the treatment of breast cancer." *Br J Surg* **73**(7): 580–584.

Kolb, H.J. and C. Poetscher (1997). "Late effects after allogeneic bone marrow transplantation." *Curr Opin Hematol* **4**(6): 401–407.

Kosuda, S., M. Satoh, et al. (1999). "Assessment of salivary gland dysfunction following chemoradiotherapy using quantitative salivary gland scintigraphy." *Int J Radiat Oncol Biol Phys* **45**(2): 379–384.

Kreuser, E.D., W.D. Hetzel, et al. (1988). "Reproductive and endocrine gonadal functions in adults following multidrug chemotherapy for acute lymphoblastic or undifferentiated leukemia." *J Clin Oncol* **6**(4): 588–595.

Krouse, R.S. (2004). "Advances in palliative surgery for cancer patients." *Journal of Supportive Oncology* **2**(1): 80–87.

Krouse, R.S., A.M. Easson, et al. (2003). "Ethical considerations and barriers to research in surgical palliative care." *J Am Coll Surg* **196**(3): 469–474.

Krouse, R.S., M. Grant, et al. (in preparation, 2004). "Colostomies: evaluation of quality of life outcomes in 599 cancer and non-cancer patients."

Krouse, R.S., K.E. Rosenfeld, et al. (2004). "Palliative care research: issues and opportunities." *Cancer Epidemiol Biomarkers Prev* **13**(3): 337–339.

Lamont, E.B. and N.A. Christakis (2001). "Prognostic disclosure to patients with cancer near the end of life." *Ann Intern Med* **134**(12): 1096–1105.

Liem, I.H., R.A. Olmos, et al. (1996). "Evidence for early and persistent impairment of salivary gland excretion after irradiation of head and neck tumours." *Eur J Nucl Med* **23**(11): 1485–1490.

Lipshultz, S.E., S.D. Colan, et al. (1991). "Late cardiac effects of doxorubicin therapy for acute lymphoblastic leukemia in childhood." *N Engl J Med* **324**(12): 808–815.

Lipshultz, S.E., S.R. Lipsitz, et al. (2002). "Long-term enalapril therapy for left ventricular dysfunction in doxorubicin-treated survivors of childhood cancer." *J Clin Oncol* **20**(23): 4517–4522.

List, M.A. and S.P. Bilir (2004). "Functional outcomes in head and neck cancer." *Semin Radiat Oncol* **14**(2): 178–189.

Locklin, J.K., A. Mannes, et al. (2004). "Palliation of soft tissue cancer pain with radiofrequency ablation." *J Support Oncol* **2**(5): 439–445.

Loescher, L.J., D. Welch-McCaffrey, et al. (1989). "Surviving adult cancers. Part 1: Physiologic effects." *Ann Intern Med* **111**(5): 411–432.

Loge, J.H., A.F. Abrahamsen, et al. (2000). "Fatigue and psychiatric morbidity among Hodgkin's disease survivors." *J Pain Symptom Manage* **19**(2): 91–99.

Mantovani, G., A. Maccio, et al. (1998). "Cytokine activity in cancer-related anorexia/cachexia: role of megestrol acetate and medroxyprogesterone acetate." *Semin Oncol* **25**(2 Suppl 6): 45–52.

Mantovani, G., A. Maccio, et al. (1995). "Megestrol acetate in neoplastic anorexia/cachexia: clinical evaluation and comparison with cytokine levels in patients with head and neck carcinoma treated with neoadjuvant chemotherapy." *Int J Clin Lab Res* **25**(3): 135–141.

Marina, N. (1997). "Long-term survivors of childhood cancer. The medical consequences of cure." *Pediatr Clin North Am* **44**(4): 1021–1042.

McCahill, L.E., R. Krouse, et al. (2002). "Indications and use of palliative surgery-results of Society of Surgical Oncology survey." *Ann Surg Oncol* **9**(1): 104–112.

McCaughan, J.S., Jr., E.C. Ellison, et al. (1996). "Photodynamic therapy for esophageal malignancy: a prospective twelve-year study." *Ann Thorac Surg* **62**(4): 1005–1009; discussion 1009–1010.

McKenna, R.J., D. Wellisch, F. Fawsy (1995). Rehabilitation and supportive care of the cancer patient. *American Cancer Society textbook of Clinical Oncology, 2nd edition.* G. P. Murphy, Lawrence, W., Lenhard, R.E. Atlanta, American Cancer Society: 635–654.

Meadows, A.T., E. Baum, et al. (1985). "Second malignant neoplasms in children: an update from the Late Effects Study Group." *J Clin Oncol* **3**(4): 532–538.

Meadows, A.T., N.L. Krejmas, J.B. Belasco (1980). The medical cost of cure: sequelae in survivors of childhood cancer. *Status of the Curability of Childhood Cancers.* J. Van Eys, Sullivan, M.P. New York, Raven Press: 263–376.

Meric, F., T.A. Buchholz, et al. (2002). "Long-term complications associated with breast-conservation surgery and radiotherapy." *Ann Surg Oncol* **9**(6): 543–549.

Meuleman, E.J. and P.F. Mulders (2003). "Erectile function after radical prostatectomy: a review." *Eur Urol* **43**(2): 95–101; discussion 101–102.

Mukherjee, S., D. Aston, et al. (2003). "The significance of cardiac doses received during chemoradiation of oesophageal and gastro-oesophageal junctional cancers." *Clin Oncol (R Coll Radiol)* **15**(3): 115–120.

Mullan, F. (1985). "Seasons of survival: reflections of a physician with cancer." *N Engl J Med* **313**(4): 270–273.

Nagel, P.H., E.D. Bruggink, et al. (2003). "Arm morbidity after complete axillary lymph node dissection for breast cancer." *Acta Chir Belg* **103**(2): 212–216.

Neri, B., V.L. Garosi, et al. (1997). "Effect of medroxyprogesterone acetate on the quality of life of the oncologic patient: a multicentric cooperative study." *Anticancer Drugs* **8**(5): 459–465.

Nieuw Amerongen, A.V. and E.C. Veerman (2003). "Current therapies for xerostomia and salivary gland hypofunction associated with cancer therapies." *Support Care Cancer* **11**(4): 226–231.

Ochs, J., R. Mulhern, et al. (1991). "Comparison of neuropsychologic functioning and clinical indicators of neurotoxicity in long-term survivors of childhood leukemia given cranial radiation or parenteral methotrexate: a prospective study." *J Clin Oncol* **9**(1): 145–151.

Ogilvy-Stuart, A.L., P.E. Clayton, et al. (1994). "Cranial irradiation and early puberty." *J Clin Endocrinol Metab* **78**(6): 1282–1286.

Osipo, C., H. Liu, et al. (2004). "The consequences of exhaustive antiestrogen therapy in breast cancer: estrogen-induced tumor cell death." *Exp Biol Med (Maywood)* **229**(8): 722–731.

Ottery, F.D. (1994). "Cancer cachexia: prevention, early diagnosis, and management." *Cancer Pract* **2**(2): 123–131.

Overholt, B.F. and M. Panjehpour (1996). "Photodynamic therapy for Barrett's esophagus: clinical update." *Am J Gastroenterol* **91**(9): 1719–1723.

Palmer, J.A. and R.S. Bush (1976). "Radiation injuries to the bowel associated with the treatment of carcinoma of the cervix." *Surgery* **80**(4): 458–464.

Petrek, J.A., R.T. Senie, et al. (2001). "Lymphedema in a cohort of breast carcinoma survivors 20 years after diagnosis." *Cancer* **92**(6): 1368–1377.

Reid, R.I. (2001). "Acute postoperative pain management: a review." *Can J Urol* **8**(6): 1394–1400.

Rowland, J., A. Mariotto, et al. (2004). "Cancer survivorship – United States, 1971–2001." *Morbidity and Mortality Weekly Report* **53**(24): 526–529.

Ryttov, N., N.V. Holm, et al. (1988). "Influence of adjuvant irradiation on the development of late arm lymphedema and impaired shoulder mobility after mastectomy for carcinoma of the breast." *Acta Oncol* **27**(6A): 667–670.

Sankila, R., S. Garwicz, et al. (1996). "Risk of subsequent malignant neoplasms among 1,641 Hodgkin's disease patients diagnosed in childhood and adolescence: a population-based cohort study in the five Nordic countries. Association of the Nordic Cancer Registries and the Nordic Society of Pediatric Hematology and Oncology." *J Clin Oncol* **14**(5): 1442–1446.

Savarese, D.M., G. Savy, et al. (2003). "Prevention of chemotherapy and radiation toxicity with glutamine." *Cancer Treat Rev* **29**(6): 501–513.

Schagen, S.B., M.J. Muller, et al. (2002). "Late effects of adjuvant chemotherapy on cognitive function: a follow-up study in breast cancer patients." *Ann Oncol* **13**(9): 1387–1397.

Schagen, S.B., F.S. van Dam, et al. (1999). "Cognitive deficits after postoperative adjuvant chemotherapy for breast carcinoma." *Cancer* **85**(3): 640–650.

Schijven, M.P., A.J. Vingerhoets, et al. (2003). "Comparison of morbidity between axillary lymph node dissection and sentinel node biopsy." *Eur J Surg Oncol* **29**(4): 341–350.

Schwartz, C.L. (1999). "Long-term survivors of childhood cancer: the late effects of therapy." *Oncologist* **4**(1): 45–54.

Schwartz, C.L., W.L. Hobbie, et al. (1993). "Corrected QT interval prolongation in anthracycline-treated survivors of childhood cancer." *J Clin Oncol* **11**(10): 1906–1910.

Serpell, J.W., P.W. Carne, et al. (2003). "Radical lymph node dissection for melanoma." *ANZ J Surg* **73**(5): 294–299.

Servaes, P., S. Verhagen, et al. (2002). "Determinants of chronic fatigue in disease-free breast cancer patients: a cross-sectional study." *Ann Oncol* **13**(4): 589–598.

Shahin, M.S. and E. Puscheck (1998). "Reproductive sequelae of cancer treatment." *Obstet Gynecol Clin North Am* **25**(2): 423–433.

Simbre, I.V., M.J. Adams, et al. (2001). "Cardiomyopathy caused by antineoplastic therapies." *Curr Treat Options Cardiovasc Med* **3**(6): 493–505.

Sixel, K.E., M.C. Aznar, et al. (2001). "Deep inspiration breath hold to reduce irradiated heart volume in breast cancer patients." *Int J Radiat Oncol Biol Phys* **49**(1): 199–204.

Sklar, C., A. Mertens, et al. (1993). "Final height after treatment for childhood acute lymphoblastic leukemia: comparison of no cranial irradiation with 1800 and 2400 centigrays of cranial irradiation." *J Pediatr* **123**(1): 59–64.

Sklar, C.A. (1999). "Overview of the effects of cancer therapies: the nature, scale and breadth of the problem." *Acta Paediatr Suppl* **88**(433): 1–4.

Splinter, T.A. (1992). "Cachexia and cancer: a clinician's view." *Ann Oncol* **3 Suppl 3**: 25–27.

Steward, W.P., J. von Pawel, et al. (1998). "Effects of granulocyte-macrophage colony-stimulating factor and dose intensification of V-ICE chemotherapy in small-cell lung cancer: a prospective randomized study of 300 patients." *J Clin Oncol* **16**(2): 642–650.

Stoudemire, A., T. Techman, et al. (1985). "Sexual assessment of the urologic oncology patient." *Psychosomatics* **26**(5): 405–408, 410.

Terrell, J.E., D.L. Ronis, et al. (2004). "Clinical predictors of quality of life in patients with head and neck cancer." *Arch Otolaryngol Head Neck Surg* **130**(4): 401–408.

Theuws, J.C., S.L. Kwa, et al. (1998). "Dose-effect relations for early local pulmonary injury after irradiation for malignant lymphoma and breast cancer." *Radiotherapy & Oncology* **48**(1): 33–43.

Theuws, J.C., Y. Seppenwoolde, et al. (2000). "Changes in local pulmonary injury up to 48 months after irradiation for lymphoma and breast cancer." *Int J Radiat Oncol Biol Phys* **47**(5): 1201–1208.

Tisdale, M.J. (1999). "Wasting in cancer." *J Nutr* **129**(1S Suppl): 243S–246S.

Trotti, A. (2002). "The evolution and application of toxicity criteria." *Semin Radiat Oncol* **12**(1 Suppl 1): 1–3.

van Dam, F.S., S.B. Schagen, et al. (1998). "Impairment of cognitive function in women receiving adjuvant treatment for high-risk breast cancer: high-dose versus standard-dose chemotherapy." *J Natl Cancer Inst* **90**(3): 210–218.

Varricchio, C.V. and N.M. Aziz (2000). Survivorship and rehabilitation. *Textbook of Clinical Oncology*. R. E. Lenhard, R.T. Osteen, T. Gansler, Blackwell Scientific Publications.

Verger, E., C. Conill, et al. (1992). "[Palliative care in cancer patients. Frequency and priority of symptoms]." *Med Clin (Barc)* **99**(15): 565–567.

Ververs, J.M., R.M. Roumen, et al. (2001). "Risk, severity and predictors of physical and psychological morbidity after axillary lymph node dissection for breast cancer." *Eur J Cancer* **37**(8): 991–999.

von der Weid, N., D. Beck, et al. (1996). "Standardized assessment of late effects in long-term survivors of childhood cancer in Switzerland: results of a Swiss Pediatric Oncology Group (SPOG) study." *Int J Pediatr Hematol Oncol* **3**: 483–490.

Von Hoff, D.D. (1998). "Asthenia." *Cancer Therapeutics* **1**(3): 184–197.

Voogd, A.C., J.M. Ververs, et al. (2003). "Lymphoedema and reduced shoulder function as indicators of quality of life after axillary lymph node dissection for invasive breast cancer." *Br J Surg* **90**(1): 76–81.

Vuong, T., E. Franco, et al. (2004). "Silver leaf nylon dressing to prevent radiation dermatitis in patients undergoing chemotherapy and external beam radiotherapy to the perineum." *Int J Radiat Oncol Biol Phys* **59**(3): 809–814.

Welch-McCaffrey, D., B. Hoffman, et al. (1989). "Surviving adult cancers. Part 2: Psychosocial implications." *Ann Intern Med* **111**(6): 517–524.

Wickline, M.M. (2004). "Prevention and treatment of acute radiation dermatitis: a literature review." *Oncol Nurs Forum* **31**(2): 237–247.

Yancik, R., P.A. Ganz, et al. (2001). "Perspectives on comorbidity and cancer in older patients: approaches to expand the knowledge base." *J Clin Oncol* **19**(4): 1147–1151.

Zimm, S., J.M. Collins, et al. (1983). "Inhibition of first-pass metabolism in cancer chemotheramy: interaction of 6-mercaptopurine and allopurinol." *Clin Pharmacol Ther* **34**(6): 810–817.

Subject Index

Printing: Krips bv, Meppel
Binding: Litges & Dopf, Heppenheim